Auditory Information Processing

Auditory Information Processing

Editor: Josue Yonge

AMERICAN
MEDICAL PUBLISHERS
www.americanmedicalpublishers.com

AMERICAN
MEDICAL PUBLISHERS
www.americanmedicalpublishers.com

Cataloging-in-Publication Data

Auditory information processing / edited by Josue Yonge.
p. cm.
Includes bibliographical references and index.
ISBN 978-1-63927-899-2
1. Auditory pathways. 2. Auditory perception. 3. Auditory adaptation. 4. Hearing. I. Yonge, Josue.
QP461 .A83 2023
612.85--dc23

American Medical Publishers,
41 Flatbush Avenue,
1st Floor, New York,
NY 11217, USA

ISBN 978-1-63927-899-2 (Hardback)

Contents

Preface VII

Chapter 1 **Glycinergic transmission modulates GABAergic inhibition in the avian auditory pathway** 1
Matthew J. Fischl and R. Michael Burger

Chapter 2 **The natural history of sound localization in mammals – A story of neuronal inhibition** 14
Benedikt Grothe and Michael Pecka

Chapter 3 **VGLUT3 does not synergize GABA/glycine release during functional refinement of an inhibitory auditory circuit** 33
Daniel T. Case, Javier Alamilla and Deda C. Gillespie

Chapter 4 **Cell-type specific short-term plasticity at auditory nerve synapses controls feed-forward inhibition in the dorsal cochlear nucleus** 41
Miloslav Sedlacek and Stephan D. Brenowitz

Chapter 5 **The relative contributions of MNTB and LNTB neurons to inhibition in the medial superior olive assessed through single and paired recordings** 53
Michael T. Roberts, Stephanie C. Seeman and Nace L. Golding

Chapter 6 **Developmental expression of inhibitory synaptic long-term potentiation in the lateral superior olive** 67
Vibhakar C. Kotak and Dan H. Sanes

Chapter 7 **Interplay between low threshold voltage-gated K^+ channels and synaptic inhibition in neurons of the chicken nucleus laminaris along its frequency axis** 75
William R. Hamlet, Yu-Wei Liu, Zheng-Quan Tang and Yong Lu

Chapter 8 **Linear coding of complex sound spectra by discharge rate in neurons of the medial nucleus of the trapezoid body (MNTB) and its inputs** 90
Kanthaiah Koka and Daniel J. Tollin

Chapter 9 **Neuronal specializations for the processing of interaural difference cues in the chick** 109
Harunori Ohmori

Chapter 10 **Inhibitory projections from the ventral nucleus of the trapezoid body to the medial nucleus of the trapezoid body in the mouse** 117
Otto Albrecht, Anna Dondzillo, Florian Mayer, John A. Thompson and Achim Klug

Chapter 11 **Inhibitory glycinergic neurotransmission in the mammalian auditory brainstem upon prolonged stimulation: Short-term plasticity and synaptic reliability** 132
Florian Kramer, Désirée Griesemer, Dennis Bakker, Sina Brill, Jürgen Franke, Erik Frotscher and Eckhard Friauf

Chapter 12 **Distribution of glycine receptors on the surface of the mature calyx of Held nerve terminal** 154
Johana Trojanova, Akos Kulik, Jiri Janacek, Michaela Kralikova, Josef Syka and Rostislav Turecek

Chapter 13 **Superficial stellate cells of the dorsal cochlear nucleus** 166
Pierre F. Apostolides and Laurence O. Trussell

Chapter 14 **Activity-dependent modulation of inhibitory synaptic kinetics in the cochlear nucleus** 175
Jana Nerlich, Christian Keine, Rudolf Rübsamen, R. Michael Burger and Ivan Milenkovic

Chapter 15 **Development of glycinergic innervation to the murine LSO and SPN in the presence and absence of the MNTB** 189
Stefanie C. Altieri, Tianna Zhao, Walid Jalabi and Stephen M. Maricich

Chapter 16 **GABAergic and glycinergic inhibitory synaptic transmission in the ventral cochlear nucleus studied in VGAT channelrhodopsin-2 mice** 197
Ruili Xie and Paul B. Manis

Chapter 17 **Nitric oxide signaling modulates synaptic inhibition in the superior paraolivary nucleus (SPN) via cGMP-dependent suppression of KCC2** 212
Lina Yassin, Susanne Radtke-Schuller, Hila Asraf, Benedikt Grothe, Michal Hershfinkel, Ian D. Forsythe and Cornelia Kopp-Scheinpflug

Permissions

List of Contributors

Index

Preface

Auditory information processing refers to the capability of interpreting sounds heard by an individual. Central auditory processing plays an important role in recognizing incoming sounds, analyzing them and assigning meaning to them. Comprises steps related to information processing, which includes mechanical, electrical, chemical and central processing. The auditory system comprises the sensory organs, such as ears, as well as the auditory components of the sensory system. Excitatory neurons have a dominant function in the auditory cortex that transfers sensory information within and across brain areas. Inhibitory interneurons on the other hand, perform a variety of modulatory activities that determine how information is represented and processed. Inhibition has long been a characteristic of neuronal circuits. It helps to generate rhythms and is even capable of activating ion channels, which mediates an inward current that leads to the generation of action potentials. This book contains some path-breaking studies on auditory information processing. It will serve as a valuable source of reference for graduate and post graduate students. The readers would gain knowledge that would broaden their perspective about this area of study.

After months of intensive research and writing, this book is the end result of all who devoted their time and efforts in the initiation and progress of this book. It will surely be a source of reference in enhancing the required knowledge of the new developments in the area. During the course of developing this book, certain measures such as accuracy, authenticity and research focused analytical studies were given preference in order to produce a comprehensive book in the area of study.

This book would not have been possible without the efforts of the authors and the publisher. I extend my sincere thanks to them. Secondly, I express my gratitude to my family and well-wishers. And most importantly, I thank my students for constantly expressing their willingness and curiosity in enhancing their knowledge in the field, which encourages me to take up further research projects for the advancement of the area.

Editor

1

Glycinergic transmission modulates GABAergic inhibition in the avian auditory pathway

Matthew J. Fischl and R. Michael Burger*

Department of Biological Sciences, Lehigh University, Bethlehem, PA, USA

Correspondence:
R. Michael Burger, Department of Biological Sciences, Lehigh University, 111 Research Drive, Bethlehem, PA 18015, USA
e-mail: burger@lehigh.edu

For all neurons, a proper balance of synaptic excitation and inhibition is crucial to effect computational precision. Achievement of this balance is remarkable when one considers factors that modulate synaptic strength operate on multiple overlapping time scales and affect both pre- and postsynaptic elements. Recent studies have shown that inhibitory transmitters, glycine and GABA, are co-released in auditory nuclei involved in the computation of interaural time disparities (ITDs), a cue used to process sound source location. The co-release expressed at these synapses is heavily activity dependent, and generally occurs when input rates are high. This circuitry, in both birds and mammals, relies on inhibitory input to maintain the temporal precision necessary for ITD encoding. Studies of co-release in other brain regions suggest that GABA and glycine receptors (GlyRs) interact via cross-suppressive modulation of receptor conductance. We performed *in vitro* whole-cell recordings in several nuclei of the chicken brainstem auditory circuit to assess whether this cross-suppressive phenomenon was evident in the avian brainstem. We evaluated the effect of pressure-puff applied glycine on synaptically evoked inhibitory currents in nucleus magnocellularis (NM) and the superior olivary nucleus (SON). Glycine pre-application reduced the amplitude of inhibitory postsynaptic currents (IPSCs) evoked during a 100 Hz train stimulus in both nuclei. This apparent glycinergic modulation was blocked in the presence of strychnine. Further experiments showed that this modulation did not depend on postsynaptic biochemical interactions such as phosphatase activity, or direct interactions between GABA and GlyR proteins. Rather, voltage clamp experiments in which we manipulated Cl^- flux during agonist application suggest that activation of one receptor will modulate the conductance of the other via local changes in Cl^- ion concentration within microdomains of the postsynaptic membrane.

Keywords: glycine, GABA, inhibition, cross-suppression, interaural time disparities

INTRODUCTION

Inhibitory input plays an integral role in the maintenance of temporal precision in the avian sound localization circuit (Funabiki et al., 1998; Yang et al., 1999; Lu and Trussell, 2000; Monsivais et al., 2000; Fukui et al., 2010; Burger et al., 2011; Coleman et al., 2011). Recent work revealed a novel form of inhibition in this circuit that results from the co-release of GABA and glycine from the same vesicles. This mode of transmission occurs in some synapses at the nucleus angularis (NA; Kuo et al., 2009) and superior olivary nucleus (SON; Coleman et al., 2011) where GABA and glycine each account for approximately 50% of the total amplitude of evoked inhibitory postsynaptic currents (IPSCs). Glycinergic transmission was also observed in the nucleus magnocellularis (NM) and nucleus laminaris (NL), where stimulation at high but physiologically relevant rates evoked a slowly emerging glycinergic component of the inhibition (Fischl et al., 2014). This glycinergic component was functionally important, as blocking glycinergic transmission reduced the efficacy of inhibition in the NM. We have also shown that GlyR block reduced the ability of SON neurons to phase-lock to pure tone stimuli near best frequency *in vivo* (Coleman et al., 2011). Despite this recent progress, the function of glycine and its co-release with GABA is not well understood in this circuit.

Synaptic inhibition is a ubiquitous feature of neurons that process sound localization cues from the brainstem to the cortex. In both mammals and avians, these inputs are subject to modulatory mechanisms that confer plasticity to the strength of inhibition. These mechanisms influence both GABAergic and glycinergic synapses at either pre- or postsynaptic loci. Some of these mechanisms include suppression of release via $GABA_BR$ activation (Lu et al., 2005; Magnusson et al., 2008; Tang et al., 2009; Hassfurth et al., 2010; Takesian et al., 2010; Fischl et al., 2012) or metabotropic glutamate receptor activation (Lu, 2007; Tang et al., 2009), retrograde GABAergic signaling (Magnusson et al., 2008) and cannabinoid receptor activation (Trattner et al., 2013). Activation of various postsynaptic signaling cascades may also affect conductances in the postsynaptic cell (Kotak and Sanes, 2002, 2003; Chang et al., 2003). This striking diversity of mechanisms amongst various neurons along the auditory pathway suggests that modulation of inhibition is integral for processing at all levels of the system. In the avian brainstem, the recent discovery of functionally relevant glycinergic transmission warrants exploration of mechanisms that may shape this conductance and characterization of glycine and GABA interactions given their similar ion permeability.

Co-release of GABA and glycine originating from single vesicles is possible because these transmitters share a vesicular transport molecule (vesicular inhibitory amino acid transporter, VIAAT or VGAT; Burger et al., 1991; McIntire et al., 1997; Sagné et al., 1997; Wojcik et al., 2006). Loading of neurotransmitters into vesicles depends on their concentration in the axon terminals (Eulenburg et al., 2005; Apostolides and Trussell, 2013). Co-release of GABA and glycine in the mammalian auditory brainstem has been observed in developing neurons (Awatramani et al., 2005; Gillespie et al., 2005), however, in the avian brainstem, hallmarks of both GABA and glycinergic signaling persist at ages where synapses are considered to be mature (Fischl et al., 2014).

In other systems where both modes of transmission are present and proximal to one another, reception of GABA or glycine has been shown to modulate the complementary neurotransmitter's action. Several experiments indicate that there is a cross-suppressive effect when both receptors are activated simultaneously. Studies in spinal cord neurons of rat (Li et al., 2003) and frog (Kalinina et al., 2009) indicate an asymmetry of occlusion where activation of GlyRs prior to GABAergic transmission yields a greater degree of suppression than the opposite condition (GABA preceding glycine). In one of these studies, the mechanism of this suppression was dependent on a signaling cascade involving phosphatase activity (Li et al., 2003). A study in rat olfactory bulb neurons showed a variety of occlusion phenotypes including neurons for which cross-suppression was either bi-directional, unidirectional, or absent (Trombley et al., 1999). Others have suggested that these results are a consequence of alteration in driving force by changes in Cl^- flux during receptor activation (Grassi, 1992; Karlsson et al., 2011). The wide range of observations regarding the cross-suppression between GABA and glycine suggests that the mechanisms involved may be specific to particular brain regions.

Given recent data suggesting that glycinergic transmission is more ubiquitous in the avian auditory circuitry than previously thought, we investigated how inhibitory synaptic transmission is affected by GlyR activation. We demonstrate that activation of GlyRs occludes synaptically evoked IPSCs in both NM and the SON. In our system, this interaction did not depend on phosphatase activity, but rather appeared to depend on local changes in Cl^- driving force. By manipulating or limiting the movement of Cl^- ions with voltage clamp, we show that ligand binding and activation of GlyRs is not sufficient to induce suppression. Further, by driving Cl^- into the neuron during glycine application (thereby increasing the Cl^- driving force) results in an enhanced evoked response. These data indicate that activation of GlyRs during inhibitory transmission provides an additional mechanism for modulation of inhibition and that titration of specific neurotransmitters at co-release terminals may influence synaptic integration at the postsynaptic membrane.

METHODS

All protocols and procedures were approved by the Lehigh University Institutional Animal Care and Use Committee.

IN VITRO BRAIN SLICE PREPARATION

For *in vitro* physiology, 56 white leghorn chickens aged E17-P5 of either sex were rapidly decapitated and the brainstem containing auditory nuclei was removed, blocked, and submerged in oxygenated artificial cerebrospinal fluid (ACSF) (containing in mM: 130 NaCl, 3 KCl, 10 glucose, 1.25 NaH_2PO_4, 26 $NaHCO_3$, 3 $CaCl_2$, 1 $MgCl_2$) at 22°C. The brainstem was placed rostral surface down on the stage of a vibrating microtome (HM650V, Microm). Coronal sections (150–200 μm) containing the auditory brainstem nuclei were collected, submerged in an incubation chamber of continuously oxygenated ACSF and incubated at 37°C for approximately 1 h. Slices were then maintained at room temperature until used for recording.

Brainstem slices were placed in a custom recording chamber on a retractable chamber shuttle system (Siskiyou Design Instruments) and neurons were visualized with a Nikon FN-1 Physiostation microscope using infrared differential interference contrast optics. Video images were captured using a CCD camera (Hammamatsu C7500-50) coupled to a video monitor. The recording chamber (volume ~1 ml) was continuously perfused with ACSF at a rate of 2–4 ml/min. An inline feedback temperature controller and heated stage were used to maintain chamber temperature at 35 ± 1°C (TC344B, Warner Instruments, Hamden, CT).

IN VITRO WHOLE-CELL RECORDINGS

Patch pipettes were pulled from thick walled borosilicate glass capillary tubes (WPI 1B120F-4) to a resistance of 4–8 MΩ using a two-stage puller (Narishige PC-10, Tokyo, Japan) and back-filled with internal solution (containing in mM: 105 $CsMeSO_3$, 35 CsCl, 5 EGTA, 10 HEPES, 1 $MgCl_2$, 4 ATP-Mg, and 0.3 GTP-Na, pH 7.2 adjusted with KOH). 5 mM QX314 was added to the internal solution to prevent antidromic action potentials. In experiments where phosphatase 2B activity was blocked, cyclosporin A (0.5–1.5 μm) was added to the internal solution. In voltage clamp, series resistance was compensated at 60–80%. Membrane voltage was clamped using a Multiclamp 700B amplifier. The signal was digitized with a Digidata 1440 data acquisition board and recorded using Clampex software (Molecular Devices, Sunnyvale, CA).

EFFECT OF GLYCINE RECEPTOR (GlyR) ACTIVATION ON INHIBITORY POSTSYNAPTIC CURRENTS (IPSCs)

Inhibitory transmission was pharmacologically isolated by using a control bath solution containing ACSF with 6,7-dinitroquinoxaline-2,3-dione (DNQX) (40 μm) and D-2-amino-5-phosphonopentanoic acid (AP5) (50 μm) to block AMPA and NMDA glutamatergic transmission. Pipettes for pressure application of glycine were pulled to a resistance of ~1 MΩ (when filled with glycine solution [500 μm in ACSF containing DNQX and AP5]) and were visually guided near (~50 μm) the surface of a patched cell. Glycine was applied using ~2.5 psi pressure injection with a PLI 100A picoliter injector (Warner Instruments). Glycine application ranged

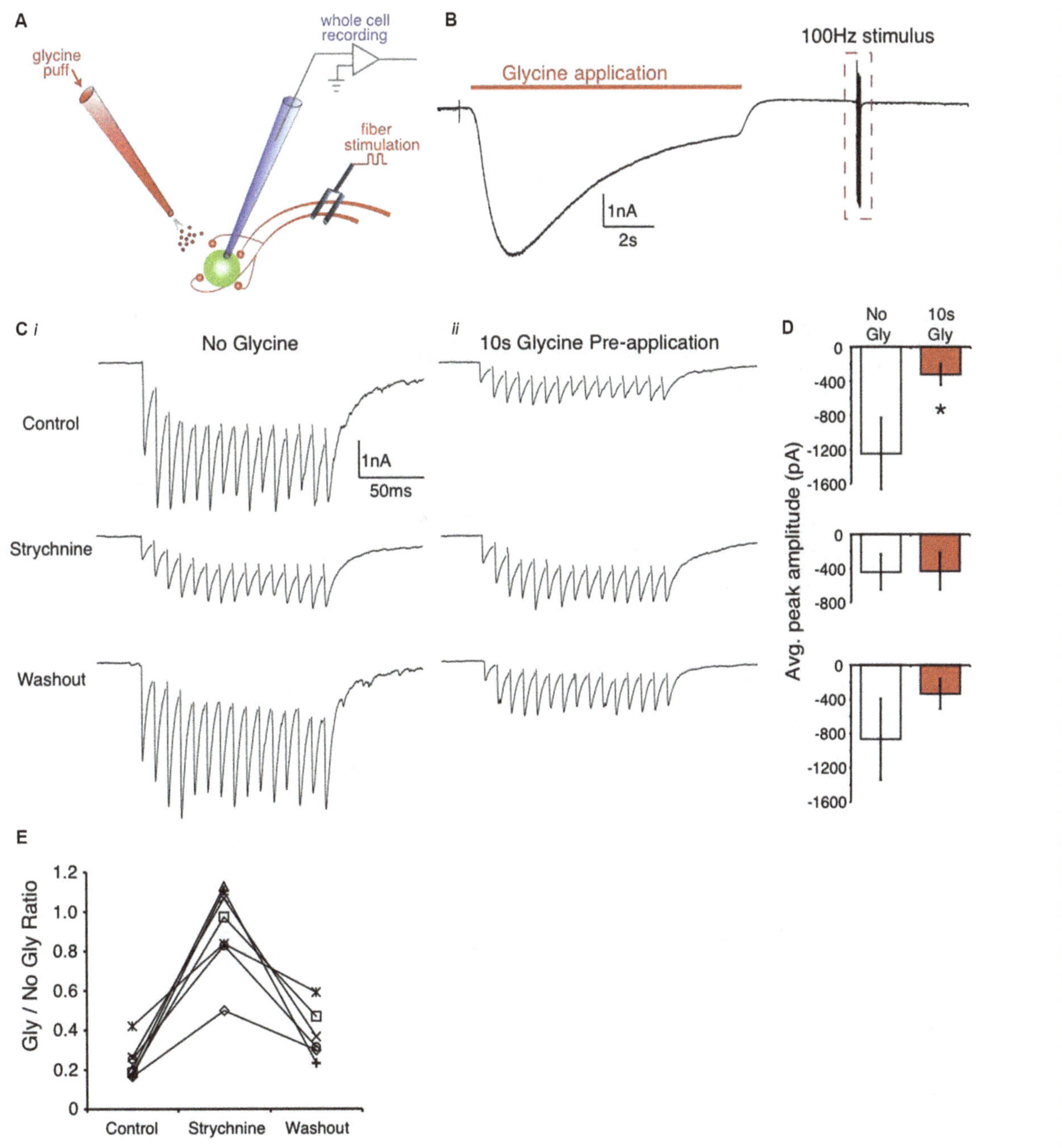

FIGURE 1 | Pre-application of glycine suppresses evoked IPSC trains in the SON. **(A)** Schematic of the recording arrangement. **(B)** Representative trace from an E18 SON neuron during the 10 s glycine application. **(C)** Expanded view of the dashed box in **(B)** showing evoked responses. **(Ci)** Evoked responses in control, strychnine, and washout conditions with no glycine pre-application. **(Cii)** Evoked IPSCs following the glycine pre-application show amplitude suppression that is blocked by strychnine. **(D)** Population data values for the IPSC amplitudes in each condition (* indicates significant difference, $p < 0.01$). **(E)** Ratio of evoked amplitudes between glycine pre-application and no glycine in each condition reveals a decrease in the suppression (ratio near 1) in strychnine.

from 10 ms to 10 s depending on the protocol. Pressure application of bath solution (ACSF) at 5 psi did not induce currents, suggesting mechanical artifacts did not contaminate recorded currents. For a few experiments, GABA was applied in the same manner (500 μm in ACSF containing DNQX and AP5).

IPSCs were evoked with 50 μs stimulus pulses with a stimulus isolation unit (Isoflex, A.M.P.I. Inc., Israel) through a concentric bipolar electrode with tungsten core (WPI TM53CCINS, Sarasota, FL). For recordings in the NM, the stimulation electrode was placed on fiber bundles adjacent to the nuclei in a ventrolateral location, and for the SON, a dorsomedial location was used.

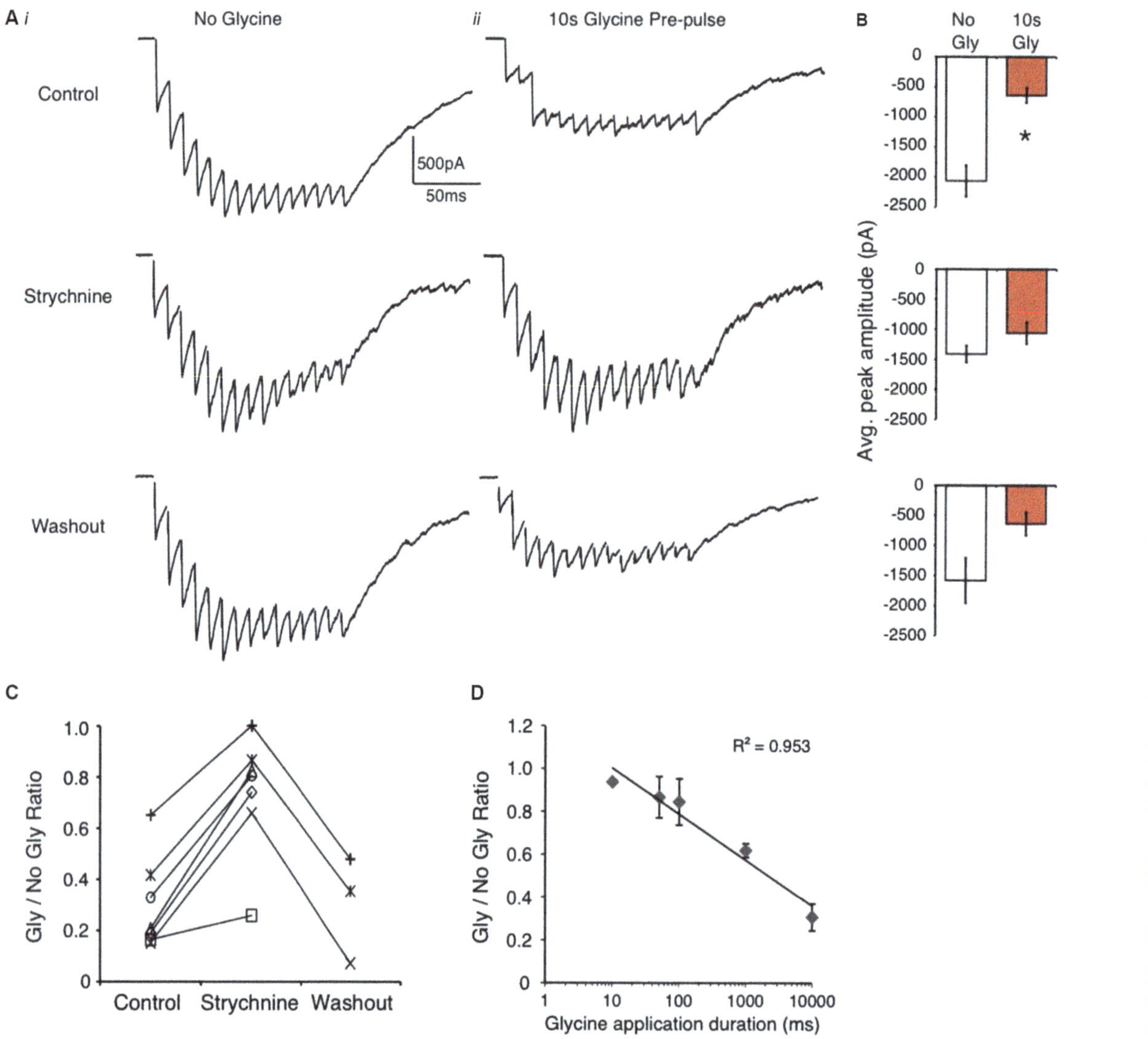

FIGURE 2 | Evoked IPSCs are suppressed by glycine pre-application in NM. (A) Representative traces from an E18 neuron showing evoked responses without glycine **(Ai)** and with glycine pre-pulse **(Aii)** in control, strychnine and washout. **(B)** Population data of peak amplitude in the absence and presence of glycine pre-application in each condition (* indicates significant difference, $p < 0.01$). **(C)** Ratio of peak amplitude between Gly/no Gly shows an increased ratio value (less suppression) during GlyR block (strychnine). **(D)** Plot illustrates that IPSC suppression increases with increasing glycine application duration ($R^2 = 0.953$, $p < 0.001$, Pearson's Correlation).

Presynaptic fibers were stimulated with pulse trains consisting of 15 pulses at 100 Hz. Stimulus magnitude (range 10–90 V) was gradually increased until IPSC amplitudes plateaued. The start of the 100 Hz train began when the current response to the 10 s glycine puff returned to baseline (usually within 5–8 s). After data were collected in the control condition, GlyRs were blocked by bath application of strychnine (1 μm) and data were collected again. Recovery of control values was attempted by washout of strychnine. This often took >20 min and full recovery was sometimes not attainable due to the high affinity binding of strychnine to the receptor. Peak IPSC amplitude during the train was used to compare treatment groups. In control, test (1 μm strychnine) and washout, evoked responses were compared between the no glycine condition and the glycine pre-pulse condition using the equation:

$$\left(1 - (\text{evoked amplitude with gly pre-pulse}/\text{evoked amplitude no gly})\right) \times 100 = \%\ \text{suppression}$$

This protocol and analysis was performed while holding the membrane voltage at three different potentials: −70 mV, approximating V_{rest} (**Figures 1, 2**); the reversal potential for glycine, ranging from −20 mV to −35 mV (average: −28.3 ± 5.2 mV, $n = 6$; derived empirically during the experiment) (**Figure 5**); and +10 mV, to drive the flux of Cl^- ions into the neuron (**Figure 7**). For these figures, data points are plotted as the quotient of the IPSC amplitude in the presence of glycine pre-application divided

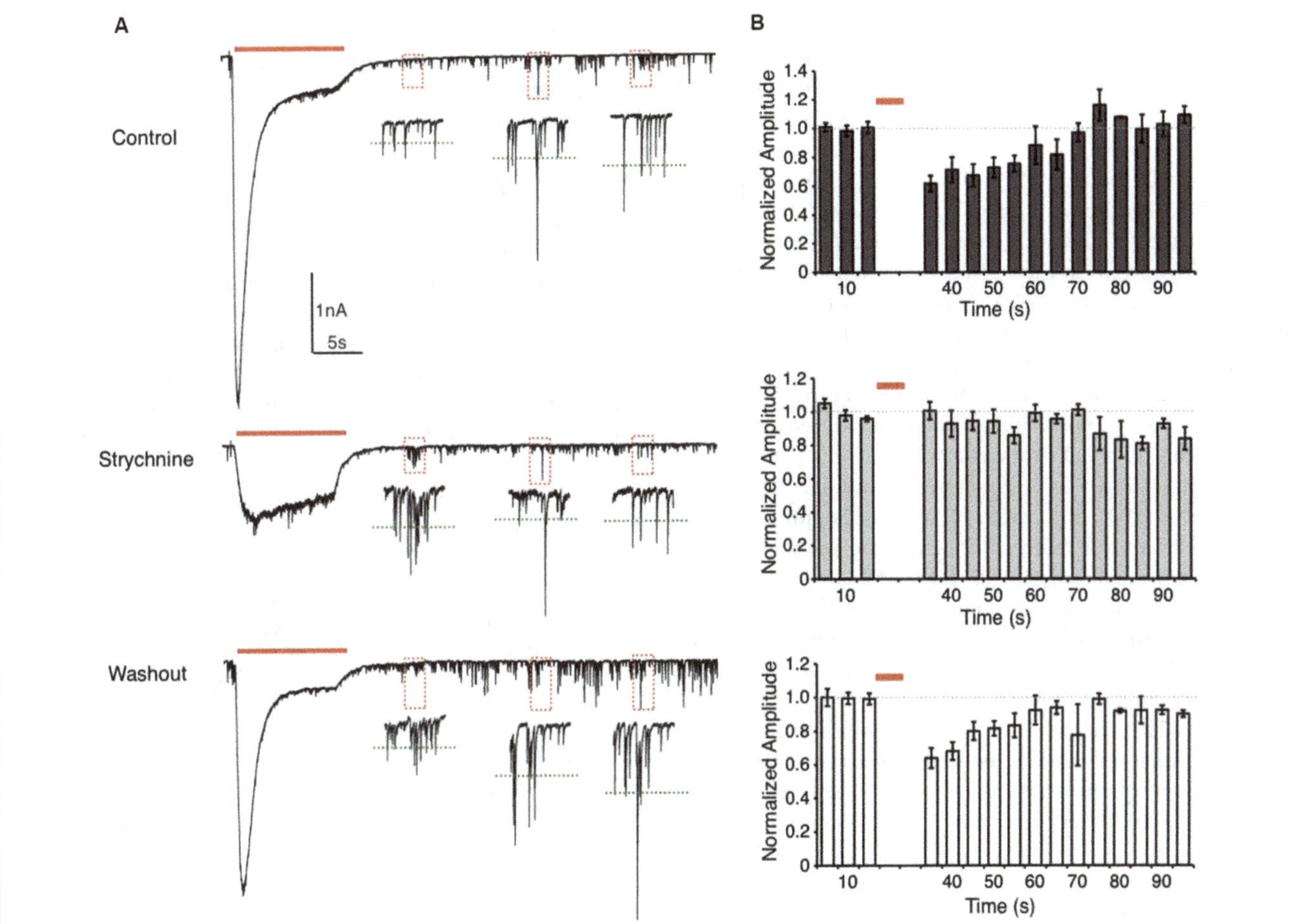

FIGURE 3 | Suppression of spontaneous IPSC (sIPSC) amplitudes after glycine application is eliminated by GlyR block. (A) Representative traces from an E20 NM neuron showing sIPSCs recorded during a glycine application protocol. Insets are expanded views of the sIPSCs in each dashed box. The green dashed lines represent the average sIPSC amplitude of the events within this two-second window. In the control condition (top) sIPSC amplitude is suppressed for a short time after glycine application. This effect was not observed during GlyR block (strychnine) but recovered after washout. Note that in the strychnine condition the GlyR block was often incomplete, but the large onset current was eliminated. **(B)** Histograms representing the normalized population data for the sIPSC amplitude analysis. Dashed line represents the average sIPSC amplitude before the glycine application. Each bin represents the average sIPSC amplitude during a 5 s time window. In the control and washout condition, sIPSC amplitude recovered to baseline values after approximately 35 s.

by IPSC amplitude in the absence of glycine (Gly/No Gly Ratio) in each condition.

The effect of GlyR activation on the amplitude of spontaneous IPSCs (sIPSCs) was also examined (**Figure 3**). A baseline amplitude of sIPSCs was acquired either during a 15 s interval prior to the application of glycine or during a 45 s recording preceding the protocol. After a 10 s glycine application, the current was allowed to return to baseline and then the amplitude of sIPSCs was measured. sIPSC amplitude was obtained for each event using a search template in Clampfit. sIPSC amplitudes were averaged during 5 s bins and compared to the pre-pulse average.

The magnitude of charge transfer ($I \times t$) was measured during the glycine application using the area under the trace and analyzed using Clampfit. Reversal potential (V_{rev}) of inhibition was computed by measuring the amplitude of evoked IPSCs at different voltages (range, −65 to −5 mV, protocol depicted in **Figure 8A**) and constructing an IV plot. V_{rev} was estimated by using a linear regression between the two voltages where the polarity of the IPSC changed from inward current to outward current. V_{rev} was calculated with and without a 10 s glycine pre-application.

Statistical significance was determined using one-way repeated measures ANOVA (Sigmaplot) unless otherwise stated. Data in the text is presented and mean ± SD. Error bars in figures are shown as SEM. Pearson's correlation was used to determine significance for **Figures 2D** and **6**.

RESULTS

GLYCINE RECEPTOR (GlyR) TRANSMISSION SUPPRESSES INHIBITORY POSTSYNAPTIC CURRENT (IPSC) AMPLITUDE

The effect of GlyR activation on evoked IPSCs in the brainstem was evaluated by applying an exogenous puff of glycine preceding presynaptic fiber stimulation. The protocol consisted of a 10 s application of glycine (via a picoliter injector) followed by a 15 pulse, 100 Hz train of inhibitory presynaptic fiber stimulation with a bipolar tungsten electrode (**Figure 1A** depicts the recording arrangement). First, we performed this protocol on SON neurons where glycine represents about 1/2 of the IPSC amplitude and is co-released with GABA from inhibitory terminals (Coleman et al., 2011). **Figure 1B** shows an averaged response (3 traces) to glycine application. We compared the amplitude of the peak synaptically evoked IPSC with (**Figure 1Cii**), and without (**Figure 1Ci**), the glycine pre-application in control, and in the presence of the glycine antagonist, strychnine (example traces shown in **Figure 1C**). In the SON, a 10 s glycine pre-application resulted in approximately 75% suppression in the control condition (76.3 ± 8.9% suppression, mean ± SD, $n = 7$, $p < 0.01$, **Figures 1C, D**, *top*). The raw data averages for the evoked IPSC amplitudes are shown for each condition in **Figure 1D**. In every neuron tested, bath application of strychnine reduced the amount of suppression observed in the control condition (8.0 ± 22.2% suppression, $n = 7$, $p > 0.05$ vs. no glycine condition, **Figures 1C, D**, *middle*; $p < 0.001$ vs. control, **Figure 1E**). Suppression levels returned near control values after strychnine washout (62.2 ± 13.0% suppression, $n = 6$, $p > 0.05$, **Figure 1E**).

Next, we performed the same experiments in NM where glycinergic transmission is recruited during high frequency stimulation (Fischl et al., 2014). The results obtained using this protocol were similar to those observed in the SON (**Figure 2**) in most regards. The glycine pre-application significantly suppressed evoked IPSCs, a result that was reduced by blockade of GlyRs with strychnine in every neuron tested (control: 68.2 ± 15.8% suppression, $n = 9$, $p < 0.001$; strychnine: 26.3 ± 23.6% suppression, $n = 7$, $p > 0.05$ vs. no glycine condition, $p < 0.001$ vs. control; washout: 69.8 ± 20.9% suppression, $n = 3$, $p > 0.05$; **Figures 2A, C**). Average traces from a representative NM neuron are shown in **Figure 2A**. Population data averages for IPSC peak amplitudes are shown in **Figure 2B**. These results taken together with those obtained from SON neurons suggest that activation of GlyRs occludes inhibition mediated by $GABA_A$ receptors.

In NM, also we investigated the time dependence of suppression by varying the duration of the agonist application from 10 ms to 10 s. **Figure 2D** shows that the degree of suppression was roughly linear with the log of the application duration, where longer application times lead to increased suppression (**Figure 2D**, $R^2 = 0.953$, Pearson's correlation, $p < 0.001$).

To further explore the temporal characteristics of this suppression, we measured the effect of prolonged glycine application on the amplitude of spontaneous IPSCs (sIPSCs) by comparing events pre- and post- glycine application (10 s pulse). This technique allowed us to evaluate the time course of recovery from suppression. In the control condition, sIPSC amplitude was suppressed by 38.2 ± 11.0% ($n = 5$) of pre-pulse levels when measured 10 s after the pulse. This was the earliest time point when the IPSCs could be accurately measured following the glycine response's return to baseline (**Figure 3**). sIPSC amplitude recovered to 90% of pre-pulse amplitude after approximately 35 s (34.0 ± 11.4 s, $n = 5$). In contrast, in the presence of bath applied strychnine, there was no systematic change in sIPSC amplitude ($n = 5$). In several cells, the glycinergic response was not completely blocked with 1 μm strychnine (**Figure 3A**, *middle*). However, strychnine did eliminate the large amplitude onset current and minimized glycinergic currents resulting in unmodulated sIPSC amplitude for the population of cells tested (**Figure 3B**, *middle*). After washout, sIPSC amplitude suppression and recovery time course mirrored that of the control condition (36.0 ± 8.4% of pre-pulse levels, $n = 4$; recovery, 27.5 ± 10.4 s).

MECHANISM OF SUPPRESSION

In previous studies, several mechanisms have been shown to mediate GABA/glycine interactions at the postsynaptic neuron. Our results show that the suppression and recovery of IPSCs occurs over tens of seconds, suggesting that second messenger systems may influence receptor conductance. Li et al. (2003) found that phosphatase 2B activity was driven by GlyR activation and suppressed $GABA_AR$ currents in rat spinal cord neurons. We therefore tested whether the suppression that we observed

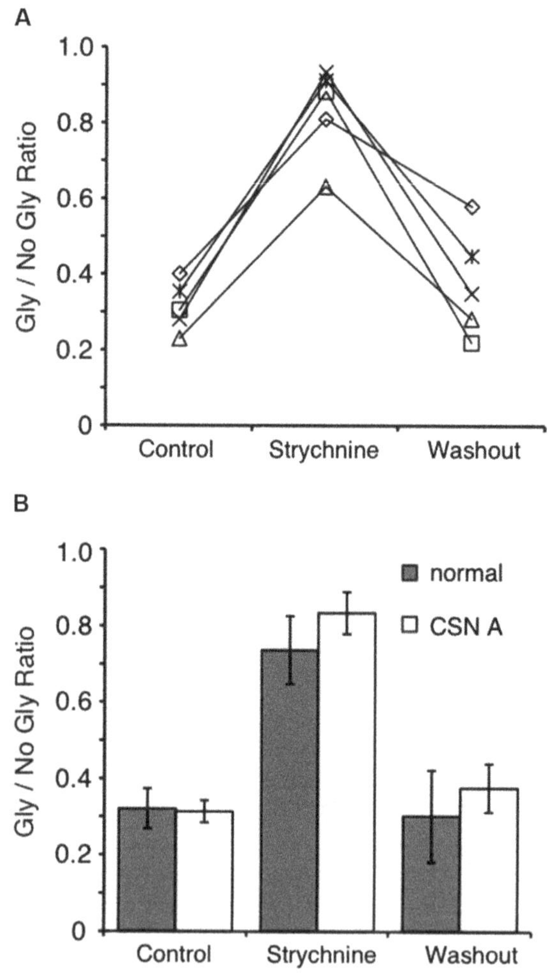

FIGURE 4 | Blocking phosphatase 2B activity does not affect suppression in the NM. (A) Ratio of peak amplitude between Gly/no Gly in each condition reveals that inclusion of cyclosporin A in the recording pipette does not prevent suppression. **(B)** Population data comparing the results using internal solution with cyclosporin A (CSN A) and the normal internal (**Figure 2C**). Phosphatase 2B activity does not play a role in the observed suppression.

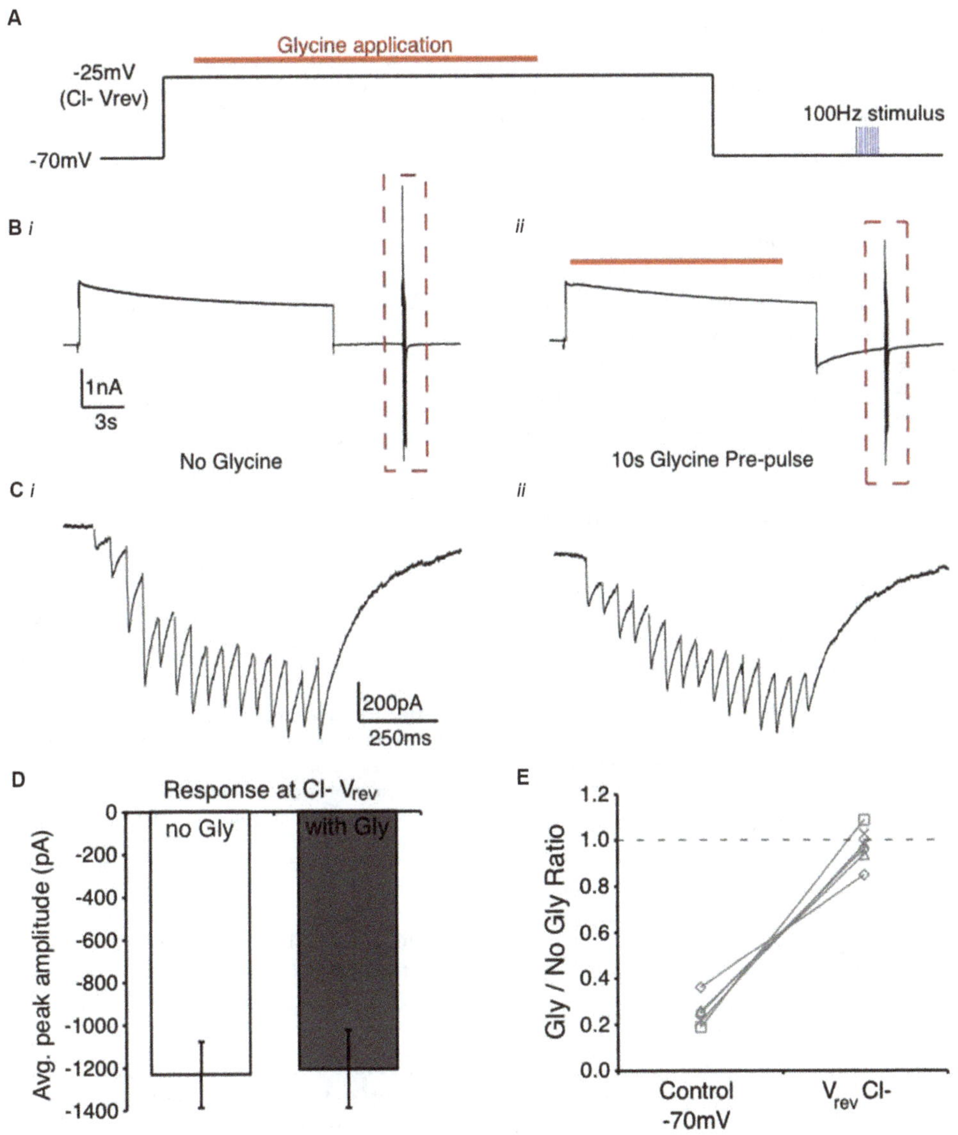

FIGURE 5 | Manipulation of Cl⁻ ion flux alters the suppression profile of glycine pre-application in the NM. (A) Schematic of voltage clamp protocol where Cl⁻ flux is minimized by holding the membrane at the reversal potential for Cl⁻ during the glycine application. **(B)** Current response from protocol in **(A)** in the absence **(Bi)** and presence **(Bii)** glycine pre-application (red line). Note the similarity between the traces in **(Bi)** and **(Bii)**, suggesting minimal current due to glycine application. **(C)** Expanded view of evoked current responses from the boxed region in **(B)**. **(D)** Average peak amplitude of the evoked current for the population of cells tested at V_{rev} Cl^-. **(E)** Ratio of peak amplitude between Gly/no Gly conditions in control and when glycine pre-application occurred at V_{rev} Cl^-. Results were similar to glycine block (no suppression observed, **Figure 2C**). Dashed line represents a ratio of 1, indicating no suppression.

was dependent on the phosphorylation state of the receptors by including cyclosporin A in the recording pipette to block phosphatase 2B activity. We observed the same suppression profile (**Figure 4A**) and no significant difference in suppression in the presence of cyclosporin A compared to the control internal solution (68.6 ± 6.6%, $n = 5$, $p > 0.05$, **Figure 4**).

Next, we determined if glycine binding to its receptor was sufficient to generate suppression, suggesting a biochemical process, or alternatively, if receptor binding and Cl^- flux was required. Neurons in NM maintain a high Cl^- concentration internally into maturity (~37 mM) yielding a Cl^- reversal potential around −34 mV (Monsivais and Rubel, 2001). For each neuron, we empirically derived the glycinergic reversal potential (average: −28.3 ± 5.2 mV, $n = 6$) using a brief (10 ms) glycine puff while manipulating the holding voltage to determine where the current was zero. To prevent Cl^- flux, we stepped the membrane voltage to the glycine conductance's reversal potential during the glycine puff application (protocol shown in **Figure 5A**). This allowed receptor binding, but prevented transmembrane Cl^- movement (representative traces, **Figures 5B, C**). In this condition, the average IPSC response amplitude was nearly identical with or without glycine pre-pulse (**Figure 5D**, $n = 6$, $p > 0.05$) and suppression was eliminated (2.7 ± 8.1% suppression, $n = 6$, $p < 0.001$ vs. control [$V_{hold} = -70$ mV], **Figure 5E**). These results suggest that the glycine-induced suppression in this system likely depends on biophysical rather than biochemical factors. Specifically, they suggest that the glycine exerts its influence by disrupting the local Cl^- concentration gradient.

To evaluate whether the Cl^- gradient was disrupted by the GlyR activation, we measured the charge transfer during glycine puff application and compared it to the subsequent suppression. We predicted that if Cl^- flux were necessary for suppression, then greater charge transfer across the membrane would yield stronger suppression. **Figure 6** shows glycine current area plotted against normalized evoked IPSC amplitude (Gly/No Gly ratio) for each cell tested in both NM and the SON. Similar to the results shown in **Figure 2D**, suppression was correlated to the log of the charge transfer (**Figure 6**, $R^2 = 0.629$, $p < 0.0001$). An additional five cells are included for which GABA was used as the agonist. Puff application of GABA induced a similar amount of suppression (**Figure 6**, + and – symbols).

Given these results together with those observed in **Figure 5**, we hypothesized that manipulation of the driving force of Cl^- ions during the glycine application would directly influence the magnitude of suppression. We employed a voltage step protocol where Cl^- ion flux direction was inverted by holding the postsynaptic cell at a voltage positive to the predicted Cl^- reversal potential. We predicted that in this condition, since Cl^- flux would be inward, the glycine application would potentiate the evoked IPSCs. Indeed, when the membrane voltage was held at +10 mV during the glycine pulse, evoked IPSC amplitude increased significantly (62.6 ± 37.1% increase, $n = 5$, $p < 0.05$, **Figures 7C–E**). These results further implicate changes in the driving force of Cl^- ions as the most likely mechanism of glycinergic modulation of inhibitory current in this system.

Finally, these changes in driving force were confirmed by measuring the reversal potential of inhibitory conductances before and after agonist application (**Figure 8**). For this protocol, we first determined the reversal potential in the control condition by measuring the amplitude of evoked IPSCs at a range of holding voltages spanning the predicted Cl^- reversal potential (protocol depicted in **Figure 8A**). The response from a representative neuron is illustrated in **Figure 8B**. **Figure 8Bi** shows the response at each voltage when glycine was applied for 10 s preceding the voltage steps. An expansion of the absolute response magnitude is shown in **Figure 8Ci** where a V_{rev} around −45 mV (red trace) was observed for this neuron in this condition. **Figures 8Bii** and Cii show the response when no glycine was applied. Here, the V_{rev} was close to −34 mV (the predicted value with this internal solution). V_{rev} was interpolated for each cell, based on linear regression fits to the IV plot. For the population, the average V_{rev} for the evoked responses in the control condition was −32.1 ± 3.9 mV (**Figures 8D, E**; $n = 7$). When a 10 s glycine pulse preceded the voltage steps, a shift in the V_{rev} was observed in the negative direction (**Figures 8Cii, D**). The average V_{rev} in the test condition with glycine pre-application was −43.9 ± 3.3 mV ($n = 7$, $p < 0.001$). This shift was in the predicted direction following the

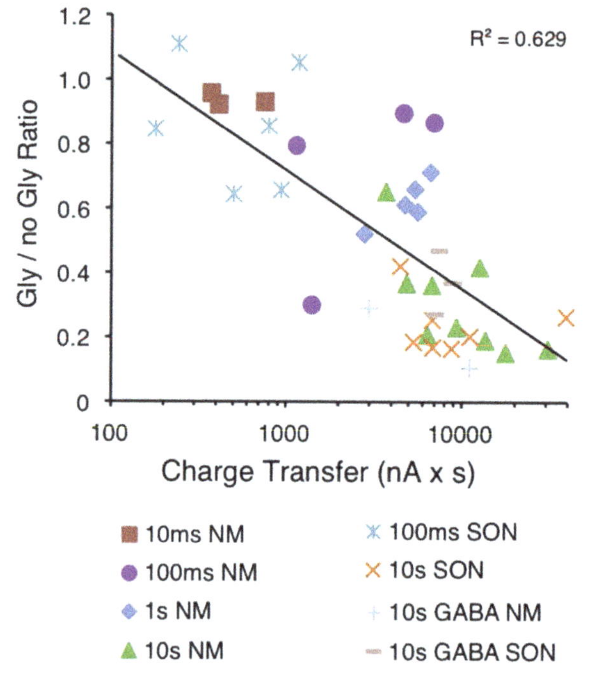

FIGURE 6 | Magnitude of suppression is correlated to the amount of charge transferred during puff application of glycine. Graph depicting the normalized amplitude of the evoked IPSC (gly/no gly ratio) in relation to the amount of charge transferred in response to the glycine pre-application. A significant correlation was observed between the log of the charge transfer and suppression ($R^2 = 0.629$, $p < 0.0001$, $n = 40$).

outward flux of Cl^- in response to the glycine puff. These results indicate that GlyR activation and the resulting Cl^- flux alters the driving force of evoked IPSCs by shifting the reversal potential.

DISCUSSION

OCCLUSION OF INHIBITORY SYNAPTIC INPUT BY GLYCINE RECEPTOR (GlyR) ACTIVATION

Our data show that activation of GlyRs suppresses the amplitude of synaptically evoked IPSCs in NM and the SON. GABA and GlyRs are both permeable to Cl^- ions, and interactions between the two receptors have been documented in areas where both receptor types are present and activated via presynaptic transmitter release. Several studies have reported a similar occlusive effect that shows the amplitude of simultaneous application of GABA and glycine is less than the predicted summed amplitude of responses to each transmitter when applied individually (Trombley et al., 1999; Li et al., 2003). Further, in some cases, the occlusion is asymmetric between the transmitters. In two studies, pre-application of glycine occluded GABAergic currents to a greater degree than for the reverse (Li et al., 2003; Kalinina et al., 2009).

The proposed mechanisms that lead to such occlusion are diverse and include receptor level interactions (Barker and McBurney, 1979; Baev et al., 1992; Lewis and Faber, 1993; Trombley et al., 1999) and biochemical signaling cascades (Li et al., 2003). Alternatively, Karlsson et al. (2011) recently proposed

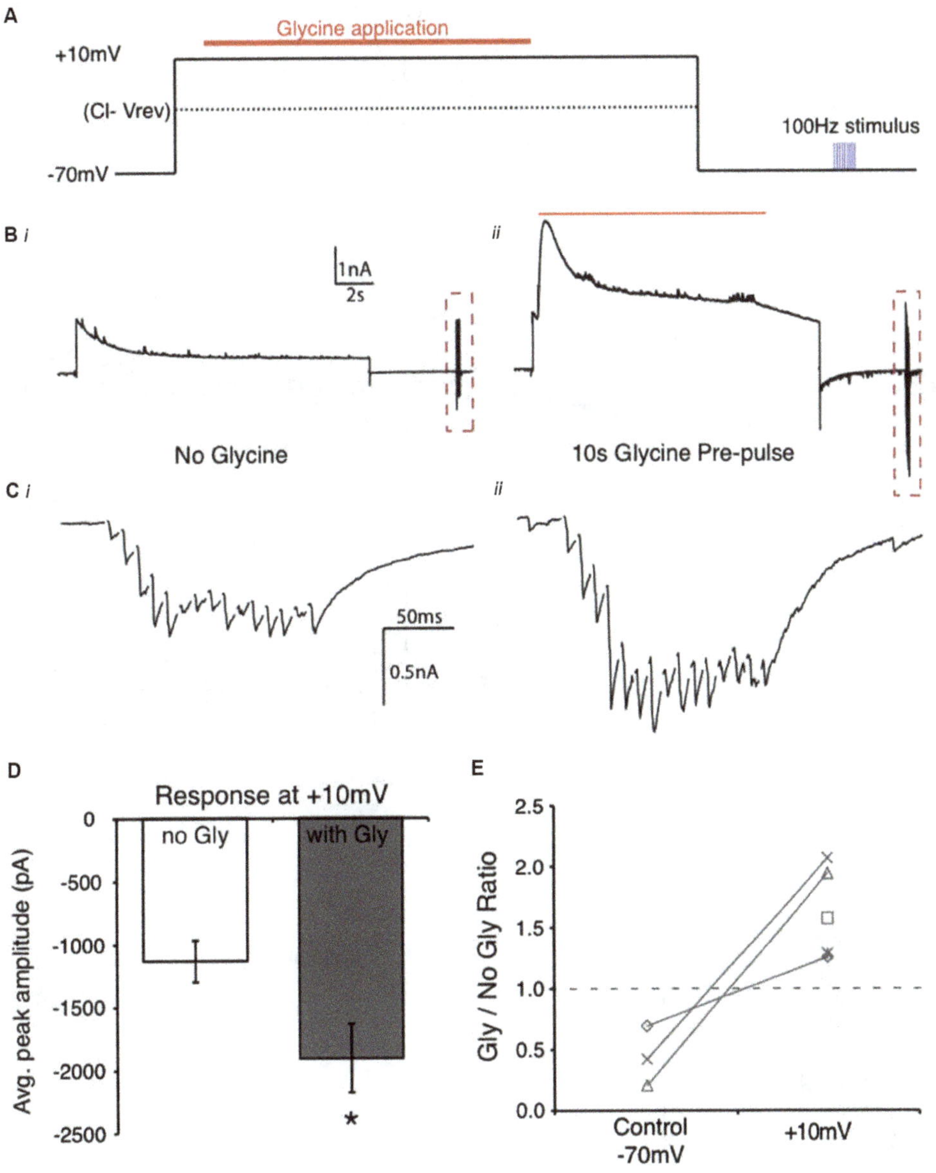

FIGURE 7 | Reversal of Cl⁻ ion flow results in an enhanced evoked IPSC in NM. (A) Schematic of the flux reversal voltage clamp protocol. The membrane was held at approximately 45 mV positive to the V_{rev} Cl⁻. **(B)** Current response from an NM cell during the protocol in **(A)**. **(C)** Expanded view of evoked responses from **(B)** (dashed box, stimulus artifacts blanked for clarity). **Cii** shows the increase in evoked response after glycine application while holding at +10 mV. **(D)** Average peak amplitudes of the evoked IPSCs in the control (no gly) and in the presence of glycine pre-application (* indicates significant difference, $p < 0.01$). **(E)** Ratio of peak amplitude between Gly/no Gly conditions in control and when glycine pre-pulse occurred at +10 mV. The ratios were >1 in each cell when glycine application occurred during the +10 mV voltage step. Dashed line represents a ratio of 1, indicating no change in evoked amplitude.

that the occlusion is only an *apparent* cross-desensitization, and that the cross-suppression does not result from a change in channel conductance, but rather from local changes in the trans-membrane Cl⁻ distribution (also concluded by Grassi, 1992). In our system, the changes in Cl⁻ ion concentration were sufficient to explain the observed occlusion. We saw no suppression when Cl⁻ flux was prevented and driving Cl⁻ flux into the cell resulted in increased evoked IPSC amplitudes, presumably due to increased driving force of Cl⁻. This conclusion was supported by the result that GABA and glycine pre-application were each similarly effective at generating suppression (**Figure 6**). However, this does not adequately explain asymmetric cross-inhibition seen in other studies where occlusion is attributed to the phosphorylation state of the receptors (Li et al., 2003). While we were unable to test the symmetry of the occlusion directly due to our study's reliance on physiologically evoked IPSCs, our results ruled out phosphatase 2B activity as the mechanism of the observed suppression.

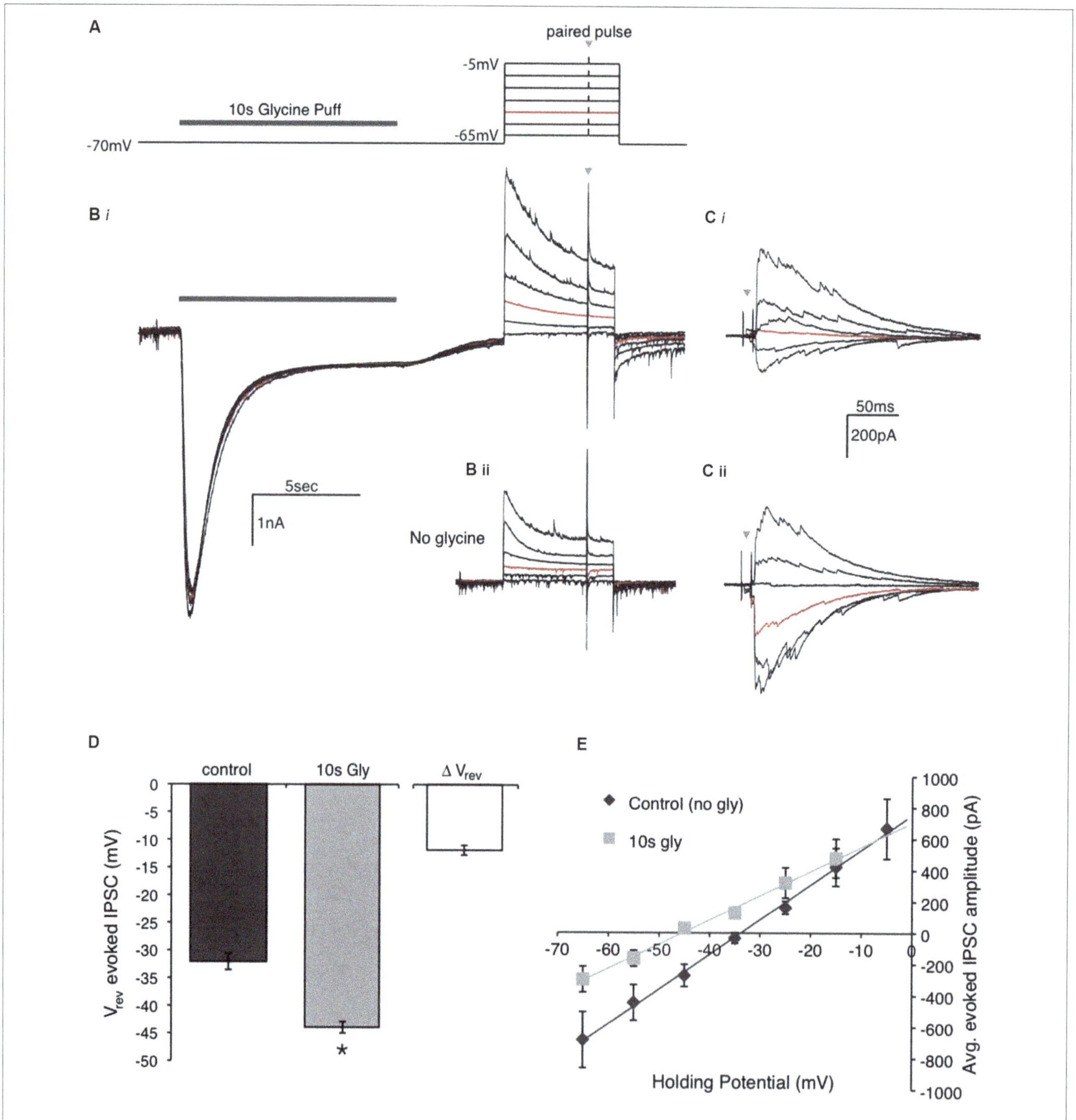

FIGURE 8 | Glycine application affects the driving force of evoked IPSCs by shifting the reversal potential. (A) Schematic of the voltage clamp protocol used to compute reversal potential of evoked IPSCs. The protocol consisted of a paired pulse stimulus (gray arrow) to evoke IPSCs at various holding voltages in the presence or absence of the glycine pre-application. The highlighted (red) step at −45 mV is the voltage used for comparison in the Panels **(B)** and **(C)**. **(B)** Raw data traces recorded during the protocol in **(A)** in the presence **(Bi)** and absence **(Bii)** the glycine pre-application. **(C)** Expanded view of the IPSCs evoked with a paired pulse stimulus during each voltage step. Note that the red trace (V_{hold} = −45 mV) in **Ci** has an evoked IPSC with outward current, while the IPSC in **Cii** is inward. **(D)** Population data for the average reversal potential in the control and glycine pre-application conditions (* indicates significant difference, $p < 0.001$, $n = 7$) as well as the average change in reversal potential between the conditions. **(E)** IV plot constructed by averaging the absolute peak IPSC amplitude of the paired pulse at each voltage step for the population of neurons tested.

ROLE OF GLYCINE IN THE AVIAN BRAINSTEM

While a biochemical interaction between glycine and GABA receptors was not supported by our data, the hypothesis that glycinergic transmission in NM and the SON shapes overall inhibitory transmission remains a compelling possibility. Many studies in the avian sound localization circuit demonstrate modulatory mechanisms that dynamically alter inhibitory transmission. These mechanisms include activation of $GABA_B$ receptors (Lu et al., 2005; Tang et al., 2009), metabotropic glutamate receptors (Lu, 2007; Okuda et al., 2013), and cooperation of both tonic and phasic inhibition (Tang et al., 2011; Yamada et al., 2013). GlyR activation could similarly modulate overall inhibitory strength.

GABA and glycine, either co-released or present at the same synapses, are also known to influence the kinetics of inhibition through a number of mechanisms. Postsynaptic activation of GlyRs and subsequent Cl^- movement would likely affect the Cl^- concentration gradient across the membrane. Changes in Cl^- concentration proximal to GABA and GlyR channel pores can modulate the temporal and voltage dependent properties of Cl^- currents (Moroni et al., 2011). Co-transmission of GABA with glycine has also been shown to speed up the decay kinetics of IPSCs in the mammalian cochlear nucleus (Lu et al., 2008). In the auditory brainstem, signal propagation is dependent on microsecond scale interaural differences in the arrival time of acoustic stimuli. The kinetics of both excitatory and inhibitory input to neurons that process these cues have an impact on their temporal selectivity (Kuba et al., 2005; Jercog et al., 2010; Fischl et al., 2012; Roberts et al., 2013). Therefore, small changes in kinetics caused by changes in local Cl^- gradients could modulate the integration of inputs that rely on precise timing in order to accurately localize sounds.

Glycinergic activity will also affect neurons differently depending on the physiology of the target cell. Physiological heterogeneity is a characteristic of neurons in both NA (Köppl and Carr, 2003; Kuo et al., 2009) and the SON (Coleman et al., 2011). In NA, the reversal potential for Cl^- is variable, such that some neurons were found to have a relatively depolarized V_{rev}, and some, a hyperpolarized V_{rev} (Kuo et al., 2009). This suggests that the polarity of glycinergic transmission will also be dependent on neuron type. The Cl^- V_{rev} of SON neurons has not been thoroughly characterized, but one study using gramicidin perforated patch recordings observed an average Cl^- V_{rev} of −61 mV from data collected in three neurons (Monsivais and Rubel, 2001). Given the heterogeneity of response properties observed in the SON (Carr et al., 1989; Lachica et al., 1994; Coleman et al., 2011), a more thorough investigation of Cl^- regulation seems necessary to fully understand the role of inhibition in this circuit.

Our experiments add to the insights provided by several very recent studies that strive to understand the role of glycine in avian auditory processing. Glycine puff application may only approximate the physiological conditions that occur with intense, prolonged stimuli, where transmitters build up in the synapse and spillover into the extrasynaptic space. In our previous study, we found that glycine recruitment was highly dependent on input rate where the highest rate (200 Hz) resulted in the largest recruitment of glycinergic current in NM (Fischl et al., 2014). Whether this recruitment generally strengthens overall inhibition to maintain inhibitory tone (Fischl et al., 2014), or alternatively limits inhibition through occlusion as the current results suggest, requires further, *in vivo* experimentation.

SUMMARY

Numerous mechanisms have been identified that modulate inhibitory synaptic strength and influence computation in neural circuitry. These mechanisms are diverse in mode, site of action, and influence on signal propagation. One known mechanism of interest for synapses that co-release inhibitory transmitters, is the cross-modulatory suppression between GABA and GlyRs. In some cases, this suppression is clearly mediated by biochemical signaling pathways, while in other systems, the modulation appears to be related to biophysical mechanisms. We explored the nature of interactions between GABA- and glycinergic transmission in neurons that rely heavily on inhibition for precise computation, and for which glycinergic input has only recently been confirmed. We showed the influence of preceding receptor activation on evoked inhibitory transmission, where preceding GlyR activation consistently occluded evoked inhibitory transmission. The magnitude of the suppression was dependent on both the duration of agonist application and magnitude of charge transfer induced by glycine, or in a few cases, GABA. The glycine dependent occlusion was blocked in the presence of strychnine. Cl^- flux was necessary for occlusion suggesting that local changes in the Cl^- driving force resulted from the glycine treatment. Cross-suppressive interactions between GABA and GlyR channels at these synapses may provide an additional modulatory influence regulating inhibition in the avian sound localization circuit. Investigation of the role of glycine in NM and NL *in vivo* is necessary to determine whether these mechanisms impact transmission during sound evoked stimuli and if these modulations influence sound localization ability.

AUTHOR CONTRIBUTIONS

Matthew J. Fischl and R. Michael Burger contributed to the conception and design of experiments as well as drafting and revising the manuscript. Matthew J. Fischl performed the experiments and analyzed the data. Matthew J. Fischl and R. Michael Burger approved the final version to be published.

ACKNOWLEDGMENTS

This work is funded by the National Institute of Health (R01 DC 008989). The authors would like to acknowledge Stefan Oline and Sonia Weimann for their comments on the manuscript.

REFERENCES

Apostolides, P. F., and Trussell, L. O. (2013). Rapid, activity-independent turnover of vesicular transmitter content at a mixed glycine/GABA synapse. *J. Neurosci.* 33, 4768–4781. doi: 10.1523/jneurosci.5555-12.2013

Awatramani, G. B., Turecek, R., and Trussell, L. O. (2005). Staggered development of GABAergic and glycinergic transmission in the MNTB. *J. Neurophysiol.* 93, 819–828. doi: 10.1152/jn.00798.2004

Baev, K. V., Rusin, K. I., and Safrono, B. V. (1992). Primary receptor for inhibitory transmitters in lamprey spinal cord neurons. *Neuroscience* 46, 931–941. doi: 10.1016/0306-4522(92)90195-8

Barker, J. L., and McBurney, R. N. (1979). GABA and glycine may share the same conductance channel on cultured mammalian neurones. *Nature* 277, 234–236. doi: 10.1038/277234a0

Burger, R. M., Fukui, I., Ohmori, H., and Rubel, E. W. (2011). Inhibition in the balance: binaurally coupled inhibitory feedback in sound localization circuitry. *J. Neurophysiol.* 106, 4–14. doi: 10.1152/jn.00205.2011

Burger, P. M., Hell, J., Mehl, E., Krasel, C., Lottspeich, F., and Jahn, R. (1991). GABA and glycine in synaptic vesicles: storage and transport characteristics. *Neuron* 7, 287–293. doi: 10.1016/0896-6273(91)90267-4

Carr, C. E., Fujita, I., and Konishi, M. (1989). Distribution of GABAergic neurons and terminals in the auditory system of the barn owl. *J. Comp. Neurol.* 286, 190–207. doi: 10.1002/cne.902860205

Chang, E. H., Kotak, V. C., and Sanes, D. H. (2003). Long-term depression of synaptic inhibition is expressed postsynaptically in the developing auditory system. *J. Neurophysiol.* 90, 1479–1488. doi: 10.1152/jn.00386.2003

Coleman, W. L., Fischl, M. J., Weimann, S. R., and Burger, R. M. (2011). GABAergic and glycinergic inhibition modulate monaural auditory response properties in the avian superior olivary nucleus. *J. Neurophysiol.* 105, 2405–2420. doi: 10.1152/jn.01088.2010

Eulenburg, V., Armsen, W., Betz, H., and Gomeza, J. (2005). Glycine transporters: essential regulators of neurotransmission. *Trends Biochem. Sci.* 30, 325–333. doi: 10.1016/j.tibs.2005.04.004

Fischl, M. J., Combs, T. D., Klug, A., Grothe, B., and Burger, R. M. (2012). Modulation of synaptic input by GABAB receptors improves coincidence detection for computation of sound location. *J. Physiol.* 590, 3047–3066. doi: 10.1113/jphysiol.2011.226233

Fischl, M. J., Weimann, S. R., Kearse, M. G., and Burger, R. M. (2014). Slowly emerging glycinergic transmission enhances inhibition in the sound localization pathway of the avian auditory system. *J. Neurophysiol.* 111, 565–572. doi: 10.1152/jn.00640.2013

Fukui, I., Burger, R. M., Ohmori, H., and Rubel, E. W. (2010). GABAergic inhibition sharpens the frequency tuning and enhances phase locking in chicken nucleus magnocellularis neurons. *J. Neurosci.* 30, 12075–12083. doi: 10.1523/jneurosci.1484-10.2010

Funabiki, K., Koyano, K., and Ohmori, H. (1998). The role of GABAergic inputs for coincidence detection in the neurones of nucleus laminaris of the chick. *J. Physiol.* 508, 851–869. doi: 10.1111/j.1469-7793.1998.851bp.x

Gillespie, D. C., Kim, G., and Kandler, K. (2005). Inhibitory synapses in the developing auditory system are glutamatergic. *Nat. Neurosci.* 8, 332–338. doi: 10.1038/nn1397

Grassi, F. (1992). Cl(-)-mediated interaction between GABA and glycine currents in cultured rat hippocampal neurons. *Brain Res.* 594, 115–123. doi: 10.1016/0006-8993(92)91035-d

Hassfurth, B., Grothe, B., and Koch, U. (2010). The mammalian interaural time difference detection circuit is differentially controlled by GABAB receptors during development. *J. Neurosci.* 30, 9715–9727. doi: 10.1523/jneurosci.1552-10.2010

Jercog, P. E., Svirskis, G., Kotak, V. C., Sanes, D. H., and Rinzel, J. (2010). Asymmetric excitatory synaptic dynamics underlie interaural time difference processing in the auditory system. *PLoS Biol.* 8:e1000406. doi: 10.1371/journal.pbio.1000406

Kalinina, N. I., Kurchavyi, G. G., Amakhin, D. V., and Veselkin, N. P. (2009). Differences in the activation of inhibitory motoneuron receptors in the frog Rana ridibunda by GABA and glycine and their interaction. *Neurosci. Behav. Physiol.* 39, 775–783. doi: 10.1007/s11055-009-9192-9

Karlsson, U., Druzin, M., and Johansson, S. (2011). Cl(-) concentration changes and desensitization of GABA(A) and glycine receptors. *J. Gen. Physiol.* 138, 609–626. doi: 10.1085/jgp.201110674

Köppl, C., and Carr, C. E. (2003). Computational diversity in the cochlear nucleus angularis of the barn owl. *J. Neurophysiol.* 89, 2313–2329. doi: 10.1152/jn.00635.2002

Kotak, V. C., and Sanes, D. H. (2002). Postsynaptic kinase signaling underlies inhibitory synaptic plasticity in the lateral superior olive. *J. Neurobiol.* 53, 36–43. doi: 10.1002/neu.10107

Kotak, V. C., and Sanes, D. H. (2003). Gain adjustment of inhibitory synapses in the auditory system. *Biol. Cybern.* 89, 363–370. doi: 10.1007/s00422-003-0441-7

Kuba, H., Yamada, R., Fukui, I., and Ohmori, H. (2005). Tonotopic specialization of auditory coincidence detection in nucleus laminaris of the chick. *J. Neurosci.* 25, 1924–1934. doi: 10.1523/jneurosci.4428-04.2005

Kuo, S. P., Bradley, L. A., and Trussell, L. O. (2009). Heterogeneous kinetics and pharmacology of synaptic inhibition in the chick auditory brainstem. *J. Neurosci.* 29, 9625–9634. doi: 10.1523/jneurosci.0103-09.2009

Lachica, E. A., Rubsamen, R., and Rubel, E. W. (1994). GABAergic terminals in nucleus magnocellularis and laminaris originate from the superior olivary nucleus. *J. Comp. Neurol.* 348, 403–418. doi: 10.1002/cne.903480307

Lewis, C. A., and Faber, D. S. (1993). GABA responses and their partial occlusion by glycine in cultured rat medullary neurons. *Neuroscience* 52, 83–96. doi: 10.1016/0306-4522(93)90184-h

Li, Y., Wu, L. J., Legendre, P., and Xu, T. L. (2003). Asymmetric cross-inhibition between GABAA and glycine receptors in rat spinal dorsal horn neurons. *J. Biol. Chem.* 278, 38637–38645. doi: 10.1074/jbc.m303735200

Lu, Y. (2007). Endogenous mGluR activity suppresses GABAergic transmission in avian cochlear nucleus magnocellularis neurons. *J. Neurophysiol.* 97, 1018–1029. doi: 10.1152/jn.00883.2006

Lu, Y., Burger, R. M., and Rubel, E. W. (2005). GABA(B) receptor activation modulates GABA(A) receptor-mediated inhibition in chicken nucleus magnocellularis neurons. *J. Neurophysiol.* 93, 1429–1438. doi: 10.1152/jn.00786.2004

Lu, T., Rubio, M. E., and Trussell, L. O. (2008). Glycinergic transmission shaped by the corelease of GABA in a mammalian auditory synapse. *Neuron* 57, 524–535. doi: 10.1016/j.neuron.2007.12.010

Lu, T., and Trussell, L. O. (2000). Inhibitory transmission mediated by asynchronous transmitter release. *Neuron* 26, 683–694. doi: 10.1016/s0896-6273(00)81204-0

Magnusson, A. K., Park, T. J., Pecka, M., Grothe, B., and Koch, U. (2008). Retrograde GABA signaling adjusts sound localization by balancing excitation and inhibition in the brainstem. *Neuron* 59, 125–137. doi: 10.1016/j.neuron.2008.05.011

McIntire, S. L., Reimer, R. J., Schuske, K., Edwards, R. H., and Jorgensen, E. M. (1997). Identification and characterization of the vesicular GABA transporter. *Nature* 389, 870–876. doi: 10.1038/39908

Monsivais, P., and Rubel, E. W. (2001). Accommodation enhances depolarizing inhibition in central neurons. *J. Neurosci.* 21, 7823–7830.

Monsivais, P., Yang, L., and Rubel, E. W. (2000). GABAergic inhibition in nucleus magnocellularis: implications for phase locking in the avian auditory brainstem. *J. Neurosci.* 20, 2954–2963.

Moroni, M., Biro, I., Giugliano, M., Vijayan, R., Biggin, P. C., Beato, M., et al. (2011). Chloride ions in the pore of glycine and GABA channels shape the time course and voltage dependence of agonist currents. *J. Neurosci.* 31, 14095–14106. doi: 10.1523/jneurosci.1985-11.2011

Okuda, H., Yamada, R., Kuba, H., and Ohmori, H. (2013). Activation of metabotropic glutamate receptors improves the accuracy of coincidence detection by presynaptic mechanisms in the nucleus laminaris of the chick. *J. Physiol.* 591(Pt. 1), 365–378. doi: 10.1113/jphysiol.2012.244350

Roberts, M. T., Seeman, S. C., and Golding, N. L. (2013). A mechanistic understanding of the role of feedforward inhibition in the mammalian sound localization circuitry. *Neuron* 78, 923–935. doi: 10.1016/j.neuron.2013.04.022

Sagné, C., El Mestikawy, S., Isambert, M. F., Hamon, M., Henry, J. P., Giros, B., et al. (1997). Cloning of a functional vesicular GABA and glycine transporter by screening of genome databases. *FEBS Lett.* 417, 177–183. doi: 10.1016/s0014-5793(97)01279-9

Takesian, A. E., Kotak, V. C., and Sanes, D. H. (2010). Presynaptic GABA(B) receptors regulate experience-dependent development of inhibitory short-term plasticity. *J. Neurosci.* 30, 2716–2727. doi: 10.1523/jneurosci.3903-09.2010

Tang, Z. Q., Dinh, E. H., Shi, W., and Lu, Y. (2011). Ambient GABA-activated tonic inhibition sharpens auditory coincidence detection via a depolarizing shunting mechanism. *J. Neurosci.* 31, 6121–6131. doi: 10.1523/jneurosci.4733-10.2011

Tang, Z. Q., Gao, H., and Lu, Y. (2009). Control of a depolarizing GABAergic input in an auditory coincidence detection circuit. *J. Neurophysiol.* 102, 1672–1683. doi: 10.1152/jn.00419.2009

Trattner, B., Berner, S., Grothe, B., and Kunz, L. (2013). Depolarization-induced suppression of a glycinergic synapse in the superior olivary complex by endocannabinoids. *J. Neurochem.* 127, 78–90. doi: 10.1111/jnc.12369

Trombley, P. Q., Hill, B. J., and Horning, M. S. (1999). Interactions between GABA and glycine at inhibitory amino acid receptors on rat olfactory bulb neurons. *J. Neurophysiol.* 82, 3417–3422.

Wojcik, S. M., Katsurabayashi, S., Guillemin, I., Friauf, E., Rosenmund, C., Brose, N., et al. (2006). A shared vesicular carrier allows synaptic corelease of GABA and glycine. *Neuron* 50, 575–587. doi: 10.1016/j.neuron.2006.04.016

Yamada, R., Okuda, H., Kuba, H., Nishino, E., Ishii, T. M., and Ohmori, H. (2013). The cooperation of sustained and phasic inhibitions increases the contrast of ITD-tuning in low-frequency neurons of the chick nucleus laminaris. *J. Neurosci.* 33, 3927–3938. doi: 10.1523/jneurosci.2377-12.2013

Yang, L., Monsivais, P., and Rubel, E. W. (1999). The superior olivary nucleus and its influence on nucleus laminaris: a source of inhibitory feedback for coincidence detection in the avian auditory brainstem. *J. Neurosci.* 19, 2313–2325.

2

The natural history of sound localization in mammals – A story of neuronal inhibition

Benedikt Grothe* and Michael Pecka

Division of Neurobiology, Department of Biology II, Ludwig Maximilians University Munich, Munich, Germany

***Correspondence:**
Benedikt Grothe, Division of Neurobiology, Department of Biology II, Ludwig Maximilians University Munich, Grosshaderner Strasse 2, 82152 Planegg-Martinsried, Munich, Germany
e-mail: grothe@lmu.de

Our concepts of sound localization in the vertebrate brain are widely based on the general assumption that both the ability to detect air-borne sounds and the neuronal processing are homologous in archosaurs (present day crocodiles and birds) and mammals. Yet studies repeatedly report conflicting results on the neuronal circuits and mechanisms, in particular the role of inhibition, as well as the coding strategies between avian and mammalian model systems. Here we argue that mammalian and avian phylogeny of spatial hearing is characterized by a convergent evolution of hearing air-borne sounds rather than by homology. In particular, the different evolutionary origins of tympanic ears and the different availability of binaural cues in early mammals and archosaurs imposed distinct constraints on the respective binaural processing mechanisms. The role of synaptic inhibition in generating binaural spatial sensitivity in mammals is highlighted, as it reveals a unifying principle of mammalian circuit design for encoding sound position. Together, we combine evolutionary, anatomical and physiological arguments for making a clear distinction between mammalian processing mechanisms and coding strategies and those of archosaurs. We emphasize that a consideration of the convergent nature of neuronal mechanisms will significantly increase the explanatory power of studies of spatial processing in both mammals and birds.

Keywords: MSO, LSO, evolution, glycine, GABA, archosaurs, birds, binaural hearing

THE EVOLUTIONARY ORIGIN OF HEARING

It has been established for all groups of gnathostomes (jawed vertebrates) that hearing via secondary receptor types, namely hair-cells in the inner ear is directly related to or derived from the same primary substrate – vestibular sensory epithelia (Fritzsch et al., 2002). This strongly supports an early date for the primordial origin of hearing in vertebrates in relation to the encoding of substrate sounds or sounds conducted via bones (e.g., the jaws, jaw joint and the joint-supporting structure, the hyomandibular bone, Manley, 1973). A common origin of substrate hearing is also supported by the overall similarity between the auditory pathways in different vertebrate groups and their close kinship to the similarly hair-cell-driven lateral-line system pathway found in fish. This assertion is amply supported by molecular and developmental studies that underline the overall similarity between these systems, implying that all hearing originated with the detection of aquatic particle motion or substrate sound by mechanical stimulation of vestibular (or lateral-line) hair-cells (Striedter, 1991; Fritzsch et al., 2002; Manley et al., 2004). Therefore, the hair-cell-based reception of non-air-born sound can be considered as basically homologous across all jawed vertebrates.

However, the issue becomes much more complex when we consider the localization of air-borne sounds. Here the concept of general homology is of no help, simply because several prerequisites have to be taken into account. In particular, efficient detection of air-borne sound requires impedance-matching devices (e.g., middle-ear bones, because jaw bones are too big to vibrate in response to air-borne sounds) and imposes specific evolutionary constraints on all neuronal structures and subsequent encoding strategies. Only in very small animals, e.g., some minute frogs, can bony elements that lack a tympanum be mechanically stimulated by air-borne sounds, and thereby directly activate the inner ear (Boistel et al., 2013). Early amniotes were not as diminutive as that. Hence, their bones were too large and massive to be displaced by air-borne pressure waves. Consequently, tympani and specialized middle-ears evolved to detect air-borne sounds. Moreover, these structures developed several times independently, namely in frogs (or some of their ancestors), sauropsids (reptiles and birds), and in mammals (Allin, 1975; Clack, 1997; **Figure 1**). In all these lineages, middle-ears derived from the same precursors, namely from the paired structure that supported the jaw joints: solely from the hyomandibular bone in non-mammals, and from three bones in mammals, specifically the "primary" jaw joint comprising the articular, quadratum, and hyomandibular bones (Reichert, 1837; Gaupp, 1913). These bones originally served both as jaws and to transmit sounds from the jaw via the hyomandibular bone, which supported the jaw joint at the otic region of the skull, by means of bone conduction. At least for mammals, this evolutionary pathway is clearly evidenced in the fossil record. Nevertheless, there is ongoing debate over how often tympanic ears might have evolved independently within the sauropsids (Clack, 2002). Moreover, some authors suggest an independent origin in monotremes and therian mammals (Rich et al., 2005) – a contention which is disputed by others (Rowe et al., 2008). In any case, evolution of the tympanic ear for transmission of air-borne sounds did not follow a single trajectory from a common origin, but represents a classic example of parallel evolution in response to a common selection pressure.

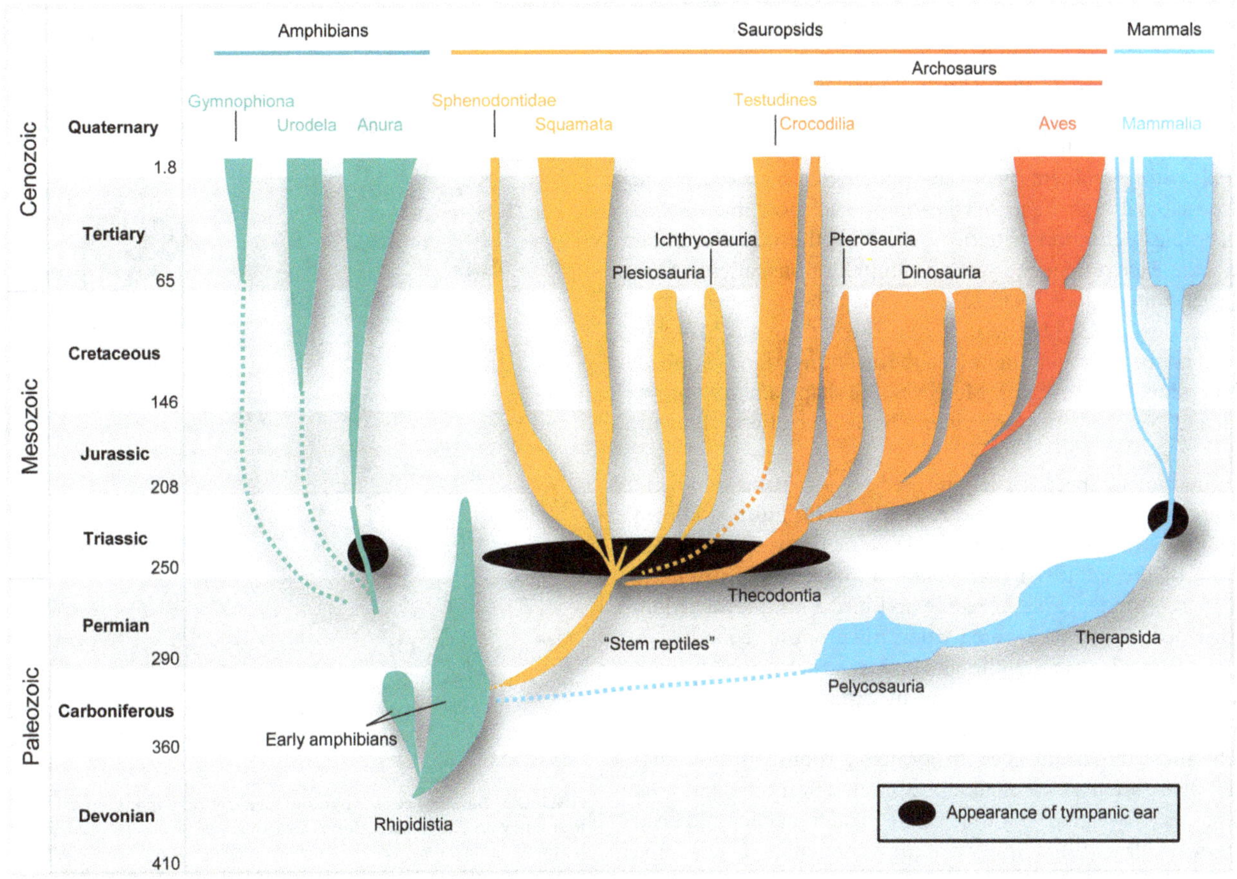

FIGURE 1 | Parallel evolution of vertebrate ears. Tympanic middle-ears capable of receiving air-borne sound evolved separately among the ancestors of mammals (blue), modern frogs ("Anura," green), "reptiles" (yellow), and birds ("Archosaurs," orange/red) in the Triassic ~210–230 million years ago (indicated by black closed circles/oval). Note that no common ancestor with tympanic ears had existed.

It is therefore safe to assume as a basis for this review that the mammalian tympanic ear evolved independently of those found in all other tetrapods – most importantly in this context, the archosaurs (crocodiles, pterosaurs, dinosaurs and their descendants, birds; **Figure 1** presents a simplified scenario). This picture is supported by the fossil record which confirms that the relevant ancestors (for instance, the predecessors of pelycosaurs, therapsids, and mammals) did not have tympanic ears (Hotton, 1959; Hopson, 1966; Clack, 1997). Further confirmation is provided by comparative anatomy, classical embryology (Rodríguez-Vázquez, 2005) and, more recently, evidence from comparative gene expression studies (reviewed by Sienknecht, 2013) and the role of the neural crest in inserting the bones into the middle-ear cavity (Thompson and Tucker, 2013).

Given that hearing of air-borne sounds evolved more than once, we have to take its evolutionary starting point and the subsequent phylogenetic events into account if we wish to reconstruct the evolution of binaural hearing in different lineages. This approach will also help us to understand and appreciate differences in the structures and processing strategies utilized for this purpose by birds and mammals. Importantly, a precise concept of homology is essential, and we therefore will employ the term "homology" only where it is clear that the structures or functions in question (like specific groups of neurons or pathways) have a common developmental origin and served the same function in the last common ancestor. Otherwise we use the term "analogy." Note that this distinction does not call into question the overall homology of hair-cell based sound reception *per se*, as mentioned above.

THE ORIGINS OF SPATIAL HEARING

Binaural sound localization circuits have developed in the context of the processing of air-borne sounds – be it for the purpose of localizing sources, segregating concurrent sounds, or distinguishing primary sounds from echoes. Their development does not exclude the possible use of common ancestral circuits, albeit not specialized for processing binaural cues (see below).

In this context we need to consider the types of spatial acoustic cues to which a given group of animals that developed middle-ears would have been exposed in significant magnitude. This issue relates directly to the anatomy of the skull and the tympanic ear itself. Thus, we first have to take into account what animals were like when they "invented" middle-ears.

We first briefly turn to the three classes of acoustic cues that animals can theoretically use (for a more detailed description see Grothe et al., 2010). First there are *spectral cues* that change when a sound-source moves from one position in space to another. Such changes are most prominent when a sound moves in the vertical plane and thus thought of as monaural. Particularly in animals with prominent outer ears (pinnae), long ear canals and well-developed high-frequency hearing – i.e., most mammals – the complex reflection patterns created by the pinna and ear canal can lead to frequency-specific amplifications, attenuations and even cancelations (defined as so-called "head-related transfer functions," HRTFs). These effects, however, are not fixed but depend on the direction from which the incoming sounds impinge on the pinna and ear canal. Moreover, the shape and size of the head, and even body posture, can modulate such effects (Blauert, 1997).

In mammals, spectral cues are used for localizing sounds in the vertical plane, where they change most. Not much is known about the use of spectral cues in non-mammalian vertebrates, but because of the nature of their skulls, such signals are unlikely to play a prominent role in reptile and bird sound localization. Furthermore, spectral cues are particularly pronounced at higher frequencies, which most reptiles and birds cannot hear (see below). However, they are of particular relevance to mammals, especially early in their evolution (see below).

The most important cues for localizing sounds in the horizontal plane are the two binaural cues, interaural time and level differences (Rayleigh, 1907) which depend on frequency and head features (Erulkar, 1972). Interaural time differences (ITDs) – the difference in the time-of-arrival of a sound at the two ears – occurs when the sound-source is not equidistant from both ears. ITDs increase with increasing lateral displacement from the sagittal plane, i.e., to the left or right. Maximal ITDs occur when a sound comes from 90° to the left or right (**Figure 2**). Since in most animals the maximal durations of ITDs are far down in the sub-millisecond range (compare this to the average duration of action potentials of about 1 ms), ITD processing requires either dedicated anatomical specializations – including acoustic/mechanical interferences [as in some insects (Michelsen, 1994) but also in frogs and to some degree in sauropsids (Christensen-Dalsgaard, 2011)]– and/or very specific neuronal adaptations at the level of nerve-cell membranes, synapses, axons, and entire circuits (for review: Grothe et al., 2010).

Finally, the head has a shadowing effect on sound coming from off the sagittal plane. For instance, a sound originating in the horizontal plane but 90° to the left will reach the right ear only after having been attenuated by the head, which lies between the contralateral ear and the sound-source. This shadowing effect results in an interaural level difference (ILD) between the sounds reaching the two ears (**Figure 2**). ILDs are frequency dependent, with high frequencies being affected most and low frequencies being almost unaffected (Rayleigh, 1907) – at least for sounds in the far field (note that in the near range, ILDs can occur even for lower frequencies; Shinn-Cunningham et al., 2000). Head width determines the frequency at which ILDs become relevant (as a rule of thumb: if the wavelength is shorter than the head width, significant ILDs will occur; for humans this corresponds to frequencies >1.3 kHz). Therefore, even very small animals can experience large ILDs at high frequencies (**Figure 2**; Erulkar, 1972; Harnischfeger et al., 1985). On the other hand, even large animals cannot exploit ILDs if they can hear only low frequencies. The former group does not need to process ITDs of only a few 10s of μs, since they can avail of the ILD information. In contrast, the latter have to use ITDs – albeit ITDs that extend to a few 100 μs, and thus these ITDs will have been potentially capable of affecting the response properties of auditory neurons when these systems evolved (Grothe, 2000).

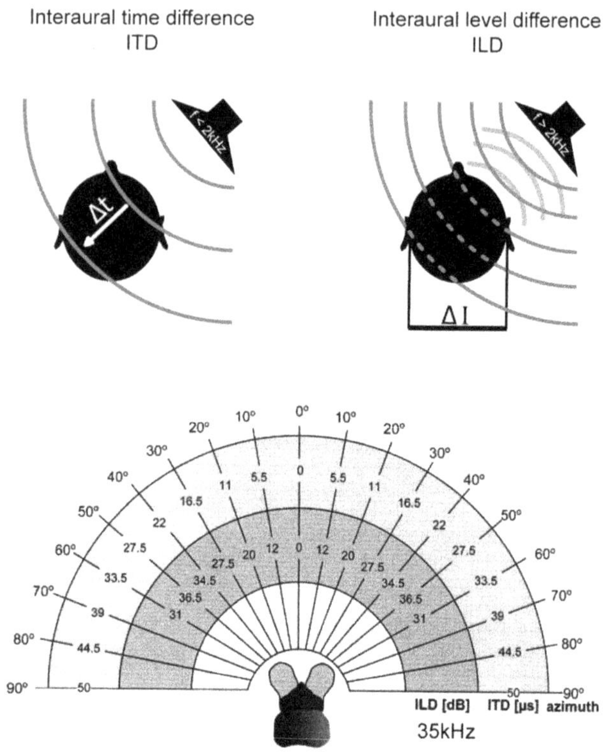

FIGURE 2 | Binaural cues for sound localization depend on sound frequency and head size. Upper left: interaural time differences (ITDs): for frequencies below ~2 kHz, the difference in the arrival time (Δt) of a sound wave (gray lines) at the two ears is used to localize a sound-source in the horizontal plane. ITDs depend on the angle of the sound-source relative to the head axis and the interaural distance (i.e., head size) of the individual. **Upper right**: interaural level differences (ILDs): for frequencies higher than ~2 kHz, the shadowing effect of the head creates differences in the intensity of the sounds at the two ears (ΔI) that are utilized for sound localization in the horizontal plane. ILDs for a particular sound-source position increase with increasing frequencies. **Lower**: range of ILDs (inner hemicycle) and ITDs (middle hemicycle) are illustrated across the range of azimuthal sound-source positions (outer hemicycle) for a small mammal (the bat *Molussus ater*). While ITDs are minute even for the most lateralized sound-source positions (±50 μs), sizable ILDs are generated by the relatively small head already at moderately high frequencies (35 kHz for this example). Modified with permission from Harnischfeger et al. (1985).

Hence, which cue an animal uses depends on its head size as well as its hearing range. Given that features of the head differed among the early tetrapods that developed tympanic ears (see below), it would not be surprising if different structural and circuit adaptations were to develop in different lineages. Moreover, different evolutionary starting points, in terms of which binaural cue was used first (and why), inevitably should have impacted on the neuronal coding strategy in a given group of animals. This is why understanding spatial hearing depends on taking the evolutionary history of hearing into account.

For reasons that are not yet understood, tympanic ears in tetrapods appeared during an – evolutionarily speaking – rather short time span of 10, maybe 20 million years in the Triassic Period (Clack, 1997). This was only some 150 million years after their amphibian ancestors had first moved onto land and probably only 100 million years after our lineage (the synapsid line leading to Pelycosauria, then Therapsida and finally Mammalia; **Figure 1**) diverged from all other land vertebrates, and apparently also after the Diapsida (most reptiles including archosaurs) had split into several subgroups (see **Figure 1**). The various groups that independently developed tympanic ears in the Triassic were very different, both in terms of anatomy and lifestyle (Tucker and Benton, 1982; Golonka, 2007; Ezcurra, 2010). Moreover, the anatomy of the middle-ear differed significantly between these groups (Manley, 2010). This difference is highly significant for the understanding of the evolution of air-born hearing, because middle-ear anatomy not only is crucial for matching the difference in sound impedance between the outer air and the fluid in the inner ear, but also defines the frequency range transmitted to the sensory epithelium. Frogs and all sauropsids only use one middle-ear bone whose size, mass and mechanics favor low-frequency conduction (see below). In contrast, the mammalian middle-ear evolved right from the start as a very small, low-mass, three-boned structure that favored higher frequency sound conduction. This has significant consequences for their original hearing range and, hence, for the "starting point" at which the evolution of their detection systems for air-borne sounds began. The original hearing range, in turn, had a major impact on the "choice" of binaural cue to be utilized for sound localization. This should be reflected in the neurobiology of hearing of recent animals. We now consider the different combinations of anatomical factors that would be expected to favor the exploitation of a specific spatial cue.

(1) The mechanics of the early middle-ears determined the frequency range of air-borne sounds that could be detected (Fleischer, 1978; Rosowski et al., 1999; Huang et al., 2000). Middle-ear systems that preferentially transmit low-frequency sounds would suggest high selection pressures for ITDs, simply because ILDs are not relevant in that context. In contrast, middle-ears that can transmit high frequencies would favor ILD processing systems (Erulkar, 1972; see above).
(2) The overall size of the animals that first acquired the capacity to use air-borne sound and, hence, that of their skulls, is particularly relevant for assessing how likely or unlikely it is that ITDs were used. Larger heads normally imply larger interaural distances and hence longer ITDs (Kuhn, 1977; Brown and May, 2005). This is relevant since ITD processing involves microsecond precision, which is rather unusual given that action potential duration (on average 1 ms), synaptic delays (>0.5 ms) and jitter (± 100s of μs) significantly compromise the acuity required, as circuits built of neurons with highly specialized membrane properties, synapses and axonal features had not yet evolved. Therefore, it seems plausible to assume that animals developed ITD coding only if ILDs were not significant and if the dimensions of their skulls allowed for ITDs that were long enough to be registered by some neurons in the early auditory pathways (>several 100s of μs). This, of course, does not preclude the evolution of ITD processing in small mammals (reviewed in Grothe, 2000; Köppl, 2009; Manley, 2010) that need to process low frequencies (and such mammals will be discussed later). It is rather a question of likelihood and feasibility.
(3) It also matters whether the original tympanic ears functioned as isolated pressure receivers or whether the two middle-ear cavities were acoustically connected and functioned as a pressure-gradient receiver (Christensen-Dalsgaard, 2005; Köppl, 2009; Manley, 2010). In the former case, the maximal ITD is roughly defined by the absolute interaural distance (i.e., the width of the skull). In the latter, interferences between sounds propagating from one middle-ear cavity to the other can magnify ITDs (Hyson et al., 1994) which helps small animals that strongly rely in low-frequency hearing to gain at least some spatial information from ITDs.
(4) In addition, acoustic and social context, e.g., acoustic communication, either as evolutionary driving force or simply as a co-evolved feature, may have been relevant (Endler, 1993). Larger animals, particularly animals with a larynx (like mammals), are likely to produce call signals at lower frequencies, owing to the resonance frequencies of their sound-producing systems. Although secondary by definition (they can only develop after hearing has been established), such contextual elements can function as an evolutionary feedback system, potent driving force, and selection pressure.

Taking all of these factors into account and combining them with knowledge available from comparative neuroanatomy and physiology, we draw a number of plausible inferences as to how a given group was equipped for the development of spatial hearing and how the initial system evolved further within the group itself. The general concept herein is the following (see also **Figure 9**): physical configurations (head size and hearing range) during the time of the middle-ear development determine the cue that can most easily be exploited for sound localization for a given taxon. The binaural cue in turn shapes the emergence of distinct neuronal mechanisms that are optimized for the processing and encoding of the particular cue. Subsequent evolutionary changes in physical configurations (i.e., changes in head size and/or hearing range) might force the use of additional cues. However, the neuronal mechanisms and coding principles that will be employed to process the additional binaural cue is determined by the original mechanisms/principles that are already in place. Thus, while the same binaural cues (e.g., ITD) are used for sound localization by birds and mammals, their evolutionary histories – and hence neuronal mechanisms – are of different origin.

A SCENARIO FOR THE EVOLUTION OF SOUND LOCALIZATION IN BIRDS: ITD AS THE ORIGINAL BINAURAL CUE

As pointed out above, we cannot yet say with certainty how often tympanic ears evolved in sauropsids. Currently, there is conflicting evidence between morphological and molecular studies on whether testudines represents a sister group of archosaurs or whether they are more remote and thus developed tympanic ears independently (Hedges, 2012). Moreover, if tympanic ears evolved only in the Triassic (Clack, 1997) and archosaurs first appeared in the Late Permian or Early Triassic (Gower and Sennikov, 1996), their organs for detecting air-borne sounds may even have been acquired separately from other diapsids in that group. In any case, almost all early archosaurs were quite large (compared to early mammals, see below) and increased in size during the Triassic (e.g., crocodiles and dinosaurs) to give rise to the largest land-dwelling tetrapods (Gower and Weber, 1998). Birds inherited their tympanic ears from them (e.g., dinosaurs). Like all archosaurs they possessed only one middle-ear bone, the columella (derived from the hyomandibular bone, like the stapes in mammals), a fact which, by and large, limits their audiograms to relatively low frequencies (from a few 10s of Hz to a few kHz; green shaded area in **Figure 3**; Fleischer, 1978; Rosowski and Saunders, 1980). Additionally, a connection between the two middle-ear cavities via a thin tube makes their hearing system a kind of pressure-gradient receiver (reviewed in Manley, 2010) that creates interferences and thereby moderately enhances ITDs. For instance, in young chicks maximal ITDs can be enhanced to reach up to 180us for low-frequency sounds, whereas maximal ITDs reach only 100 μs at frequencies of 2–4 kHz and thus appear to rely solely on the interaural distance (Hyson et al., 1994). Hence, Triassic archosaurs perceived low frequencies associated with only minimal ILDs, but experienced comparatively large ITDs (up to several 100 μs, in some dinosaurs well above 1 ms). It is therefore not surprising that these animals developed a sophisticated neuronal ITD coding system [e.g., the nucleus laminaris, NL; (Carr, 1993; Carr et al., 2001)]. Interestingly, testudines (turtles) possess a prominent NL (Willis et al., 2013), corroborating the molecular evidence that they might be closely related to archosaurs (Shen et al., 2011; Chiari et al., 2012; Lu et al., 2013; Field et al., 2014). The situation is less clear for other diapsids, apart from the fact that they have a true pressure-gradient receiving system (the middle-ear cavities are continuous with the oral cavity), which introduces significant binaural interference patterns that will generate a mixture of ITDs and ILDs of their own (Christensen-Dalsgaard and Manley, 2008; Christensen-Dalsgaard, 2011; Christensen-Dalsgaard et al., 2011). To summarize, the sound localization system in birds most likely evolved to process low-frequency signals and thus is specialized for ITD detection.

A SCENARIO FOR THE EVOLUTION OF SOUND LOCALIZATION IN MAMMALS: ILD AS THE ORIGINAL BINAURAL CUE

The ancestors of mammals, which belonged to the late therapsids, were probably the last to develop tympanic ears in the Late Triassic (Allin, 1975; Clack, 1997). Two factors distinguish their evolution from all others. Firstly, they developed a secondary jaw joint, probably due to a change of diet to seeds, which required crushing (Crompton, 1963; Kemp, 1982). This deprived all three original jaw ossicles of their former primary function – cutting and tearing – and allowed them to take on a secondary function, the transmission of sounds (substrate sound/bone conductance from the lower jaw). Secondly, at this point, therapsids – the hitherto dominant group of tetrapods – were being pushed aside by the rapidly evolving dinosaurs, and were facing extinction. The only clade that survived did so by rapidly decreasing in size, ultimately giving rise to animals smaller than laboratory mice. Interestingly, during this phase, the originally much larger middle-ear bones shrank isometrically with the rest of the skull to a size suitable for transmitting sounds [for instance *Thrinaxodon* (Estes, 1961)], – and they have allometrically remained in this state despite the ensuing changes

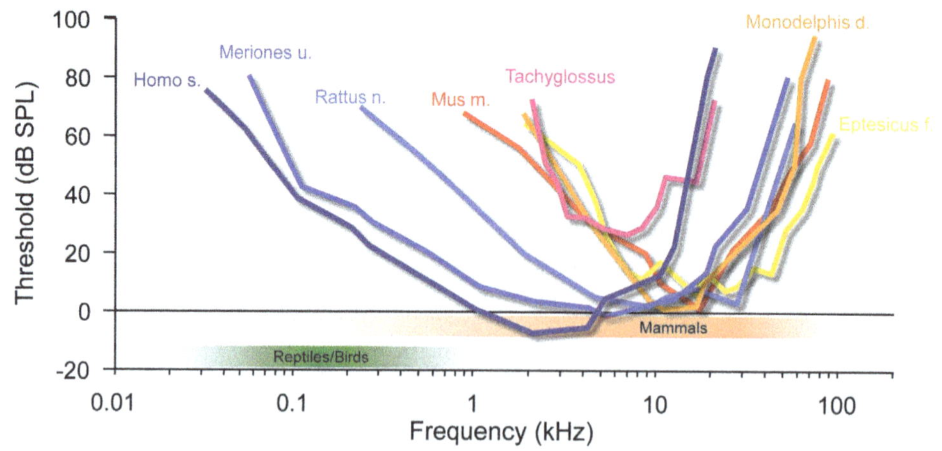

FIGURE 3 | Mammalian hearing originated in the ILD-dominated range. A hallmark of mammalian audiograms is that they are centered in the high-frequency range (>10 kHz), where ILDs are the dominant cue for sound localization. Many recent mammalian species like mice (*Mus m.*), bats (*Eptesicus f.*), rats (*Rattus n.*) and short-tailed opossums (*Monodelphis d.*) even expanded the high-frequency hearing compared to early mammals (*Tachyglossus*), allowing for an increase in obtainable ILDs. Only few species including Gerbils (*Meriones u.*) and man (*Homo s.*) expanded their hearing range into the low-frequency range, where ITD is an attainable sound localization cue (<2 kHz). Audiograms modified from: Echidna/Tachyglossus: Mills and Shepherd (2001); *Monodelphis*: Reimer (1995); Mouse: Heffner and Masterton (1980), Radziwon et al. (2009); Bat (*Eptesicus fuscus*): Koay et al. (1997); Rat (hooded rat): Heffner et al. (1994); Gerbil: Ryan (1976).

in overall body size (Crompton and Hylander, 1986; Maier, 1990). Early mammals like *Morganucodon* (early Jurassic) give us insight into their nocturnal life in the shadow of the dinosaurs. They possessed the new three-ossicle middle-ear, which was basically identical to that of today's echidnas (*Tachyglossus*, one of the two recent monotremes). Theoretical considerations had already suggested that this ear does not efficiently transmit low frequencies, but responds well to mid-range frequencies from a few up to maximally 20 kHz (**Figure 3**; Rosowski and Graybeal, 1991). More recent psychoacoustic evaluations and auditory brainstem potential measurements in echidna support this assumption (Mills and Shepherd, 2001). Hence, early mammals like *Morganucodon* lived in a different acoustic world from that inhabited by the dominating diurnal reptiles. This is also suggested by their small size and that of a potential larynx, which would have produced high-frequency sounds and is supported by the fact that most small mammals still use communications calls in a frequency range beyond that of reptilian and bird hearing (e.g., mother – pup communication, Liu et al., 2003; Ehret, 2005). This separation between reptilian (and later, bird) hearing and that of mammals has apparently tended to increase rather than diminish during evolution. Small marsupials (like *Monodelphis*) or placental mammals (mice, bats etc.) extended their hearing range, as evident from fossils showing the coiled cochlea as a result of lengthening (Fernández and Schmidt, 1963). Comparing the audiograms of recent mammals of various groups indicates that their hearing range almost exclusively extended into the high-frequency range (**Figure 3**). Bat echolocation calls mostly fall within the hearing range of small mammals and should not be considered as unusual – "ultrasound" is a purely anthropocentric, not a mammaliocentric term (**Figure 3**, although this does not imply that bats are not highly specialized in other ways, and some species further extended their hearing range even above 100 kHz). Notably, such extension of hearing range to ever higher frequencies significantly improves the use of HRTFs in the vertical plane. Since localization in the vertical is of the utmost importance for small prey animals (Wallace et al., 2013), reliable HRTF-based localization may well have been a crucial evolutionary pressure on the hearing range of small early mammals. The second advantage of mainly high-frequency hearing is that even the smallest mammals have always experienced significant ILDs (**Figure 2**; Erulkar, 1972; Harnischfeger et al., 1985). On the other hand, their tiny heads produced ITDs of maximally a few 10s of μs (**Figure 2**, <50 μs in animals like *Morganucodon*). There is ongoing debate about whether early mammalian ears also acted as pressure receivers, which could have increased the range of ITDs by a few 10s of μs (Köppl, 2009; Manley, 2010). Whether this would have been significant enough to justify the use of ITDs (despite the availability of large ILDs) seems doubtful. And even if it were, one may ask why such a useful feature would have disappeared in all mammals (including monotremes)? In both cases, the conclusion appears obvious: mammals simply did not need to process ITDs.

Even today, most small mammals rely almost entirely on ILDs, and the neuronal structure responsible for the initial processing of ILDs, the lateral superior olive (LSO), is homogenous in all terrestrial mammals investigated (Tollin, 2003; Grothe et al., 2010). In contrast, the ITD processing structure, the medial superior olive (MSO) exhibits significant differences in shape and size, which are likely to be related to the hearing range in the respective species (low- versus high-frequency sensitivity; Grothe, 2000). Significant selection pressure to use ITDs existed only relatively late during the evolution mammals, probably in relation to increasing body size, which not only conditioned production of low-frequency communication calls, but also necessitated larger territories and long-distance communications – and low frequencies travel further.

THE FUNCTION OF INHIBITION IN ILD PROCESSING CAN EXPLAIN ITS ROLE IN ITD PROCESSING

ILDs AS A STARTING POINT FOR A POPULATION CODE OF SPATIAL POSITION

As outlined above, early mammals most probably could hear high-frequency sounds and had relatively small heads. Hence, ILDs were the only binaural cues available to them for azimuthal sound localization. This suggests that the ancestral neuronal structure used to process binaural spatial information was devoted to ILD detection. It is well established that ILD sensitivity is generated by the LSO in the brainstem, whose bipolar neurons are the initial site of binaural convergence (Galambos et al., 1959; Boudreau and Tsuchitani, 1968; Tsuchitani and Boudreau, 1969). They integrate excitatory (glutamatergic) inputs from the ipsilateral antero-ventral cochlear nucleus (AVCN) with inhibitory (glycinergic) inputs coming from the ipsilateral medial nucleus of the trapezoid body (MNTB), which itself is innervated by the contralateral AVCN (**Figure 4**). This integration process can be thought of as a comparative mechanism that gages the relative sound levels at the two ears (within a particular spectral bandwidth at a given time point), which are encoded in the respective activity levels of the two LSO inputs (Moore and Caspary, 1983; Finlayson and Caspary, 1989; Sanes, 1990; Tollin, 2003). Accordingly, LSO response rates (measured as the number of action potentials elicited per unit time) are highest for ipsilateral sound-source locations that create positive ILDs, i.e., high sound level at the ipsilateral ear allows the excitatory pathway to be fully activated, whereas the sound level at the farther ear is greatly attenuated by the skull, and thus activation of the contralateral inhibitory pathway is minimal. More importantly, response rates are faithfully modulated as a function of the ILD, and most LSO neurons are completely inhibited from spiking at ILDs favoring the contralateral ear (negative ILDs). Such ILD response functions typically take the shape of a sigmoid, generating high sensitivity for small changes in ILD along the slope of the function (**Figure 4**). Note that any ILD sensitivity found in downstream brain areas crucially depends on an LSO input, be it excitatory or inhibitory. This is most probably attributable to neuronal specialization necessary for ILD extraction (see below).

The LSO has no homolog in other vertebrates. In birds, ILD sensitivity is generated by convergence of contralateral excitatory and ipsilateral inhibitory inputs at the level of the lateral lemniscus (Moiseff and Konishi, 1983; Takahashi and Keller, 1992). This connectivity therefore represents a rather complex reciprocal ILD processing circuit that does not reflect the integration mechanism

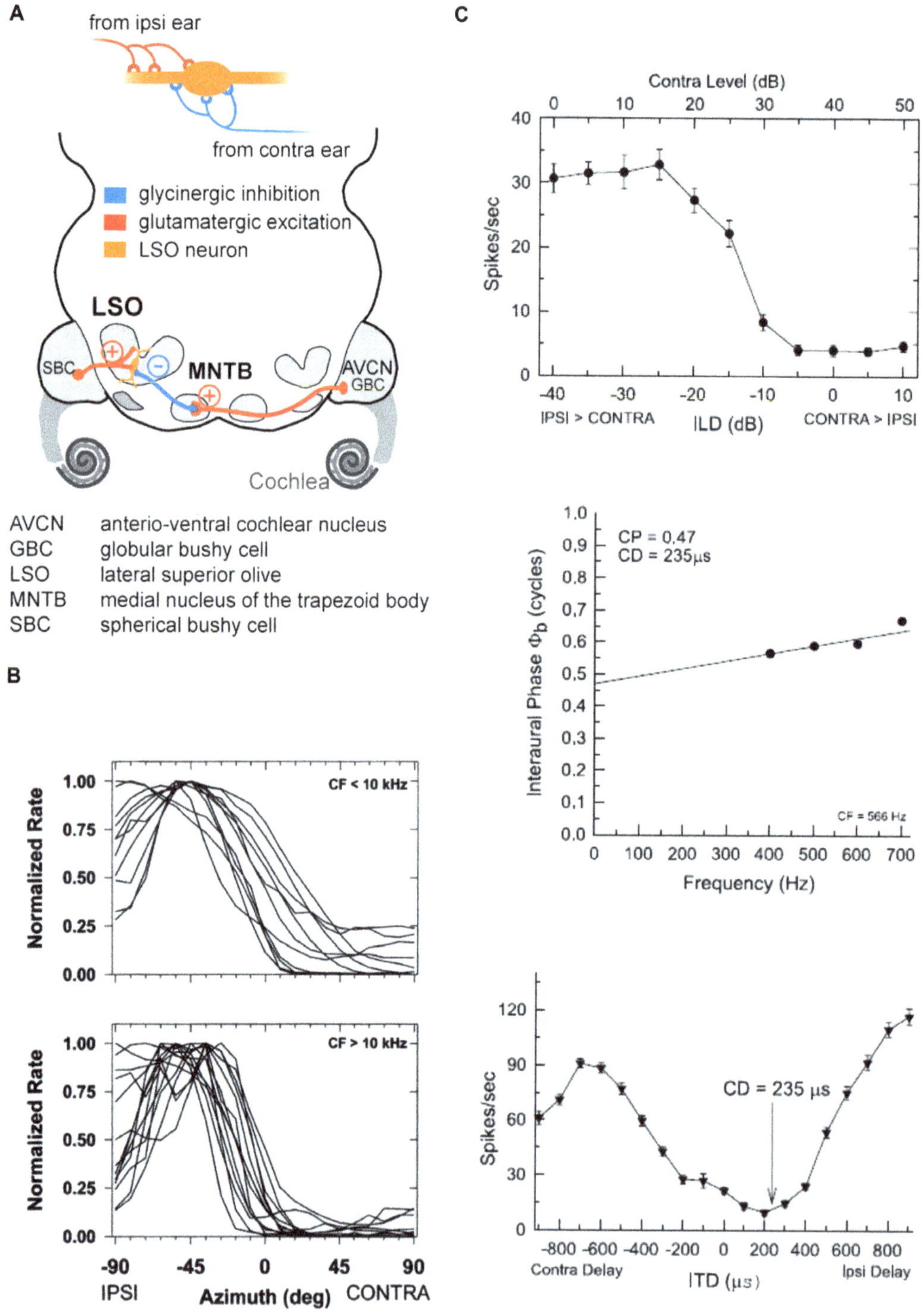

FIGURE 4 | The coincidence mechanism of LSO neurons allows both as ILD and ITD detection. (A) LSO neurons receive excitatory inputs from SBCs in the ipsilateral AVCN and inhibitory inputs from the MNTB that is innervated from by GBCs from the contralateral AVCN. **(B)** The spatial tuning functions of LSO neurons take a hemispheric shape with the slope of the functions crossing frontal azimuthal positions. Upper and lower panels show normalized tuning functions for LSO neurons in cat with CFs below and above 10 kHz, respectively, recorded under virtual acoustic space stimulation that incorporates the HRTFs. Re-printed with permission from Tollin and Yin (2002). **(C)** Low CF neurons in the LSO are both ILD and ITD sensitive: upper panel shows ILD tuning function of a cat LSO neuron (CF = 566Hz), while the lower two panels illustrate the ITD-sensitivity of the same neuron. Note that the characteristic delay (CD) for this neuron, i.e., the delay of coincidence of excitatory and inhibitory inputs, results in a minimal response rate. Re-printed with permission from Tollin and Yin (2005).

of monaural inhibition and excitation of the mammalian LSO: first, inhibitory and excitatory ear are reversed. Second, the ipsilateral inhibition is conveyed by the lateral lemniscus of the other hemisphere, hence by a binaural nucleus. Third, because it is conveyed via an additional synaptic station through the binaural detector of the other hemisphere, inhibition is significantly delayed relative to excitation and seems to serve a response gain modulation (Steinberg et al., 2013). As we will explain in the following and in 3.2., inhibition in the LSO has purposes directly related to establishing binaural sensitivity.

The LSO is well-developed in all terrestrial mammals, including echo-locating bats and humans (Moore, 2000). The overall size of the LSO in a particular species seems to correlate with the range of frequencies to which that species is sensitive (Moore, 2000), most probably owing to the tonotopic organization of the nucleus. All mammals appear to use the same neural mechanism for processing ILDs in the LSO, namely the integration of ipsilateral excitatory inputs from the AVCN and contralateral, inhibitory inputs via the MNTB (see below, Grothe, 2000; Yin, 2002; reviewed in Grothe et al., 2010). Hence, they employ similar coding strategies for high-frequency sound-source localization at the level of the LSO. This coding strategy can be described as a roughly hemispheric code in which individual neurons encode a range of ILDs through response-rate modulation along the slope of their ILD functions (Tollin and Yin, 2002). The LSO neurons studied to date exhibit rather similar ranges of sensitivity to ILDs: the slope of LSO ILD functions is typically centered close to 0 dB ILD (Park et al., 1997, 2004; Park, 1998; Tollin and Yin, 2002). Interestingly, in a study of the cat LSO using virtual space stimuli (i.e., incorporating monaural spectral effects of sound-source location), Tollin and Yin (2002) observed that the tuning of LSO neurons is remarkably stereotypic, as the slope of most spatial-response functions covered a similar range of azimuthal space around the midline and the nearby ipsilateral areas (**Figure 4**). Together, these findings suggest an overrepresentation of near-midline locations, in agreement with the reported maximal psychophysical resolution of ILDs around the midline (Blauert, 1997). However, the interpretation of characteristics of ILD functions in general is difficult, as the peak and slope positions of ILD functions are markedly affected (shifted) by previous activity levels (Park et al., 2008). These shifts are mediated by, among other mechanisms, the retrograde release of GABA from LSO cells onto their own presynaptic inputs (Magnusson et al., 2008), which suggests high plasticity of ILD coding based on recent stimulus history. Hence, even at the level of single binaural comparator neurons, representations of spatial positions are likely to change according to the current auditory context rather than being inflexibly coded. This use of inhibition to generate flexible representations, and their implications for downstream coding, are discussed in more detail in Section "Dynamics of ILD and ITD Processing: $GABA_B$-Mediated Inhibition" below.

ILD PROCESSING – THE ROLE OF THE MNTB AND GLYCINERGIC INHIBITION

The integration of inhibitory and excitatory inputs by LSO cells is often informally referred to as subtraction. This overly simplistic analogy should be treated with caution, insofar as it tends to imply the comparison of net activity levels in the ipsi- and contralateral input integrated over the entire duration of a given acoustic stimulus. In fact, essentially the opposite is true, as timing information – more specifically, information relating to temporal fluctuations in stimulus amplitude – is highly conserved within the LSO circuit. Indeed, neurons involved in ILD detection, including the components of the inhibitory MNTB pathway, are among the most temporally precise in the brain. Two key demands on the system impose the need for high temporal acuity.

The first is the general functional requirement for high temporal resolution in sound localization circuits. These systems cannot afford to integrate over long intervals to produce an average intensity difference, because the source of this average signal might well have changed in the meantime. Moreover, in the presence of multiple, concurrently active sound-sources, short integration times are crucial for discrimination between individual sounds (Meffin and Grothe, 2009; Khouri et al., 2011). Natural signals (communication calls, speech, rustling noises generated by moving prey, etc.) are characterized by prominent and rapid amplitude modulations. Hence, to faithfully detect and track the site of origin of such signals, the LSO circuit must be able to resolve ILDs on very short temporal scales (Joris and Yin, 1995; Tollin, 2003). This is accomplished by the well-known phenomenon of phase-locking, which describes the ability of auditory (brainstem) neurons to lock the timing of their spiking activity to a particular phase of the stimulus (Joris et al., 1994). Phase-locking is commonly invoked in the context of low-frequency carrier or envelope sinusoidal signals, but can (and should) be generalized to the encoding of the rising slopes or transients in any complex signal, irrespective of its frequency (Dietz et al., 2014). Accordingly, phase-locking allows for the precise encoding of a particular time of occurrence in the auditory nerve and downstream pathways. The classical work of Joris et al. (1994) has demonstrated that the quality of phase-locking (measured in terms of vector strength) is actually maintained or even enhanced in the post-synaptic target of the auditory nerve fibers of the binaural system, namely the spherical and globular bushy cells (SBCs and GBCs) of the AVCN, which provide the input to MNTB and LSO, respectively (Warr, 1966; Spangler et al., 1985; Cant and Casseday, 1986; Friauf and Ostwald, 1988; Sanes, 1990). In particular, synaptic transmission between GBC axon and MNTB soma has been studied extensively because of the large size of the pre-synaptic structure (Schneggenburger and Neher, 2005; Kopp-Scheinpflug et al., 2011; Borst and Soria van Hoeve, 2012), and this synaptic relay is one of the fastest and temporally most precise known in the brain (von Gersdorff and Borst, 2002). Evidently, MNTB neurons exhibit similar phase-locking precision to GBCs, while LSO cells – the post-synaptic targets of both MNTB and SBCs – themselves exhibit fast membrane kinetics that allow for exquisite temporal sensitivity to the arrival time and duration of incoming synaptic events (Tollin, 2003). Taken together, these properties of the LSO circuit allow for highly precise and independent ILD processing of each fast transient or onset in a signal.

The second functional demand that necessitates the extreme temporal sensitivity of the LSO circuit is directly linked to the previous argument and explains the specific morphological and physiological adaptations for temporal fidelity and transmission speed that are found within the inhibitory sub-circuit involving the MNTB. A faithful representation of amplitude-modulated signals requires not only that both the excitatory and inhibitory inputs should reliably encode the precise time of occurrence of transient events, but also that both inputs should arrive in close coincidence at the LSO cell to allow for interaction of the two. Clearly, this poses a challenge for the inhibitory input, as it must somehow compensate for the longer axonal pathway from the contralateral AVCN, as well as for the additional synapse between GBC and MNTB, which will introduce a further delay. Indeed, a detailed anatomical examination of the MNTB pathway reveals particular specializations for high conduction velocity, as both axon diameter and myelin thickness are larger in GBCs than in SBCs (Morest, 1968; Schwartz, 1992). Moreover, synaptic delays at the calyx of Held are among to the shortest that have been measured in the CNS (von Gersdorff and Borst, 2002; Kopp-Scheinpflug et al., 2011). Accordingly, physiological evidence shows that inhibition is capable of suppressing even the first spike of LSO responses (Tsuchitani, 1988; Tollin, 2003), demonstrating (at least) coincident arrival of contralateral inhibition and ipsilateral excitation.

In summary, the ILD circuit represents the ancestral binaural sound localization circuit of mammals. LSO neurons detect ILDs via a coincidence detector mechanism of ipsilateral excitation and contralateral inhibition. All components of the LSO circuit are tuned for temporal fidelity, and the inhibitory pathway of the MNTB in particular has evolved anatomical and physiological adaptations to compensate for the longer pathway and additional synaptic delay.

ITD PROCESSING IS DERIVED FROM ILD PROCESSING IN MAMMALS

Shared components of ILD and ITD circuits

The evolutionary and anatomical evidence suggests that, as a nucleus for highly precise binaural discrepancy detection in the time domain, the MSO might have evolved in response to other morphological adaptations that occurred within Mammalia (see The Origins of Spatial Hearing). Increased body (and head) size resulted in a larger interaural distance and a larger larynx, and made it possible to communicate over larger distances (which are best bridged by low-frequency signals). These constraints in turn exerted a selective pressure which favored adaptations that allowed for processing of ITDs (Grothe, 2000; Schnupp and Carr, 2009), as more informative and reliable cues with which to localize relevant sounds or communication calls (since ILDs are negligible at low frequencies). Coincidentally, the "subtraction" mechanism embodied in the LSO, which had developed for ILD detection, is already equipped (pre-adapted) for ITD detection. As has been demonstrated by studies in both cats and chinchillas (**Figure 4**; Finlayson and Caspary, 1991; Joris and Yin, 1995; Tollin and Yin, 2002, see also Park et al., 1996), response rates of low-frequency LSO neurons are strongly modulated by microsecond changes in ITD. These data therefore clearly establish that the temporal fidelity of the glycinergic MNTB input is sufficient to generate ITD sensitivity in LSO neurons tuned to low frequencies by modulating the excitatory inputs excitatory post-synaptic potentials (EPSPs) in response to fast transients. Hence, the MSO circuit which, in mammals specialized for hearing low-frequency sounds, is dedicated to ITD processing only, can be conceptually regarded as a refined LSO circuit (**Figure 5**). Interestingly, mammals with good low-frequency hearing typically possess both a large low-frequency limb of the LSO and a well-developed MSO (Grothe, 2000; Grothe et al., 2010). Potentially their combined output is beneficial to the reliable encoding of sound-source positions, because the spatial tuning functions in the two nuclei are mirror images of each other: a purely suppressive coincidence mechanism (i.e., spiking occurs *unless* binaural coincidence exists) in the LSO is converted into an essentially excitatory coincidence mechanism for the MSO (spiking occurs *only if* binaural coincidence exists). This conversion is achieved by the addition of two more inputs onto MSO neurons. First, a second excitatory input from the contralateral side is required to allow for binaural excitatory coincidence detection. Second there is also an additional inhibitory ipsilateral input via the LNTB (**Figures 5** and **6**). Thus, synaptic inhibition represents an essential feature of the MSO circuit. Anatomical and physiological studies have demonstrated that MSO neurons receive relatively few, but unusually strong, glycinergic inputs (Clark, 1969; Grothe and Sanes, 1993, 1994; Kapfer et al., 2002; Werthat et al., 2008; Couchman et al., 2012) that are well balanced in quantity and quantal size with the excitatory MSO inputs (Couchman et al., 2010). Consequently, the MSO must integrate excitatory and inhibitory inputs from both sides, and is not a simple excitatory coincidence detection circuit. The evolutionary pressure that favored such an arrangement is unclear, but it is reasonable to speculate that the system requires a delicate balance of excitation and inhibition in order to accomplish precise temporal integration (see below). Functionally speaking, the two inhibitory inputs may have important implications for the specific ITD tuning of MSO neurons, a topic that is still being debated today. Initially, research focused on the contralateral source of inhibition via the MNTB, as it had been much more extensively characterized (see above). We suggested earlier that the basic role of phase-locked inhibition might actually be the fine-tuning of best delays (ITD of maximal spiking response) in MSO neurons by modulating the time window for binaural excitatory inputs (**Figure 6**; Brand et al., 2002; Pecka et al., 2008). Specifically, it was suggested that contralateral inhibitory post-synaptic potentials (IPSPs) might arrive at the MSO cell soma slightly in advance of the contralateral EPSPs (**Figure 5**). This would result in a delay of the net excitatory potential, and thus explain the clustering of contralateral best delays in MSO neurons, which has been observed experimentally and across species (McAlpine et al., 2001; Hancock and Delgutte, 2004; Pecka et al., 2008). This scenario might seem to impose significant temporal demands on the MNTB input, but – as described earlier – it is well established that the same MNTB input suppresses the onset of LSO responses, i.e., that contralateral inhibition arrives simultaneously with the ipsilateral excitation. Thus, it seems plausible that contralateral inhibition should actually be slightly faster than contralateral excitation, and both older and recent work with acute brain slice preparations has confirmed that IPSPs can precede EPSPs at MSO cell somata after contralateral AVCN stimulation (Grothe and Sanes, 1994; Roberts et al., 2013). However, the influence of contralateral inhibition alone is insufficient to explain the extent of modulation suggested by *in vivo* pharmacological experiments (Zhou et al.,

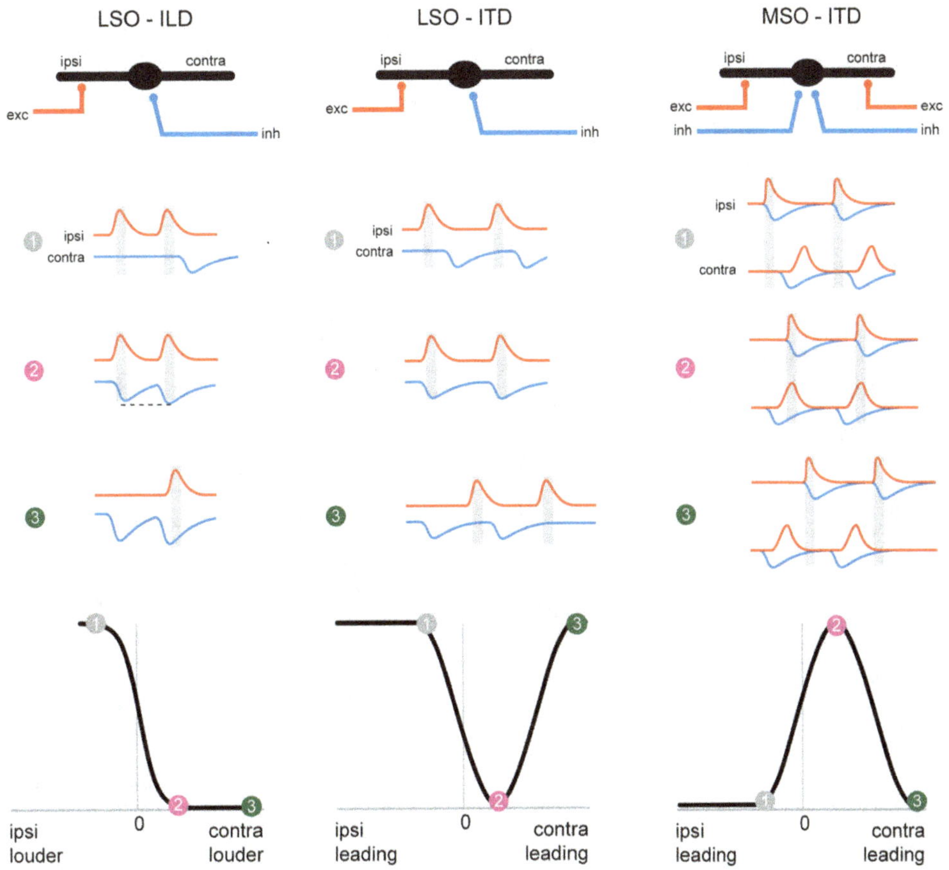

FIGURE 5 | The MSO coincidence mechanism is derived from the LSO coincidence mechanism. The schematic depicts temporal relationships of EPSPs and IPSPs, (red and blue traces, respectively) during ipsi-favoring (1, gray), slightly contra-favoring (2, magenta) and strongly contra-favoring (3, green) input combinations. The left-hand and middle column illustrates processing of these synaptic inputs in the LSO for ILDs and ITDs respectively, and ITD processing in the MSO is shown in the right-hand panel. Note that the MSO integrates EPSPs and IPSPs from both the ipsi- and contralateral side, because of the additional excitatory (contralateral) and inhibitory (ipsilateral) inputs compared to the LSO. The panel in the lower row explains how conditions 1–3 affect spatial tuning functions in the respective nuclei.

2005; Jercog et al., 2010; Roberts et al., 2013; van der Heijden et al., 2013). To clarify this issue, we recently investigated the ability of the ipsilateral source of inhibition to modulate coincidence detection in the MSO, and found that it had a marked capacity to modulate the timing of binaural coincidence (**Figure 6**; Myoga et al., 2014). Although more research is required to thoroughly understand the ipsilateral source of inhibition (Leibold, 2010), it is becoming increasingly clear that having two sources of inhibition (instead of just the contralateral source) provides for greater flexibility in modulating the circuit (**Figure 6**). Thus, while inhibition in the MSO circuit remains a topic of debate, it is reasonable to assume that it serves a central function in the circuit: compared to the ITD-sensitive archetype (i.e., the LSO), an additional (ipsilateral) inhibitory input has evolved in the MSO circuit.

Dedicated inhibitory pathways also exist within the NL-circuit in chicks and owls that seems to serve multiple functions related to ITD processing (Burger et al., 2011). Neurons of the superior olivary nucleus (SON) provide GABAergic inputs to the NL and form a gain control circuit by reducing the amplitude of excitatory inputs and shortening their duration, thereby ensuring consistent ITD sensitivity across intensity levels (Peña et al., 1996; Dasika et al., 2005; Nishino et al., 2008). SON-mediated inhibition also improves phase-locking precision of both the excitatory inputs and NL responses (Nishino et al., 2008; Burger et al., 2011). Importantly, the inhibition from SON onto NL neurons is not timed (it is decoupled from the phase-locked excitation; Yang et al., 1999), and it actually has a depolarizing effect on the NL cells (due to a high intracellular Cl^- concentration), which in turn activates low-threshold potassium-channels that lead to shunting of the cell (Hyson et al., 1995; Yang et al., 1999; Burger et al., 2005a). Interestingly, phase-locked GABAergic inhibition that is conveyed by a feed-forward circuit outside the SON has been found to act on NL neurons tuned to very low frequencies to cooperatively enhance ITD tuning together with tonic inhibition (Yamada et al., 2013). It follows that, analogs to the mammalian system, ITD processing at low frequencies requires the (co)-action of timed inhibition. Hence, both in the mammalian and avian ITD system, inhibition serves a prominent function toward refining the ITD sensitivity of the detector neurons. However, the respective neurotransmitters

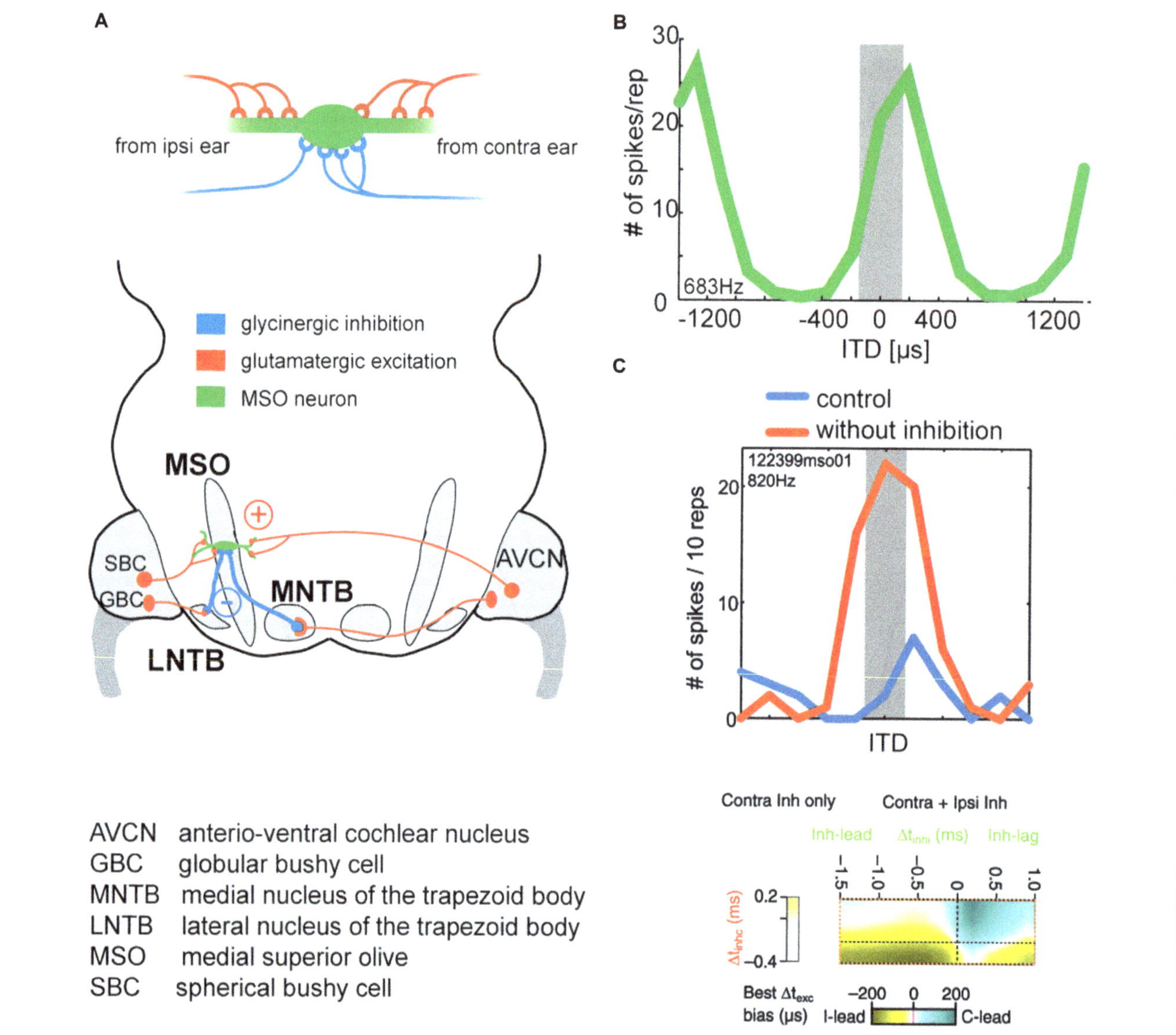

FIGURE 6 | Binaural excitation and inhibition of the MSO circuit allows fine-tuning of the coincidence mechanism. (A) MSO neurons receive binaural excitatory inputs from SBCs in the AVCN of either side and binaural inhibitory inputs from LNTB and MNTB, which are innervated by GBCs of the ipsilateral and contralateral AVCN, respectively. **(B)** ITD tuning function of a gerbil MSO neuron (CF = 683Hz). Note that the peak of the function ("best ITD") is positioned at a contralateral leading ITD outside of the range of physiological ITDs (gray area), while the slope spans the entire range of physiological ITDs. **(C) Upper panel**: blocking inhibition in MSO cells *in vivo* shifts the best ITD toward 0 ITD. Thus, inhibitory inputs tune the ITD of coincidence in MSO cells. Taken from Pecka et al. (2008). **Lower panel**: combination of ipsi- and contralateral inhibitory inputs (right-sided box) allow for both larger shifts of the best ITD (color-coded) than contralateral inhibition alone (left-sided box). Modified from Myoga et al. (2014).

and their associated mode of action and functional time scales are different.

Shared components in ILD and ITD circuits lead to shared coding principles

So far, we have discussed the similar roles of MSO and LSO as binaural discrepancy detectors that share many of their circuit components and design principles. Consequently, similarities are also found in the ways in which particular ITDs and ILDs are reflected in the spiking responses of the respective neurons. Both MSO and LSO neurons exhibit broad, hemispheric tuning to sound-source location, i.e., response rates change monotonically over a large range of azimuthal space (Grothe et al., 2010). Importantly, spatial tuning in both nuclei appears to be more or less stereotypical, with the majority of neurons having their highest spatial sensitivity (the slope of their tuning functions, which conveys most information about changes in location) at frontal positions (**Figures 4** and **6**; Tollin, 2003; Harper and McAlpine, 2004). For ILDs, this stereotypical arrangement becomes most apparent when (virtual) free-field stimulation is used, suggesting a crucial role for spectral composition of the stimuli in azimuthal sound localization at higher frequencies (Tollin and Yin, 2002).

Furthermore, the peak positions of ITD tuning functions have been found to depend on stimulation frequency in many species, irrespective of the head sizes of the species studied (Middlebrooks et al., 1994; McAlpine et al., 2001; Hancock and Delgutte, 2004; Pecka et al., 2008; Werner-Reiss and Groh, 2008). These data have multiple crucial implications: first, that hearing range and the presence of a well-developed MSO, and not body or head size (i.e., physiological ITD range), determines whether a particular species exploits ITDs for sound localization. Since the MSO circuitry is similar in all mammals with low-frequency hearing (Grothe, 2000), neuronal microsecond ITD sensitivity (not spatial acuity in degree, which is a function of interaural size) is also similar across species (Phillips et al., 2012). Second, the frequency-dependence of ITD tuning refutes the notion of a distributed labeled-line representation of azimuthal space (i.e., in which the activity of individual neurons represents the reception of a signal from a fixed direction in space), and have led to numerous speculations on the nature of the underlying coding strategy. The broad tuning functions stimulated the idea of hemispheric, oppositely coding channels on each side of the brain that might be compared upstream of the MSO and LSO (McAlpine et al., 2001; Stecker and Middlebrooks, 2003; Hancock and Delgutte, 2004; Harper and McAlpine, 2004; **Figure 7**). Note that the MSO output – but not the LSO output – to the midbrain crosses the midline, which unifies the hemispheric polarity of the two within each midbrain side (**Figure 7**). While the particular nature of this code is currently under debate (Day and Delgutte, 2013; Goodman et al., 2013), one compelling concept relies on the idea that similar activity levels in each channel represent sound-source position at the midline, such that a relative increase in activity in one of the two brain hemispheres would indicate a proportionally contralateral location with respect to the more active brain hemisphere (**Figure 7**). Psychophysical and functional imaging studies corroborate this scenario of hemispheric coding also in humans (Thompson et al., 2006; von Kriegstein et al., 2008; Magezi and Krumbholz, 2010; Salminen et al., 2010). In particular, using elegant adaptation paradigms, Phillips and Hall (2005), Vigneault-MacLean et al. (2007) have confirmed the presence of a population code that underlies sound localization in humans and also showed that prior stimulation influences subsequent spatial perception. These data pointed the way to more recent discoveries pertaining to how spatial tuning functions can be strongly modulated according to their recent acoustic context. Physiologically, such activity-dependent effects have been demonstrated in the cortex and midbrain (Dahmen et al., 2010; Lee and Middlebrooks, 2011), and even in the MSO and LSO (Magnusson et al., 2008; Park et al., 2008; Stange et al., 2013), suggesting that the primary role of MSO and LSO might not be the encoding of absolute sound-source positions in space (in contrast to the avian system, which employs a labeled line code with a consequently sparse output corresponding to any one position in space), but rather of their relative locations compared to other sound-sources. Similar adaptive coding concepts

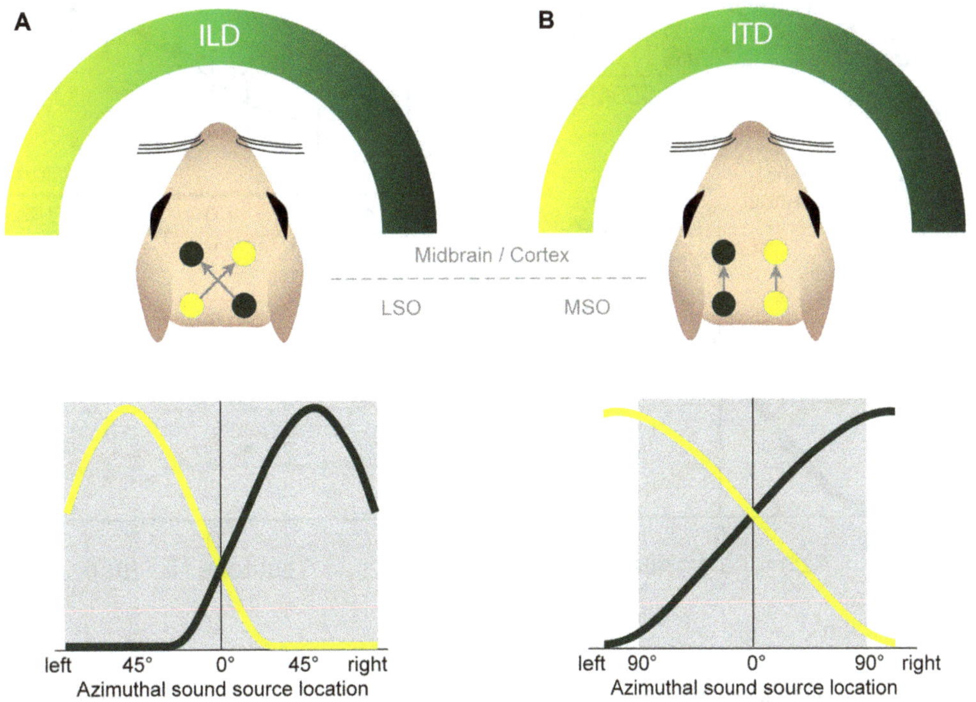

FIGURE 7 | Both the ILD and ITD code is based on hemispheric tuning functions. The azimuthal tuning function of both LSO and MSO span a wide range of azimuthal space. **(A)** LSO neurons respond best to ipsilateral sound-source positions (compare **Figure 4B**). This ipsi-preference is flipped to a contra-preference upstream of the LSO because of the contralateral projections of LSO neurons to the midbrain. **(B)** MSO neurons respond best to contralateral sound-source positions. This contra-preference is maintained upstream of the LSO because of the ipsilateral projections of MSO neurons to the midbrain.

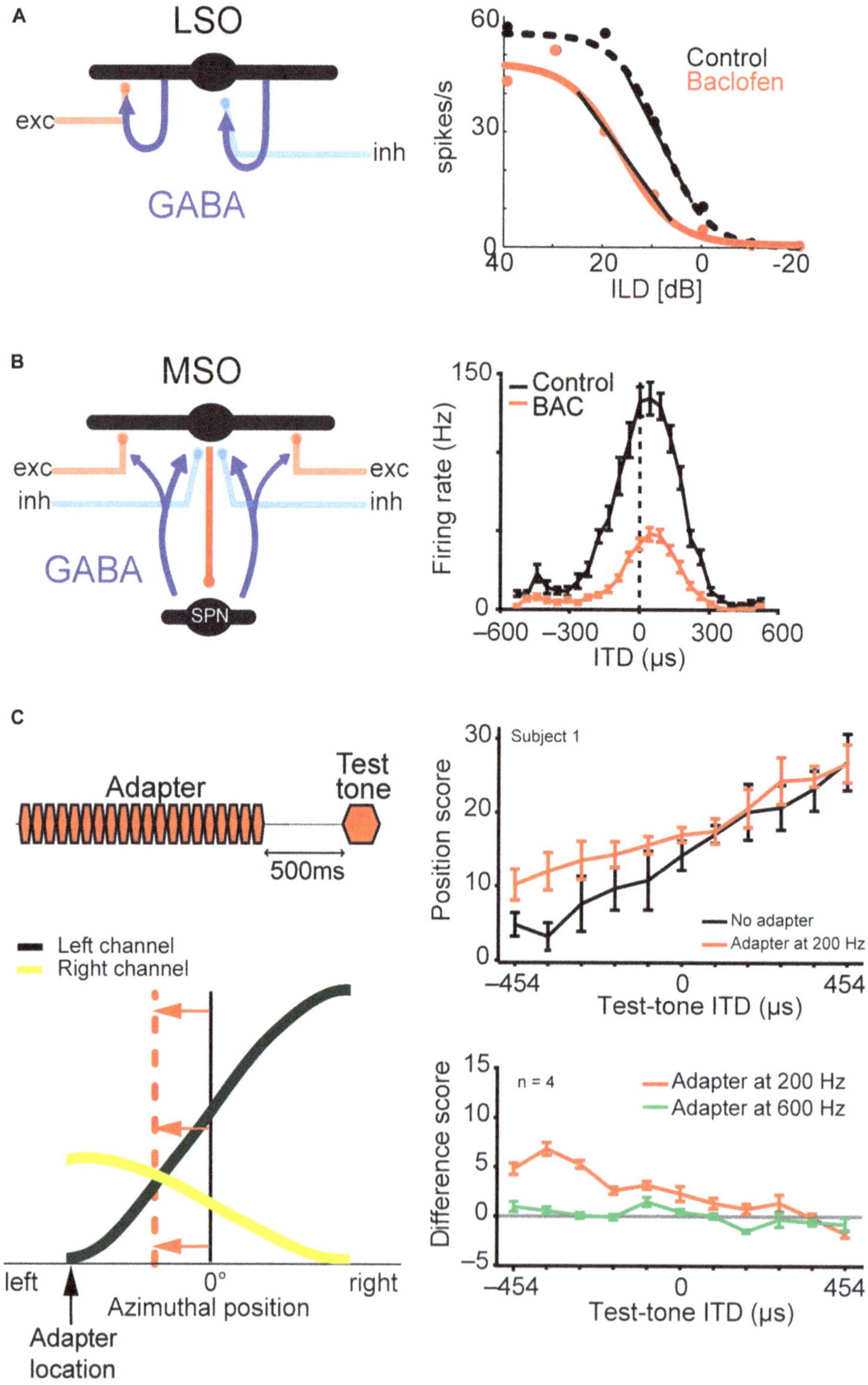

FIGURE 8 | LSO and MSO responses are modulated by prior activity and thus encode relative sound-source positions. The firing rates of both LSO and MSO neurons are controlled in an activity-dependent manner via GABAergic inhibition. **(A)** In the LSO, GABA is released retrogradly by dendritic release from LSO neurons onto their synaptic partners. **(B)** In the MSO, GABA is released via a di-synaptic feedback loop including the SPN (superior para-olivary nucleus). Both mechanisms generate levels of GABA-mediated inhibition that are proportional to the prior activity of the respective LSO/MSO neuron. In both cases, the firing activity is modulated by $GABA_B$-receptors, resulting in a divisive gain control mechanism. Data modified from Magnusson et al. (2008) **(A)** and Stange et al. (2013) **(B)**.

(Continued)

FIGURE 8 | Continued
(C) *In vivo* recordings in gerbils showed that upon prolonged presentation of an Adapter stimulus from a very lateralized sound-source position (stimulus paradigm is schematized in upper left), the GABAergic gain control results in asymmetric changes in the two coding channels (ipsi- and contralateral MSOs or LSOs) due to the asymmetric activity profile between the two channels and the activity dependence of the gain control mechanism. Particularly, the cross-point between left and right coding channel is shifted away from the actual midline (indicated by red horizontal arrows) and toward the location of the Adapter location (indicated by black vertical arrow). In accordance with the hypothesis of hemispheric coding channels of sound localization, this stimulation paradigm leads to systematic shifts of the perception of test tone positions in human listeners (right column). The result from a single subject is shown in the upper panel, the average from four subjects is shown in the lower panel. A difference score of 5 approximates a shift in lateral perception of 30°. As predicted from the activity-dependence of the GABAergic gain control circuit, the presentation of an Adapter stimulus at a different frequency than the test tone (green line) did not affect the localization percept. Data taken from Stange et al. (2013).

are well-known in other sensory modalities and will be considered in the context of sound localization in the following section.

DYNAMICS OF ILD AND ITD PROCESSING: GABA$_B$-MEDIATED INHIBITION

Across sensory modalities, the representation of stimulus features in an individual coding element may depend on the global distribution of that feature across the population of coding channels. For example, for a given magnitude of a feature, the response rate of individual neurons is modulated by the overall distribution of response rates in the entire population of neurons. This adaptation principle, in which the tuning of single neurons is normalized to the population average, serves to prevent response saturation and thereby increases coding efficiency (Wark et al., 2007; Carandini and Heeger, 2012). Traditionally, such adaptive strategies have not been associated with sound localization. However, recent results from both human psychophysics (Getzmann, 2004; Phillips and Hall, 2005; Vigneault-MacLean et al., 2007; Maier et al., 2009; Dahmen et al., 2010) and animal physiology (Park et al., 2008; Dahmen et al., 2010) have clearly demonstrated a dependency of ITD and ILD tuning, and even spatial perception, on the prior stimulation (specifically, on the stimulus properties and their temporal profile). We have recently discovered similar dynamic adaptation mechanisms in both the LSO and MSO directly (Magnusson et al., 2008; Stange et al., 2013). In both nuclei, the response magnitude of individual neurons is causally correlated with its prior spiking activity. High prior activity leads to strong response adaptation (decreased rates) and *vice versa*. Notably this particular response modulation, which acts on time scales of 10s of ms and can last for seconds, is mediated by similar mechanisms but employs different circuits in MSO and LSO. In each case, GABA$_B$ receptor signaling is involved, albeit in distinct ways (**Figure 8**). In the LSO, GABA is released in activity-dependent manner directly from principal LSO neurons and differentially activates GABA$_B$ receptors that are located on its presynaptic inputs (Magnusson et al., 2008, the effect is stronger on excitatory than on inhibitory inputs). Thus, the strength of inputs to a given LSO cell is controlled by its own spiking activity. In contrast, MSO cells are not themselves GABAergic. Instead, a di-synaptic feedback-loop exists, in which MSO neurons innervate GABAergic neurons in a nearby nucleus that subsequently feed back onto the MSO (Stange et al., 2013; **Figure 8**). While it is not known how specific the projections, and thus the adaptation effects, are between the two nuclei, one-to-one cell connectivity seems improbable (GABA is most probably released via volume transmission). Hence this circuit design is more reminiscent of the classical concept of divisive normalization, which includes averaging of activity levels over multiple neurons (Carandini and Heeger, 2012). Nevertheless, frequency specificity of GABA$_B$-mediated adaptation is apparently maintained (Stange et al., 2013).

GABA-mediated control of input strength can also be found in the avian NL circuit: SON shares the input source with NL and is additionally also innervated by NL neurons, creating a differential gain control circuit for the NL (Monsivais and Rubel, 2001; Burger et al., 2005a). Moreover, GABA$_B$-receptors are present pre-synaptically on neurons in NL and its excitatory input source, allowing for complex modulation of the ITD circuit depending on the activity level (Burger et al., 2005b; Tang et al., 2009).

In contrast to the avian system, in mammals, the activity-dependent rate adaptations in ILD and ITD coding will ultimately lead to a change in the tuning to the respective parameter, which is a consequence of the specific coding strategy of mammals (**Figure 8**). In the LSO, ILD functions of individual neurons will shift significantly, changing the range of ILDs to which they are sensitive. In contrast, the tuning functions of MSO neurons are not shifted at the single-cell level, as mainly the response gain is modulated. However, these modulations have significant consequences at the level of population coding, particularly in the case of the hemispheric channel model. Since response rates are activity dependent, a lateralized sound-source will generate unequal adaptation in the two hemispheres (with pronounced rate adaptation only in the contralateral channel). This asymmetric change in response rates will therefore shift the intersection of the two tuning channels away from the midline toward the adapting sound-source (**Figure 8C**). Given that the intersection of the two hemispheric channels encodes the perceived (subjective) midline, one would expect that such a lateralized adapting source would shift the perceived location of a subsequently presented sound-source. As noted above, Phillips and Hall (2005), Vigneault-MacLean et al. (2007) first tested this hypothesis in a number of psychophysical paradigms and were able to demonstrate a pronounced shift in the perceived location of sound-sources after prior presentation of a lateralized adapter in human listeners. Our lab has more recently demonstrated that GABA$_B$-mediated rate adaptation in the MSO is sufficient to explain these shifts in human perception (Stange et al., 2013).

The primary function of these perceptual shifts seems to be the relative segregation of the adapting and subsequent sound-source, as the reported shifts in location are directed away from the adapter location, i.e., the perceived distance between the sound-sources is increased relative to the actual distance. This interpretation is supported by the finding that the presence of adapting sound-sources increases spatial resolution at the adapter position (Getzmann, 2004).

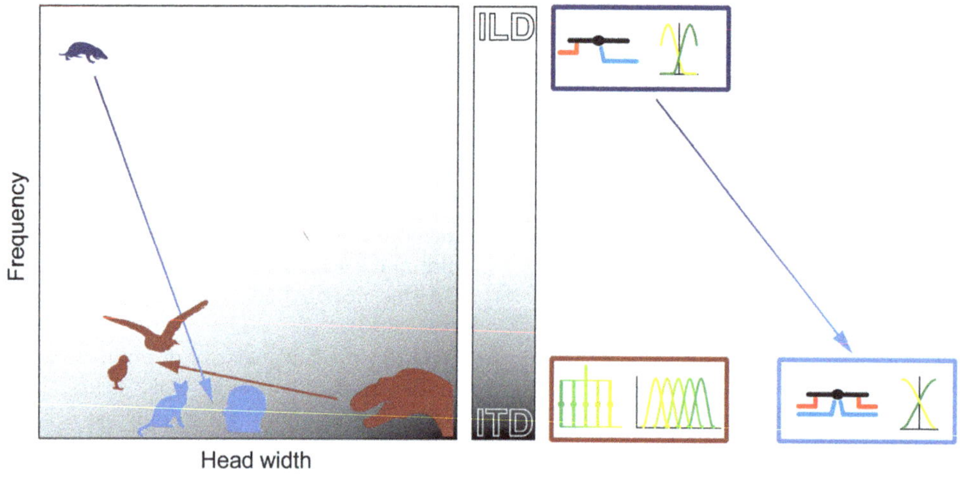

FIGURE 9 | Physical prerequisites shaped distinct binaural processing and coding strategies in mammals and birds. Head size (abscissa) and hearing range (ordinate) during the time of the middle-ear development define the binaural cue (gray scale: white = ILD; gray = ITD) that is most easily exploitable for horizontal sound localization by mammals (blue) and archosaurs/birds (brown). The binaural cue in turn shaped the emergence of distinct neuronal mechanisms that are optimized for the processing and encoding of the particular cue (boxes on right-hand side of panel). Early mammals (*Morganucodon*, dark blue) were very small and had high-frequency hearing. Therefore, they used ILDs as original binaural cue. Subsequent evolutionary changes in head size and/or hearing range (e.g., cats or humans, light blue) allowed the use of ITDs. However, the neuronal mechanisms (precise temporal integration of excitatory and inhibitory inputs) and coding principles (population code) remained similar to early, high-frequency hearing mammals (dark and light blue boxes on right-hand side of panel). Early archosaurs (brown) were very large and had low-frequency hearing. Therefore, they used ITDs as original binaural cue. Subsequent evolutionary changes in head size and/or hearing range in birds (e.g., chicks or barn owls, brown) allowed the continued use of ITDs. Thus, the neuronal mechanisms (delay-lines) and coding principles (labeled line) remained the same as in early archosaurs (brown box on right-hand side of panel).

Taken together, these findings strongly suggest that the binaural system serves to encode the relative separation of concurrent or subsequent sound-sources rather than to provide an absolute representation of position in space.

CONCLUSION

It is clear from the fossil record that spatial processing of airborne sound in mammals evolved independently of comparable systems in other vertebrates. Moreover, the electrophysiological circumstances in which such systems emerged were quite diverse, leading sauropsids and frogs into a low-frequency and mammals into a high-frequency world.

Therefore, from the beginning, mammals could make use of ample spectral information for vertical localization using HRTFs, and for lateralization using ILDs.

Interaural level differences as the original binaural cue for mammals are encoded via a population code, which largely derives from binaural interactions of excitation and inhibition (**Figure 9**). Later, those mammals that developed low-frequency hearing based their ITD processing, at least partially, on the same neuronal structures (including glycinergic inhibition as an important parameter for tuning ILD/ITD sensitivity in LSO und MSO), similar computations and coding strategies (e.g., a population code at the binaural comparator level, **Figure 9**). This leads to compatible representations of ILDs and ITDs at higher neuronal levels.

In contrast to mammals, archosaurs used ITDs as original binaural cue, because their heads were large and their hearing range was restricted to lower frequencies (**Figure 9**). Birds extended the hearing range only slightly compared to early archosaurs and thus maintained the original neuronal processing mechanisms (based on delay-lines) and coding strategy (**Figure 9**). Thus, physical restrictions shaped different processing mechanisms and coding strategies of binaural cues in birds and mammals.

The mammalian population code is modulated by context even at the binaural detector level. Again, inhibitory inputs (here: GABAergic feedback activating pre-synaptic $GABA_B$ receptors) play a major role in adjusting the population output of LSO and MSO. As a consequence, the system serves relative rather than absolute sound localization. This suggests that the main evolutionary constraint in (originally nocturnal) mammals was sound segregation rather than sound localization. More importantly, it suggests a paradigm shift beyond the current understanding of sound localization principles. For several decades the paradigm stated that binaural computations should transform auditory information in a manner similar to how retinotopic processing transforms visual information. In light of the more recent findings of constant remapping in both the auditory (Lee and Middlebrooks, 2011; Maddox et al., 2014) and visual system (Rolfs et al., 2011), we propose instead that the major challenge of localization and orientation is to overcome receptor-surface-bound information encoded via labeled-lines in order to create a flexible representation of external objects in the context of active movement in space and time.

ACKNOWLEDGMENTS

We thank Dr. M. H. Myoga for helpful comments on the manuscript and Dr. T. R. Jennings for help with figure design.

This work was supported by the German Science Foundation Collaborative Research Centre (CRC) 870.

REFERENCES

Allin, E. F. (1975). Evolution of the mammalian middle ear. *J. Morphol.* 147, 403–437. doi: 10.1002/jmor.1051470404

Blauert, J. (1997). *Spatial Hearing: The Psychophysics of Human Sound Localization.* Cambridge: MIT Press.

Boistel, R., Aubin, T., Cloetens, P., Peyrin, F., Scotti, T., Herzog, P., et al. (2013). How minute sooglossid frogs hear without a middle ear. *Proc. Natl. Acad. Sci. U.S.A.* 110, 15360–15364. doi: 10.1073/pnas.1302218110

Borst, J. G. G., and Soria van Hoeve, J. (2012). The calyx of held synapse: from model synapse to auditory relay. *Annu. Rev. Physiol.* 74, 199–224. doi: 10.1146/annurev-physiol-020911-153236

Boudreau, J. C., and Tsuchitani, C. (1968). Binaural interaction in the cat superior olive S segment. *J. Neurophysiol.* 31, 442–454. doi: 10.1121/1.2144209

Brand, A., Behrend, O., Marquardt, T., McAlpine, D., and Grothe, B. (2002). Precise inhibition is essential for microsecond interaural time difference coding. *Nature* 417, 543–547. doi: 10.1038/417543a

Brown, C. H., and May, B. J. (2005). "Comparative mammalian sound localization," in *Sound Source Localization Springer Handbook of Auditory Research,* eds A. N. Popper and R. R. Fay (New York: Springer), 124–178.

Burger, R. M., Fukui, I., Ohmori, H., and Rubel, E. W. (2011). Inhibition in the balance: binaurally coupled inhibitory feedback in sound localization circuitry. *J. Neurophysiol.* 106, 4–14. doi: 10.1152/jn.00205.2011

Burger, R. M., Pfeiffer, J. D., Westrum, L. E., Bernard, A., and Rubel, E. W. (2005a). Expression of GABA(B) receptor in the avian auditory brainstem: ontogeny, afferent deprivation, and ultrastructure. *J. Comp. Neurol.* 489, 11–22. doi: 10.1002/cne.20607

Burger, R. M., Cramer, K. S., Pfeiffer, J. D., and Rubel, E. W. (2005b). Avian superior olivary nucleus provides divergent inhibitory input to parallel auditory pathways. *J. Comp. Neurol.* 481, 6–18. doi: 10.1002/cne.20334

Cant, N. B., and Casseday, J. H. (1986). Projections from the anteroventral cochlear nucleus to the lateral and medial superior olivary nuclei. *J. Comp. Neurol.* 247, 457–476. doi: 10.1002/cne.902470406

Carandini, M., and Heeger, D. J. (2012). Normalization as a canonical neural computation. *Nat. Rev. Neurosci.* 13, 51–62. doi: 10.1038/nrn3136

Carr, C. E. (1993). Processing of temporal information in the brain. *Annu. Rev. Neurosci.* 16, 223–243. doi: 10.1146/annurev.ne.16.030193.001255

Carr, C. E., Soares, D., Parameshwaran, S., and Perney, T. (2001). Evolution and development of time coding systems. *Curr. Opin. Neurobiol.* 11, 727–733. doi: 10.1016/S0959-4388(01)00276-8

Chiari, Y., Cahais, V., Galtier, N., and Delsuc, F. (2012). Phylogenomic analyses support the position of turtles as the sister group of birds and crocodiles (*Archosauria*). *BMC Biol.* 10:65. doi: 10.1186/1741-7007-10-65

Christensen-Dalsgaard, J. (2005). "Directional hearing in nonmammalian tetrapods," in *Sound Source Localization Springer Handbook of Auditory Research,* eds A. N. Popper and R. R. Fay (New York: Springer), 67–123.

Christensen-Dalsgaard, J. (2011). Vertebrate pressure-gradient receivers. *Hear. Res.* 273, 37–45. doi: 10.1016/j.heares.2010.08.007

Christensen-Dalsgaard, J., and Manley, G. A. (2008). Acoustical coupling of lizard eardrums. *J. Assoc. Res. Otolaryngol. JARO* 9, 407–416. doi: 10.1007/s10162-008-0130-2

Christensen-Dalsgaard, J., Tang, Y., and Carr, C. E. (2011). Binaural processing by the gecko auditory periphery. *J. Neurophysiol.* 105, 1992–2004. doi: 10.1152/jn.00004.2011

Clack, J. A. (1997). The evolution of tetrapod ears and the fossil record. *Brain Behav. Evol.* 50, 198–212. doi: 10.1159/000113334

Clack, J. A. (2002). Patterns and processes in the early evolution of the tetrapod ear. *J. Neurobiol.* 53, 251–264. doi: 10.1002/neu.10129

Clark, G. M. (1969). Vesicle shape versus type of synapse in the nerve endings of the cat medial superior olive. *Brain Res.* 15, 548–551. doi: 10.1016/0006-8993(69)90181-4

Couchman, K., Grothe, B., and Felmy, F. (2010). Medial superior olivary neurons receive surprisingly few excitatory and inhibitory inputs with balanced strength and short-term dynamics. *J. Neurosci.* 30, 17111–17121. doi: 10.1523/JNEUROSCI.1760-10.2010

Couchman, K., Grothe, B., and Felmy, F. (2012). Functional localization of neurotransmitter receptors and synaptic inputs to mature neurons of the medial superior olive. *J. Neurophysiol.* 107, 1186–1198. doi: 10.1152/jn.00586.2011

Crompton, A. W. (1963) The evolution of the mammalian jaw. *Evolution* 17, 431–439. doi: 10.2307/2407093

Crompton, A. W., and Hylander, W. L. (1986). "Changes in the mandibular function following the acquisition of a dentary squamosal articulation," in *The Ecology and Biology of Mammal-like Reptiles,* eds N. Hotton, P. D. Maclean, J. J. Roth, and E. C. Roth (Washington, DC: Smithsonian Institution Press), 263–282.

Dahmen, J. C., Keating, P., Nodal, F. R., Schulz, A. L., and King, A. J. (2010). Adaptation to stimulus statistics in the perception and neural representation of auditory space. *Neuron* 66, 937–948. doi: 10.1016/j.neuron.2010.05.018

Dasika, V. K., White, J. A., Carney, L. H., and Colburn, H. S. (2005). Effects of inhibitory feedback in a network model of avian brain stem. *J. Neurophysiol.* 94, 400–414. doi: 10.1152/jn.01065.2004

Day, M. L., and Delgutte, B. (2013). Decoding sound source location and separation using neural population activity patterns. *J. Neurosci.* 33, 15837–15847. doi: 10.1523/JNEUROSCI.2034-13.2013

Dietz, M., Marquardt, T., Stange, A., Pecka, M., Grothe, B., and McAlpine, D. (2014). Emphasis of spatial cues in the temporal fine-structure during the rising segments of amplitude modulated sounds II: single neuron recordings. *J. Neurophysiol.* 111, 1973–1985. doi: 10.1152/jn.00681.2013

Ehret, G. (2005). Infant rodent ultrasounds – a gate to the understanding of sound communication. *Behav. Genet.* 35, 19–29. doi: 10.1007/s10519-004-0853-8

Endler, J. A. (1993). Some general comments on the evolution and design of animal communication systems. *Philos. Trans. R. Soc. Lond. B Biol. Sci.* 340, 215–225. doi: 10.1098/rstb.1993.0060

Erulkar, S. D. (1972). Comparative aspects of spatial localization of sound. *Physiol. Rev.* 52, 237–360.

Estes, R. (1961). Cranial anatomy of the cynodont reptile *Thrinaxodon liorhinus. Bull. Mus. Comp. Zool.* 125, 165–180.

Ezcurra, M. D. (2010). Biogeography of Triassic tetrapods: evidence for provincialism and driven sympatric cladogenesis in the early evolution of modern tetrapod lineages. *Proc. Biol. Sci.* 277, 2547–2552. doi: 10.1098/rspb.2010.0508

Fernández, C., and Schmidt, R. S. (1963). The opossum ear and evolution of the coiled cochlea. *J. Comp. Neurol.* 121, 151–159. doi: 10.1002/cne.901210111

Field, D. J., Gauthier, J. A., King, B. L., Pisani, D., Lyson, T. R., and Peterson, K. J. (2014). Toward consilience in reptile phylogeny: miRNAs support an archosaur, not lepidosaur, affinity for turtles. *Evol. Dev.* 16, 189–196. doi: 10.1111/ede.12081

Finlayson, P. G., and Caspary, D. M. (1989). Synaptic potentials of chinchilla lateral superior olivary neurons. *Hear. Res.* 38, 221–228. doi: 10.1016/0378-5955(89)90067-1

Finlayson, P. G., and Caspary, D. M. (1991). Low-frequency neurons in the lateral superior olive exhibit phase-sensitive binaural inhibition. *J. Neurophysiol.* 65, 598–605.

Fleischer, G. (1978). Evolutionary principles of the mammalian middle ear. *Adv. Anat. Embryol. Cell Biol.* 55, 7–60. doi: 10.1007/978-3-642-67143-2_1

Friauf, E., and Ostwald, J. (1988). Divergent projections of physiologically characterized rat ventral cochlear nucleus neurons as shown by intra-axonal injection of horseradish peroxidase. *Exp. Brain Res.* 73, 263–284. doi: 10.1007/BF00248219

Fritzsch, B., Beisel, K. W., Jones, K., Fariñas, I., Maklad, A., Lee, J., et al. (2002). Development and evolution of inner ear sensory epithelia and their innervation. *J. Neurobiol.* 53, 143–156. doi: 10.1002/neu.10098

Galambos, R., Schwartzkopf, J., and Rupert, A. (1959). Microelectrode study of superior olivary nuclei. *Am. J. Physiol.* 197, 527–536.

Gaupp, E. W. T. (1913). *Die Reichertsche theorie: Hammer-, Amboss- und Kieferfrage.* Leipzig: Veit & Comp.

Getzmann, S. (2004). Spatial discrimination of sound sources in the horizontal plane following an adapter sound. *Hear. Res.* 191, 14–20. doi: 10.1016/j.heares.2003.12.020

Golonka, J. (2007). Late Triassic and Early Jurassic palaeogeography of the world. *Palaeogeogr. Palaeoclimatol. Palaeoecol.* 244, 297–307. doi: 10.1016/j.palaeo.2006.06.041

Goodman, D. F., Benichoux, V., and Brette, R. (2013). Decoding neural responses to temporal cues for sound localization. *Elife* 2:e01312. doi: 10.7554/eLife.01312

Gower, D. J., and Sennikov, A. G. (1996). Morphology and phylogenetic informativeness of early archosaur braincases. *Palaeontology* 39, 883–906.

Gower, D. J., and Weber, E. (1998). The braincase of Euparkeria, and the evolutionary relationships of birds and crocodilians. *Biol. Rev.* 73, 367–411. doi: 10.1017/S0006323198005222

Grothe, B. (2000). The evolution of temporal processing in the medial superior olive, an auditory brainstem structure. *Prog. Neurobiol.* 61, 581–610. doi: 10.1016/S0301-0082(99)00068-4

Grothe, B., Pecka, M., and McAlpine, D. (2010). Mechanisms of sound localization in mammals. *Physiol. Rev.* 90, 983–1012. doi: 10.1152/physrev.00026.2009

Grothe, B., and Sanes, D. H. (1993). Bilateral inhibition by glycinergic afferents in the medial superior olive. *J. Neurophysiol.* 69, 1192–1196.

Grothe, B., and Sanes, D. H. (1994). Synaptic inhibition influences the temporal coding properties of medial superior olivary neurons: an in vitro study. *J. Neurosci.* 14, 1701–1709.

Hancock, K. E., and Delgutte, B. (2004). A physiologically based model of interaural time difference discrimination. *J. Neurosci.* 24, 7110–7117. doi: 10.1523/JNEUROSCI.0762-04.2004

Harnischfeger, G., Neuweiler, G., and Schlegel, P. (1985). Interaural time and intensity coding in superior olivary complex and inferior colliculus of the echolocating bat *Molossus ater*. *J. Neurophysiol.* 53, 89–109.

Harper, N. S., and McAlpine, D. (2004). Optimal neural population coding of an auditory spatial cue. *Nature* 430, 682–686. doi: 10.1038/nature02768

Hedges, S. B. (2012). Amniote phylogeny and the position of turtles. *BMC Biol.* 10:64. doi: 10.1186/1741-7007-10-64

Heffner, H. E., Heffner, R. S., Contos, C., and Ott, T. (1994). Audiogram of the hooded Norway rat. *Hear. Res.* 73, 244–247. doi: 10.1016/0378-5955(94)90240-2

Heffner, H. E., and Masterton, B. (1980). Hearing in glires: domestic rabbit, cotton rat, feral house mouse, and kangaroo rat. *J. Acoust. Soc. Am.* 68, 1584–1599. doi: 10.1121/1.385213

Hopson, J. A. (1966). The origin of the mammalian middle ear. *Am. Zool.* 6, 437–450. doi: 10.1093/icb/6.3.437

Hotton, N. H. (1959). The pelycosaur tympanum and early evolution of the middle ear. *Evolution* 13, 99–121. doi: 10.2307/2405947

Huang, G. T., Rosowski, J. J., and Peake, W. T. (2000). Relating middle-ear acoustic performance to body size in the cat family: measurements and models. *J. Comp. Physiol. A* 186, 447–465. doi: 10.1007/s003590050444

Hyson, R. L., Overholt, E. M., and Lippe, W. R. (1994). Cochlear microphonic measurements of interaural time differences in the chick. *Hear. Res.* 81, 109–118. doi: 10.1016/0378-5955(94)90158-9

Hyson, R. L., Reyesm, A. D., and Rubel, E. W. (1995). A depolarizing inhibitory response to GABA in brainstem auditory neurons of the chick. *Brain Res.* 677, 117–126. doi: 10.1016/0006-8993(95)00130-I

Jercog, P. E., Svirskis, G., Kotak, V. C., Sanes, D. H., and Rinzel, J. (2010). Asymmetric excitatory synaptic dynamics underlie interaural time difference processing in the auditory system. *PLoS Biol.* 8:e1000406. doi: 10.1371/journal.pbio.1000406

Joris, P. X., Carney, L. H., Smith, P. H., and Yin, T. C. (1994). Enhancement of neural synchronization in the anteroventral cochlear nucleus. I. Responses to tones at the characteristic frequency. *J. Neurophysiol.* 71, 1022–1036.

Joris, P. X., and Yin, T. C. (1995). Envelope coding in the lateral superior olive. I. Sensitivity to interaural time differences. *J. Neurophysiol.* 73, 1043–1062.

Kapfer, C., Seidl, A. H., Schweizer, H., and Grothe, B. (2002). Experience-dependent refinement of inhibitory inputs to auditory coincidence-detector neurons. *Nat. Neurosci.* 5, 247–253. doi: 10.1038/nn810

Kemp, T. S. (1982). *Mammal-Like Reptiles and the Origin of Mammals.* London: Academic Press.

Khouri, L., Lesica, N. A., and Grothe, B. (2011). Impaired auditory temporal selectivity in the inferior colliculus of aged *Mongolian gerbils*. *J. Neurosci.* 31, 9958–9970. doi: 10.1523/JNEUROSCI.4509-10.2011

Koay, G., Heffner, H. E., and Heffner, R. S. (1997). Audiogram of the big brown bat (*Eptesicus fuscus*). *Hear. Res.* 105, 202–210. doi: 10.1016/S0378-5955(96)00208-0

Köppl, C. (2009). Evolution of sound localisation in Land vertebrates. *Curr. Biol.* 19, R635–R639. doi: 10.1016/j.cub.2009.05.035

Kopp-Scheinpflug, C., Steinert, J. R., and Forsythe, I. D. (2011). Modulation and control of synaptic transmission across the MNTB. *Hear. Res.* 279, 22–31. doi: 10.1016/j.heares.2011.02.007

Kuhn, G. F. (1977). Model for the interaural time differences in the azimuthal plane. *J. Acoust. Soc. Am.* 62, 157–167. doi: 10.1121/1.381498

Lee, C.-C., and Middlebrooks, J. C. (2011). Auditory cortex spatial sensitivity sharpens during task performance. *Nat. Neurosci.* 14, 108–114. doi: 10.1038/nn.2713

Leibold, C. (2010). Influence of inhibitory synaptic kinetics on the interaural time difference sensitivity in a linear model of binaural coincidence detection. *J. Acoust. Soc. Am.* 127, 931–942. doi: 10.1121/1.3282997

Liu, R. C., Miller, K. D., Merzenich, M. M., and Schreiner, C. E. (2003). Acoustic variability and distinguishability among mouse ultrasound vocalizations. *J. Acoust. Soc. Am.* 114, 3412–3422. doi: 10.1121/1.1623787

Lu, B., Yang, W., Dai, Q., and Fu, J. (2013). Using genes as characters and a parsimony analysis to explore the phylogenetic position of turtles. *PLoS ONE* 8:e79348. doi: 10.1371/journal.pone.0079348

Maddox, R. K., Pospisil, D. A., Stecker, G. C., and Lee, A. K. C. (2014). Directing eye gaze enhances auditory spatial cue discrimination. *Curr. Biol.* 24, 748–752. doi: 10.1016/j.cub.2014.02.021

Magezi, D. A., and Krumbholz, K. (2010). Evidence for opponent-channel coding of interaural time differences in human auditory cortex. *J. Neurophysiol.* 104, 1997–2007. doi: 10.1152/jn.00424.2009

Magnusson, A. K., Park, T. J., Pecka, M., Grothe, B., and Koch, U. (2008). Retrograde GABA signaling adjusts sound localization by balancing excitation and inhibition in the brainstem. *Neuron* 59, 125–137. doi: 10.1016/j.neuron.2008.05.011

Maier, J. K., McAlpine, D., Klump, G. M., and Pressnitzer, D. (2009). Context effects in the discriminability of spatial cues. *J. Assoc. Res. Otolaryngol.* 11, 319–328. doi: 10.1007/s10162-009-0200-200

Maier, W. (1990). Phylogeny and ontogeny of mammalian middle ear structures. *Neth. J. Zool.* 40, 55–74. doi: 10.1163/156854289X00183

Manley, G. A. (1973). A review of some current concepts of the functional evolution of the ear in terrestrial vertebrates. *Evolution* 26, 608–621.

Manley, G. A. (2010). An evolutionary perspective on middle ears. *Hear. Res.* 263, 3–8. doi: 10.1016/j.heares.2009.09.004

Manley, G. A., Popper, A. N., and Fay, R. R. (2004). *Evolution of the Vertebrate Auditory System.* New York: Springer.

McAlpine, D., Jiang, D., and Palmer, A. R. (2001). A neural code for low-frequency sound localization in mammals. *Nat. Neurosci.* 4, 396–401. doi: 10.1038/86049

Meffin, H., and Grothe, B. (2009). Selective filtering to spurious localization cues in the mammalian auditory brainstem. *J. Acoust. Soc. Am.* 126, 2437–2454. doi: 10.1121/1.3238239

Michelsen, A. (1994). "Directional hearing in crickets and other small animals," in *Neural Basis of Behavioural Adaptations*, eds K. Schildberger and N. Elsner (Stuttgart: Fischer), 253–284.

Middlebrooks, J. C., Clock, A. E., Xu, L., and Green, D. M. (1994). A panoramic code for sound location by cortical neurons. *Science* 264, 842–844. doi: 10.1126/science.8171339

Mills, D. M., and Shepherd, R. K. (2001) Distortion product otoacoustic emission and auditory brainstem responses in the echidna (*Tachyglossus aculeatus*). *J. Assoc. Res. Otolaryngol.* 2, 130–146. doi: 10.1007/s101620010059

Moiseff, A., and Konishi, M. (1983). Binaural characteristics of units in the owl's brainstem auditory pathway: precursors of restricted spatial receptive fields. *J. Neurosci.* 3, 2553–2562.

Monsivais, P., and Rubel, E. W. (2001). Accommodation enhances depolarizing inhibition in central neurons. *J. Neurosci.* 21, 7823–7830.

Moore, J. K. (2000). Organization of the human superior olivary complex. *Microsc. Res. Tech.* 51, 403–412. doi: 10.1002/1097-0029(20001115)51:4<403::AID-JEMT8>3.0.CO;2-Q

Moore, M. J., and Caspary, D. M. (1983). Strychnine blocks binaural inhibition in lateral superior olivary neurons. *J. Neurosci.* 3, 237–242.

Morest, D. K. (1968). The collateral system of the medial nucleus of the trapezoid body of the cat, its neuronal architecture and relation to the olivo-cochlear bundle. *Brain Res.* 9, 288–311. doi: 10.1016/0006-8993(68)90235-7

Myoga, M. H., Lehnert, S., Leibold, C., Felmy, F., and Grothe, B. (2014). Glycinergic inhibition tunes coincidence detection in the auditory brainstem. *Nat. Commun.* 5:3790. doi: 10.1038/ncomms4790

Nishino, E., Yamada, R., Kuba, H., Hioki, H., Furuta, T., Kaneko, T., et al. (2008). Sound-intensity-dependent compensation for the small interaural time difference cue for sound source localization. *J. Neurosci.* 28, 7153–7164. doi: 10.1523/JNEUROSCI.4398-07.2008

Park, T. J. (1998). IID sensitivity differs between two principal centers in the interaural intensity difference pathway: the LSO and the IC. *J. Neurophysiol.* 79, 2416–2431.

Park, T. J., Brand, A., Koch, U., Ikebuchi, M., and Grothe, B. (2008). Dynamic changes in level influence spatial coding in the lateral superior olive. *Hear. Res.* 238, 58–67. doi: 10.1016/j.heares.2007.10.009

Park, T. J., Grothe, B., Pollak, G. D., Schuller, G., and Koch U. (1996). Neural delays shape selectivity to interaural intensity differences in the lateral superior olive. *J. Neurosci.* 16, 6554–6566.

Park, T. J., Klug, A., Holinstat, M., and Grothe, B. (2004). Interaural level difference processing in the lateral superior olive and the inferior colliculus. *J. Neurophysiol.* 92, 289–301. doi: 10.1152/jn.00961.2003

Park, T. J., Monsivais, P., and Pollak, G. D. (1997). Processing of interaural intensity differences in the LSO: role of interaural threshold differences. *J. Neurophysiol.* 77, 2863–2878.

Pecka, M., Brand, A., Behrend, O., and Grothe, B. (2008). Interaural time difference processing in the mammalian medial superior olive: the role of glycinergic inhibition. *J. Neurosci.* 28, 6914–6925. doi: 10.1523/JNEUROSCI.1660-08.2008

Peña, J. L., Viete, S., Albeck, Y., and Konishi, M. (1996). Tolerance to sound intensity of binaural coincidence detection in the nucleus laminaris of the owl. *J. Neurosci.* 16, 7046–7054.

Phillips, D. P., and Hall, S. E. (2005). Psychophysical evidence for adaptation of central auditory processors for interaural differences in time and level. *Hear. Res.* 202, 188–199. doi: 10.1016/j.heares.2004.11.001

Phillips, D. P., Quinlan, C. K., and Dingle, R. N. (2012). Stability of central binaural sound localization mechanisms in mammals, and the Heffner hypothesis. *Neurosci. Biobehav. Rev.* 36, 889–900. doi: 10.1016/j.neubiorev.2011.11.003

Radziwon, K. E., June, K. M., Stolzberg, D. J., Xu-Friedman, M. A., Salvi, R. J., and Dent, M. L. (2009). Behaviorally measured audiograms and gap detection thresholds in CBA/CaJ mice. *J. Comp. Physiol. A Neuroethol. Sens. Neural Behav. Physiol.* 195, 961–969. doi: 10.1007/s00359-009-0472-1

Rayleigh, L. (1907). On our perception of sound direction. *Philos. Mag.* 13:232.

Reichert, K. B. (1837). *Ueber die Visceralbogen der Wirbelthiere im Allgemeinen und deren Metamorphose bei den Säugethieren und Vögeln.* Berlin: Sittenfeld.

Reimer, K. (1995). Hearing in the marsupial *Monodelphis domestica* as determined by auditory-evoked brainstem responses. *Audiology* 34, 334–342. doi: 10.3109/00206099509071923

Rich, T. H., Hopson, J. A., Musser, A. M., Flannery, T. F., and Vickers-Rich, P. (2005). Independent origins of middle ear bones in monotremes and therians. *Science* 307, 910–914. doi: 10.1126/science.1105717

Roberts, M. T., Seeman, S. C., and Golding, N. L. (2013). A mechanistic understanding of the role of feedforward inhibition in the mammalian sound localization circuitry. *Neuron* 78, 923–935. doi: 10.1016/j.neuron.2013.04.022

Rodríguez-Vázquez, J. F. (2005). Development of the stapes and associated structures in human embryos. *J. Anat.* 207, 165–173. doi: 10.1111/j.1469-7580.2005.00441.x

Rolfs, M., Jonikaitis, D., Deubel, H., and Cavanagh, P. (2011). Predictive remapping of attention across eye movements. *Nat. Neurosci.* 14, 252–256. doi: 10.1038/nn.2711

Rosowski, J. J., and Graybeal, A. (1991). What did *Morganucodon* hear? *Zool. J. Linn. Soc.* 101, 131–168. doi: 10.1111/j.1096-3642.1991.tb00890.x

Rosowski, J. J., Ravicz, M. E., Teoh, S. W., and Flandermeyer, D. (1999). Measurements of middle-ear function in the *Mongolian gerbil*, a specialized mammalian ear. *Audiol. Neurootol.* 4, 129–136. doi: 10.1159/000013831

Rosowski, J. J., and Saunders, J. C. (1980). Sound transmission through the avian interaural pathways. *J. Comp. Physiol.* 136, 183–190. doi: 10.1007/BF00657532

Rowe, T., Rich, T. H., Vickers-Rich, P., Springer, M., and Woodburne, M. O. (2008). The oldest platypus and its bearing on divergence timing of the platypus and echidna clades. *Proc. Natl. Acad. Sci. U.S.A.* 105, 1238–1242. doi: 10.1073/pnas.0706385105

Ryan, A. (1976). Hearing sensitivity of the *Mongolian gerbil, Meriones unguiculatis. J. Acoust. Soc. Am.* 59, 1222–1226. doi: 10.1121/1.380961

Salminen, N. H., Tiitinen, H., Yrttiaho, S., and May, P. J. C. (2010). The neural code for interaural time difference in human auditory cortex. *J. Acoust. Soc. Am.* 127, EL60–EL65. doi: 10.1121/1.3290744

Sanes, D. H. (1990). An in vitro analysis of sound localization mechanisms in the gerbil lateral superior olive. *J. Neurosci.* 10, 3494–3506.

Schneggenburger, R., and Neher, E. (2005). Presynaptic calcium and control of vesicle fusion. *Curr. Opin. Neurobiol.* 15, 266–274. doi: 10.1016/j.conb.2005.05.006

Schnupp, J. W. H., and Carr, C. E. (2009). On hearing with more than one ear: lessons from evolution. *Nat. Neurosci.* 12, 692–697. doi: 10.1038/nn.2325

Schwartz, I. R. (1992). "The superior olivary complex and lateral lemniscal nuclei," in *The Mammalian Auditory Pathway: Neuroanatomy Springer Handbook of Auditory Research*, eds D. B. Webster, A. N. Popper, and R. R. Fay (New York: Springer), 117–167.

Shen, X. X., Liang, D., Wen, J. Z., and Zhang, P. (2011). Multiple genome alignments facilitate development of NPCL markers: a case study of tetrapod phylogeny focusing on the position of turtles. *Mol. Biol. Evol.* 28, 3237–3252. doi: 10.1093/molbev/msr148

Shinn-Cunningham, B. G., Santarelli, S., and Kopco, N. (2000). Tori of confusion: binaural localization cues for sources within reach of a listener. *J. Acoust. Soc. Am.* 107, 1627–1636 doi: 10.1121/1.428447

Sienknecht, U. J. (2013). Developmental origin and fate of middle ear structures. *Hear. Res.* 301, 19–26. doi: 10.1016/j.heares.2013.01.019

Spangler, K. M., Warr, W. B., and Henkel, C. K. (1985). The projections of principal cells of the medial nucleus of the trapezoid body in the cat. *J. Comp. Neurol.* 238, 249–262. doi: 10.1002/cne.902380302

Stange, A., Myoga, M. H., Lingner, A., Ford, M. C., Alexandrova, O., Felmy, F., et al. (2013). Adaptation in sound localization: from GABAB receptor-mediated synaptic modulation to perception. *Nat. Neurosci.* 16, 1840–1847. doi: 10.1038/nn.3548

Stecker, G. C., and Middlebrooks, J. C. (2003). Distributed coding of sound locations in the auditory cortex. *Biol. Cybern.* 89, 341–349. doi: 10.1007/s00422-003-0439-431

Steinberg, L. J., Fischer, B. J., and Peña, J. L. (2013). Binaural gain modulation of spectrotemporal tuning in the interaural level difference-coding pathway. *J. Neurosci.* 33, 11089–11099. doi: 10.1523/JNEUROSCI.4941-12.2013

Striedter, G. F. (1991). Auditory, electrosensory, and mechanosensory lateral line pathways through the forebrain in channel catfishes. *J. Comp. Neurol.* 312, 311–331. doi: 10.1002/cne.903120213

Takahashi, T. T., and Keller, C. H. (1992). Commissural connections mediate inhibition for the computation of interaural level difference in the barn owl. *J. Comp. Physiol. A* 170, 161–169. doi: 10.1007/BF00196898

Tang, Z. Q., Gao, H., and Lu, Y. (2009). Control of a depolarizing GABAergic input in an auditory coincidence detection circuit. *J. Neurophysiol.* 102, 1672–1683. doi: 10.1152/jn.00419.2009

Thompson, H., and Tucker, A. S. (2013). Dual origin of the epithelium of the mammalian middle ear. *Science* 339, 1453–1456. doi: 10.1126/science.1232862

Thompson, S. K., von Kriegstein, K., Deane-Pratt, A., Marquardt, T., Deichmann, R., Griffiths, T. D., et al. (2006). Representation of interaural time delay in the human auditory midbrain. *Nat. Neurosci.* 9, 1096–1098. doi: 10.1038/nn1755

Tollin, D. J. (2003). The lateral superior olive: a functional role in sound source localization. *Neuroscientist* 9, 127–143. doi: 10.1177/1073858403252228

Tollin, D. J., and Yin, T. C. T. (2002). The coding of spatial location by single units in the lateral superior olive of the cat. I. Spatial receptive fields in azimuth. *J. Neurosci.* 22, 1454–1467.

Tollin D. J., and Yin T. C. T. (2005). Interaural phase and level difference sensitivity in low-frequency neurons in the lateral superior olive. *J. Neurosci.* 25, 10648–10657. doi: 10.1523/JNEUROSCI.1609-05.2005

Tsuchitani, C. (1988). The inhibition of cat lateral superior olive unit excitatory responses to binaural tone bursts. II. The sustained discharges. *J. Neurophysiol.* 59, 184–211.

Tsuchitani, C., and Boudreau, J. C. (1969). Stimulus level of dichotically presented tones and cat superior olive S-segment cell dcharge. *J. Acoust. Soc. Am.* 46, 979–988. doi: 10.1121/1.1911818

Tucker, M. E., and Benton, M. J. (1982). Triassic environments, climates and reptile evolution. *Palaeogeogr. Palaeoclimatol. Palaeoecol.* 40, 361–379. doi: 10.1016/0031-0182(82)90034-90037

van der Heijden, M., Lorteije, J. A. M., Plauška, A., Roberts, M. T., Golding, N. L., and Borst, J. G. G. (2013). Directional hearing by linear summation of binaural inputs at the medial superior olive. *Neuron* 78, 936–948. doi: 10.1016/j.neuron.2013.04.028

Vigneault-MacLean, B. K., Hall, S. E., and Phillips, D. P. (2007). The effects of lateralized adaptors on lateral position judgements of tones within and across frequency channels. *Hear. Res.* 224, 93–100. doi: 10.1016/j.heares.2006.12.001

von Gersdorff, H., and Borst, J. G. G. (2002). Short-term plasticity at the calyx of held. *Nat. Rev. Neurosci.* 3, 53–64. doi: 10.1038/nrn705

von Kriegstein, K., Griffiths, T. D., Thompson, S. K., and McAlpine, D. (2008). Responses to interaural time delay in human cortex. *J. Neurophysiol.* 100, 2712–2718. doi: 10.1152/jn.90210.2008

Wallace, D. J., Greenberg, D. S., Sawinski, J., Rulla, S., Notaro, G., and Kerr, J. N. D. (2013). Rats maintain an overhead binocular field at the expense of constant fusion. *Nature* 498, 65–69. doi: 10.1038/nature12153

Wark, B., Lundstrom, B. N., and Fairhall, A. (2007). Sensory adaptation. *Curr. Opin. Neurobiol.* 17, 423–429. doi: 10.1016/j.conb.2007.07.001

Warr, W. B. (1966). Fiber degeneration following lesions in the anterior ventral cochlear nucleus of the cat. *Exp. Neurol.* 14, 453–474. doi: 10.1016/0014-4886(66)90130-0

Werner-Reiss, U., and Groh, J. M. (2008). A rate code for sound azimuth in monkey auditory cortex: implications for human neuroimaging studies. *J. Neurosci.* 28, 3747–3758. doi: 10.1523/JNEUROSCI.5044-07.2008

Werthat, F., Alexandrova, O., Grothe, B., and Koch, U. (2008). Experience-dependent refinement of the inhibitory axons projecting to the medial superior olive. *Dev. Neurobiol.* 68, 1454–1462. doi: 10.1002/dneu.20660

Willis, K. L., Christensen-Dalsgaard, J., Ketten, D. R., and Carr, C. E. (2013). Middle ear cavity morphology is consistent with an aquatic origin for testudines. *PLoS ONE* 8:e54086. doi: 10.1371/journal.pone.0054086

Yamada, R., Okuda, H., Kuba, H., Nishino, E., Ishii, T. M., and Ohmori, H. (2013). The cooperation of sustained and phasic inhibitions increases the contrast of ITD-tuning in low-frequency neurons of the chick nucleus laminaris. *J. Neurosci.* 33, 3927–3938. doi: 10.1523/JNEUROSCI.2377-12.2013

Yang, L. C., Monsivais, P., and Rubel, E. W. (1999). The superior olivary nucleus and its influence on nucleus laminaris: a source of inhibitory feedback for coincidence detection in the avian auditory brainstem. *J. Neurosci.* 19, 2313–2325.

Yin, T. C. T. (2002). "Neural mechanisms of encoding binaural localization cues in the auditory brainstem," in *Integrative Functions in the Mammalian Auditory Pathway,* eds R. R. Fay and A. N. Popper (New York: SpringerVerlag), 99–159.

Zhou, Y., Carney, L. H., and Colburn, H. S. (2005). A model for interaural time difference sensitivity in the medial superior olive: interaction of excitatory and inhibitory synaptic inputs, channel dynamics, and cellular morphology. *J. Neurosci.* 25, 3046–3058. doi: 10.1523/JNEUROSCI.3064-04.2005

3

VGLUT3 does not synergize GABA/glycine release during functional refinement of an inhibitory auditory circuit

Daniel T. Case[1‡], Javier Alamilla[2†‡] and Deda C. Gillespie[1,2]*

[1] Neuroscience Graduate Program, McMaster University, Hamilton, ON, Canada
[2] Department of Psychology, Neuroscience and Behaviour, McMaster University, Hamilton, ON, Canada

***Correspondence:**
Deda C. Gillespie, Department of Psychology, Neuroscience and Behaviour, McMaster University, 1280 Main St W, Hamilton, ON L8S 4K1, Canada
e-mail: dgillespie@mcmaster.ca

[†]Present address:
Daniel T. Case and Javier Alamilla, Centro Universitario de Investigaciones Biomédicas, Universidad de Colima, Colima, Col. México

[‡]These authors have contributed equally to this work.

The vesicular glutamate transporter 3 (VGLUT3) is expressed at several locations not normally associated with glutamate release. Although the function of this protein has been generally elusive, when expressed in non-glutamatergic synaptic terminals, VGLUT3 can not only allow glutamate co-transmission but also synergize the action of non-glutamate vesicular transporters. Interestingly, in the immature glycinergic projection between the medial nucleus of the trapezoid body (MNTB) and the lateral superior olive (LSO) of auditory brainstem, the transient early expression of VGLUT3 is required for normal developmental refinement. It has however been unknown whether the primary function of VGLUT3 in development of these inhibitory synapses is to enable glutamate release or to promote loading of inhibitory neurotransmitter through vesicular synergy. Using tissue from young mice in which *Vglut3* had been genetically deleted, we evaluated inhibitory neurotransmission in the MNTB-LSO pathway. Our results show, in contrast to what has been seen at adult synapses, that VGLUT3 expression has little or no effect on vesicular synergy at the immature glycinergic synapse of brainstem. This finding supports the model that the primary function of increased VGLUT3 expression in the immature auditory brainstem is to enable glutamate release in a developing inhibitory circuit.

Keywords: co-transmission, lateral superior olive, medial nucleus of trapezoid body, vesicular transport proteins, inhibitory synapses, development

INTRODUCTION

The glycinergic projection from the medial nucleus of the trapezoid body (MNTB) to lateral superior olive (LSO) is a critical component of the neural circuit for localizing higher frequency sound sources (for review, see Tollin, 2003, though see also Jalabi et al., 2013). Although the MNTB-LSO pathway, with its precise, tonotopically organized circuitry and well-defined inputs, has been a model system for understanding inhibitory circuit refinement, the mechanisms of this synaptic refinement have yet to be elucidated, in part because immature MNTB-LSO synapses exhibit a complex neurotransmitter phenotype. First, as is common at other immature glycinergic synapses, MNTB terminals in the LSO use GABA transmission (Kotak et al., 1998; Nabekura et al., 2004), for unknown reasons (Gillespie and Kandler, 2009). Second, due to the transient expression of vesicular glutamate transporter 3 (VGLUT3), MNTB terminals also release glutamate during the first postnatal week (Gillespie et al., 2005), a period characterized by major synaptic refinement (Kim and Kandler, 2003). As hearing onset does not occur until about postnatal day 10 (P10), this circuit refinement is understood to be directed by neural activity spontaneously generated in the cochlea (Tritsch et al., 2007), and the expression of VGLUT3 is required for normal refinement (Noh et al., 2010). The precise role of VGLUT3 in this refinement has not been elucidated.

The function of VGLUT3 in the nervous system generally has been elusive. Although originally identified by sequence homology with its more common family members *Vglut1 and Vglut2, Vglut3* has a distinctly different expression pattern and likely function. First, VGLUT3 exhibits a biphasic temporal expression pattern, with intense, transient expression in immature cerebellum and brainstem. Additionally, in both neonatal and adult tissue, VGLUT3 is notably expressed at "non-glutamatergic" release sites (Fremeau et al., 2002; Gras et al., 2002, 2005; Herzog et al., 2004). This seemingly ectopic expression of VGLUT3 naturally led to an initial hypothesis that a primary function might be to enable glutamate release from non-canonical glutamate synapses and/or from astrocytes. More recently, however, another role has come to light. In particular, in the striatum and raphe nucleus of adult, VGLUT3 is targeted to cholinergic and serotonergic vesicles where it synergizes the action of vesicular transporters for acetylcholine and serotonin, increasing both rate and degree of vesicle filling (Gras et al., 2008; Amilhon et al., 2010; for review, see El Mestikawy et al., 2011).

In the MNTB-LSO pathway, the working model for the role of VGLUT3 in functional refinement has been that depolarizing GABA and/or glycine at the immature MNTB-LSO synapse relieves Mg^{++}-block at NMDA receptors that, upon their activation by glutamate co-transmission, mediate activity-dependent plasticity (Kandler and Friauf, 1995; Kotak et al., 1998; Ehrlich et al., 1999; Kalmbach et al., 2010; Case and Gillespie, 2011). A central assumption of this model is that VGLUT3 is expressed in the developing auditory brainstem primarily to enable glutamate release from immature glycinergic synapses. The possibility that VGLUT3 could synergize packaging of GABA/glycine vesicles in immature MNTB terminals, however, gives rise to an alternate hypothesis for why developmental refinement here requires VGLUT3. In the alternate model, at what would otherwise be a sluggish immature synapse, VGLUT3 boosts GABA/glycinergic transmission, activating L-type voltage-gated Ca^{++} channels (Kullmann et al., 2002) that could lead to downstream plasticity.

If VGLUT3 permits or directs refinement of MNTB-LSO synapses by boosting GABA/glycinergic vesicle loading, we would expect loss of VGLUT3 to cause abnormal GABA/glycinergic transmission during the period of major circuit refinement. Using whole-cell recordings in tissue from genetically altered mice, we found that VGLUT3 expression does not synergize GABA/glycine vesicle loading in the developing MNTB-LSO circuit.

MATERIALS AND METHODS

All procedures adhered to Canadian Council on Animal Care guidelines and were previously approved by the Animal Research Ethics Board of McMaster University. Mice heterozygous (+/−) for *Vglut3* (gift of S. El Mestikawy) were bred on site to yield litters containing wild-type (WT), heterozygous (het), and knockout (KO) mice. Genotypes were determined after all other procedures had been performed, to ensure that slice preparation and electrophysiology were always performed blind to *Vglut3* expression.

Pups age postnatal day 4–5 (P4–5; day of birth is P0) were anesthetized and quickly decapitated, and the brains were removed into ice-cold artificial cerebrospinal fluid (ACSF, pH 7.2) containing (in mM): 125 NaCl, 1 $MgSO_4$, 5 KCl, 1.25 KH_2PO_4, 10 dextrose, 26 $NaHCO_3$, 2 $CaCl_2$, 1 ascorbic acid, 1 kynurenic acid. Tail tissue for subsequent genotype determination was collected at sacrifice. Brainstem slices (300 μm) containing the MNTB and LSO were allowed to recover at room temperature for ≥1 h in a humidified, oxygenated, interface chamber. Slices were transferred to a recording chamber where they were continuously perfused with ACSF at elevated temperature (32–35°C) and superfused with 95% O_2/5% CO_2. Perfusion ACSF was identical to slicing ACSF, with the addition of 0.3 mM ascorbic acid and 0.5 mM D-glutamine.

Recording electrodes (1–4 MΩ) were filled with a Cs-gluconate solution containing (in mM): 64 D-gluconic acid, 64 CsOH, 11 EGTA, 56 CsCl, 1 $MgCl_2$, 1 $CaCl_2$, 10 HEPES, 0.3 GTP-Na, 4 ATP-Mg, 0.1 mM spermine (Acros Organics). In several cases, the internal solution also contained 0.5% biocytin for histological verification of cell type; in some instances QX-314 (5 mM; Tocris) was added to the internal solution to increase patch stability. Principal cells in the medial and middle limbs of the LSO were visually identified under IR-DIC by their morphology and orientation and were patched in whole-cell mode. Recordings were sampled at 10 kHz, and filtered at 5 kHz. Series resistance was compensated by 80% with < 10 μs lag, and recordings were discarded if series resistance changed by ≥15%. All recordings were made at a holding potential of −60 mV. Data were saved for offline analysis using MiniAnalysis (Synaptosoft), Clampfit (Molecular Devices) or custom Matlab programs, and are presented as mean +/− S.E.M.

In each slice, a stimulating electrode was placed at the lateral edge of the MNTB, the minimum intensity that reliably elicited a response was determined, and stimulus intensity thereafter was unaltered throughout the experiment. Within pulse trains, the peak current amplitude for each pulse was measured relative to current immediately before the pulse; all paired-pulse ratios (PPRs) are reported with the amplitude of the first response in the denominator.

To estimate quantal content and probability of release, we delivered 20 electrical stimuli at 100 Hz and normalized the amplitude of each response in the train to the amplitude of the first response. We then performed a linear regression on the last 6 points in the cumulative response amplitude curve and extrapolated to time = 0 (response 1) to estimate the size of the readily releasable pool of vesicles multiplied by quantal amplitude (N_q) (Inchauspe et al., 2007), and thence to estimate probability of release.

Spontaneous miniature GABA/glycinergic events are uncommon in the immature LSO. To increase the probability of observing miniature GABA/glycinergic events, we delivered high-frequency stimulation (20 pulses at 100 Hz) to MNTB fibers, or replaced $CaCl_2$ in the ACSF with $SrCl_2$ (2 mM) to promote asynchronous vesicular release. Miniature events were identified, individually verified, and analyzed in MiniAnalysis. For comparison and verification, a subset of miniature events was also analyzed in Clampfit. As results from the two analyses showed no differences, all results shown here were analyzed in MiniAnalysis.

DNA was isolated from tail tissue obtained at sacrifice, and polymerase chain reaction (PCR) reactions using *VGlut3* WT (278 bp) and *VGlut3* KO cassette (604 bp) primers (Gras et al., 2008; Mobix Lab, McMaster University) were completed in separate tubes in a Peltier Thermal Cycler (Dyad DNA Engine). Following the PCR reaction, primer bands were identified using gel electrophoresis.

RESULTS

If the vesicular synergy model holds true in the immature MNTB-LSO pathway, we would expect differing levels of *Vglut3* to correlate with differences in GABA/glycinergic transmission, in particular for measures of short-term plasticity, recovery from short-term depression, and quantal size. For example, if VGLUT3 promotes faster vesicle reloading, VGLUT3-expressing synapses might be expected to recover more quickly from short-term depression. More specifically, we predicted that quantal size and hence the amplitude of miniature synaptic events would be larger at MNTB-LSO synapses expressing VGLUT3.

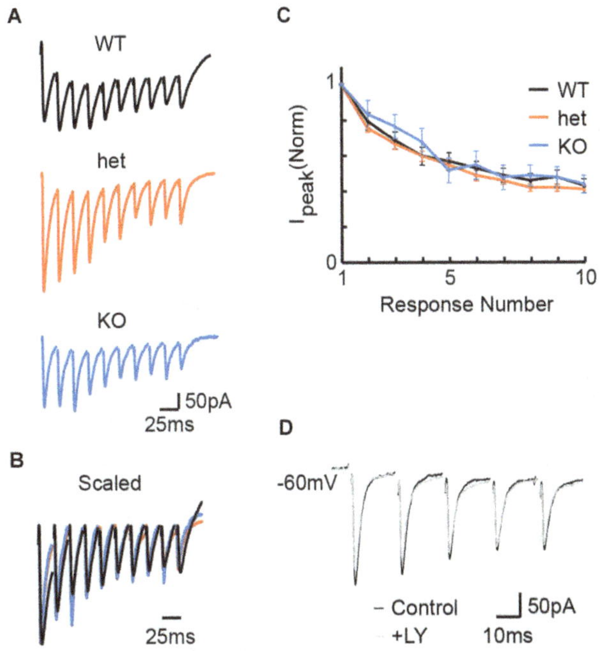

FIGURE 1 | Stimulation at 50 Hz in the MNTB revealed no effect of genotype on release properties in the LSO. (A) Representative responses to 50 Hz stimulation for WT (P4), het (P5), and KO (P4) tissue. **(B)** Example traces from **(A)**, scaled for comparison. Traces were first scaled to force all genotypes to have the same value for the amplitude of the first response; then, within each train, the baseline for each response was reset to zero (i.e., baseline for first-response). **(C)** No differences appeared between WT (n = 20), het (n = 49), and KO (n = 9) mice for paired-pulse ratios (**C**; p = 0.32, see text). **(D)** Application of the mGluR antagonist LY 341 495 had no effect on PPR in slices expressing VGLUT3. Example P5 WT slice.

Normal developmental refinement in the murine MNTB-LSO pathway, which is characterized by changes in quantal size, quantal content, and probability of release (Kim and Kandler, 2010), is perturbed in *VGlut3*$^{-/-}$ mice (Noh et al., 2010). Therefore, to minimize the likelihood of measuring differences that had resulted from an ultimate effect of VGLUT3 on synaptic refinement rather than a proximal effect on vesicular synergy, we restricted our recordings to tissue from animals P4-P5. At this age in LSO, VGLUT3 levels and glutamate release are relatively high and the synaptic changes associated with the major period of developmental refinement have just begun. To avoid possible bias, all tissue collection, recordings, and analyses were performed blind to genotype.

VGLUT3 EXPRESSION DOES NOT AFFECT GABA/GLYCINE RELEASE UPON 50 HZ STIMULATION

We first wanted to determine whether PPRs differ between *VGlut3* WT, heterozygous (het), and KO mice. We made whole-cell recordings in the LSO while delivering pulse trains to MNTB fibers at frequencies previously shown to cause short-term depression at immature MNTB-LSO synapses (Kim and Kandler, 2010; Case and Gillespie, 2011). Most cells exhibited depression consistent with previous results; the small number of anomalous cells that exhibited facilitation (n = 1 WT, 4 het, 2 KO) were excluded from analysis. Representative responses (for PPR) to stimulation at 50 Hz in the MNTB (**Figures 1A,B**) show no influence of genotype on PPR. We note that the responses depicted here were chosen by selecting for each condition the response with median PPR. It happens that the WT recording with median PPR response (shown) exhibited a background tonic current not seen in the median responses for the het and KO conditions. However, this tonic current is atypical; it was not characteristic, it did not occur more often in any particular genotype, and it did not affect PPR (data not shown). For the population of cells stimulated at 50 Hz, we found no effect of genotype on PPR (**Figure 1C**; PPRs: WT = 0.79 +/− 0.05, n = 21; het = 0.75 +/− 0.02, n = 49; KO = 0.83 +/− 0.08, n = 9; Kruskal-Wallis test: p = 0.32). Co-expression of VGLUT3 with other vesicular transporters has been shown to increase the rate and extent to which synaptic vesicles are filled (Gras et al., 2008; Amilhon et al., 2010). If VGLUT3 synergizes vesicle filling and if vesicle filling is a rate-limiting step, we would expect synapses from KO tissue to follow high frequency stimulation less well than those from WT or het tissue. Thus, these results do not support vesicular synergy between VGLUT3 and the GABA/glycine vesicular transporter (VIAAT/VGAT).

In the neonatal rat LSO, repetitive stimulation of the glutamatergic afferents from the ipsilateral cochlear nucleus can cause mGluR-mediated modulation of inhibitory neurotransmission at MNTB terminals (Nishimaki et al., 2007). To ask whether the presumably smaller amount of glutamate released by MNTB terminals could similarly modulate release properties, we compared pulse trains before and after the application of the mGluR2/3 antagonist LY 341 495 (Tocris) in a separate set of 3 WT slices (example shown in **Figure 1D**). Because blocking mGluRs did not affect paired pulse ratios or current amplitudes in any instance, we did not include the antagonist in further studies.

VGLUT3 EXPRESSION DOES NOT AFFECT GABA/GLYCINE RELEASE UPON 100 HZ STIMULATION

Adult neurons in the auditory brainstem achieve high rates of neural activity, and so, even in young tissue, it is possible that 50 Hz stimulation is simply too slow to test the system. In a new set of slices, we therefore stressed the synapse further by delivering stimuli at 100 Hz to the MNTB while recording in the LSO. Representative recordings from WT, het, and KO mice following 100 Hz stimulation are shown in **Figure 2A**, and these traces are shown overlaid in **Figures 2B,C** (normalized to the highest amplitude recording, the WT cell, in **Figure 2A**). With the faster 100 Hz stimulation, we still found no effect of genotype on paired-pulse depression (**Figure 2D**; PPRs: WT = 0.68 +/− 0.09, n = 8; het = 0.68 +/− 0.08, n = 9; KO = 0.64 +/− 0.09, n = 8; Kruskal-Wallis: p = 0.75), or on cumulative normalized amplitude of the pulse train (**Figure 2E**; cumulative amplitudes of 20 responses: WT = 8.06 +/− 0.86, n = 8; het = 7.43 +/− 0.74, n = 9; KO = 6.68 +/− 0.81, n = 8; Kruskal-Wallis: p = 0.28).

From the same cells, using cumulative amplitude to estimate quantal content N_q and probability of release (see Methods), we

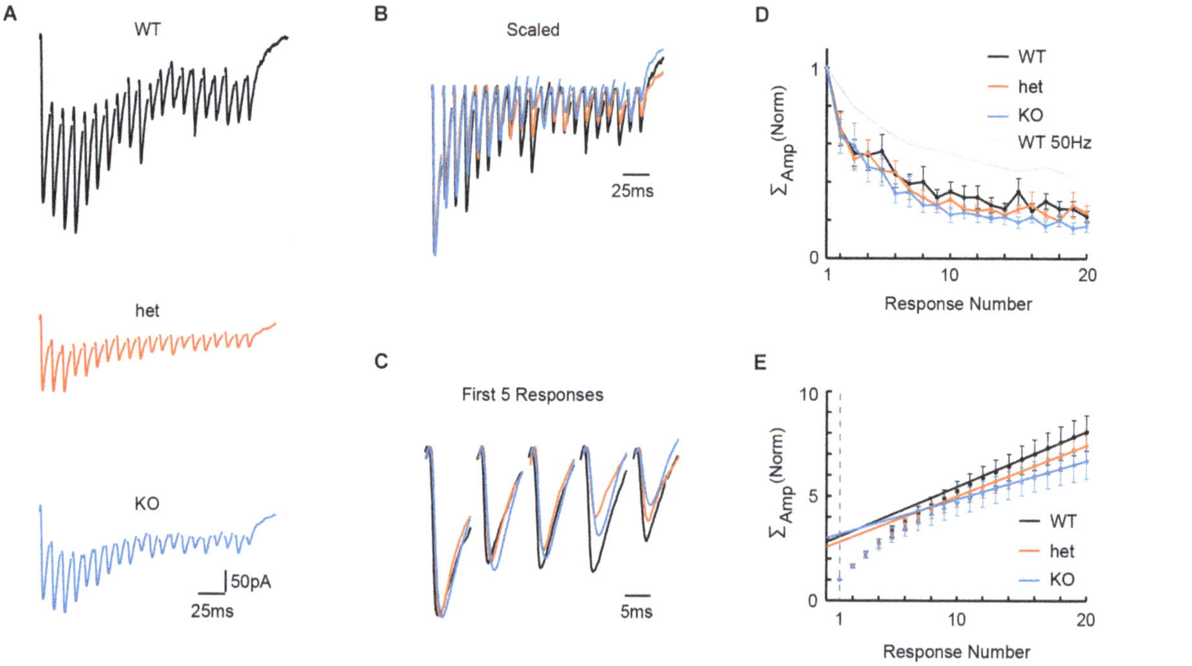

FIGURE 2 | Stimulation at 100 Hz in the MNTB revealed no effect of genotype on release properties in the LSO. To more stringently test for differences in release properties, we delivered 20 pulses at 100 Hz in tissue from WT ($n = 8$), het ($n = 9$), and KO ($n = 8$) mice. **(A)** Representative responses to 100 Hz trains of 20 pulses for WT (P4), het (P4), and KO (P4) tissue. **(B)** Example traces from **(A)**, scaled for comparison. Traces were first scaled to force all genotypes to have the same value for first-response-amplitude; then, within each train, the baseline for each response was reset to zero (i.e., baseline for first-response). **(C)** First 5 responses from examples in **(B)**, enlarged for clarity. **(D,E)** No differences were apparent between WT ($n = 8$), het ($n = 9$) and KO ($n = 8$) tissue for paired-pulse ratios (**D**; $p = 0.75$, see text) or cumulative event amplitudes (**E**; $p = 0.28$, see text). Probability of release, as estimated using these cumulative amplitude functions, was also similar among genotypes (see text).

found similar estimates for N_q and release probability between genotypes (**Figure 2E**; N_q: WT = 3.1 +/− 0.3; het = 2.8 +/− 0.3; KO = 3.2 +/− 0.4; Kruskal-Wallis test, $p = 0.74$; release probability: WT = 0.35 +/− 0.04; het = 0.39 +/− 0.05; KO = 0.35 +/− 0.05; Kruskal-Wallis test, $p = 0.71$). Together, these results argue that *VGlut3* expression does not affect release properties for GABA/glycine at MNTB terminals.

VGLUT3 EXPRESSION DOES NOT AFFECT RECOVERY FROM DEPRESSION FOLLOWING 50 HZ STIMULATION

Though our pulse train experiments had failed to show obvious effects of *VGlut3* expression on release properties, we considered the possibility that differences in vesicle re-filling might affect synaptic transmission on a longer timescale, and that this might be observed as an effect on recovery from depression. To test this model, we delivered two 50 Hz 10-pulse trains, separating by varying intervals (Dittman and Regehr, 1998) in order to estimate the time required for neurotransmission to recover to its original level (**Figure 3A**).

Cells were included in this analysis if we were able to test at least 8 recovery intervals, including one of at least 4 s. In practice, using these criteria ensured that 90% or greater recovery was attained for all cells analyzed. Percent depression as a function of recovery interval was then fit to an exponential (individual cells, **Figure 3B**; averages, **Figure 3C**). Neither average time to 90% recovery (WT: 3.2 +/− 0.7 s, $n = 5$; het: 2.9 +/− 0.2 s, $n = 12$; KO: 3.0 +/− 1.0 s, $n = 6$; Kruskal-Wallis test, $p = 0.76$) nor exponential time constants for recovery (recovery time constants: WT = 2.4 +/− 0.7 s, het = 1.7 +/− 0.2 s, KO = 1.9 +/− 0.8 s; Kruskal-Wallis test, $p = 0.32$) differed among genotypes.

VGLUT3 EXPRESSION DOES NOT AFFECT SIZE OF GABA/GLYCINE MINIATURE EVENTS

VGLUT3 has been shown to increase not only the rate, but also the amount of transmitter loading into synaptic vesicles (Gras et al., 2008). If VGLUT3 increases the concentration of GABA/glycine in vesicles at MTNB terminals, we would expect KO tissue to exhibit smaller responses to quantal release. To test this model, we compared the amplitudes of miniature GABA/glycinergic events recorded from WT and KO tissue. Because spontaneous vesicular release is uncommon in the immature LSO, we artificially increased release of single vesicles by either (1) first delivering brief high frequency stimulation to the MNTB-LSO pathway, or (2) adding Sr^{++} to the perfusate to desynchronize vesicular release in response to single stimuli (Bekkers and Clements, 1999). Miniature events were collected in the 20 s following the stimulus, and the individual events were analyzed. Cells were always allowed to recover at least 20 s before a new stimulus. In the examples of **Figure 4A**, no effect of genotype on mean event amplitude is seen (WT: 537 events, mean amplitude = 25.9 +/− 0.4 pA,

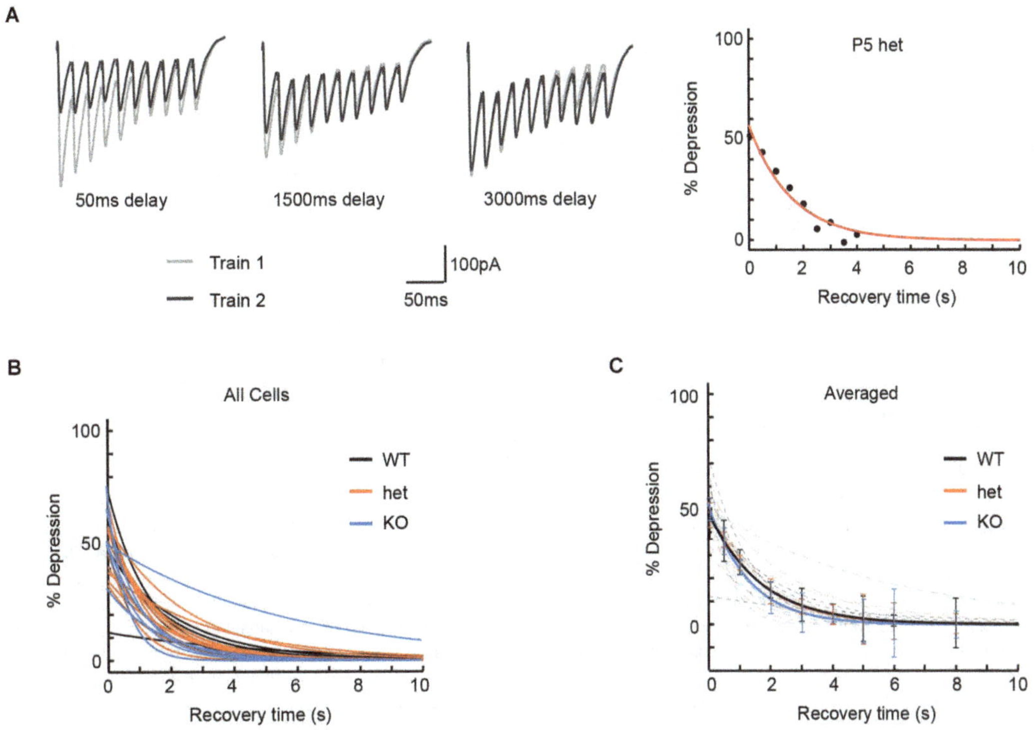

FIGURE 3 | Recovery from paired-pulse depression was unaffected by genotype. To determine the time required for MNTB-LSO synapses to recover from paired-pulse depression, we delivered pairs of 50 Hz trains of 10 pulses each, with each pair of trains separated by intervals ranging from 50 ms to 12 s. **(A)** Left: Three representative responses used to determine recovery time for a P5 het neuron. In each panel, Train 1 comprises the responses to the initial pulse train, and Train 2 the responses to the second pulse train of the pair, delivered after the interval shown. Right: Percent depression as a function of recovery interval (8 intervals, 50 ms to 4 s) for the cell shown at the left. Recovery time constant = 1.56 s; R-square of curve fit = 0.94. **(B)** Exponential fits for recovery from depression are shown for each cell thus examined (*n* values: WT = 5, het = 12, KO = 6). **(C)** Average of recovery curves (bold) for each genotype, with individual recovery curves from **(B)** in background (dashed, desaturated curves). Genotype had no effect on time to recovery from paired-pulse depression (Recovery time constant: WT = 2.4 +/− 0.7 s, het = 1.7 +/− 0.2 s, KO = 1.9 +/− 0.8 s; Kruskal-Wallis test, $p = 0.32$).

median amplitude = 25.0 pA; KO: 326 events, mean amplitude = 22.1 +/− 0.5 pA, median amplitude = 20.8 pA). This similarity in event amplitude held true across all cells (**Figure 4B**; WT: average mean amplitude = 31.8 +/− 2.4 pA, average median amplitude = 29.0 pA+/− 2.2 pA, $n = 22$; KO: average mean amplitude = 31.6 +/− 4.3 pA, average median amplitude = 29.2 pA+/− 3.8 pA, $n = 9$; t-test for means, $p = 0.98$; t-test for medians, $p = 0.95$). Comparison of current decay times also yielded no significant difference between genotypes (**Figure 4C**; WT: average mean decay = 10.3 +/− 1.5 ms, average median decay = 7.8 +/− 1.1 ms; KO: average mean decay = 11.7 +/− 2.5 ms, average median decay = 10.6 +/− 2.4 ms; t-test for means, $p = 0.65$; t-test for medians, $p = 0.23$), and even the cumulative probabilities found by pooling all miniatures within genotype showed only the suggestion of a difference (**Figure 4D**). Together, these results provide further evidence that *VGlut3* expression does not appreciably influence GABA/glycine vesicle loading at immature MNTB terminals.

DISCUSSION

VGlut3 is expressed in select populations of typically non-glutamatergic neurons. At adult synaptic terminals, VGLUT3 can increase both rate and level of neurotransmitter packing in cholinergic, serotonergic, and GABAergic vesicles in the striatum, raphe nuclei and hippocampus (Gras et al., 2008; Amilhon et al., 2010; Zander et al., 2010), and at least in the striatum VGLUT3 is required for normal cholinergic transmission (Nelson et al., 2014). To ask whether the transient expression of *VGlut3* during early postnatal development plays a similar role in synergizing GABA/glycine transmission at immature MNTB terminals in the LSO, we made whole-cell patch-clamp recordings from *VGlut3* WT, heterozygous and KO mice. The similarity among tissue from WT, het, and KO mice for PPRs and time to recovery from synaptic depression argues against a primary effect of VGLUT3 on rate of vesicle filling. The similarity in amplitude of miniature GABA/glycinergic events across genotype further argues against a model in which VGLUT3 increases level of vesicle filling. As the only other known function for VGLUT3 is to enable glutamate release, our results lend further support to the model that normal developmental refinement in the MNTB-LSO pathway requires VGLUT3 because refinement requires glutamate release. This model still needs to be tested explicitly.

We note that VGLUT3 may have exerted a nuanced effect on GABA/glycine transmission in our samples (e.g., **Figure 4D**),

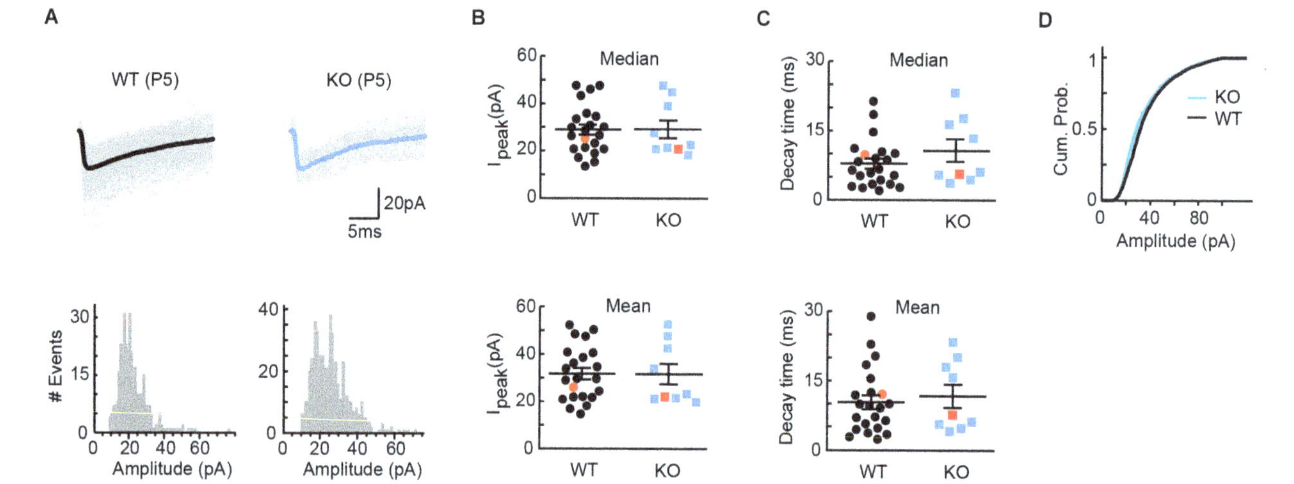

FIGURE 4 | Quantal size, as assessed by miniature events, was unaffected by genotype. **(A)** Example miniature events for cells from WT (left, P5, 537 events, mean = 25.9 +/– 0.4 pA, median = 25.0 pA) and KO (right, P5, 326 events, mean = 22.1 +/– 0.5 pA, median = 20.8 pA) tissue. Bold trace is the average miniature event for each cell. Event histograms for each cell are included below the example traces. **(B)** No differences were observed between WT ($n = 22$) and KO ($n = 9$) tissue for either mean or median peak amplitude (means: WT = 31.8 +/– 2.4 pA, KO = 31.6 +/– 4.3 pA; *t*-test $p = 0.98$; medians: WT = 29.0 +/– 2.2 pA, KO = 29.2 +/– 3.8 pA; *t*-test $p = 0.95$). Red markers indicate example cells in **(A)**. **(C)** For the cells shown in **(B)**, no differences were observed between WT and KO tissue for either mean or median decay times (means: WT = 10.3 +/– 1.5 ms, KO = 11.7 +/– 2.5 ms; *t*-test, $p = 0.65$; medians: WT = 7.8 +/– 1.1 ms, KO = 10.6 +/– 2.4 ms; *t*-test, $p = 0.23$). Red markers indicate example cells in **(A)**. **(D)** Cumulative probabilities for all miniature amplitudes, pooled within genotype, for the cells shown in **(B,C)**.

but if so, it was a small effect, and one that might well have occurred if already by P4–5 a subset of synapses had undergone more maturation in WT than in KO mice (Kim and Kandler, 2010; Noh et al., 2010). It has been nicely demonstrated that the window for synaptic refinement in the rat MNTB-LSO pathway is between P3 and P8 (Kim and Kandler, 2003), and in mice, we expect this period to be the same or perhaps shifted a day earlier. While in theory our question could be addressed by analyzing tissue collected before the synaptic refinement begins, VGLUT3 expression increases enough between P1 and P5 to cause problems for such an analysis. We note also that if VGLUT3 normally induces vesicular synergy that is followed by a compensatory reduction in quantal content (Daniels et al., 2004) we might miss an effect of VGLUT3 on miniature synaptic events. Nevertheless, whatever advantage VGLUT3 may provide to GABA/glycine neurotransmission, clearly that effect is small relative to the transformative effect of enabling glutamate release from immature inhibitory terminals. In sum, these results suggest that VGLUT3 plays qualitatively different roles at neonatal and adult inhibitory synapses, and in the immature auditory brainstem the likely primary function of VGLUT3 is to enable glutamate release.

Although *VGlut3* is already highly expressed in the superior olive at P4–5, its expression continues to increase until about P9–10, after which it declines rapidly (Gras et al., 2005). This raises the question of whether VGLUT3-induced vesicular synergy could be more prominent at P9–P10 and we did not observe it simply because we tested at P4–5. In fact, it would be difficult to disentangle demonstrated differences in miniature event amplitudes between WT and *VGlut3* KO mice at P9–12 (Noh et al., 2010), which are understood to reflect normal developmental strengthening due to postsynaptic effects (Kim and Kandler, 2010), from a synergistic effect. Nevertheless, even if any part of these differences at P9–12 could be attributed to a larger role for VGLUT3 in vesicular synergy, P9 is already past the window for functional refinement in the MNTB-LSO pathway (Kim and Kandler, 2003); hence, vesicular synergy found at P9 could not be a significant contributor to refinement.

Another possibility that could have obscured a vesicular synergy effect in our study is if loss of VGLUT3 results in compensatory presynaptic expression of VGLUT1 or VGLUT2 or increased postsynaptic expression of $GABA_A$ and/or glycine receptors. This seems unlikely. In vesicular synergy studies with *VGlut3* KO mice, compensatory increases in glutamate transporters have not been seen (Gras et al., 2008). Furthermore, if another vesicular glutamate transporter were upregulated, glutamate release should still be seen in the MNTB-LSO pathway of *VGlut3* KO mice, whereas in fact it disappears (Noh et al., 2010). Finally, while it is possible that compensatory changes in the expression of other, unidentified, synaptic proteins could have prevented our identification of a vesicular synergy effect, once again, that hypothetical compensatory effect is insufficient to rescue refinement (Noh et al., 2010), which further supports the conclusion that supporting vesicular synergy is not the critical role VGLUT3 plays in MNTB-LSO pathway refinement.

Normally considered a rare protein, VGLUT3 exhibits a striking expression profile in the developing superior olive, increasing dramatically from birth until about P10 and then declining to nearly undetectable levels (Blaesse et al., 2005; Cooper and Gillespie, 2011). As this transient expression most probably reflects a distinctly developmental role for VGLUT3 at immature inhibitory synapses in the superior olive, our results do not contradict but rather complement those reported at adult synapses. Indeed, whereas mature expression of VGLUT3 can suppress excitability (Zander et al., 2010) and support synergistic packaging of other neurotransmitters (Gras et al., 2008; Amilhon et al., 2010), the early expression of VGLUT3 in the auditory brainstem is required for normal developmental circuit refinement (Noh et al., 2010).

The refinement for which VGLUT3 is required in the rodent LSO occurs during the first postnatal week (Kim and Kandler, 2003, 2010), a period during which the brainstem receives no acoustically driven inputs. Activity-dependent refinement must therefore rely upon the activity generated spontaneously in the developing cochlea (Tritsch et al., 2007, 2010), and indeed it has recently been shown that altering the temporal statistics of this activity affects circuit refinement (Clause et al., 2014). As the mechanisms underlying refinement in this inhibitory circuit are still unknown, the role of VGLUT3 has inspired speculation. In one proposed role, VGLUT3 enables glutamate co-transmission to activate NMDA receptors. In the alternate proposed role, VGLUT3 boosts GABA/glycinergic transmission, which in turn depolarizes NMDA receptors or activates voltage-gated Ca^{++} channels. Our results argue against a primary function of VGLUT3 in promoting loading of GABA/glycine into synaptic vesicles in the developing brainstem and highlight the importance of establishing a robust model for mechanistic studies of synaptic plasticity and the role of VGLUT3 at this glycinergic synapse.

ACKNOWLEDGMENTS

The authors thank S. El Mestikawy for the gift of mice, C. Fasano for advice on colony management and genotyping, and J. A. Foster for genotyping equipment and technical expertise. This work was supported by the NSERC (grant to Deda C. Gillespie) and the CONACyT (postdoctoral award to Javier Alamilla).

REFERENCES

Amilhon, B., Lepicard, E., Renoir, T., Mongeau, R., Popa, D., Poirel, O., et al. (2010). VGLUT3 (vesicular glutamate transporter type 3) contribution to the regulationof serotonergic transmission and anxiety. *J. Neurosci.* 30, 2198–2210. doi: 10.1523/jneurosci.5196-09.2010

Bekkers, J. M., and Clements, J. D. (1999). Quantal amplitude and quantal variance of strontium-induced asynchronous EPSCs in rat dentate granule neurons. *J. Physiol.* 516, 227–248. doi: 10.1111/j.1469-7793.1999.227aa.x

Blaesse, P., Ehrhardt, S., Friauf, E., and Nothwang, H. G. (2005). Developmental pattern of three vesicular glutamate transporters in the rat superior olivary complex. *Cell Tissue Res.* 320, 33–50. doi: 10.1007/s00441-004-1054-8

Case, D. T., and Gillespie, D. C. (2011). Pre- and postsynaptic properties of glutamatergic transmission in the immature inhibitory MNTB-LSO pathway. *J. Neurophysiol.* 106, 2570–2579. doi: 10.1152/jn.00644.2010

Clause, A., Kim, G., Sonntag, M., Weisz, C. J., Vetter, D. E., Rbsamen, R., et al. (2014). The precise temporal pattern of prehearing spontaneous activity is necessary for tonotopic map refinement. *Neuron* 82, 822–835. doi: 10.1016/j.neuron.2014.04.001

Cooper, A. P., and Gillespie, D. C. (2011). Synaptotagmins I and II in the developing rat auditory brainstem: synaptotagmin I is transiently expressed in glutamate-releasing immature inhibitory terminals. *J. Comp. Neurol.* 519, 2417–2433. doi: 10.1002/cne.22634

Daniels, R. W., Collins, C. A., Gelfand, M. V., Dant, J., Brooks, E. S., Krantz, D. E., et al. (2004). Increased expression of the Drosophila vesicular glutamate transporter leads to excess glutamate release and a compensatory decrease in quantal content. *J. Neurosci.* 24, 10466–10474. doi: 10.1523/jneurosci.3001-04.2004

Dittman, J. S., and Regehr, W. G. (1998). Calcium dependence and recovery kinetics of presynaptic depression at the climbing fiber to Purkinje cell synapse. *J. Neurosci.* 18, 6147–6162.

Ehrlich, I., Lohrke, S., and Friauf, E. (1999). Shift from depolarizing to hyperpolarizing glycine action in rat auditory neurones is due to age-dependent Cl- regulation. *J. Physiol.* 520, 121–137. doi: 10.1111/j.1469-7793.1999.00121.x

El Mestikawy, S., Wallén-Mackenzie, A., Fortin, G. M., Descarries, L., and Trudeau, L. E. (2011). From glutamate co-release to vesicular synergy: vesicular glutamate transporters. *Nat. Rev. Neurosci.* 12, 204–216. doi: 10.1038/nrn2969

Fremeau, R. T. Jr., Burman, J., Qureshi, T., Tran, C. H., Proctor, J., Johnson, J., et al. (2002). The identification of vesicular glutamate transporter 3 suggests novel modes of signaling by glutamate. *Proc. Natl. Acad. Sci. U S A* 99, 14488–14493. doi: 10.1073/pnas.222546799

Gillespie, D. C., and Kandler, K. (2009). "GABA, glycine and glutamate co-release at developing inhibitory synapses," in *Co-Existence and Co-Release of Classical Neurotransmitters*, ed R. Gutierrez (New York: Springer Verlag), 55–80.

Gillespie, D. C., Kim, G., and Kandler, K. (2005). Inhibitory synapses in the developing auditory system are glutamatergic. *Nat. Neurosci.* 8, 332–338. doi: 10.1038/nn1397

Gras, C., Amilhon, B., Lepicard, E. M., Poirel, O., Vinatier, J., Herbin, M., et al. (2008). The vesicular glutamate transporter VGLUT3 synergizes striatal acetylcholine tone. *Nat. Neurosci.* 11, 292–300. doi: 10.1038/nn2052

Gras, C., Herzog, E., Bellenchi, G. C., Bernard, V., Ravassard, P., Pohl, M., et al. (2002). A third vesicular glutamate transporter expressed by cholinergic and serotoninergic neurons. *J. Neurosci.* 22, 5442–5451.

Gras, C., Vinatier, J., Amilhon, B., Guerci, A., Christov, C., Ravassard, P., et al. (2005). Developmentally regulated expression of VGLUT3 during early post-natal life. *Neuropharmacology* 49, 901–911. doi: 10.1016/j.neuropharm.2005.07.023

Herzog, E., Gilchrist, J., Gras, C., Muzerelle, A., Ravassard, P., Giros, B., et al. (2004). Localization of VGLUT3, the vesicular glutamate transporter type 3, in the rat brain. *Neuroscience* 123, 983–1002. doi: 10.1016/j.neuroscience.2003.10.039

Inchauspe, C. G., Forsythe, I. D., and Uchitel, O. D. (2007). Changes in synaptic transmission properties due to the expression of N-type calcium channels at the calyx of Held synapse of mice lacking P/Q-type calcium channels. *J. Physiol.* 584, 835–851. doi: 10.1113/jphysiol.2007.139683

Jalabi, W., Kopp-Scheinpflug, C., Allen, P. D., Schiavon, E., DiGiacomo, R. R., Forsythe, I. D., et al. (2013). Sound localization ability and glycinergic innervation of the superior olivary complex persist after genetic deletion of the medial nucleus of the trapezoid body. *J. Neurosci.* 33, 15044–15049. doi: 10.1523/jneurosci.2604-13.2013

Kalmbach, A., Kullmann, P. H., and Kandler, K. (2010). NMDAR-mediated calcium transients elicited by glutamate co-release at developing inhibitory synapses. *Front. Synaptic Neurosci.* 2:27. doi: 10.3389/fnsyn.2010.00027

Kandler, K., and Friauf, E. (1995). Development of glycinergic and glutamatergic synaptic transmission in the auditory brainstem of perinatal rats. *J. Neurosci.* 15, 6890–6904.

Kim, G., and Kandler, K. (2003). Elimination and strengthening of glycinergic/GABAergic connections during tonotopic map formation. *Nat. Neurosci.* 6, 282–290. doi: 10.1038/nn1015

Kim, G., and Kandler, K. (2010). Synaptic changes underlying the strengthening of GABA/glycinergic connections in the developing lateral superior olive. *Neuroscience* 171, 924–933. doi: 10.1016/j.neuroscience.2010.09.054

Kotak, V. C., Korada, S., Schwartz, I. R., and Sanes, D. H. (1998). A developmental shift from GABAergic to glycinergic transmission in the central auditory system. *J. Neurosci.* 18, 4646–4655.

Kullmann, P. H., Ene, F. A., and Kandler, K. (2002). Glycinergic and GABAergic calcium responses in the developing lateral superior olive. *Eur. J. Neurosci.* 15, 1093–1104. doi: 10.1046/j.1460-9568.2002.01946.x

Nabekura, J., Katsurabayashi, S., Kakazu, Y., Shibata, S., Matsubara, A., Jinno, S., et al. (2004). Developmental switch from GABA to glycine release in single central synaptic terminals. *Nat. Neurosci.* 7, 17–23. doi: 10.1038/nn1170

Nelson, A. B., Bussert, T. G., Kreitzer, A. C., and Seal, R. P. (2014). Striatal cholinergic neurotransmission requires VGLUT3. *J. Neurosci.* 34, 8772–8777. doi: 10.1523/jneurosci.0901-14.2014

Nishimaki, T., Jang, I. S., Ishibashi, H., Yamaguchi, J., and Nabekura, J. (2007). Reduction of metabotropic glutamate receptor-mediated heterosynaptic inhibition of developing MNTB-LSO inhibitory synapses. *Eur. J. Neurosci.* 26, 323–330. doi: 10.1111/j.1460-9568.2007.05656.x

Noh, J., Seal, R. P., Garver, J. A., Edwards, R. H., and Kandler, K. (2010). Glutamate co-release at GABA/glycinergic synapses is crucial for the refinement of an inhibitory map. *Nat. Neurosci.* 13, 232–238. doi: 10.1038/nn.2478

Tollin, D. J. (2003). The lateral superior olive: a functional role in sound source localization. *Neuroscientist* 9, 127–143. doi: 10.1177/1073858403252228

Tritsch, N. X., Rodríguez-Contreras, A., Crins, T. T., Wang, H. C., Borst, J. G., and Bergles, D. E. (2010). Calcium action potentials in hair cells pattern auditory neuron activity before hearing onset. *Nat. Neurosci.* 13, 1050–1052. doi: 10.1038/nn.2604

Tritsch, N. X., Yi, E., Gale, J. E., Glowatzki, E., and Bergles, D. E. (2007). The origin of spontaneous activity in the developing auditory system. *Nature* 450, 50–55. doi: 10.1038/nature06233

Zander, J. F., Münster-Wandowski, A., Brunk, I., Pahner, I., Gómez-Lira, G., Heinemann, U., et al. (2010). Synaptic and vesicular coexistence of VGLUT and VGAT in selected excitatory and inhibitory synapses. *J. Neurosci.* 30, 7634–7645. doi: 10.1523/jneurosci.0141-10.2010

4

Cell-type specific short-term plasticity at auditory nerve synapses controls feed-forward inhibition in the dorsal cochlear nucleus

***Miloslav Sedlacek*[†] *and Stephan D. Brenowitz* ***

Section on Synaptic Transmission, National Institute on Deafness and Other Communication Disorders, National Institutes of Health, Bethesda, MD, USA

***Correspondence:**
Stephan D. Brenowitz, Janelia Farm Research Campus, Howard Hughes Medical Institute, 19700 Helix Drive, Ashburn, VA 20147, USA
e-mail: brenowitzs@janelia.hhmi.org

[†]**Present address:**
Miloslav Sedlacek, Laboratory of Cell Structure and Dynamics, National Institute on Deafness and Other Communication Disorders, National Institutes of Health, Bethesda, MD, USA

Feed-forward inhibition (FFI) represents a powerful mechanism by which control of the timing and fidelity of action potentials in local synaptic circuits of various brain regions is achieved. In the cochlear nucleus, the auditory nerve provides excitation to both principal neurons and inhibitory interneurons. Here, we investigated the synaptic circuit associated with fusiform cells (FCs), principal neurons of the dorsal cochlear nucleus (DCN) that receive excitation from auditory nerve fibers and inhibition from tuberculoventral cells (TVCs) on their basal dendrites in the deep layer of DCN. Despite the importance of these inputs in regulating fusiform cell firing behavior, the mechanisms determining the balance of excitation and FFI in this circuit are not well understood. Therefore, we examined the timing and plasticity of auditory nerve driven FFI onto FCs. We find that in some FCs, excitatory and inhibitory components of FFI had the same stimulation thresholds indicating they could be triggered by activation of the same fibers. In other FCs, excitation and inhibition exhibit different stimulus thresholds, suggesting FCs and TVCs might be activated by different sets of fibers. In addition, we find that during repetitive activation, synapses formed by the auditory nerve onto TVCs and FCs exhibit distinct modes of short-term plasticity. Feed-forward inhibitory post-synaptic currents (IPSCs) in FCs exhibit short-term depression because of prominent synaptic depression at the auditory nerve-TVC synapse. Depression of this feedforward inhibitory input causes a shift in the balance of fusiform cell synaptic input towards greater excitation and suggests that fusiform cell spike output will be enhanced by physiological patterns of auditory nerve activity.

Keywords: dorsal cochlear nucleus, auditory nerve, synaptic transmission, synaptic plasticity, feedforward inhibition

INTRODUCTION

In many regions of the mammalian brain, feed-forward inhibition (FFI) represents a complex synaptic arrangement in neuronal networks that results from parallel activation of principal cells and inhibitory interneurons by the same excitatory input (Buzsaki, 1984; Pouille and Scanziani, 2001; Blitz and Regehr, 2005; Gabernet et al., 2005; Mittmann et al., 2005; Cruikshank et al., 2007; Torborg et al., 2010; Ellender et al., 2011; Kuo and Trussell, 2011; Najac et al., 2011; Zhou et al., 2012). Activation of inhibitory interneurons consequently provides inhibition to principal cells to reduce their excitability. The temporal resolution of integration of synaptic inputs depends on the time window within which excitatory inputs can be summated and reach the threshold for firing an action potential in the postsynaptic neuron (Pouille and Scanziani, 2001). The precise timing of excitation and inhibition plays a significant role during high frequency repetitive neuronal activity and has been shown previously to control short-term synaptic plasticity of excitatory and inhibitory inputs (Gabernet et al., 2005; Torborg et al., 2010).

The dorsal cochlear nucleus (DCN) integrates non-auditory and auditory information and plays a role in localization of sound sources and filtering self-generated noise (Shore and Zhou, 2006; Requarth and Sawtell, 2011). Fusiform cells (FCs) are the principal neurons of the DCN that integrate multiple excitatory and inhibitory synaptic inputs onto their apical and basal dendrites (Voigt and Young, 1980, 1990; Blackstad et al., 1984; Oertel and Wu, 1989; Berrebi and Mugnaini, 1991; Zhang and Oertel, 1994). Excitatory inputs contacting apical dendrites of FCs come from granule cell parallel fibers located in the superficial molecular layer. These fibers also innervate cartwheel cells, local glycinergic interneurons that also provide inhibition to FC apical dendrites (Roberts and Trussell, 2010; Kuo and Trussell, 2011). Excitatory inputs onto basal dendrites are conveyed via auditory nerve fibers that carry precisely timed, tonotopically organized acoustic information. Additional excitatory input is formed by the T-stellate cells that send their axons from the ventral cochlear nucleus to the deep layer of the DCN (Oertel and Young, 2004; Oertel et al., 2010). Predominantly glycinergic inhibition terminating onto the basal dendrite of FCs is represented by inputs from the tuberculoventral cells (TVCs), also referred to as vertical cells, and D-stellate cells (Zhang and Oertel, 1994), which share the same auditory nerve input with FCs. This complex synaptic arrangement associated with the basal dendrite forms the basis for a feed-forward inhibitory circuit associated with transmission of acoustic information via FCs. Moreover, TVCs form inhibitory synapses onto each other (Kuo et al., 2012). TVCs lie in bands parallel to isofrequency laminae, and their targets, including FCs in the DCN, are innervated by the same auditory nerve fibers (Wickesberg and Oertel, 1988; Voigt and Young, 1990). Moreover, TVCs are sensitive to narrowband stimuli, as only a small number of auditory nerve fibers provide excitation to these interneurons, distinguishing them from D-stellate cells that are sensitive to broadband sounds and are innervated by auditory nerve fibers tuned to a wider frequency range (Voigt and Young, 1990; Winter and Palmer, 1995; Palmer and Winter, 1996). Therefore, inhibition of FCs by TVCs can regulate firing behavior of FCs (Nelken and Young, 1994; Oertel and Young, 2004), although recent evidence indicates the strength of individual connections might be rather weak (Kuo et al., 2012).

To examine the basis for feed-forward inhibitory control and plasticity of auditory processing in the DCN, we determined the synaptic mechanisms that control the balance of excitation and inhibition and affect the output from the nucleus. In this study, we show that short-term synaptic plasticity of auditory nerve-evoked disynaptic inhibition onto FCs exhibits facilitation when activated directly by stimulating inhibitory inputs onto FCs, similar to what has been shown previously using paired recordings from fusiform and TVCs (Kuo et al., 2012). In addition, we show that short-term synaptic plasticity, that is cell type specific in this synaptic circuit, controls FFI received by FCs. We demonstrate that facilitation of TVC-mediated inhibition of FCs shifts to significant depression when driven by the auditory nerve. This shift in synaptic plasticity and excitation-inhibition balance in FCs during repetitive auditory nerve stimulation results from pronounced activity-dependent short-term depression of auditory nerve synapses onto TVCs.

MATERIALS AND METHODS

COCHLEAR NUCLEUS SLICE PREPARATION

All experiments were conducted in accordance with animal protocols approved by the NIH Animal Care and Use Committee. P17–P22 C57BL/6 mice of either sex were deeply anesthetized with isoflurane before decapitation and parasagittal brainstem slices containing the cochlear nucleus were cut using a ceramic blade mounted on a vibrating microtome (Leica VT1200S, Leica Microsystems). In order to preserve the complex circuitry and long-distance synaptic connections necessary to study FFI, a midline cut was made, the brainstem was cut into two halves and the medial surface of the right half was glued down to the slicing platform. Then, the first cut was made right above the lateral surface of the cochlear nucleus without touching the surface of the nucleus or the auditory nerve root. A second cut was made to obtain a thick (380–450 μm) slice containing most of the cochlear nucleus. Using a thick slice preparation allowed us to preserve the auditory nerve inputs to the DCN which is critical for studying disynaptic inhibition. Dissections were performed in an ice-cold, sucrose-based extracellular solution that contained the following (in mM): 75 NaCl, 26 $NaHCO_3$, 75 sucrose, 25 glucose, 2.5 KCl, 1.25 NaH_2PO_4, 7 $MgCl_2$, 0.5 $CaCl_2$, 2 Na-pyruvate, 3 myo-inositol, 0.4 Na-ascorbate (pH 7.35, ~325 mOsm). Slices were then incubated in the same solution for 20 min at 34°C, transferred to saline solution that contained the following (in mM): 125 NaCl, 26 $NaHCO_3$, 25 glucose, 2.5 KCl, 1.25 NaH_2PO_4, 1 $MgCl_2$, 2 $CaCl_2$, 2 Na-pyruvate, 0.4 Na-ascorbate (pH 7.35, ~315 mOsm) and were incubated for additional 20 min at 34°C. All solutions were bubbled with 5% O_2/95% CO_2.

ELECTROPHYSIOLOGY

Slices were placed in a recording chamber in a way that the intact lateral surface of the nucleus faced the bottom of the chamber and all recordings were made from the medial surface of the DCN. Slices were continuously perfused (2–3 ml/min) with saline extracellular solution. Fusiform and TVCs were visually identified using a 60 × 0.9 NA objective (Olympus) and infrared differential interference contrast. Recording electrodes (2.2–4 MΩ) pulled from thick-walled borosilicate glass (Sutter Instruments) were filled with intracellular solution that contained (in mM): 120 $CsMeSO_4$, 10 HEPES, 5 NaCl, 3 $MgSO_4$, 2 QX-314, 4 Mg-ATP, 0.4 Na-GTP, 14 Tris-phosphocreatine for voltage-clamp experiments, or (in mM): 125 $KMeSO_4$, 10 HEPES, 5 NaCl, 1 $MgCl_2$, 4 Mg-ATP, 0.4 Na-GTP, 14 Tris-phosphocreatine for current-clamp experiments. To verify the identity of recorded fusiform and tuberculoventral neurons, all intracellular solutions were supplemented with Alexa Fluor 594 hydrazide (20 μM). Cell morphology was visualized using a two-photon laser scanning microscope and a Ti:sapphire pulsed laser (Chameleon, Coherent) tuned to 840 nm for excitation. Data were filtered at 3 or 6 kHz using a Multiclamp 700B amplifier (Molecular Devices) and sampled at 10 or 20 kHz, respectively. Series resistance (7–18 MΩ) was compensated by 75% and experiments in which the series resistance increased by >20% were excluded from further analysis. To evoke synaptic responses, a tungsten bipolar stimulating electrode with 140 μm tip spacing and with tips bent at a 45° angle (FHC, Bowdoin, ME) was placed in the auditory nerve root (for FFI and direct stimulation of excitatory inputs), or in the deep layer of the DCN (for direct stimulation of inhibitory inputs). Because FCs also receive excitatory granule cell inputs in addition to the auditory nerve inputs, care was taken to directly stimulate auditory nerve fibers in region of the nerve root attached to the ventral region of the cochlear nucleus. The nerve root was readily identified with transmitted light under a 4x objective, as well as auditory nerve fibers within the root, and could be visually traced beyond the ascending/descending auditory nerve branch bifurcation. However, the placement of the stimulating electrode within the auditory nerve root did not prevent the activation of T-stellate cell excitatory inputs onto FCs in some cases, which could be seen as disynaptic excitation in fusiform cell recordings (for example see **Figure 2A**). We observed the disynaptic excitation in ~35% of FCs while recording auditory nerve (AN) evoked EPSCs. These recordings were used for further analyses since the later, presumably T-stellate cell-mediated peak did not interfere with the first peak in any way. Moreover, during the FFI trials, the fast kinetics and fast onset of AN evoked inhibitory post-synaptic currents (IPSCs) eliminated the T-stellate cell mediated peak completely. To further ensure and verify that excitation of FCs originated from activation of the auditory nerve fibers, we tested short-term synaptic plasticity of the recorded excitatory responses and verified that excitatory responses were evoked by stimulation of the auditory nerve inputs by the presence of short-term synaptic depression. In contrast. stimulation of parallel fiber synapses evoked synaptic responses that strongly facilitate (Tzounopoulos et al., 2004; Roberts and Trussell, 2010) and can therefore be distinguished from auditory nerve stimulation. Synaptic responses were evoked with 0.2 ms current pulses (0–100 μA) delivered by an isolated stimulus unit (World Precision Instruments). To record FFI consisting of an EPSC-IPSC sequence, FCs were voltage clamped at −40 mV, a holding potential between the reversal potentials for excitatory and inhibitory transmission, and no synaptic blockers were added to the perfusion solution. Direct auditory nerve-evoked EPSCs were recorded at −60 mV with strychnine (2 μM) and picrotoxin (40 μM) in the bath. Direct IPSCs were recorded at −40 mV with 6,7-dinitrodihydroquinoxaline-2,3-dione (DNQX) (20 μM) and R-CPP (5 μM) in the bath. To analyze timing of FFI, EPSCs were recorded at the chloride reversal potential (E_{Cl} = −59 to −65 mV), IPSCs were recorded at the reversal potential for glutamatergic transmission (E_{glu} = +5 to +12 mV), and no synaptic blockers were present in the bath. Recordings were not corrected for the liquid junction potential. Picrotoxin was from Tocris Cookson, DNQX and R-CPP were from Abcam, Alexa Fluor 594 hydrazide was from Invitrogen, all other chemicals were from Sigma. All recordings were performed at 33–35°C.

DATA ANALYSIS

All data were acquired and analyzed using custom routines written in Matlab (MathWorks) and IgorPro (WaveMetrics), respectively. Averages are presented as means ± SEM. To distinguish between facilitating and depressing synapses, the ratio of the 10th stimulus to the 1st stimulus (S10/S1) was calculated. Recordings with S10/S1>1 were considered facilitating, while those with S10/S1<1 were considered to be depressing. Latencies were calculated as the time between the beginning of the stimulus artifact and the onset of excitatory/inhibitory synaptic event.

RESULTS

AUDITORY NERVE ACTIVITY TRIGGERS FEED-FORWARD INHIBITION IN FUSIFORM CELLS

Basal dendrites of FCs in the DCN receive direct excitatory inputs from the auditory nerve and inhibitory synaptic inputs from TVCs in the deep layer of the DCN (Zhang and Oertel, 1993; Rhode, 1999; Oertel and Young, 2004; Kuo et al., 2012). To further investigate the roles of synaptic excitation and inhibition in auditory processing by FCs, we used parasagittal slices of the cochlear nucleus (see Materials and Methods) that preserve components of the synaptic circuit associated with the fusiform cell basal dendrites (**Figure 1**).

Whole-cell voltage clamp recordings were made from visually identified FCs. The membrane potential of the fusiform cell was clamped at −40 mV, which is above the reversal potential for inhibitory synaptic currents (E_{Cl}, ~−60 mV) and below the reversal for excitatory synaptic currents (E_{Glu}, ~0 mV). Synaptic responses were evoked from a distance of several hundred micrometers from the target postsynaptic neurons. Stimulation of auditory nerve fibers evoked postsynaptic currents in FC (**Figure 1A**) that consisted of a sequence of inward excitatory (EPSC) and outward inhibitory (IPSC) components (**Figure 1B**). Subsequent bath application of the glycine receptor antagonist strychnine (2 μM) completely blocked the outward component of the synaptic current (**Figure 1B**, top $n = 3$ cells). These results indicate that the inward EPSCs recorded from the FC were evoked directly by stimulation of the auditory nerve fibers.

In separate experiments, application of the AMPA receptor antagonist DNQX (20 μM) completely abolished both the inward and outward component. The blockade was partially reversible (**Figure 1B**, bottom $n = 5$ cells). Sensitivity of inhibitory synaptic transmission to a blocker of excitatory transmission demonstrates that the IPSCs were evoked by auditory nerve stimulation rather than by direct activation of inhibitory fibers and were therefore disynaptic in nature. Interneurons providing inhibition to FCs in the deep layer of the DCN have been identified as TVCs (Zhang and Oertel, 1993; Rhode, 1999; Oertel and Young, 2004; Kuo et al., 2012). We conclude that auditory nerve activity drives a feed-forward inhibitory circuit in the DCN that includes tuberculoventral cells, DCN interneurons that provide inhibition to FCs in the deep layer of the DCN.

TIMING OF FEED-FORWARD INHIBITION ONTO BASAL DENDRITES OF FUSIFORM CELLS

Timing of excitatory and inhibitory inputs can have significant consequences for the generation of action potentials in postsynaptic neurons both in the auditory system (Oertel, 1999; Brand et al., 2002), as well as in other brain regions (Buzsaki, 1984; Gil and Amitai, 1996; Borg-Graham et al., 1998). Therefore, having demonstrated the presence of disynaptic inhibition onto fusiform cells evoked by auditory nerve stimulation, we next examined the relative timing of individual components of the feed-forward EPSC-IPSC sequence. We recorded synaptic responses from fusiform cells, and by voltage clamping the cells at different holding potentials we isolated individual components without having to use pharmacological tools. First, we recorded the control FFI sequence at −40 mV with both inward and outward components present (**Figure 2A**, top). To isolate the inhibitory component of the sequence, fusiform cells were voltage clamped at the reversal potential for excitatory transmission (E_{glu}, +8.25 ± 1.5 mV; $n = 4$ cells) and we recorded IPSCs triggered by auditory nerve stimulation. Then, the membrane potential was hyperpolarized to the reversal potential for chloride ions (E_{Cl}, −60 ± 0.7 mV; $n = 4$ cells) to isolate EPSCs evoked by auditory nerve stimulation. We analyzed latencies of EPSCs and IPSCs after the stimulus, as well as the interval between the EPSC and IPSC in the sequence. We refer to the beginning of the stimulation artifact as t0, and to the onsets of EPSC and IPSC as t1 and t2, respectively (**Figure 2A**, bottom).

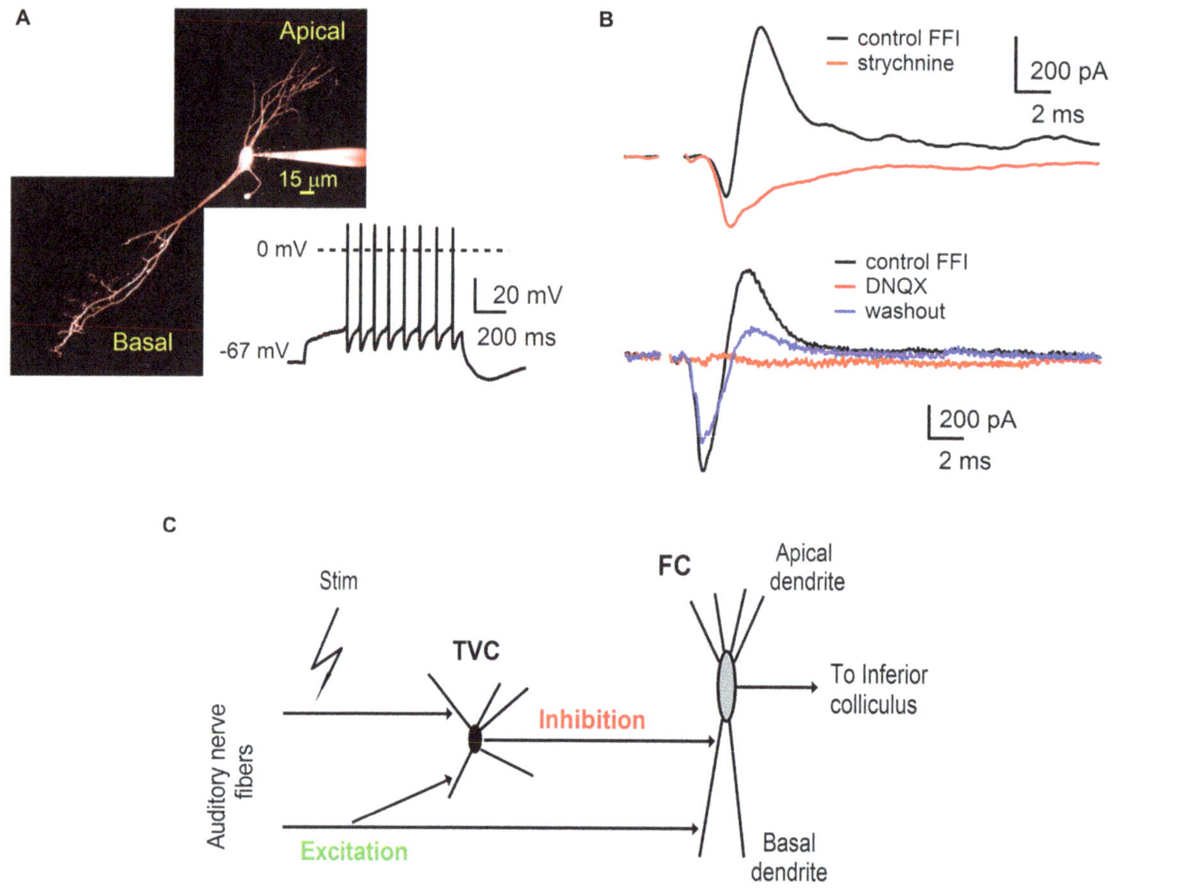

FIGURE 1 | Auditory nerve drives feed-forward inhibition onto fusiform cells in the DCN. (A) A two-photon laser scanning microscopy image of a fusiform cell loaded with Alexa Fluor 594 showing apical and basal dendritic branching. The trace shows a representative example of firing properties of fusiform cells (FCs). Note the delayed spiking pattern (build up) while the cell was held at hyperpolarized membrane potentials. **(B)** Voltage clamp recordings of feed-forward inhibition from FCs evoked by extracellular stimulation of the auditory nerve. Inhibitory component of the EPSC-IPSC sequence (outward deflection of the black trace) was completely blocked with 2 µM strychnine (top traces, n = 3 cells). Application of AMPA receptor antagonist 6,7-dinitrodihydroquinoxaline-2,3-dione (DNQX) (20 µM) reversibly blocked both components of the sequence (bottom traces, n = 5 cells). Stimulation artifacts were removed for clarity. Traces represent averages of 5–10 trials. **(C)** A schematic of the feed-forward inhibitory circuit driven by the auditory nerve in the dorsal cochlear nucleus. Auditory nerve fibers synapse onto FC, as well as onto tuberculoventral cells (TVC) which further provide inhibition to the FC.

We found that the timing for activation of the feed-forward inhibitory circuit was very precise with latencies of EPSCs, IPCSs and relative EPSC-IPSC sequences of 1.50 ± 0.16 ms, 2.68 ± 0.13 ms and 1.18 ± 0.09 ms, respectively (n = 4 cells, **Figure 2B**).

INNERVATION PATTERNS OF FUSIFORM CELLS AND INTERNEURONS BY AUDITORY NERVE FIBERS

Auditory nerve fibers innervate both fusiform and TVCs (Wickesberg and Oertel, 1988; Zhang and Oertel, 1994; Fujino and Oertel, 2003). However, the pattern of innervation is not known: disynaptic inhibition in FCs may arise from the activation of the same auditory nerve fibers that form synapses onto both the fusiform and the tuberculoventral cell, or fibers innervating FCs may be different from those innervating tuberculoventral cells. Even though evidence from previous anatomical studies exists that some of the fusiform cell targets of TVCs are innervated by the same auditory nerve fibers as the TVCs themselves (Wickesberg and Oertel, 1988), no physiological evidence exists to support this innervation pattern.

To address this, we recorded FFI in FCs using increasing stimulation intensity to evoke auditory nerve-mediated synaptic responses (Chen and Regehr, 2000; Blitz and Regehr, 2005; Cao and Oertel, 2010; **Figure 3**). We predicted that if the same set of auditory nerve fibers innervates both the fusiform and the TVCs in the disynaptic circuit, then both the excitatory and inhibitory components would have the same activation threshold. Alternatively, EPSCs and IPSCs could have distinct thresholds, indicative of innervation by different sets of auditory nerve fibers. To distinguish between these possibilities, we used low stimulation intensities (0–25 µA) incremented in 1–5 µA steps to record both EPSC/IPSC failures and successes. As the stimulation

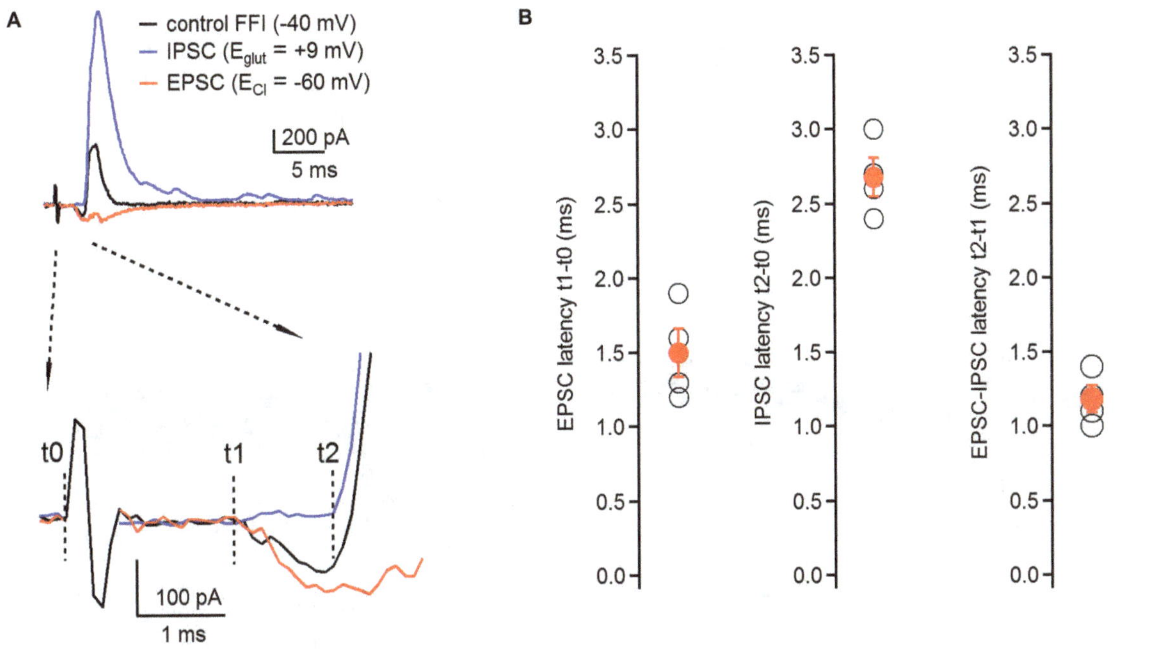

FIGURE 2 | Timing of feed-forward inhibition onto fusiform cells. (A) Latencies of individual components of the EPSC-IPSC sequence (black trace) were examined at respective reversal potentials for excitatory and inhibitory transmission. EPSCs (red trace) were recorded at E_{Cl} (−60 ± 0.7 mV, *n* = 4 cells); IPSCs (blue trace) were recorded at E_{glut} (8.25 ± 1.5 mV, *n* = 4 cells) (top traces). No synaptic blockers were added to the perfusion solution. Timing of individual components was analyzed using the time difference between the beginning of the stimulating artifact (t0) and the onset of synaptic events (t1 for EPSCs, t2 for IPSCs). EPSC-IPSC latency was calculated as t2 − t1 (bottom traces). Traces represent averages of 5–10 trials. Only stimulation artifact in the control FFI (black) trace is shown, the other two were removed from EPSC and IPSC traces for clarity. **(B)** Plots of latencies of EPSCs and IPSCs from the stimulation artifact, and timing of EPSC-IPSC sequence. Each black data point represents one neuron; red data points represent averages ± SEM; *n* = 4 cells.

intensity increased in subsequent trials, successful synaptic events started to appear (**Figure 3**). We consider the constant stimulation intensity that gave rise to failures and successes to be the minimal stimulation in these experiments.

We found that in a subset of cells, the threshold for evoking both EPSC and IPSC in the disynaptic sequence was different (**Figures 3A–E**). In this example, the first successful synaptic events recorded were IPSCs without any EPSCs. The latency of these inhibitory responses corresponded to the disynaptic latencies shown in **Figure 2**, confirming they were not evoked by direct stimulation. As the stimulation intensity increased, the excitatory component appeared as well. This innervation pattern represented ~54% (7/13 FCs). The remaining ~46% of FCs exhibited an innervation pattern in which thresholds for evoking excitatory and inhibitory components in disynaptic circuit were the same (**Figures 3F–J**). In this example, both components were recruited at the same level of stimulation intensity. With further increase in the stimulation intensity, the amplitudes of EPSCs remained unchanged, or slightly increased with further stimulation, and the IPSC amplitudes further increased until they reached their maximum value (**Figure 3G**). We further analyzed the correlation between IPSC/EPSC amplitudes in individual trials to examine whether these are interdependent and possibly activated by the same or different sets of fibers. **Figure 3D** shows a plot where there is a weak correlation between the IPSC and EPSC amplitudes (R = 0.20), whereas in the case of recordings where both EPSCs and IPSCs have the same activation thresholds, strong correlation (R = 0.87) between IPSC and EPSC amplitudes was observed (**Figure 3I**). Several possible explanations exist for the observed results, although clear and precise conclusions about the innervating pattern by the auditory nerve fibers are difficult to draw. Our results show that distinct auditory nerve fibers may innervate fusiform and TVCs separately, or the same fiber can innervate both cell types. However, since there is no direct evidence for innervation by single auditory nerve fibers, due to insufficient resolution of the stimulation technique, our minimal stimulation trials can also represent activation of multiple weak auditory nerve fibers as with the same activation threshold. Challenging experiments such as simultaneous recordings from fusiform and tuberculoventral cells, while stimulating auditory nerve could eventually provide more insight into the issue.

An interesting and important finding of the presented study is the TVC-mediated amount of inhibition onto FCs. In contrast to previously published results (Kuo et al., 2012) describing unitary TVC to FC connections as weak, we show that increasing intensity of stimulation results in large amount of auditory nerve driven inhibition that is received by FCs. In our FFI experiments, we also analyzed the IPSC amplitudes in order to estimate the minimal and maximal number of TVCs innervating a single FC. Our results show that the minimal amplitude of IPSCs when

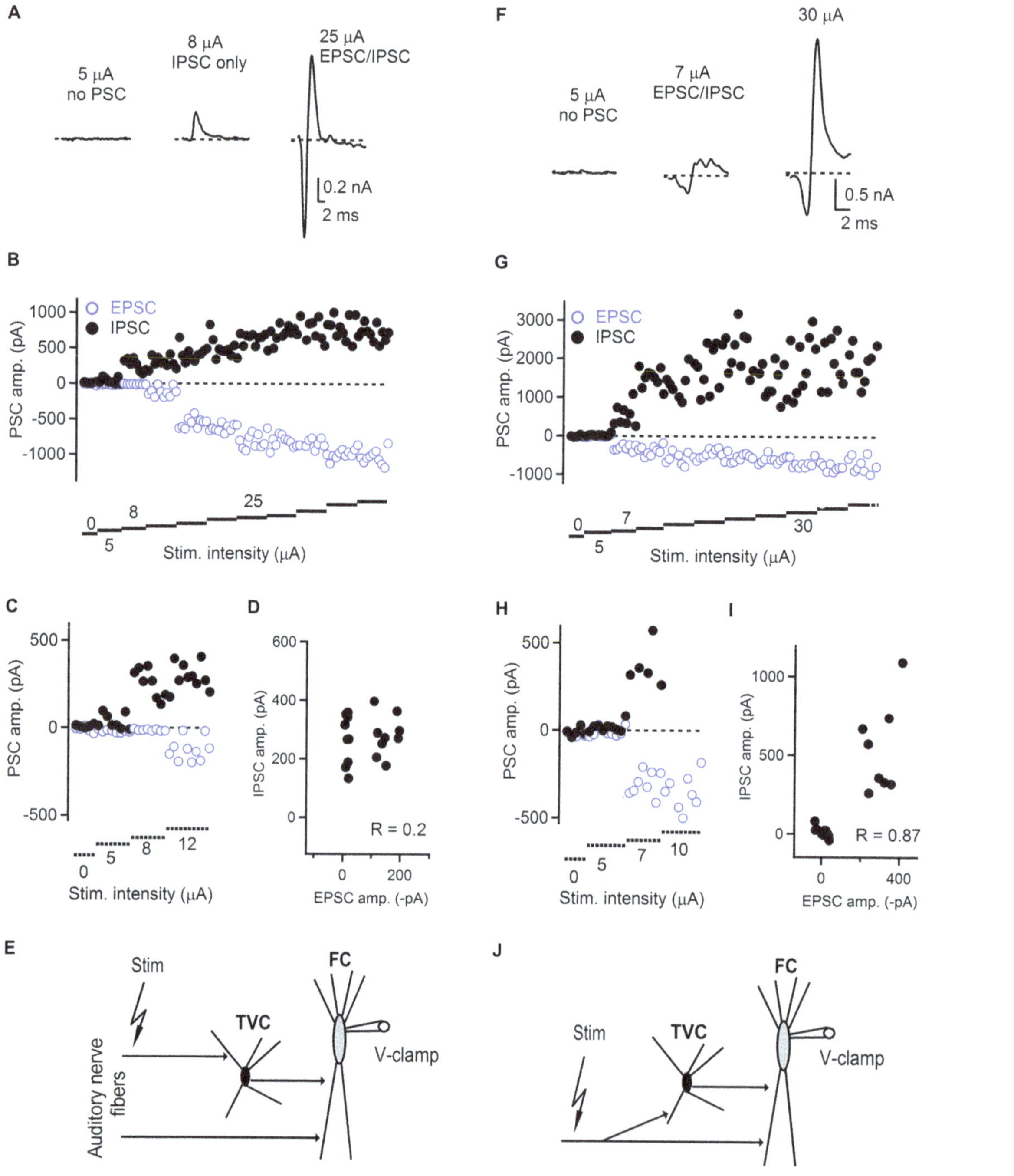

FIGURE 3 | Innervation pattern of the auditory nerve fibers in the dorsal cochlear nucleus. (A) Representative examples of feed-forward inhibition evoked by auditory nerve stimulation and recorded from FCs. At low stimulation intensity, no postsynaptic currents were recorded (left trace). When the stimulation was increased, only an IPSC appeared with a latency that was characteristic for a disynaptic connection (middle trace). With further increase of the stimulation intensity, EPSCs appeared while the amplitude of IPSCs increased (right trace) and amplitudes of both components later saturated. Trials that were evoked with the lowest stimulation intensity evoked both successes and failures of synaptic events that can be seen in the plot shown in **(B)**. **(C)** Plot of low stimulation evoked EPSC/IPSC amplitudes shown at expanded scale. **(D)** Plot of IPSC vs. EPSC amplitudes showing low correlation ($R = 0.2$) between IPSCs and EPSCs. **(E)** Schematic drawing of the innervation pattern described in **A–D**. Separate auditory nerve fibers innervate the fusiform (FC) and tuberculoventral (TVC) cells. ~54% (7/13) of FCs tested exhibited this type of innervation. **(F)** Representative examples of FFI and innervation pattern in which the same set of auditory nerve fibers innervates both tuberculoventral and FCs. Following failures in both EPSCs and IPSCs, both components appeared with the same threshold. Stimulation artifacts in **A** and **F** were removed for clarity and all traces represent averages of 5–10 trials. **(G)** With increasing stimulation intensity both components increased in their amplitude until both of them reached saturation. **(H)** Plot of low stimulation evoked EPSC/IPSC amplitudes shown at expanded scale. **(I)** Plot of IPSC vs. EPSC amplitudes showing high correlation ($R = 0.87$) between IPSCs and EPSCs. **(J)** A schematic drawing of the innervation pattern shown in **F–I**. ~46% (6/13) of FCs tested exhibited this type of innervation.

we recorded failures and successes during FFI trials was 163 ± 25 pA (n = 10 cells), which corresponds to average conductance 4 nS (range 2–7 nS) at −40 mV. The mean saturating amplitude of IPSCs during same FFI trials was 1594 ± 365 pA (n = 10 cells), corresponding to an average conductance of 40 nS (range 9–105 nS) when recorded at −40 mV. Based on the previously reported data on unitary TVC-FC conductance (approximately 2.1 nS at −60 mV) (Kuo et al., 2012), our results suggest that the estimated average number of TVCs innervating a single FC is between 2 (activated by a single auditory nerve fiber) and 20 with saturating stimulation intensity. However, the range of unitary conductances that Kuo et al. (2012) report is 0.7–10.3 nS, as well as the range of conductances reported in the present study mean that the exact and accurate number of TVCs may vary by several fold. One of the explanations of the discrepancy between our study and Kuo et al. (2012) can be divergence of auditory nerve fibers onto TVCs combined with convergence of TVC inputs to FCs, because auditory nerve fibers can activate multiple TVC inputs to FCs and, moreover, multiple TVCs could innervate a single FC. Also, recording and stimulation conditions in the two studies are markedly different which contributes to the differences in the amount of inhibition observed.

DYNAMICS OF FEED-FORWARD INHIBITORY CIRCUIT DURING REPETITIVE AUDITORY NERVE ACTIVITY

Excitatory synapses formed by the auditory nerve onto various postsynaptic targets in all three subdivisions of the cochlear nucleus exhibit short-term synaptic plasticity with varying amounts of synaptic depression related to their specific postsynaptic target, including FCs in the DCN (Wu and Oertel, 1987; Cao et al., 2008; Yang and Xu-Friedman, 2008; Cao and Oertel, 2010; Chanda and Xu-Friedman, 2010; Kuo et al., 2012). Relatively less is known about the short-term synaptic plasticity of inhibitory inputs that contact basal dendrites of FCs (Kuo et al., 2012). Also, little is known about the temporal dynamics of FFI with both excitation and inhibition intact.

Therefore, to ask how repetitive activity of the auditory nerve affects the FFI onto the FCs, we first recorded mixed excitatory and inhibitory responses in response to stimulus trains delivered to the auditory nerve. FCs were voltage clamped at −40 mV and FFI was evoked by repetitive stimulation of the auditory nerve (10 stimuli) at 20, 50 and 100 Hz. We found that the feed-forward inhibitory circuit associated with basal dendrites of FCs undergoes short-term synaptic plasticity at all frequencies tested (**Figure 4**). However, plasticity of excitation and inhibition differed. After 10 stimuli delivered to the auditory nerve, the amplitude of the last EPSC in the train was not significantly different from the first EPSC at the frequencies tested (94 ± 9%, 115 ± 11% and 104 ± 4%, at 20, 50, and 100 Hz respectively, **Figures 4A–D**, n = 6 cells). In contrast to the excitation, the inhibitory component of FFI exhibited significant depression at all frequencies tested (S10/S1 of 48 ± 9%, 57 ± 10%, and 59 ± 11% at 20, 50 and 100 Hz stimulation, respectively, **Figure 4E**). In sum, these results show that repetitive auditory nerve stimulation generates mixed excitatory-inhibitory responses. The excitatory component exhibits little short-term plasticity when activated at 20–100 Hz. In contrast the inhibitory component exhibits moderate depression of 40–50%.

Recently it has been shown that IPSCs evoked in FCs by stimulation of TVCs exhibit mild facilitation when activated at 100 Hz in paired recordings (Kuo et al., 2012), which is in contrast with our observation of IPSC depression. One factor that can influence the amplitudes of EPSCs and IPSCs in FCs during the biphasic response to auditory nerve stimulation is temporal overlap of the synaptic conductances. Although IPSCs are disynaptic and therefore have a longer latency, FCs exhibit relatively slow EPSC kinetics compared to other auditory nerve targets (Gardner et al., 1999) and therefore the inward peak of the biphasic response can be truncated by onset of the fast IPSC. An additional factor that can influence IPSC amplitudes during FFI is plasticity at the auditory nerve to tuberculoventral cell synapse. Either of these factors could explain differences in short-term plasticity of IPSCs when evoked by direct activation of inhibitory axons compared to those evoked by feed-forward activation of interneurons by auditory nerve fibers. We therefore performed experiments to test these possibilities.

In the first set of experiments we examined short-term plasticity of pharmacologically-isolated excitatory and inhibitory inputs onto FCs. By blocking GABA and glycine receptors (with picrotoxin and strychnine, respectively) we recorded isolated auditory nerve EPSCs evoked at 20–100 Hz. Under conditions where FFI is blocked (**Figure 5A**), auditory nerve-evoked EPSCs undergo slight depression (S10/S1 of 83 ± 6%, 93 ± 4% and 86 ± 11% at 20, 50 and 100 Hz, respectively, **Figures 5A,B**, n = 5 cells).

Next, we recorded IPSCs from FCs in the presence of DNQX and R-CPP, blockers of excitatory transmission, to investigate whether the amount of IPSC synaptic depression would be the same as during the FFI trials. FCs were voltage clamped at −40 mV and IPSCs were evoked by direct stimulation of inhibitory inputs in the deep layer of the DCN (**Figure 5C**). Surprisingly, IPSC trains exhibited slight synaptic depression at 20 Hz (S10/S1 was 82 ± 1%), and slight facilitation at 50 and 100 Hz, respectively (S10/S1 at 50 Hz was 103 ± 5%, S10/S1 at 100 Hz was 119 ± 13%; n = 6 cells, **Figure 5D**). These results are consistent with previously reported data from paired recordings between tuberculoventral and FCs (Kuo et al., 2012). However, the comparatively moderate short-term plasticity of directly evoked and pharmacologically isolated IPSCs seems unlikely to explain the pronounced short-term depression of inhibition during FFI when excitation and inhibition are intact.

Therefore, we next investigated whether short-term plasticity at the auditory nerve to tuberculoventral cell synapse accounts for the strong IPSC depression during FFI. For this purpose, we recorded auditory nerve-evoked EPSCs from TVCs visually identified in the slice (**Figure 6A**). One characteristic of TVCs is that they exhibit fast EPSCs with sub-millisecond decay kinetics (Gardner et al., 1999; Kuo et al., 2012). In our experiments, we confirmed this (**Figure 6B**) and used the rapidly decaying spontaneous synaptic events as a criteria for distinguishing TVCs from other cell types in the deep layer of the DCN (Gardner et al., 1999). Another distinguishing characteristic is that TVCs are mostly electrically silent (Shofner and Young, 1985; Spirou et al., 1999), and in slices rarely spike spontaneously (Kuo et al.,

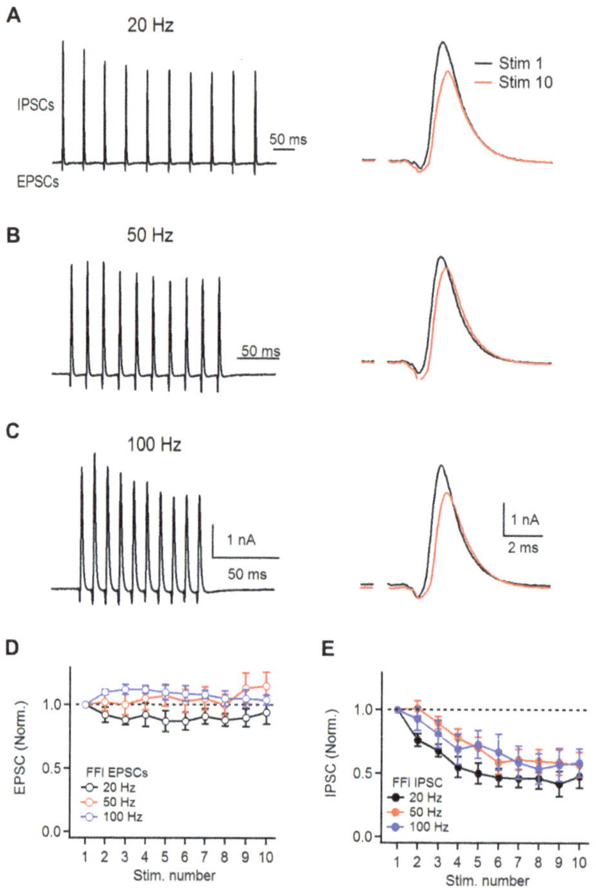

FIGURE 4 | Dynamics of feed-forward inhibitory circuit during repetitive auditory nerve activity. (A) Representative recordings of feed-forward inhibition. 10 stimuli were delivered to the auditory nerve at 20 Hz and short-term plasticity of both the excitatory and the inhibitory components was analyzed. Stimulation artifacts were removed for clarity from all traces shown. Response to the first (Stim 1) and 10th (Stim 10) are superimposed on the right. **(B,C)** Recordings of feed-forward inhibition in FCs at 50 and 100 Hz. **(D)** Plot of EPSC short-term plasticity in the EPSC-IPSC sequence at 20, 50 and 100 Hz. Amplitudes were normalized to the first EPSC in the train. **(E)** Plot of IPSC short-term plasticity during FFI trials at 20, 50 and 100 Hz showing pronounced depression. IPSCs were normalized to the first PSC in the train **(B and C**, $n = 6$ cells).

2012), which we confirmed by recording in cell-attached mode before breaking into the whole-cell configuration (data not shown). Finally, we confirmed the cell identity by inspecting their morphology using fluorescent dye in the recording pipette (**Figure 6A**). EPSCs recorded from TVCs were evoked by extracellular stimulation of the auditory nerve (**Figure 6C**), similar to EPSCs recorded from the FCs. Repetitive stimulation of the auditory nerve with 10 stimuli evoked a train of EPSCs that exhibited pronounced short-term synaptic depression (**Figure 6D**). At all frequencies tested (20, 50 and 100 Hz), EPSCs significantly depressed with S10/S1 of 48 ± 1%, 41 ± 3% and 35 ± 4% at 20, 50 and 100 Hz, respectively (**Figure 6E**, $n = 6$ cells). These values match very closely with the amount of depression of IPSCs evoked during FFI recorded from the FCs (see **Figure 4**). Therefore, these results, together with our previous findings strongly indicate that short-term depression at the synapse between the auditory nerve and tuberculoventral cell accounts for the activity dependent change in excitation-inhibition balance in a synapse specific manner. It also accounts for the observed shift in short-term synaptic plasticity of fusiform cell deep-layer inhibition, from facilitation when IPSCs are directly stimulated, to strong depression when FFI is intact.

DISCUSSION

In the current study, we investigated the properties and mechanisms of FFI in the DCN driven by the auditory nerve. We used patch clamp recordings from fusiform and TVCs to provide evidence that synapse specific and activity dependent synaptic plasticity regulates the balance of excitation and inhibition in a feed-forward inhibitory synaptic circuit associated with basal dendrites of FCs in the DCN.

Our results show that auditory nerve fibers activate both FCs and TVCs that represent the DCN principal neurons and local interneurons, respectively. TVCs further provide strong FFI to FCs. The strong inhibition of FCs that we observe differs from what has recently been shown by Kuo et al. (2012), who demonstrate that connections between TVCs and FCs are rather weak. One explanation that can account for this discrepancy

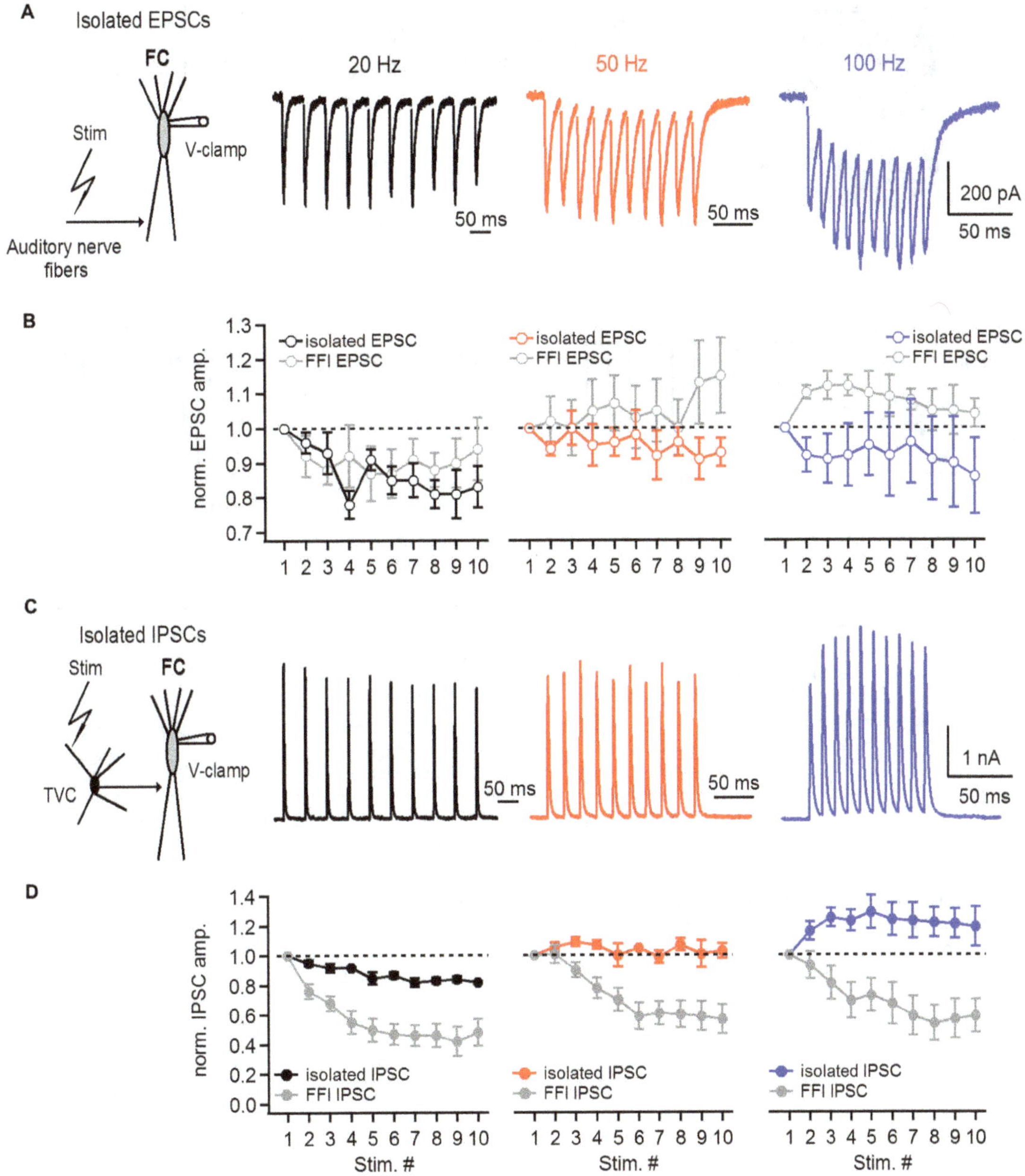

FIGURE 5 | Short-term plasticity of directly stimulated excitatory and inhibitory inputs onto basal dendrites of fusiform cells. (A) Representative examples of EPSCs recorded from a fusiform cell evoked by 20, 50 and 100 Hz auditory nerve stimulation. Schematic in the left shows the experimental protocol. Recordings were performed with 2 μM strychnine and 40 μM picrotoxin in perfusion solution. **(B)** Plots of EPSC amplitudes at corresponding stimulation frequencies of the auditory nerve. EPSCs in the train were normalized to the first EPSC in the train. For comparison, gray data points in all three graphs represent data of EPSC short-term plasticity evoked during feed-forward inhibition trials shown in **Figure 4** ($n = 5$ cells). **(C)** Representative examples of IPSCs recorded from a fusiform cell evoked by direct stimulation of inhibitory inputs in the deep layer of the DCN at 20, 50 and 100 Hz. Schematic drawing in the left shows the experimental protocol. All recordings were done in 20 μM DNXQ and 5 μM R-CPP to block excitatory transmission. **(D)** Plots of IPSC amplitudes in the train normalized to the first IPSC at corresponding frequencies of stimulation of inhibitory inputs. Gray data of IPSC short-term plasticity recorded during feed-forward inhibition trials and shown in **Figure 4** are included for comparison. Differences in short-term plasticity of directly stimulated IPSCs and those evoked during FFI were statistically significant ($P < 0.001$, $n = 6$ cells). All stimulation artifacts in **A and C** were removed for clarity. Traces represent averages of 5–10 trials.

is that the stimulation paradigms between the two studies are different. Paired recordings that Kuo et al. (2012) used in their study represent unitary connections with only a small number of synapses being activated. In case of our experiments, bulk stimulation of the auditory nerve activates multiple auditory nerve fibers that could lead to activation of multiple TVC inputs

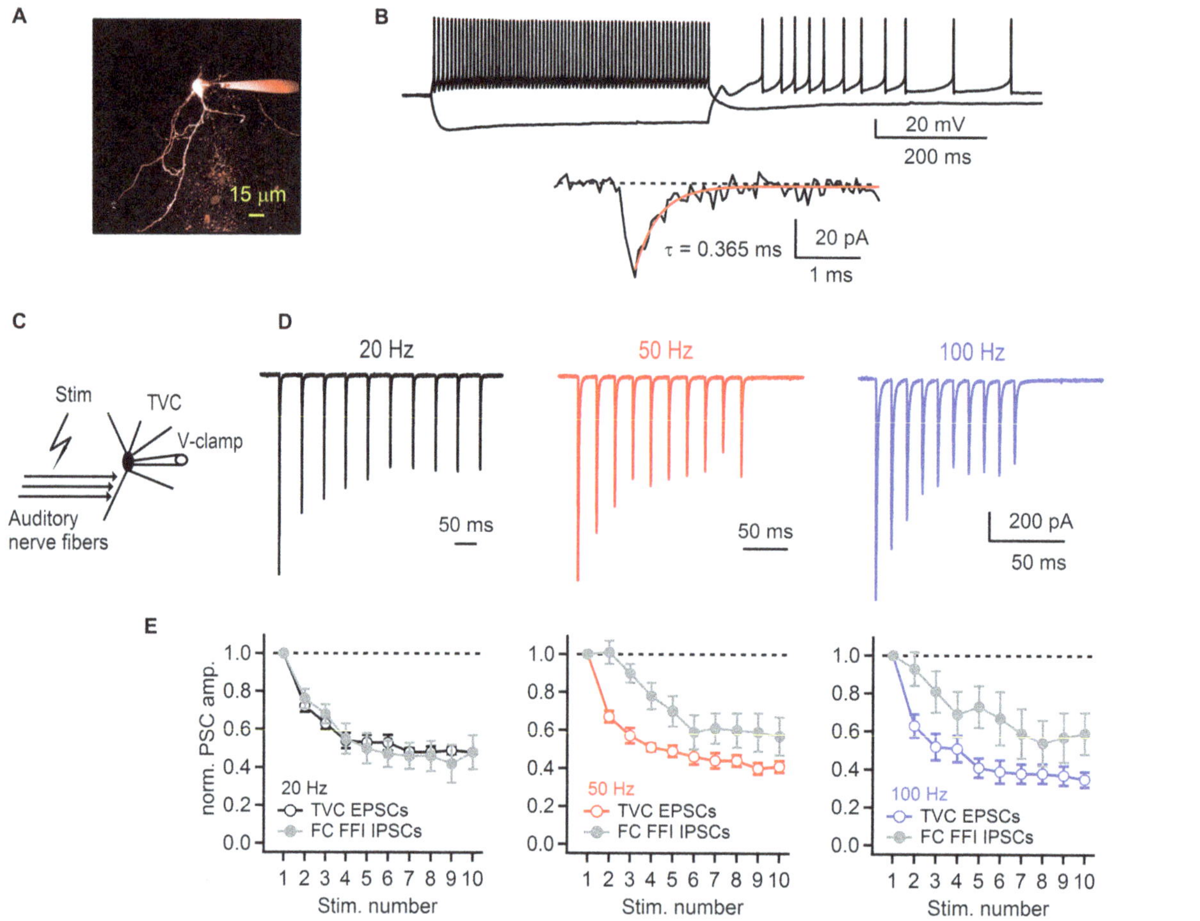

FIGURE 6 | Synaptic plasticity at the auditory nerve-tuberculoventral cell synapse regulates feed-forward inhibition onto fusiform cells. (A) A two-photon laser scanning microscopy image of a tuberculoventral cell loaded with Alexa Fluor 594. **(B)** Electrophysiological properties of tuberculoventral cells in DCN slices. Top traces show tonic firing upon prolonged depolarization, high input resistance examined with hyperpolarizing current injection that resulted in rebound firing when returned back to resting membrane potential (−66 mV). Bottom trace shows a representative example of a spontaneous EPSC (sEPSC). Single exponential fit of the rapid decay kinetics is shown in red. **(C)** Experimental protocol for recording auditory nerve evoked EPSCs from tuberculoventral cells. **(D)** Short-term plasticity of EPSCs recorded from a tuberculoventral cell during repetitive auditory nerve stimulation at 20, 50 and 100 Hz. All recordings were performed with 2 μM strychnine and 40 μM picrotoxin in the perfusion solution. Note the pronounced depression that is comparable to the amount of depression of the inhibitory component of FFI sequence recorded from FCs. Stimulation artifacts were removed for clarity. Traces represent averages of 5–10 trials. **(E)** Plots of EPSC amplitudes at corresponding stimulation frequencies of the auditory nerve. Gray data of IPSC short-term plasticity recorded from FCs during feed-forward inhibition trials and shown in **Figure 4** are included for comparison. EPSCs in the train were normalized to the first EPSC in the train (n = 6 cells).

to FCs. In addition, multiple TVCs could innervate a single FC which would further increase the amount of inhibition recorded from a single FC. A more complete understanding of the circuit mechanisms that control fusiform cell responses to sound will also require understanding of the effects of inhibitory contacts among TVCs themselves (Kuo et al., 2012).

The activation and timing of the disynaptic inhibition that we recorded was fast and very precisely timed, occurring within approximately 1 ms after auditory nerve activation. The narrow time window for summation of inputs has been shown to play a significant role in reaching action potential threshold in postsynaptic neurons (Pouille and Scanziani, 2001), and it is likely to be important in regulating the output of the DCN. Fast and consistently narrow jitter of FFI timing in our experiments provides further evidence for a disynaptic connection. The delay that we describe here is comparable with timing of FFI in the visual system (Blitz and Regehr, 2005), cerebellum (Mittmann et al., 2005) or cortex (Gabernet et al., 2005), but was shorter than in case of FFI described previously in hippocampus (Pouille and Scanziani, 2001; Torborg et al., 2010). Different needs for speed of synaptic transmission and input integration in various brain regions may account for these discrepancies. One of the mechanisms underlying the precision and accurate timing of FFI in the local DCN circuit that we studied may be the kinetics of EPSCs evoked in TVCs by stimulation of auditory nerve fibers. Previous studies (Gardner et al., 1999, 2001), and our data (**Figures 6B,D**) demonstrate that TVC EPSCs exhibit extremely fast kinetics. The rapid decay kinetics is hypothesized to be predominantly due to expression of fast AMPA receptors containing GluR4 subunits in cells receiving exclusively auditory nerve excitatory inputs (Gardner et al., 1999, 2001).

By using low-intensity stimulation of the auditory nerve we further observe that some auditory nerve fibers evoke a biphasic response in FCs that consists of a monosynaptic EPSC and a disynaptic IPSC. In other cases, EPSCs exhibited a higher threshold for activation and only IPSCs were observed. With increasing stimulation intensity, and thus recruiting more auditory nerve fibers, we observed that excitatory and/or inhibitory components of the FFI began to be recruited gradually and contributed to the overall complex responses recorded from FCs. Similar observations have been described in the visual system (Blitz and Regehr, 2005); however, unlike the mentioned study, we were not always able to distinguish activation of a single auditory nerve fiber from activation of a few weaker fibers in our experiments. Therefore, it is difficult to draw clear conclusions defining the precise innervation pattern of fusiform and TVCs by auditory nerve fibers. Using a challenging approach such as simultaneous recordings from both fusiform and TVCs while stimulating the auditory nerve could help resolve this issue.

Data from *in vivo* experiments show that FCs can be divided into two groups, intensity-selective and intensity-nonselective, based on their responses to sound of various intensities (Zhou et al., 2012). Intensity-selective neurons have a non-monotonic rate-level function and thus respond most strongly to sounds of a specific intensity, whereas intensity non-selective neurons have a monotonic rate-level function. Although the circuit mechanisms for these distinct response types are not known, an intriguing possibility is that differential patterns of FFI by TVCs could play a role. TVCs in DCN are thought to represent type II neurons (Davis and Voigt, 1997; Rhode, 1999) and are important for intensity selectivity of FCs because of their ability to suppress or even eliminate FC firing. Therefore, the innervation patterns of FCs and TVCs can play a crucial role in the output of the DCN since low sound intensities can recruit excitatory inputs onto FCs in the absence of inhibition. Further increases in sound intensity strengthens both excitatory and inhibitory components (Zhou et al., 2012). Our results demonstrate strongly increasing amplitude of inhibition as progressively more auditory nerve fibers are activated, a situation analogous to progressive recruitment of auditory nerve fibers by increasing sound intensity.

An important question related to synaptic input integration and information processing is how repetitive activity regulates the output of a synaptic circuit, especially when both excitatory and inhibitory components are involved. Excitatory synapses between the auditory nerve and its targets have been shown to exhibit various amounts of short-term synaptic depression depending on the type of postsynaptic neuron (Cao and Oertel, 2010; Kuo et al., 2012). Consistent with recent work (Kuo et al., 2012), we observe minimal depression at the auditory nerve-FC synapse and pronounced depression at the synapse between the auditory nerve and TVCs, under conditions where excitation and inhibition, respectively, were pharmacologically isolated. This indicates target-specific specializations of short-term synaptic plasticity, a phenomenon that has also been reported in other brain areas, but is not well understood (Blackman et al., 2013). However, examination of short-term plasticity of EPSCs and IPSCs recorded from FCs during FFI trials provided evidence that short-term plasticity of synaptic currents under conditions when both components are present differs from that recorded when either of the two components is isolated. Such differences may arise from temporal overlap of synaptic conductances during repetitive stimulation. In the case of DCN FCs, the combination of relatively slow EPSC kinetics (Gardner et al., 1999) and fast IPSC kinetics (Xie and Manis, 2013) results in greater summation of excitatory responses during repetitive synaptic activity and IPSC amplitudes are consequently reduced by the tonic inward current. A second factor is synaptic depression at the auditory nerve-tuberculoventral cell synapse (Kuo et al., 2012, our **Figure 6**). In DCN FCs, synaptic depression at the feed-forward synapse onto the inhibitory interneuron is of greater magnitude than the degree of summation of either excitatory or inhibitory responses during repetitive activation of the feed-forward circuit. In conclusion, our study demonstrates how FFI can regulate the balance of excitation and inhibition in FCs in a dynamic manner during repetitive auditory nerve activity, findings that may be relevant for our understanding of the role of FFI in other brain regions as well.

ACKNOWLEDGMENTS

This work was supported by the National Institute on Deafness and Other Communication Disorders Intramural Research Program.

REFERENCES

Berrebi, A. S., and Mugnaini, E. (1991). Distribution and targets of the cartwheel cell axon in the dorsal cochlear nucleus of the guinea pig. *Anat. Embryol. (Berl)* 183, 427–454. doi: 10.1007/bf00186433

Blackman, A. V., Abrahamsson, T., Costa, R. P., Lalanne, T., and Sjöström, P. J. (2013). Target-cell-specific short-term plasticity in local circuits. *Front. Synaptic Neurosci.* 5:11. doi: 10.3389/fnsyn.2013.00011

Blackstad, T. W., Osen, K. K., and Mugnaini, E. (1984). Pyramidal neurones of the dorsal cochlear nucleus: a Golgi and computer reconstruction study in cat. *Neuroscience* 13, 827–854. doi: 10.1016/0306-4522(84)90099-x

Blitz, D. M., and Regehr, W. G. (2005). Timing and specificity of feed-forward inhibition within the LGN. *Neuron* 45, 917–928. doi: 10.1016/j.neuron.2005.01.033

Borg-Graham, L. J., Monier, C., and Frégnac, Y. (1998). Visual input evokes transient and strong shunting inhibition in visual cortical neurons. *Nature* 393, 369–373. doi: 10.1038/30735

Brand, A., Behrend, O., Marquardt, T., McAlpine, D., and Grothe, B. (2002). Precise inhibition is essential for microsecond interaural time difference coding. *Nature* 417, 543–547. doi: 10.1038/417543a

Buzsaki, G. (1984). Feed-forward inhibition in the hippocampal formation. *Prog. Neurobiol.* 22, 131–153. doi: 10.1016/0301-0082(84)90023-6

Cao, X. J., McGinley, M. J., and Oertel, D. (2008). Connections and synaptic function in the posteroventral cochlear nucleus of deaf jerker mice. *J. Comp. Neurol.* 510, 297–308. doi: 10.1002/cne.21788

Cao, X. J., and Oertel, D. (2010). Auditory nerve fibers excite targets through synapses that vary in convergence, strength and short-term plasticity. *J. Neurophysiol.* 104, 2308–2320. doi: 10.1152/jn.00451.2010

Chanda, S., and Xu-Friedman, M. A. (2010). A low-affinity antagonist reveals saturation and desensitization in mature synapses in the auditory brain stem. *J. Neurophysiol.* 103, 1915–1926. doi: 10.1152/jn.00751.2009

Chen, C., and Regehr, W. G. (2000). Developmental remodeling of the retinogeniculate synapse. *Neuron* 28, 955–966. doi: 10.1016/s0896-6273(00)00166-5

Cruikshank, S. J., Lewis, T. J., and Connors, B. W. (2007). Synaptic basis for intense thalamocortical activation of feedforward inhibitory cells in neocortex. *Nat. Neurosci.* 10, 462–468. doi: 10.1038/nn1861

Davis, K. A., and Voigt, H. F. (1997). Evidence of stimulus-dependent correlated activity in the dorsal cochlear nucleus of decerebrate gerbils. *J. Neurophysiol.* 78, 229–247.

Ellender, T. J., Huerta-Ocampo, I., Deisseroth, K., Capogna, M., and Bolam, J. P. (2011). Differential modulation of excitatory and inhibitory striatal synaptic transmission by histamine. *J. Neurosci.* 31, 15340–15351. doi: 10.1523/JNEUROSCI.3144-11.2011

Fujino, K., and Oertel, D. (2003). Bidirectional synaptic plasticity in the cerebellum-like mammalian dorsal cochlear nucleus. *Proc. Natl. Acad. Sci. U S A* 100, 265–270. doi: 10.1073/pnas.0135345100

Gabernet, L., Jadhav, S. P., Feldman, D. E., Carandini, M., and Scanziani, M. (2005). Somatosensory integration controlled by dynamic thalamocortical feed-forward inhibition. *Neuron* 48, 315–327. doi: 10.1016/j.neuron.2005.09.022

Gardner, S. M., Trussell, L. O., and Oertel, D. (1999). Time course and permeation of synaptic AMPA receptors in cochlear nuclear neurons correlate with input. *J. Neurosci.* 19, 8721–8729.

Gardner, S. M., Trussell, L. O., and Oertel, D. (2001). Correlation of AMPA receptor subunit composition with synaptic input in the mammalian cochlear nuclei. *J. Neurosci.* 21, 7428–7437.

Gil, Z., and Amitai, Y. (1996). Properties of convergent thalamocortical and intracortical synaptic potentials in single neurons of neocortex. *J. Neurosci.* 16, 6567–6578.

Kuo, S. P., Lu, H. W., and Trussell, L. O. (2012). Intrinsic and synaptic properties of vertical cells of the mouse dorsal cochlear nucleus. *J. Neurophysiol.* 108, 1186–1198. doi: 10.1152/jn.00778.2011

Kuo, S. P., and Trussell, L. O. (2011). Spontaneous spiking and synaptic depression underlie noradrenergic control of feed-forward inhibition. *Neuron* 71, 306–318. doi: 10.1016/j.neuron.2011.05.039

Mittmann, W., Koch, U., and Häusser, M. (2005). Feed-forward inhibition shapes the spike output of cerebellar Purkinje cells. *J. Physiol.* 563, 369–378. doi: 10.1113/jphysiol.2004.075028

Najac, M., De Saint Jan, D., Reguero, L., Grandes, P., and Charpak, S. (2011). Monosynaptic and polysynaptic feed-forward inputs to mitral cells from olfactory sensory neurons. *J. Neurosci.* 31, 8722–8729. doi: 10.1523/jneurosci.0527-11.2011

Nelken, I., and Young, E. D. (1994). Two separate inhibitory mechanisms shape the responses of dorsal cochlear nucleus type IV units to narrowband and wideband stimuli. *J. Neurophysiol.* 71, 2442–2462.

Oertel, D. (1999). The role of timing in the brain stem auditory nuclei of vertebrates. *Annu. Rev. Physiol.* 61, 497–519. doi: 10.1146/annurev.physiol.61.1.497

Oertel, D., Wright, S., Cao, X. J., Ferragamo, M., and Bal, R. (2010). The multiple functions of T stellate/multipolar/chopper cells in the ventral cochlear nucleus. *Hear. Res.* 276, 61–69. doi: 10.1016/j.heares.2010.10.018

Oertel, D., and Wu, S. H. (1989). Morphology and physiology of cells in slice preparations of the dorsal cochlear nucleus of mice. *J. Comp. Neurol.* 283, 228–247. doi: 10.1002/cne.902830206

Oertel, D., and Young, E. D. (2004). What's a cerebellar circuit doing in the auditory system? *Trends Neurosci.* 27, 104–110. doi: 10.1016/j.tins.2003.12.001

Palmer, A. R., and Winter, I. M. (1996). The temporal window of two-tone facilitation in onset units of the ventral cochlear nucleus. *Audiol. Neurootol.* 1, 12–30. doi: 10.1159/000259199

Pouille, F., and Scanziani, M. (2001). Enforcement of temporal fidelity in pyramidal cells by somatic feed-forward inhibition. *Science* 293, 1159–1163. doi: 10.1126/science.1060342

Requarth, T., and Sawtell, N. B. (2011). Neural mechanisms for filtering self-generated sensory signals in cerebellum-like circuits. *Curr. Opin. Neurobiol.* 21, 602–608. doi: 10.1016/j.conb.2011.05.031

Rhode, W. S. (1999). Vertical cell responses to sound in cat dorsal cochlear nucleus. *J. Neurophysiol.* 82, 1019–1032.

Roberts, M. T., and Trussell, L. O. (2010). Molecular layer inhibitory interneurons provide feedforward and lateral inhibition in the dorsal cochlear nucleus. *J. Neurophysiol.* 104, 2462–2473. doi: 10.1152/jn.00312.2010

Shofner, W. P., and Young, E. D. (1985). Excitatory/inhibitory response types in the cochlear nucleus: relationships to discharge patterns and responses to electrical stimulation of the auditory nerve. *J. Neurophysiol.* 54, 917–939.

Shore, S. E., and Zhou, J. (2006). Somatosensory influence on the cochlear nucleus and beyond. *Hear. Res.* 216–217, 90–99. doi: 10.1016/j.heares.2006.01.006

Spirou, G. A., Davis, K. A., Nelken, I., and Young, E. D. (1999). Spectral integration by type II interneurons in dorsal cochlear nucleus. *J. Neurophysiol.* 82, 648–663.

Torborg, C. L., Nakashiba, T., Tonegawa, S., and McBain, C. J. (2010). Control of CA3 output by feedforward inhibition despite developmental changes in the excitation-inhibition balance. *J. Neurosci.* 30, 15628–15637. doi: 10.1523/jneurosci.3099-10.2010

Tzounopoulos, T., Kim, Y., Oertel, D., and Trussell, L. O. (2004). Cell-specific, spike timing-dependent plasticities in the dorsal cochlear nucleus. *Nat. Neurosci.* 7, 719–725. doi: 10.1038/nn1272

Voigt, H. F., and Young, E. D. (1980). Evidence of inhibitory interactions between neurons in dorsal cochlear nucleus. *J. Neurophysiol.* 44, 76–96.

Voigt, H. F., and Young, E. D. (1990). Cross-correlation analysis of inhibitory interactions in dorsal cochlear nucleus. *J. Neurophysiol.* 64, 1590–1610.

Wickesberg, R. E., and Oertel, D. (1988). Tonotopic projection from the dorsal to the anteroventral cochlear nucleus of mice. *J. Comp. Neurol.* 268, 389–399. doi: 10.1002/cne.902680308

Winter, I. M., and Palmer, A. R. (1995). Level dependence of cochlear nucleus onset unit responses and facilitation by second tones or broadband noise. *J. Neurophysiol.* 73, 141–159.

Wu, S. H., and Oertel, D. (1987). Maturation of synapses and electrical properties of cells in the cochlear nuclei. *Hear. Res.* 30, 99–110. doi: 10.1016/0378-5955(87)90187-0

Xie, R., and Manis, P. B. (2013). Target-specific IPSC kinetics promote temporal processing in auditory parallel pathways. *J. Neurosci.* 33, 1598–1614. doi: 10.1523/JNEUROSCI.2541-12.2013

Yang, H., and Xu-Friedman, M. A. (2008). Relative roles of different mechanisms of depression at the mouse endbulb of Held. *J. Neurophysiol.* 99, 2510–2521. doi: 10.1152/jn.01293.2007

Zhang, S., and Oertel, D. (1993). Tuberculoventral cells of the dorsal cochlear nucleus of mice: intracellular recordings in slices. *J. Neurophysiol.* 69, 1409–1421.

Zhang, S., and Oertel, D. (1994). Neuronal circuits associated with the output of the dorsal cochlear nucleus through fusiform cells. *J. Neurophysiol.* 71, 914–930.

Zhou, M., Tao, H. W., and Zhang, L. I. (2012). Generation of intensity selectivity by differential synaptic tuning: fast-saturating excitation but slow-saturating inhibition. *J. Neurosci.* 32, 18068–18078. doi: 10.1523/jneurosci.3647-12.2012

5

The relative contributions of MNTB and LNTB neurons to inhibition in the medial superior olive assessed through single and paired recordings

Michael T. Roberts, Stephanie C. Seeman and Nace L. Golding*

Department of Neuroscience, Center for Learning and Memory, The University of Texas at Austin, Austin, TX, USA

Correspondence:
Nace L. Golding, Department of Neuroscience, Center for Learning and Memory, The University of Texas at Austin, 1 University Station, C7000, Austin, TX 78712, USA
e-mail: golding@austin.utexas.edu

The medial superior olive (MSO) senses microsecond differences in the coincidence of binaural signals, a critical cue for detecting sound location along the azimuth. An important component of this circuit is provided by inhibitory neurons of the medial and lateral nuclei of the trapezoid body (MNTB and LNTB, respectively). While MNTB neurons are fairly well described, little is known about the physiology of LNTB neurons. Using whole cell recordings from gerbil brainstem slices, we found that LNTB and MNTB neurons have similar membrane time constants and input resistances and fire brief action potentials, but only LNTB neurons fire repetitively in response to current steps. We observed that LNTB neurons receive graded excitatory and inhibitory synaptic inputs, with at least some of the latter arriving from other LNTB neurons. To address the relative timing of inhibition to the MSO from the LNTB versus the MNTB, we examined inhibitory responses to auditory nerve stimulation using a slice preparation that retains the circuitry from the auditory nerve to the MSO intact. Despite the longer physical path length of excitatory inputs driving contralateral inhibition, inhibition from both pathways arrived with similar latency and jitter. An analysis of paired whole cell recordings between MSO and MNTB neurons revealed a short and reliable delay between the action potential peak in MNTB neurons and the onset of the resulting IPSP (0.55 ± 0.01 ms, $n = 4$, mean $\pm$ SEM). Reconstructions of biocytin-labeled neurons showed that MNTB axons ranged from 580 to 858 μm in length ($n = 4$). We conclude that while both LNTB and MNTB neurons provide similarly timed inhibition to MSO neurons, the reliability of inhibition from the LNTB at higher frequencies is more constrained relative to that from the MNTB due to differences in intrinsic properties, the strength of excitatory inputs, and the presence of feedforward inhibition.

Keywords: inhibition, auditory brainstem, timing, sound localization, axon

INTRODUCTION

To identify the origin of low frequency sounds in the azimuthal plane, animals discern microsecond-order differences in the arrival times of sounds at the two ears. In mammals, neurons in the medial superior olive (MSO) detect these interaural time differences (ITDs) by comparing the timing of excitatory inputs received from pathways that begin at the ipsilateral and contralateral cochlea (**Figure 1A**; Joris and Yin, 2007; Grothe et al., 2010). *In vivo* studies, however, have long found signs that MSO computations are also influenced by inhibition (Goldberg and Brown, 1969; Yin and Chan, 1990; Spitzer and Semple, 1995). Some studies have suggested that this influence extends to defining the temporal window for coincidence detection in the MSO (Brand et al., 2002; Pecka et al., 2008), although others have concluded that coincidence detection requires only the information provided by excitatory inputs (Day and Semple, 2011; van der Heijden et al., 2013).

The main sources of inhibitory input to the MSO are neurons in the lateral nucleus of the trapezoid body (LNTB; Cant and Hyson, 1992; Kuwabara and Zook, 1992; Spirou and Berrebi, 1996) and the medial nucleus of the trapezoid body (MNTB; Spangler et al., 1985; Banks and Smith, 1992). LNTB and MNTB neurons are glycinergic (Adams and Mugnaini, 1990; Spirou and Berrebi, 1997), and receive excitatory input from globular bushy cells in the ipsilateral and contralateral cochlear nuclei, respectively (**Figure 1A**; Tolbert et al., 1982; Friauf and Ostwald, 1988; Kuwabara et al., 1991; Smith et al., 1991; Thompson and Schofield, 2000). In the *in vitro* slice preparation, stimulation of LNTB or MNTB inputs elicits fast inhibitory responses in MSO neurons (Grothe and Sanes, 1993, 1994; Magnusson et al., 2005; Chirila et al., 2007; Couchman et al., 2010; Fischl et al., 2012).

Given the importance of timing in MSO computations, the speed and temporal precision of LNTB and MNTB neurons are critical to understanding the role of inhibition in ITD detection. It is well established that bushy cell inputs to the LNTB and MNTB preserve timing information with a high degree of precision (Spirou et al., 1990; Smith et al., 1991; Joris et al., 1994a,b; Mc Laughlin et al., 2008; Rhode, 2008; Lorteije et al., 2009; Recio-Spinoso, 2012). Recently, we showed in the cochlear nucleus-superior olive (CN-SO) slice preparation that stimulation of either the ipsilateral or contralateral auditory nerve evokes inhibitory postsynaptic potentials (IPSPs) in MSO neurons

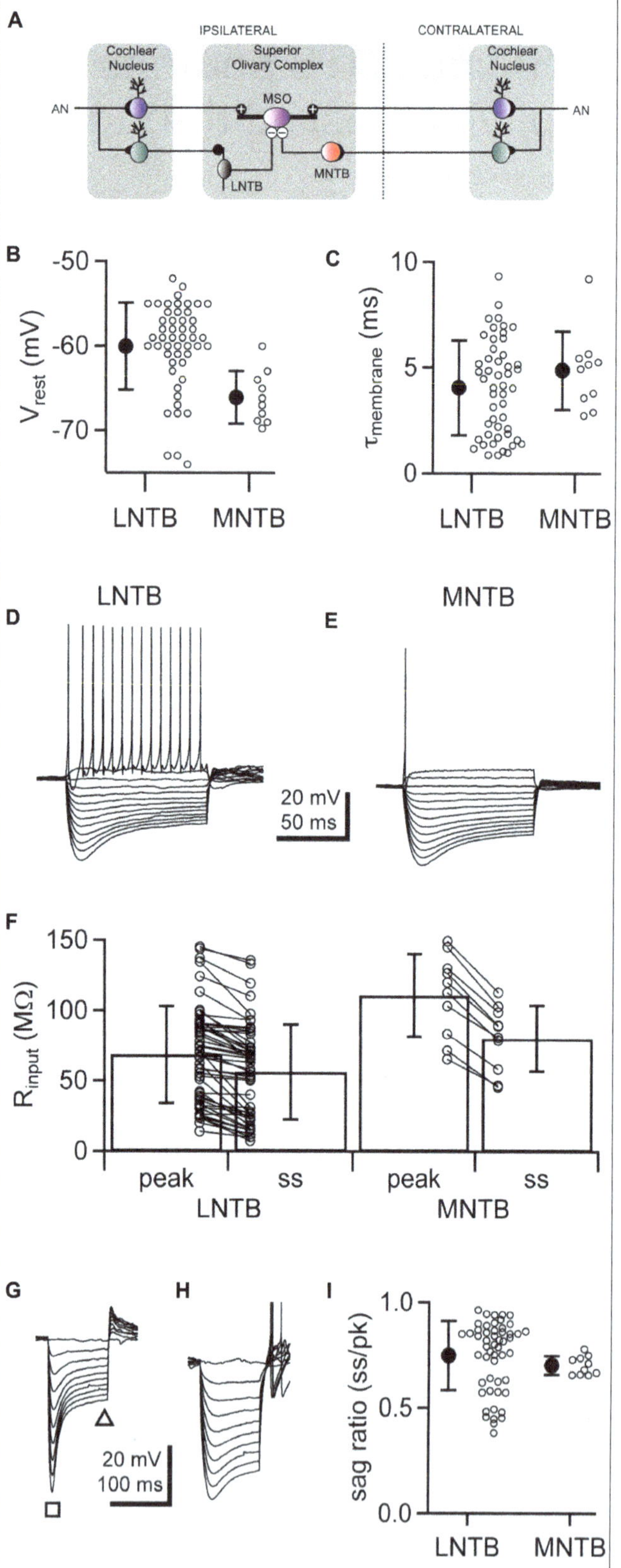

FIGURE 1 | Continued

FIGURE 1 | Continued
LNTB and MNTB neurons have similar intrinsic physiology but differ in action potential firing. (A) Cartoon illustrating circuitry from the cochlear nuclei, through the lateral and medial nuclei of the trapezoid body, to the medial superior olive. **(B,C)** Comparison of resting membrane potentials **(B)** and membrane time constants **(C)** between LNTB and MNTB neurons. **(D,E)** Responses of an LNTB **(D)** and an MNTB **(E)** neuron to a series of current steps. A suprathreshold depolarizing current step evoked repetitive firing in the LNTB neuron but only a single action potential in the MNTB neuron. **(F)** Comparison of input resistances between LNTB and MNTB neurons. Input resistances were measured at the peak and steady-state portions of the responses to a series of hyperpolarizing current steps. **(G,H)** Responses of LNTB neurons to hyperpolarizing current steps highlight the variability in I_h expression across LNTB neurons [**(G)**,sag ratio = 0.46; **(H)**, sag ratio = 0.85]. Note the presence of rebound spikes in **(H)**. The square and triangle in **(G)** indicate where peak and steady-state voltage measurements were taken, respectively. **(I)** Sag ratios measured when the peak response reached ~−80 mV show the range of I_h expression in LNTB and MNTB neurons. Open circles indicate measurements from individual cells. Error bars represent SD. $n = 50$ LNTB neurons, $n = 10$ MNTB neurons.

that arrive earlier than excitatory postsynaptic potentials (EPSPs; Roberts et al., 2013). This suggests that the inhibitory pathways to the MSO are adapted for speed. Consistent with this, MNTB neurons receive powerful excitatory drive from the calyx of Held and have intrinsic physiology that allows rapid, reliable, and temporally precise firing (Kopp-Scheinpflug et al., 2011; Borst and Soria van Hoeve, 2012). However, direct recordings between synaptically coupled MNTB and MSO neurons have not been previously reported, leaving the timing and strength of MNTB inhibition of MSO neurons unresolved. In contrast to the MNTB, only a few studies have examined the physiology of LNTB neurons, and these have focused on responses to sound *in vivo*. These studies found that neurons in and around the LNTB are driven with short latencies by ipsilateral sounds and exhibit a variety of firing patterns (Guinan et al., 1972a,b; Tsuchitani, 1977). Thus, the physiology of LNTB neurons remains largely unexplored, leaving a large gap in our understanding of how ipsilateral inhibition to the MSO is shaped.

In the present study, we hypothesized that the intrinsic and synaptic physiology of both LNTB and MNTB neurons are adapted to provide rapid and temporally precise inhibition to the MSO. With whole cell current clamp recordings from LNTB and MNTB neurons in acute brainstem slices from the Mongolian gerbil, we found that LNTB neurons share many properties with MNTB neurons, including the ability to fire high frequency trains of action potentials. We identified an inhibitory input to LNTB neurons that may derive from other LNTB neurons, suggesting a feedforward or lateral inhibitory circuit within the LNTB. Using the CN-SO slice preparation, we found that stimulation of the ipsilateral and contralateral auditory nerves elicited IPSPs in MSO neurons with similar latencies and very low jitter. Finally, recordings from synaptically coupled pairs of MNTB and MSO neurons showed that MNTB neurons provide rapid and temporally precise inhibition to the MSO. Based on computer reconstructions of MNTB neuron axons together with synaptic latency measurements, we estimate the conduction velocities along this projection to the MSO.

MATERIALS AND METHODS

SLICE ELECTROPHYSIOLOGY

All procedures were conducted in accordance with National Institutes of Health guidelines and were approved by The University of Texas at Austin IACUC. Mongolian gerbils (*Meriones unguiculatus*) were deeply anesthetized with halothane or isoflurane, then their brains were rapidly removed into 32°C artificial cerebrospinal fluid (ACSF). The brainstem was isolated and transferred to a Vibratome (Leica VT1000S or VT1200S) where 200 μm-thick slices were cut in the coronal plane for LNTB recordings or the horizontal plane for MNTB and MSO recordings. Slices were incubated in 35°C ACSF for 30–60 min, then stored at room temperature until use. ACSF was continuously bubbled with 95% O_2/5% CO_2 and was comprised of 125 mM NaCl, 25 mM glucose, 25 mM $NaHCO_3$, 2.5 mM KCl, 1.25 mM NaH_2PO_4, 2.0 mM $CaCl_2$, and 1.0 mM $MgSO_4$.

Whole cell current clamp recordings were made using a Dagan BVC-700A or Molecular Devices MultiClamp 700B amplifier. Slices were perfused with ACSF at 1–2 ml/min and visualized using differential interference contrast optics. Experiments were conducted at 35°C except for recordings between MNTB–MSO pairs, which were conducted at 37°C. Recording electrodes (2–6 MΩ) were filled with an intracellular solution comprised of 115 mM K-gluconate, 4.42 mM KCl, 0.5 mM EGTA, 10 mM HEPES, 10 mM Na_2Phosphocreatine, 4 mM MgATP, 0.3 mM NaGTP, and 0.1% biocytin, osmolality adjusted to 300 mmol/kg with sucrose, pH adjusted to 7.30 with KOH. LNTB and MNTB recordings were made from P18–22 gerbils and MNTB–MSO paired recordings from P15–16 gerbils. Data were sampled at 50–100 kHz and lowpass filtered at 3–10 kHz. Bridge balance was compensated during all experiments. Membrane potentials are corrected for a 10 mV junction potential. Four cells in the MNTB data set were included in a previous study (Scott et al., 2005). Rheobase was found by injecting a series of 100 ms depolarizing current steps and identifying the smallest amplitude current step that elicited an action potential.

THE CN-SO SLICE

The cochlear nucleus-superior olive (CN-SO) slice preparation was prepared as previously described (Roberts et al., 2013). In brief, coronal slices from P15–20 gerbils were cut at a thickness of 1.0–1.5 mm to preserve the circuitry from the cut end of the auditory nerve through the cochlear nuclei to the superior olivary complex. Slices were incubated in a custom interface chamber to improve oxygenation. During recordings, slices were perfused with 35°C ACSF at 8–10 ml/min. The ACSF for CN-SO slice experiments was the same as described above except that it contained 1.5 mM $CaCl_2$ and 1.5 mM $MgSO_4$. Stimuli to the auditory nerve stumps were delivered through suction electrodes (0.8–1.0 mm tip diameter). Whole cell current clamp recordings were made from MSO neurons visualized near the surface of the slice. IPSP onset was defined as the time at which the IPSP amplitude exceeded three times the standard deviation of the immediately preceding baseline.

IDENTIFYING MNTB–MSO PAIRS

After patching onto an MSO neuron, a puffer pipette containing a glutamate-based solution and connected to a picospritzer (Toohey Company) was placed over the adjacent MNTB. The puffing solution contained 10 mM glutamate, 125 mM NaCl, 2.5 mM KCl, 3 mM HEPES, and 0.1% fast green for visualization. The effective spread of the glutamate-based solution was controlled by varying puff duration. To coarsely survey the MNTB for candidate presynaptic neurons, 300 ms puffs (8 psi) were applied as the puffer was moved over the MNTB in a grid-like pattern. When a puff elicited a short latency train of IPSPs in the MSO neuron, the duration of the puff was systematically decreased and the search area refined. Finally, when puff duration was decreased to 3 ms, the spatial resolution of the puffer was sufficient to discriminate between two neighboring MNTB cells (somata <200 μm apart), such that puffing onto one cell body elicited IPSPs while puffing onto the other did not. The puffer pipette was then retracted away from the surface of the slice and the candidate MNTB neuron was patched with a third pipette. If action potentials evoked in the MNTB neuron with brief current steps elicited IPSPs in the MSO neuron, the pair was synaptically coupled.

ANATOMY

Cells were filled with biocytin via the recording electrode. Immediately after recording, slices were fixed in 4% formaldehyde in PBS and stored at 4°C. Tissue was treated with an avidin–biotin horseradish peroxidase complex (Vectastain Elite ABC kit, Vector Labs), stained with a nickel-enhanced DAB reaction, and mounted onto slides with Mowiol 4-88 (Calbiochem). Neurons were reconstructed with a Neurolucida system (MBF Bioscience) using a 100× oil immersion objective. Axonal path length, branching, and synaptic contacts were quantified using Neurolucida Explorer (MBF Bioscience).

DATA ANALYSIS

Data were analyzed using custom algorithms implemented in IgorPro. Action potential threshold was defined as the membrane potential at which the second time derivative of the membrane potential crossed 500 mV/ms^2. Inter-spike intervals were measured based on the time at which each spike crossed threshold. Spontaneous IPSPs were detected using a template-based algorithm (Clements and Bekkers, 1997). In brief, this method involved generating a template by fitting a bi-exponential function to a typical sIPSP. The template was then scanned across the data from a single cell, and the ability of the template to fit each consecutive set of data points equal in length to the template was assessed. When the quality of the fit exceeded a set criterion, the underlying data was considered to contain a sIPSP. Detected sIPSPs were verified by visual inspection then individually analyzed to assess sIPSP kinetics. Synaptic jitter was defined as the standard deviation of the IPSP latency for an individual cell. Mean jitter represents the average across the jitter measured for each cell in a group. Significant differences ($p < 0.05$) were detected with Student's t-tests. Data are expressed as mean ± SEM unless otherwise indicated.

RESULTS

INTRINSIC PHYSIOLOGY OF LNTB AND MNTB NEURONS

We hypothesized that LNTB neurons, like MNTB neurons, are specialized for providing rapid and reliable inhibition to the MSO (see circuitry in **Figure 1A**). To test this hypothesis, we investigated the intrinsic physiology of LNTB neurons and compared it to that of MNTB neurons. Whole cell current clamp recordings of LNTB neurons were made in coronal brainstem slices from P18–22 gerbils. The LNTB was readily identifiable under bright-field microscopy as a lightly myelinated region located along the ventro-lateral edge of the slice. Neurons were filled via the recording pipette with biocytin, and all recovered neurons ($n = 21$) were confirmed as being in the LNTB. Whole cell current clamp recordings of MNTB neurons were made in horizontal brainstem slices from P19–22 gerbils.

We found that the resting membrane potential of LNTB neurons was depolarized relative to that of MNTB neurons on average (mean ± SD: LNTB, −60.0 ± 5.2 mV versus MNTB, −66.1 ± 3.1 mV; $p < 0.001$; **Figure 1B**), although the resting potential of some LNTB neurons was more negative than the most negative MNTB neurons in our data set. Membrane time constants, which were assessed by fitting an exponential function to the rising phase of the response to small (<3 mV) hyperpolarizing current steps, did not significantly differ between LNTB and MNTB neurons (mean ± SD: LNTB, 4.04 ± 2.26 ms versus MNTB, 4.88 ± 1.87 ms; $p = 0.23$; **Figure 1C**). In response to hyperpolarizing current steps, LNTB and MNTB neurons exhibited a depolarizing sag characteristic of the expression of hyperpolarization-activated current (I_h), while depolarizing current steps elicited repetitive firing in LNTB neurons but only one to three action potentials in MNTB neurons (**Figures 1D,E**). Repetitive firing in LNTB neurons was characterized by a longer interspike interval between the first and second action potentials in a train than between subsequent action potential pairs. Action potentials in many LNTB neurons also exhibited multi-component afterhyperpolarizations. Properties of action potential firing are addressed in more detail below.

Input resistance was measured based on a linear fit to the peak and steady-state responses to current steps that hyperpolarized the membrane potential <15 mV. Both peak and steady-state input resistances were significantly lower in LNTB neurons than MNTB neurons (mean ± SD: LNTB, $R_{pk} = 68.8 \pm 34.6$ MΩ, $R_{ss} = 56.5 \pm 33.7$ MΩ; MNTB, $R_{pk} = 111.0 \pm 29.4$ MΩ, $Rss = 80.6 \pm 23.4$ MΩ; R_{pk}, $p < 0.01$; R_{ss}, $p < 0.05$; **Figure 1F**). Within each neuron type, the steady-state input resistance was significantly less than the peak input resistance (pairwise t-test: LNTB, $p < 0.001$; MNTB, $p < 0.001$). This is consistent with the expression of I_h in both neuron types. Across LNTB neurons, we noticed that the amount of sag in response to hyperpolarizing current steps could be quite large (**Figure 1G**) or more moderate (**Figure 1H**). To quantify the amount of sag, we measured the ratio of the steady-state to peak membrane potential responses to current steps that hyperpolarized the membrane potential to ∼−80 mV at the peak. These sag ratios revealed that LNTB and MNTB neurons consistently expressed I_h, but that the amount of expression varied considerably within the population of LNTB neurons (mean ± SD: LNTB, 0.75 ± 0.16; MNTB, 0.70 ± 0.04; $p = 0.10$; **Figure 1I**). The heterogeneity of intrinsic physiology across LNTB neurons suggests that different subsets of LNTB neurons may serve different computational roles.

To compare the properties of action potentials in LNTB and MNTB neurons, we examined the first action potential fired at rheobase, the most negative membrane potential at which a spike was evoked for a given cell. Both LNTB (**Figure 2A**) and MNTB (**Figure 2B**) neurons fired large amplitude action potentials that were brief in duration. Action potentials in MNTB neurons were followed by afterhyperpolarizations exhibiting a single repolarizing phase (**Figure 2B** *inset*). In contrast, in 65% of LNTB neurons the afterhyperpolarization was comprised of multiple phases: an initial rapid hyperpolarization followed after a brief delay by a second, slower hyperpolarization (**Figure 2A** *inset*). This type of multi-phasic afterhyperpolarization was termed a double undershoot when it was observed in some cochlear nucleus and dorsal nucleus of the lateral lemniscus neurons, and we adopt that terminology here (Oertel et al., 1990; Zhang and Oertel, 1993a,b; Wu and Kelly, 1995). The remaining LNTB neurons had simple afterhyperpolarizations similar to those in MNTB neurons. Besides the presence of double undershoots in the majority of LNTB neurons, the properties of action potentials in LNTB and MNTB neurons were largely similar. Action potential thresholds (**Figure 2C**) were well matched between the two cell types, while action potential amplitudes relative to threshold were on average 15% larger in LNTB neurons ($p = 0.03$; **Figure 2D**). Action potential half-widths were quite brief (**Figure 2E**) due in large part to a rapid rate of repolarization (**Figure 2F**) following the action potential peak. Despite differences in afterhyperpolarization shape, the most negative voltage reached during the afterhyperpolarization did not differ significantly between LNTB and MNTB neurons (**Figure 2G**). Together, the similarity in action potential properties between LNTB and MNTB neurons, particularly the brief duration and strong repolarization rate, suggests that LNTB neurons may share the capacity of MNTB neurons to fire at high frequencies.

Unlike MNTB neurons, LNTB neurons fire repetitively in response to depolarizing current steps (**Figures 1D,E**). To assess the properties of action potentials in LNTB neurons during repetitive firing we analyzed responses to 100 ms current steps that elicited firing at overall rates of approximately 100 and 200 Hz (**Figure 3A**). Almost all LNTB neurons (94%) could sustain 100 Hz firing in response to current steps while most (79%) could sustain 200 Hz firing. During repetitive firing at both frequencies, the interval between the first and second action potentials was significantly longer than the interval between the second and third action potentials (paired t-test: 100 Hz, $p = 0.03$; 200 Hz, $p = 0.01$; **Figure 3B**). By the third or fourth pair of action potentials, the interspike interval stabilized, indicating a lack of spike frequency adaptation. Similarly, action potential thresholds increased after the first spike in the train but stabilized by the third or fourth spike (**Figure 3C**). Action potential half-widths showed a slight trend toward lengthening (**Figure 3D**) and peak amplitudes a slight trend toward decreasing (**Figure 3E**) across the 100 and 200 Hz trains. The amplitudes of afterhyperpolarizations, measured relative to the threshold of the preceding spike, became

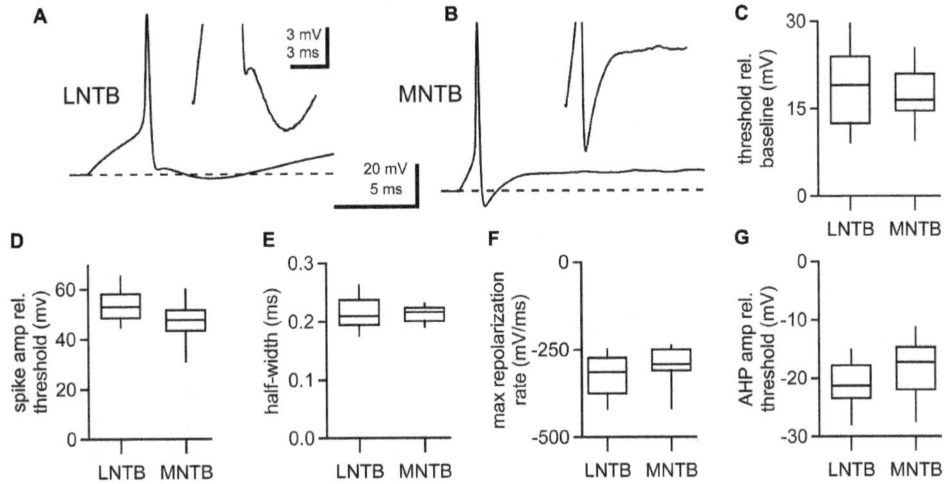

FIGURE 2 | Action potential properties assessed at rheobase in LNTB and MNTB neurons. **(A)** An action potential from an LNTB neuron exhibiting an afterhyperpolarization with a double undershoot. **(B)** An action potential from an MNTB neuron with a characteristic monophasic afterhyperpolarization. **(C–G)** Box plots comparing properties of the first action potential fired at rheobase in LNTB and MNTB neurons. Action potential amplitudes were significantly larger in LNTB neurons (**D**; $p = 0.03$), but there was no significant difference in action potential threshold **(C)**, half-width **(E)**, maximum repolarization rate **(F)**, or afterhyperpolarization amplitude **(G)** between LNTB and MNTB neurons ($p > 0.05$). Boxes mark median, 25th and 75th percentiles. Whiskers indicate 10th and 90th percentiles. $n = 52$ LNTB neurons, $n = 10$ MNTB neurons.

more negative following the first two to three spikes in a train, then stabilized for the remainder of the train (**Figure 3F**). As a group, these results show that the properties of action potentials in LNTB neurons are quite stable following the onset phase of repetitive firing. In five LNTB neurons, we explored the dynamic range of repetitive firing by eliciting action potentials with 1 s current steps over a range of amplitudes. While three neurons sustained firing in excess of 300 Hz, with one reaching 530 Hz (**Figure 3G**), the remaining two neurons exhibited more moderate firing rates. Thus, there is a diversity in input-output functions for LNTB neurons (**Figure 3H**).

Given the rapid repolarization rates and brief half-widths of action potentials in LNTB neurons, we suspected that at least some of these neurons might be able to fire at even higher rates than revealed by current steps. It has been shown that globular bushy cells, which provide excitatory drive to LNTB neurons, can phase lock to frequencies >1 kHz (Spirou et al., 1990; Smith et al., 1991; Joris et al., 1994a,b; Rhode, 2008; Recio-Spinoso, 2012). Thus, we injected trains of twenty brief current pulses into LNTB neurons to test their ability to phase lock to high frequency inputs. In five neurons, trains of 1 ms current pulses with amplitudes up to 2000 pA elicited firing with 96.1 ± 0.1% (mean ± SD) reliability at up to 600 Hz. In one of these neurons, we also injected trains of 20, 0.5 ms current pulses with amplitudes up to 4500 pA and observed firing at 1 kHz with 99.5% reliability (spikes/20 current pulses in 20 trials; **Figure 3I**). These results suggest that LNTB neurons *in vivo* might be capable of phase locking to bushy cell inputs at frequencies of 600 Hz or higher.

LNTB NEURONS RECEIVE EXCITATORY AND INHIBITORY SYNAPTIC INPUTS

During the course of recording from LNTB neurons, we frequently detected spontaneous EPSPs (**Figure 4A**) and IPSPs (**Figure 4B**). To more closely examine the properties of synaptic inputs to LNTB neurons, we used stimulating electrodes to directly evoke EPSPs (**Figure 4C**) and IPSPs (**Figure 4D**). Stimulus-evoked EPSPs had submillisecond rise times and half-widths of ~3 ms (**Table 1**). Stimulus-evoked and spontaneous IPSPs had much slower kinetics, with half-widths averaging ~4.5 and 8 ms, respectively (**Table 1**). Evoked IPSPs were completely blocked by 1 μM strychnine in 5 out of 5 cells, indicating that they were mediated by glycine receptors. In some neurons, evoked EPSPs were sufficiently large to evoke action potentials (**Figure 4E**). In other neurons, we noted that evoked EPSPs could be followed after a delay by an IPSP (**Figure 4F**). This delay suggests that inhibition onto LNTB neurons might involve a feedforward or lateral circuit. Consistent with this, in two LNTB neurons we found that IPSPs appeared during trains of stimuli, with a tendency to become stronger later in the train (**Figures 4G,H**). In one case, IPSPs followed the offset of the train by ~10 ms (**Figure 4H**). The role of inhibition in the LNTB is unknown, but its presence suggests that the LNTB is more than a sign-inverting relay for bushy cell inputs.

ANATOMY OF LNTB NEURONS

Using biocytin staining, we successfully recovered anatomy for 21 of 44 neurons in the LNTB data set. Of these, six LNTB neurons possessed axons that remained in the plane of the slice (**Figure 5**). These axons exited the LNTB heading in a dorsomedial direction and branched extensively, forming a number of collaterals. In four of the neurons, one or more axon collaterals terminated in the MSO (**Figures 5A,C,E,F**). Some axons formed terminals in a region dorsal to the MSO, possibly synapsing onto neurons in the superior periolivary nucleus (e.g., **Figures 5A,F**). Interestingly, several neurons possessed axon collaterals that projected back into the LNTB, where they formed terminal fields (**Figures 5D–F**). This suggests that at least some of the inhibitory

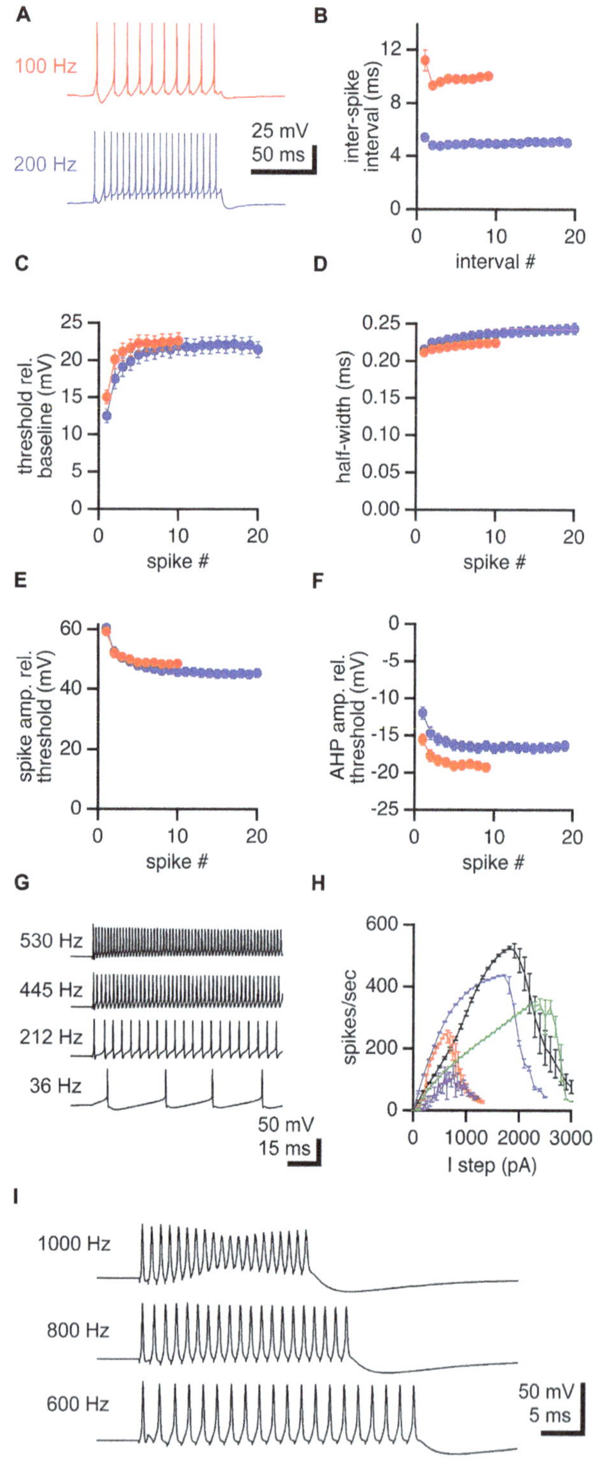

FIGURE 3 | Repetitive firing in LNTB neurons in response to current steps. (A) An LNTB neuron responded to 100 ms current steps of 400 and 900 pA with 100 Hz (red) and 200 Hz (blue) trains of action potentials. **(B)** The first inter-spike interval was longer than subsequent intervals during trains. During sustained firing, LNTB neurons did not exhibit spike frequency adaptation. **(C)** Action potential threshold was lowest at the onset of trains, but remained relatively stable after the third action potential. **(D)** Action potential half-widths remained brief

(Continued)

FIGURE 3 | Continued
throughout trains. **(E)** Action potential amplitudes were consistently large during trains. **(F)** Afterhyperpolarization amplitudes decreased during the early portion of trains. **(B–F)** 100 Hz trains (red), $n = 49$. 200 Hz trains (blue), $n = 41$. **(G)** In response to 1 second current steps of (from bottom to top) 100, 700, 1300, and 1900 pA, an LNTB neuron fired trains of action potentials at frequencies of 36–530 Hz. **(H)** Action potential firing versus current injection relationships for 5 LNTB neurons. Action potential counts indicate the average number of action potentials fired during 1 s current steps. **(I)** Action potentials elicited by trains of 20 current pulses delivered at 600 Hz (1 ms, 3000 pA pulses), 800 Hz (0.5 ms, 4000 pA pulses), or 1000 Hz (0.5 ms, 4500 pA pulses). Error bars indicate SEM.

input we observed in LNTB neurons (e.g., **Figures 4F–H**) came from other LNTB neurons. Among the axons that projected to the MSO, there was a surprising diversity in the path lengths traversed prior to terminating in the MSO. Measured from the axon hillock to the terminal, three neurons possessed collaterals that followed relatively direct paths to the MSO, with average path lengths ranging from 412 to 678 μm (mean ± SD: 544 ± 133 μm). The fourth neuron possessed an axon collateral that followed a very indirect path, traveling 978 μm dorsomedially before turning back to terminate in the ventral portion of the MSO, 1917 μm away from the axon hillock (**Figure 5E**). It is unclear whether the axonal projection pattern of this neuron represents an unusual case or if it is typical of a subset of LNTB neurons.

The dendritic arbors of LNTB neurons provide another example of morphological diversity. Some neurons possessed relatively simple dendritic arbors with little branching (**Figures 5A,B,D,E**), while others possessed larger arbors with more extensive branching (**Figures 5C,F**). The dendrites of some neurons mostly extended along an axis parallel to the long axis of the LNTB (**Figures 5B,D**), while others extended orthogonally (**Figures 5A,E**). The dendritic arbor of one neuron extended to cover much of the LNTB (**Figure 5C**). At present, there is little information about the *in vivo* tuning curves of LNTB neurons. Based on the diversity in dendritic arbor morphology shown here, we predict that some LNTB neurons may receive bushy cell inputs representing a narrow band of sound frequencies while others may be much more broadly tuned.

TIMING OF INHIBITION TO THE MSO

Studies of MNTB neurons have shown that the coupling between presynaptic input and postsynaptic spiking is highly reliable, rapid, and temporally precise (Mc Laughlin et al., 2008; Lorteije et al., 2009). Based on *in vivo* recordings in the MSO, it has also been proposed that the timing of inhibition provided by MNTB neurons to the MSO (i.e., contralaterally driven inhibition) is sufficiently precise that sound driven inhibition can arrive prior to the arrival of sound driven excitation (Brand et al., 2002; Pecka et al., 2008). Previously, we developed a novel slice preparation that retains the circuitry from the auditory nerve through the cochlear nucleus to the superior olivary complex (Roberts et al., 2013). This cochlear nucleus-superior olive (CN-SO) slice preparation allowed us to directly stimulate the auditory nerve while using whole cell current clamp recordings to assess responses elicited in MSO neurons. These experiments provided direct evidence that stimulation of

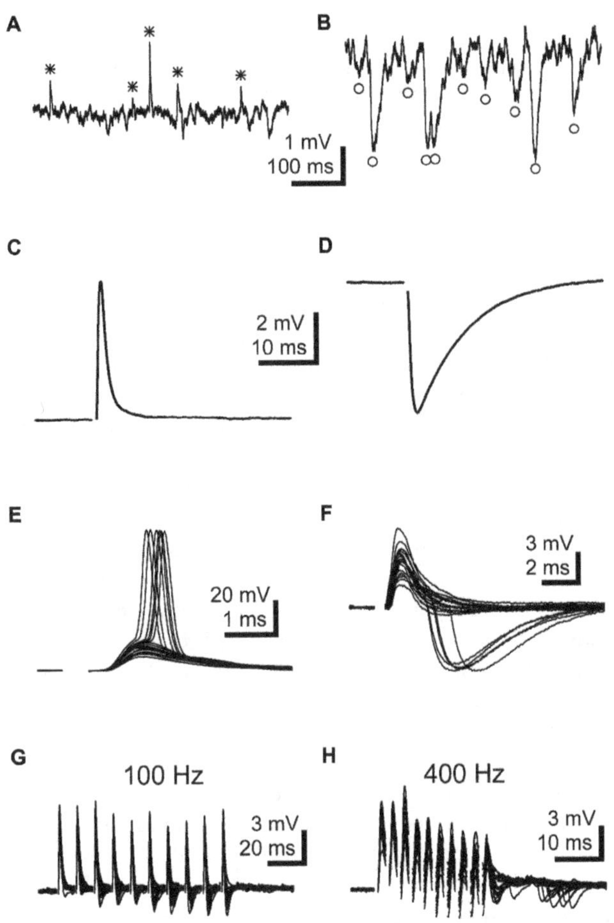

FIGURE 4 | LNTB neurons receive EPSPs and glycinergic IPSPs. **(A,B)** Spontaneous EPSPs **(A*)** and IPSPs **(B°)** were commonly observed in LNTB neurons. **(C)** An EPSP evoked in an LNTB neuron from a shock delivered in the trapezoid body dorsal to the LNTB. **(D)** An IPSP evoked in an LNTB neuron with a shock delivered in the LNTB. **(E)** Overlay of 20 responses to shocks evoking EPSPs. In 6 trials, the EPSPs elicited action potentials. **(F)** Overlay of 20 responses to shocks evoking EPSPs and, in 5 trials, delayed IPSPs. The delayed onsets of the IPSPs suggest that these were elicited through a disynaptic pathway. **(G,H)** Trains of ten stimuli at 100 **(G)** and 400 Hz **(H)** evoked EPSPs and delayed onset IPSPs. IPSPs became more prominent as the trains progressed, and at 400 Hz IPSPs continued after the train offset. Overlays of 20 trials are shown.

either the ipsilateral or contralateral auditory nerve elicited IPSPs in MSO neurons that, on average, arrived 0.32 ± 0.13 ms (ipsilateral) or 0.38 ± 0.09 ms (contralateral) prior to the arrival of EPSPs. Here, we performed additional analysis of this data set to test the hypothesis that nerve-driven inhibition to the MSO is as fast and temporally precise along the ipsilateral (LNTB) pathway as it is widely assumed to be along the contralateral (MNTB) pathway.

In five MSO neurons, we were able to evoke IPSPs by directly stimulating the ipsilateral auditory nerve. Ipsilateral IPSPs arrived with a latency of 1.69 ± 0.31 ms (**Figure 6A**) and jitter of 0.06 ± 0.02 ms (mean ± SD; jitter = SD of latency for an individual cell; **Figure 6B**). In five other neurons, IPSPs were elicited by stimulating the contralateral auditory nerve. These data showed that the latency to contralateral IPSPs (mean ± SD: 1.73 ± 0.17; **Figure 6A**) was not significantly different from the latency to ipsilateral IPSPs (t-test: $p = 0.79$), nor was there a significant difference between the contralateral jitter (mean ± SD: 0.07 ± 0.02 ms) and the ipsilateral jitter (t-test: $p = 0.37$; **Figure 6B**). Signals along both the ipsilateral and contralateral inhibitory pathways must traverse three synapses and two cell types to travel from the auditory nerve to the MSO. Given this, it is remarkable that the jitter along the ipsilateral and contralateral pathways is less than 5% of the total latency to IPSPs (mean ± SD: ipsi, 3.81 ± 1.47%; contra, 4.26 ± 0.97%; $p = 0.55$; **Figure 6C**). These results indicate that LNTB neurons in the ipsilateral inhibitory pathway can at least transiently provide inhibition to the MSO with the same high speed and precision as provided by MNTB neurons in the contralateral inhibitory pathway.

The finding that ipsilateral and contralateral inhibition is temporally well matched is surprising given the length disparity of the axons of the respective presynaptic excitatory inputs. To more directly assess the speed at which inhibition provided by the MNTB reaches the MSO, we recorded from synaptically coupled pairs of MNTB and MSO neurons. Such pairs were identified by patching onto an MSO neuron and using glutamate puffs to search the MNTB for potential presynaptic partners. When a small glutamate puff onto a visualized MNTB neuron evoked an IPSP in the MSO neuron, we patched onto the MNTB neuron. Synaptic coupling was confirmed if an action potential elicited by a brief current step in the MNTB neuron (**Figure 7B** top) was followed after a brief delay by an IPSP in the MSO neuron (**Figure 7B** bottom). IPSPs elicited in this way could be rather large (mean ± SEM: 6.94 ± 0.23 mV; **Figure 7C**), but averaged 3.90 ± 2.52 mV (mean ± SD) across the five synaptically coupled pairs we obtained. These pairs allowed us to measure the latency from the peak of an evoked action potential in an MNTB neuron to the 20% rise of the IPSP in the MSO neuron (**Figures 7D,E**). For the example cell shown in **Figures 7B–E**, the latency was 0.46 ms with a jitter of 0.02 ms. Across the five pairs in the data set, the latency averaged 0.58 ± 0.04 ms and the jitter 0.04 ± 0.01 ms (mean ± SEM; **Figure 7F**). For each pair, we successfully recovered the anatomy of the MNTB and MSO neuron (**Figure 7A**). Previous studies showed that glycinergic inhibition to the MSO undergoes a developmental shift from a uniform somatodendritic distribution to one that is biased strongly to the soma (Clark, 1969; Kapfer et al., 2002; Couchman et al., 2010, 2012). In agreement with these findings, we could visualize 1–4 putative synaptic contacts, with most located on the soma or nearby on the proximal dendrites (**Figure 7A** insets). These numbers can only be considered a minimum estimate because the black biocytin labeling of the cell obscured visualization of all contacts except those on the sides of the cell body. Reconstructions of recovered neurons revealed axon lengths from the MNTB to the MSO ranging from 580 to 858 μm and averaging 738 ± 45 μm (mean ± SEM). There was a correlation between the latency to the IPSP recorded in the MSO and axon length ($r = 0.63$; **Figure 7G**). Paired recordings between the calyx of Held and MNTB neurons have shown that the time required for synaptic transmission is ~0.2–0.3 ms at 35°C (Fedchyshyn and Wang, 2007). Assuming a synaptic delay in this

Table 1 | Properties of EPSPs and IPSPs in LNTB neurons.

	n	Mean amp. (mV)	10–90% rise time (ms)	Decay τ (ms)	Half-width (ms)
Evoked EPSP	6	6.04 ± 0.92	0.56 ± 0.10	3.84 ± 2.30	3.02 ± 1.26
Evoked IPSP	6	3.44 ± 0.60	0.94 ± 0.10	4.34 ± 1.05	4.54 ± 0.81
Spont. IPSP	8	1.47 ± 0.51	2.05 ± 0.74	13.80 ± 3.47	7.96 ± 2.01

Mean ± SEM.

range, our measurements of axon lengths and IPSP latencies predict that the axonal conduction velocity for MNTB neurons was ~1.9–2.6 m/s.

In vivo recordings have shown that MNTB neurons rarely fire isolated action potentials but instead fire repetitively, with spikes phase-locked to sound stimuli at rates that can exceed 500 Hz (Spirou et al., 1990; Kopp-Scheinpflug et al., 2008; Lorteije et al., 2009). We next asked how this high frequency activity in the MNTB affected the strength and temporal resolution of inhibition delivered to the MSO. In three of our synaptically coupled MNTB–MSO pairs we were able to examine the inhibition produced in the MSO by trains of twenty action potentials elicited in the MNTB neuron at frequencies ranging from 100 to 800 Hz. We found that two of the MNTB neurons were able to sustain firing at 600 Hz without failure (e.g., **Figure 8A**, top right), while the third achieved 800 Hz without failure. At the relatively low frequency of 100 Hz, MNTB spikes elicited IPSPs in the MSO that were distinct and clearly distinguishable (**Figure 8A**, left). At 600 Hz, however, IPSPs overlapped and exhibited temporal summation (**Figure 8A**, right). The average IPSP trains elicited across trials at a particular frequency revealed that IPSPs underwent short term depression at all frequencies and exhibited temporal summation early in the train at frequencies ≥300 Hz (**Figure 8B**). To quantify the amount of short term depression, we measured the foot-to-peak amplitude of each IPSP in an average train and compared it to the amplitude of the first IPSP (**Figure 8C**). This depression index showed that depression was evident throughout the entire frequency range. The average depression index across the last five IPSPs in each train was 44.6 ± 6.7% at 100 Hz and decreased to 20.2 ± 2.5% at 600 Hz (**Figure 8E**). To assess the extent of temporal summation during trains, we measured IPSP amplitudes relative to the resting membrane potential for each IPSP in an average train and compared these to the amplitude of the first IPSP (**Figure 8D**). This summation index revealed that IPSP amplitudes toward the end of trains were surprisingly similar across the frequencies tested. Indeed, the average summation index across the last five IPSPS in each train was 42.7 ± 5.7% at 100 Hz and remained stable at less than 50% until increasing at 600 Hz to 81.5 ± 14.6% (**Figure 8E**). The peak value of the summation index increased as a function of train frequency (**Figure 8E**), exceeding a value of 1 at 300 Hz and higher frequencies. This indicates that temporal summation countered the effects of short term depression at higher frequencies. Thus, the interplay between temporal summation and short-term depression allows MNTB neurons to provide relatively consistent levels of inhibition during the sustained portion of an inhibitory response, regardless of input frequency.

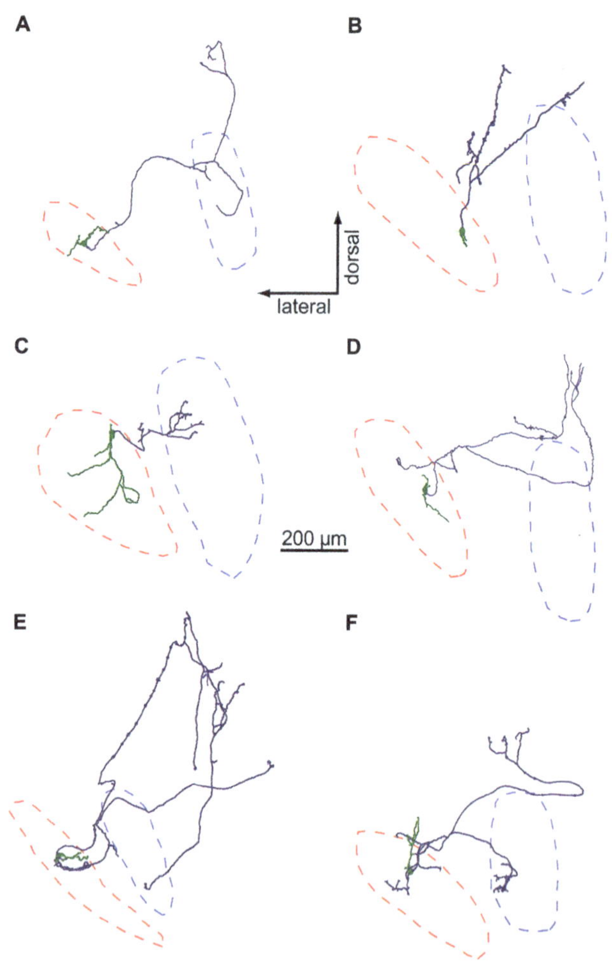

FIGURE 5 | LNTB neurons have multi-polar dendrites and axons that project to the MSO and/or periolivary nuclei. Somata and dendrites are shown in green, axons in purple. Red and blue dashed lines mark the predicted borders of the LNTB and MSO, respectively. The axons of neurons in **(A,C,E,F)** form terminals in the MSO, while the axons in **(B,D)** do not.

DISCUSSION

The physiology and temporal precision of LNTB and MNTB neurons are key determinants of how inhibition shapes coincidence detection in the MSO. Here, we investigated how LNTB and MNTB neurons are adapted for their roles in sound localization, providing the first descriptions of the intrinsic physiology of LNTB neurons

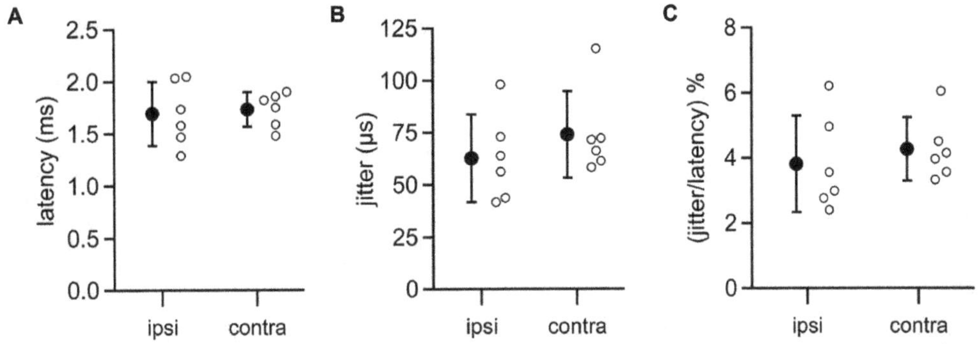

FIGURE 6 | Latencies from auditory nerve stimuli to IPSPs in MSO neurons. Recordings were made from MSO neurons in the CN-SO slice preparation, which retains circuitry from the auditory nerve to the MSO. IPSPs were evoked by direct stimulation of the auditory nerve stump on the ipsilateral or contralateral side of the slice. Neither the latency to IPSP onset **(A)** or the jitter in IPSP latencies **(B)** differed significantly between ipsilateral and contralateral pathways (*t*-tests: latency, $p = 0.79$; jitter, $p = 0.37$). **(C)** The jitter in IPSP timing represented a small percentage of the total latency to IPSP onset (*t*-test, $p = 0.55$). Open circles denote data from individual MSO neurons. Error bars show SD. Ipsilateral, $n = 6$; contralateral, $n = 6$.

and the first recordings from synaptically coupled pairs of MNTB and MSO neurons. We found that LNTB neurons share many properties with MNTB neurons, including brief action potentials and a capacity to fire at high frequencies, but differ in their ability to fire repetitively during sustained depolarizations and the strength of their excitatory inputs. We uncovered glycinergic input to LNTB neurons, suggesting a feedforward or lateral inhibitory circuit within the LNTB. Auditory nerve stimulation in CN-SO slice recordings showed that LNTB and MNTB neurons provide inhibition to the MSO with similar latencies and jitters. With paired recordings between synaptically coupled MNTB and MSO neurons, we found that propagation along MNTB axons was extremely fast and consistent across trials, providing a possible explanation for how the contralateral inhibitory pathway matches the timing of the ipsilateral pathway despite having to traverse a much longer distance. Together, these results support the hypothesis that the LNTB and MNTB provide rapid and precise inhibition to the MSO, while also suggesting that inhibition from LNTB neurons will be less reliable during sustained stimuli.

IMPLICATIONS OF LNTB PHYSIOLOGY AND MORPHOLOGY FOR IPSILATERAL INHIBITION OF THE MSO

In the absence of *in vivo* recordings of IPSPs in MSO neurons, the dynamics of sound-evoked inhibition in the MSO must largely be inferred from the properties of LNTB and MNTB neurons. For the MNTB, it is reasonable to assume that the fast and reliable conversion of calyx of Held input into action potentials, as evidenced by strong phase locking to auditory stimuli *in vivo*, enables MNTB neurons to provide reliable and temporally precise inhibition to the MSO (for reviews, see Kopp-Scheinpflug et al., 2011; Borst and Soria van Hoeve, 2012). Our results suggest three reasons why inhibition from LNTB neurons might be more nuanced, particularly during sustained stimuli.

First, input-output coupling in the MNTB is extremely powerful due to the calyx of Held synapse, which can release up to 100 vesicles in response to a single presynaptic spike (Borst and Sakmann, 1996) and which produces EPSCs in MNTB neurons that are generally much larger than what is required to exceed action potential threshold (Brew and Forsythe, 1995; Mc Laughlin et al., 2008; Lorteije et al., 2009; Berger et al., 2014). In contrast, we found that stimulus-evoked EPSPs in LNTB neurons could be small and were typically subthreshold. This suggests that synchronous synaptic input from multiple globular bushy cells, such as that presumably elicited by auditory nerve stimulation in the CN-SO slice experiment, might be required to bring an LNTB neuron to spike. In addition, the relatively extensive dendritic morphology of the LNTB neurons for which we recovered anatomy supports the idea that individual LNTB neurons receive input from multiple bushy cells. Previous anatomical studies have similarly described the dendrites of LNTB neurons as spanning significant portions of the width of the LNTB, and presumably representing a broad range of frequencies (Kuwabara and Zook, 1992; Kulesza, 2008).

Second, low voltage-activated Kv1 channels almost always limit the response of an MNTB neuron to one action potential per EPSP or depolarizing current step (Brew and Forsythe, 1995; Dodson et al., 2002; Klug and Trussell, 2006). This 1:1 relationship between input and output underlies the ability of MNTB neurons to accurately phase lock to a sound stimulus. In the LNTB, however, we found that while isolated EPSPs elicited single action potentials, sustained current steps evoked repetitive firing. This indicates that low voltage activated K^+ channels in LNTB neurons can limit excitability in response to a single EPSP but are not powerful enough to do so during a sustained depolarization, such as would be expected during periods of high frequency input when EPSPs undergo temporal summation.

Third, while action potentials in MNTB neurons are followed by brief afterhyperpolarizations (Forsythe and Barnes-Davies, 1993; Brew and Forsythe, 1995), those in LNTB neurons were typically much slower and were characterized in nearly two-thirds of cases by double undershoots. The effect of these strong afterhyperpolarizations was apparent during repetitive firing in LNTB neurons, increasing interspike intervals particularly between the first two action potentials in a train (**Figure 3**). This result suggests that the conductance responsible for the slow phase

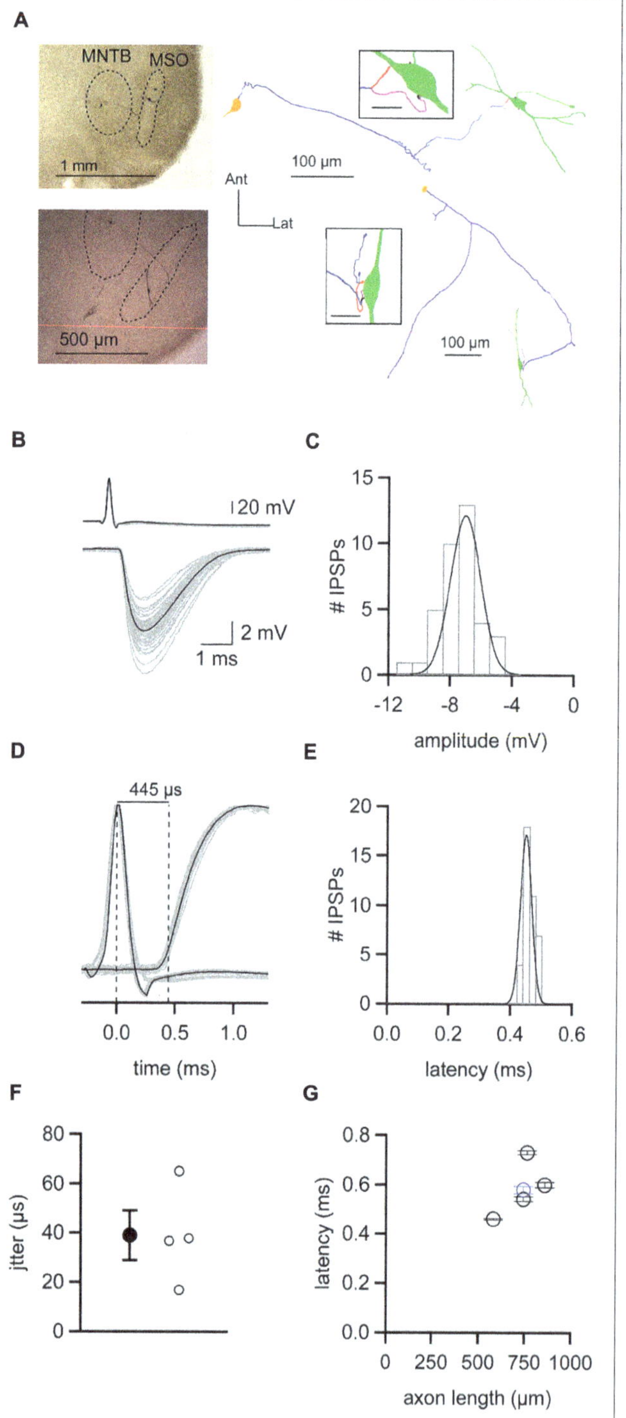

FIGURE 7 | Latencies from action potentials in MNTB neurons to IPSPs in MSO neurons (A) Left, micrographs showing staining of biocytin-filled, synaptically coupled MNTB and MSO neuron pairs. Right, reconstructions of the pairs shown on the left. MNTB somata are yellow, axons are purple. MSO neurons are green. Insets show putative synaptic contacts (magenta) between MNTB neuron terminals and MSO neurons. Inset scale bars = 20 μm. **(B)** Action potentials elicited in an MNTB neuron (top) lead to IPSPs in a postsynaptic MSO neuron (bottom). Gray data show 38 individual trials. Black data shows the average of these trials. **(C)** Histogram of IPSP amplitudes observed from the cell shown

(Continued)

FIGURE 7 | Continued
in **(B)**. Data are fit with a Gaussian function. **(D)** Plot of data shown in **(B)** with action potential and IPSP amplitudes normalized to reveal the average 445 μs latency between the peak of the presynaptic action potential and the 20% rise of postsynaptic IPSP. **(E)** Histogram of latency measurements for individual IPSPs from the cell shown in **(B–D)**. Data are fit with a Gaussian function. **(F)** Mean (filled circle) and individual (open circles) jitters in the onset of IPSPs from four MNTB–MSO pairs. **(G)** Relationship between the latency to IPSP onset and the length of the axon connecting the MNTB neuron to the MSO neuron soma. Black data are from four pairs recorded at 37°C. Blue data point is from one pair recorded at 35°C. Error bars show SEM.

of the after hyperpolarization in LNTB neurons, i.e., the second undershoot, inactivates during repetitive firing. Thus, the influence of afterhyperpolarizations on LNTB neuron excitability might vary according to the level of activity.

Despite these properties, LNTB neurons were capable of reliably sustaining firing rates of hundreds of Hz in response to sustained depolarizations, and up to 1 kHz in response to trains of brief current steps. This capacity to fire at high frequencies was aided by the brevity of action potentials in LNTB neurons, a property shared with MNTB neurons. In MNTB neurons, high voltage activated K^+ channels belonging to the Kv3 family constrain the duration of action potentials, which promotes high frequency firing by limiting inactivation of voltage gated Na^+ channels (Brew and Forsythe, 1995; Wang et al., 1998; Li et al., 2001; Klug and Trussell, 2006). Kv3 channels probably also underlie action potential repolarization in LNTB neurons. This similarity to MNTB neurons suggests that temporal coding is important to the function of LNTB neurons, but the graded EPSPs, less influential Kv1 channels, and long afterhyperpolarizations in LNTB neurons lead us to propose that LNTB neurons provide less consistent inhibition than MNTB neurons. In particular, we suspect that LNTB neurons will provide reliable and temporally precise inhibition during the onset phase of a sound, but that reliability and precision will degrade as a sound continues.

THE ROLE OF INHIBITION WITHIN THE LNTB

Our observation of glycinergic IPSPs in LNTB neurons provides functional confirmation of anatomical studies showing inhibitory terminals contacting the somata of LNTB neurons (Spirou and Berrebi, 1997; Spirou et al., 1998). These studies proposed that inhibitory terminals came from neurons within the LNTB or other periolivary nuclei. Our anatomical results support this, showing that the axon collaterals of some LNTB neurons projected back into the LNTB. In addition, given the limits of the circuitry left intact in a 200 μm-thick brain slice, our findings of putatively disynaptic IPSPs (**Figure 4F**) and instances where IPSPs were increasingly elicited in LNTB neurons during trains of stimuli (**Figures 4G,H**) also support a local source of LNTB inhibition. In such a circuit arrangement inhibition in the LNTB would function in a feedforward or lateral manner, depending on whether the presynaptic neuron receives input from the same or different globular bushy cells (Roberts and Trussell, 2010). In either case, it is possible that inhibition improves temporal precision in LNTB neurons by limiting the duration of the excitation provided by an EPSP (Pouille and Scanziani, 2001). Alternatively, our

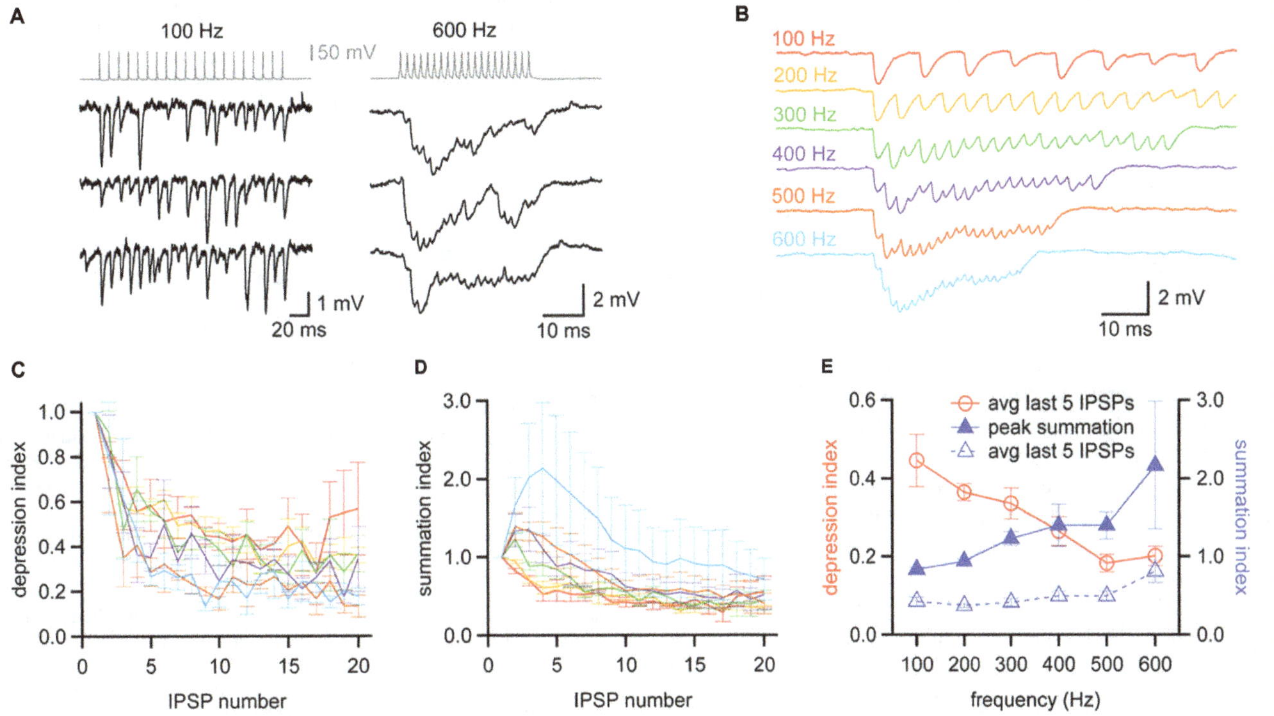

FIGURE 8 | Balanced synaptic depression and temporal summation of MNTB to MSO IPSPs during high frequency trains. (A) Trains of IPSPs observed in an MSO neuron (black data, bottom) in response to trains of 20 action potentials evoked at 100 and 600 Hz in an MNTB neuron (gray data, top). Three trials at each frequency are shown for the MSO neuron. **(B)** Average responses of the MSO neuron in **(A)** to trains of action potentials elicited at 100–600 Hz in the presynaptic MNTB neuron. $n = 7$ trials at each frequency. **(C)** The depression index reports the foot-to-peak amplitudes of each IPSP relative to the amplitude of the first IPSP in the train, revealing that depression occurred at all frequencies tested. **(D)** The summation index reports the baseline-to-peak amplitude of each IPSP as a function of the amplitude of the first IPSP in the train. **(C,D)** Colors follow the scheme in **(B)**. **(E)** The average depression index across the last 5 IPSPs of trains (red data, open circles) decreased with increasing train frequency while the peak summation index of trains (blue data, closed triangles) increased with increasing frequency. The average summation index across the last 5 IPSPs of trains was relatively insensitive to changes in train frequency (blue data, open triangles), suggesting that the effects of depression and summation counteract each other. $n = 3$. Error bars show SEM.

train data suggest that inhibition might dampen the excitability of LNTB neurons during periods of sustained activity, such as that following the onset phase of a sound. This model is particularly compelling considering the temporal summation of IPSPs expected from their relatively slow kinetics. A similar mechanism has been proposed for the role of inhibition in the MNTB (Awatramani et al., 2004).

TIMING OF IPSILATERAL VERSUS CONTRALATERAL INHIBITION TO THE MSO

The axons of globular bushy cells travel a greater distance to reach the MNTB than the LNTB (Spirou et al., 1990; Smith et al., 1991). Despite this, our CN-SO slice recordings found no significant difference in the latency to IPSPs evoked by stimulation of the ipsilateral versus the contralateral auditory nerves. In a previous study, within-cell comparisons of ipsilateral and contralateral EPSP latencies revealed a trend ($p = 0.192$) of ipsilateral EPSPs arriving 0.20 ms faster than contralateral EPSPs (Roberts et al., 2013). If a similarly small trend exists for IPSPs, it probably could not have been detected in our experiment, which involved between-cell comparisons of IPSP latencies. Nonetheless, there is ample evidence to suggest that the short latency to contralateral IPSPs may be attributed to mechanisms that speed transmission within the contralateral pathway. In particular, coupling between synaptic release at the calyx of Held and spiking in MNTB neurons is consistently fast and highly dependable. *In vivo* recordings from mice and cats have shown that the latency from a calyx of Held spike to a postsynaptic MNTB spike is ~0.40–0.50 ms (Mc Laughlin et al., 2008; Lorteije et al., 2009). This tight coupling requires large, rapidly-rising EPSCs (Taschenberger and von Gersdorff, 2000; Iwasaki and Takahashi, 2001; Joshi and Wang, 2002; Joshi et al., 2004; Koike-Tani et al., 2005; Yang et al., 2011). In contrast, stimulus-evoked EPSPs in LNTB neurons were graded in amplitude and often did not elicit action potentials. This suggests that spiking in LNTB neurons might require synchronous input from multiple bushy cell axons and that the timing of input-output coupling in LNTB neurons is slower than in MNTB neurons. The contralateral pathway may also be adapted for rapid transmission between the MNTB and the MSO. In our paired MNTB–MSO recordings, the mean latency from an MNTB spike to an MSO IPSP was 0.58 ms, and, based on anatomical reconstructions, we estimated the axonal conduction velocity to be 1.9–2.6 m/s. The conduction velocity of LNTB axons is currently unknown, but the wide range of axon lengths we observed for LNTB projections to MSO hint that, in some cases at least, axon conduction times may be longer for LNTB than MNTB.

The temporal measurements made here and those from previous studies provide a foundation for making predictions about the conduction time in globular bushy cell axons (Seidl et al., 2010, 2014; Seidl, 2013). In the CN-SO slice, the average latency from contralateral auditory nerve stimulation to IPSPs in the MSO was 1.73 ms. Given a 0.58 ms mean latency from an MNTB spike to an MSO IPSP and assuming a 0.40 ms latency from a presynaptic terminal spike to a postsynaptic spike for both the endbulb of Held synapse onto globular bushy cells and the calyx of Held synapse onto MNTB neurons, the remaining time for axonal conduction in the contralateral pathway is ~0.35 ms. If we then assume that the axon length from a globular bushy cell to an MNTB neuron is twice that of the same axon to an LNTB neuron, we see that the increased travel distance to the MNTB may only add ~0.17 ms to the contralateral transit, a time that might easily be compensated for by the calyx of Held synapse. Interestingly, anatomical studies have revealed calyceal synapses in the most ventral portion of cat LNTB (Stotler, 1953; Adams, 1983; Spirou and Berrebi, 1996; Spirou et al., 1998). While it is unknown whether calyceal synapses are present in the ventral LNTB of gerbil, none of the LNTB neurons that we found projecting to the MSO were located in the ventral region of the LNTB, suggesting that such synapses are not a requirement for LNTB neurons that inhibit MSO neurons.

ACKNOWLEDGMENTS

We thank Wen-Ke Li for contributions to the LNTB recordings and Lauren J. Kreeger and Brandy Zrubek for technical assistance with Neurolucida. This work was supported by NIDCD grants DC006877 and DC011403 to NLG.

REFERENCES

Adams, J. C. (1983). Cytology of periolivary cells and the organization of their projections in the cat. *J. Comp. Neurol.* 215, 275–289. doi: 10.1002/cne.902150304

Adams, J. C., and Mugnaini, E. (1990). Immunocytochemical evidence for inhibitory and disinhibitory circuits in the superior olive. *Hear. Res.* 49, 281–298. doi: 10.1016/0378-5955(90)90109-3

Awatramani, G. B., Turecek, R., and Trussell, L. O. (2004). Inhibitory control at a synaptic relay. *J. Neurosci.* 24, 2643–2647. doi: 10.1523/JNEUROSCI.5144-03.2004

Banks, M. I., and Smith, P. H. (1992). Intracellular recordings from neurobiotin-labeled cells in brain slices of the rat medial nucleus of the trapezoid body. *J. Neurosci.* 12, 2819–2837.

Berger, C., Meyer, E. M. M., Ammer, J. J., and Felmy, F. (2014). Large somatic synapses on neurons in the ventral lateral lemniscus work in pairs. *J. Neurosci.* 34, 3237–3246. doi: 10.1523/JNEUROSCI.3664-13.2014

Borst, J. G. G., and Soria van Hoeve, J. (2012). The calyx of held synapse: from model synapse to auditory relay. *Annu. Rev. Physiol.* 74, 199–224. doi: 10.1146/annurev-physiol-020911-153236

Borst, J. G., and Sakmann, B. (1996). Calcium influx and transmitter release in a fast CNS synapse. *Nature* 383, 431–434. doi: 10.1038/383431a0

Brand, A., Behrend, O., Marquardt, T., McAlpine, D., and Grothe, B. (2002). Precise inhibition is essential for microsecond interaural time difference coding. *Nature* 417, 543–547. doi: 10.1038/417543a

Brew, H. M., and Forsythe, I. D. (1995). Two voltage-dependent K+ conductances with complementary functions in postsynaptic integration at a central auditory synapse. *J. Neurosci.* 15, 8011–8022.

Cant, N. B., and Hyson, R. L. (1992). Projections from the lateral nucleus of the trapezoid body to the medial superior olivary nucleus in the gerbil. *Hear. Res.* 58, 26–34. doi: 10.1016/0378-5955(92)90005-8

Chirila, F. V., Rowland, K. C., Thompson, J. M., and Spirou, G. A. (2007). Development of gerbil medial superior olive: integration of temporally delayed excitation and inhibition at physiological temperature. *J. Physiol.* 584, 167–190. doi: 10.1113/jphysiol.2007.137976

Clark, G. M. (1969). The ultrastructure of nerve endings in the medial superior olive of the cat. *Brain Res.* 14, 293–305. doi: 10.1016/0006-8993(69)90111-5

Clements, J. D., and Bekkers, J. M. (1997). Detection of spontaneous synaptic events with an optimally scaled template. *Biophys. J.* 73, 220–229. doi: 10.1016/S0006-3495(97)78062-7

Couchman, K., Grothe, B., and Felmy, F. (2010). Medial superior olivary neurons receive surprisingly few excitatory and inhibitory inputs with balanced strength and short-term dynamics. *J. Neurosci.* 30, 17111–17121. doi: 10.1523/JNEUROSCI.1760-10.2010

Couchman, K., Grothe, B., and Felmy, F. (2012). Functional localization of neurotransmitter receptors and synaptic inputs to mature neurons of the medial superior olive. *J. Neurophysiol.* 107, 1186–1198. doi: 10.1152/jn.00586.2011

Day, M. L., and Semple, M. N. (2011). Frequency-dependent interaural delays in the medial superior olive: implications for interaural cochlear delays. *J. Neurophysiol.* 106, 1985–1999. doi: 10.1152/jn.00131.2011

Dodson, P. D., Barker, M. C., and Forsythe, I. D. (2002). Two heteromeric Kv1 potassium channels differentially regulate action potential firing. *J. Neurosci.* 22, 6953–6961.

Fedchyshyn, M. J., and Wang, L.-Y. (2007). Activity-dependent changes in temporal components of neurotransmission at the juvenile mouse calyx of Held synapse. *J. Physiol.* 581, 581–602. doi: 10.1113/jphysiol.2007.129833

Fischl, M. J., Combs, T. D., Klug, A., Grothe, B., and Burger, R. M. (2012). Modulation of synaptic input by GABAB receptors improves coincidence detection for computation of sound location. *J. Physiol.* 590, 3047–3066 doi: 10.1113/jphysiol.2011.226233

Forsythe, I. D., and Barnes-Davies, M. (1993). The binaural auditory pathway: membrane currents limiting multiple action potential generation in the rat medial nucleus of the trapezoid body. *Proc. Biol. Sci.* 251, 143–150. doi: 10.1098/rspb.1993.0021

Friauf, E., and Ostwald, J. (1988). Divergent projections of physiologically characterized rat ventral cochlear nucleus neurons as shown by intra-axonal injection of horseradish peroxidase. *Exp. Brain Res.* 73, 263–284. doi: 10.1007/BF00248219

Goldberg, J. M., and Brown, P. B. (1969). Response of binaural neurons of dog superior olivary complex to dichotic tonal stimuli: some physiological mechanisms of sound localization. *J. Neurophysiol.* 32, 613–636.

Grothe, B., Pecka, M., and McAlpine, D. (2010). Mechanisms of sound localization in mammals. *Physiol. Rev.* 90, 983–1012. doi: 10.1152/physrev.00026.2009

Grothe, B., and Sanes, D. H. (1993). Bilateral inhibition by glycinergic afferents in the medial superior olive. *J. Neurophysiol.* 69, 1192–1196.

Grothe, B., and Sanes, D. H. (1994). Synaptic inhibition influences the temporal coding properties of medial superior olivary neurons: an in vitro study. *J. Neurosci.* 14, 1701–1709.

Guinan, J. J., Guinan, S. S., and Norris, B. E. (1972a). Single auditory units in the superior olivary complex: I: responses to sounds and classifications based on physiological properties. *Int. J. Neurosci.* 4, 101–120. doi: 10.3109/00207457209147165

Guinan, J. J., Guinan, S. S., and Norris, B. E. (1972b). Single auditory units in the superior olivary complex: II: locations of unit categories and tonotopic organization. *Int. J. Neurosci.* 4, 147–166. doi: 10.3109/00207457209164756

Iwasaki, S., and Takahashi, T. (2001). Developmental regulation of transmitter release at the calyx of Held in rat auditory brainstem. *J. Physiol.* 534, 861–871. doi: 10.1111/j.1469-7793.2001.00861.x

Joris, P. X., Carney, L. H., Smith, P. H., and Yin, T. C. (1994a). Enhancement of neural synchronization in the anteroventral cochlear nucleus. I. Responses to tones at the characteristic frequency. *J. Neurophysiol.* 71, 1022–1036.

Joris, P. X., Smith, P. H., and Yin, T. C. (1994b). Enhancement of neural synchronization in the anteroventral cochlear nucleus. II. Responses in the tuning curve tail. *J. Neurophysiol.* 71, 1037–1051.

Joris, P., and Yin, T. C. T. (2007). A matter of time: internal delays in binaural processing. *Trends Neurosci.* 30, 70–78. doi: 10.1016/j.tins.2006.12.004

Joshi, I., Shokralla, S., Titis, P., and Wang, L.-Y. (2004). The role of AMPA receptor gating in the development of high-fidelity neurotransmission at the calyx of Held synapse. *J. Neurosci.* 24, 183–196. doi: 10.1523/JNEUROSCI.1074-03.2004

Joshi, I., and Wang, L.-Y. (2002). Developmental profiles of glutamate receptors and synaptic transmission at a single synapse in the mouse auditory brainstem. *J. Physiol.* 540, 861–873. doi: 10.1113/jphysiol.2001.013506

Kapfer, C., Seidl, A. H., Schweizer, H., and Grothe, B. (2002). Experience-dependent refinement of inhibitory inputs to auditory coincidence-detector neurons. *Nat. Neurosci.* 5, 247–253. doi: 10.1038/nn810

Klug, A., and Trussell, L. O. (2006). Activation and deactivation of voltage-dependent K+ channels during synaptically driven action potentials in the MNTB. *J. Neurophysiol.* 96, 1547–1555. doi: 10.1152/jn.01381.2005

Koike-Tani, M., Saitoh, N., and Takahashi, T. (2005). Mechanisms underlying developmental speeding in AMPA-EPSC decay time at the calyx of Held. *J. Neurosci.* 25, 199–207. doi: 10.1523/JNEUROSCI.3861-04.2005

Kopp-Scheinpflug, C., Steinert, J. R., and Forsythe, I. D. (2011). Modulation and control of synaptic transmission across the MNTB. *Hear. Res.* 279, 22–31. doi: 10.1016/j.heares.2011.02.007

Kopp-Scheinpflug, C., Tolnai, S., Malmierca, M. S., and Rübsamen, R. (2008). The medial nucleus of the trapezoid body: comparative physiology. *Neuroscience* 154, 160–170. doi: 10.1016/j.neuroscience.2008.01.088

Kulesza, R. J. (2008). Cytoarchitecture of the human superior olivary complex: nuclei of the trapezoid body and posterior tier. *Hear. Res.* 241, 52–63. doi: 10.1016/j.heares.2008.04.010

Kuwabara, N., DiCaprio, R. A., and Zook, J. M. (1991). Afferents to the medial nucleus of the trapezoid body and their collateral projections. *J. Comp. Neurol.* 314, 684–706. doi: 10.1002/cne.903140405

Kuwabara, N., and Zook, J. M. (1992). Projections to the medial superior olive from the medial and lateral nuclei of the trapezoid body in rodents and bats. *J. Comp. Neurol.* 324, 522–538. doi: 10.1002/cne.903240406

Li, W., Kaczmarek, L. K., and Perney, T. M. (2001). Localization of two high-threshold potassium channel subunits in the rat central auditory system. *J. Comp. Neurol.* 437, 196–218. doi: 10.1002/cne.1279

Lorteije, J. A. M., Rusu, S. I., Kushmerick, C., and Borst, J. G. G. (2009). Reliability and precision of the mouse calyx of Held synapse. *J. Neurosci.* 29, 13770–13784. doi: 10.1523/JNEUROSCI.3285-09.2009

Magnusson, A. K., Kapfer, C., Grothe, B., and Koch, U. (2005). Maturation of glycinergic inhibition in the gerbil medial superior olive after hearing onset. *J. Physiol.* 568, 497–512. doi: 10.1113/jphysiol.2005.094763

Mc Laughlin, M., van der Heijden, M., and Joris, P. X. (2008). How secure is in vivo synaptic transmission at the calyx of Held? *J. Neurosci.* 28, 10206–10219. doi: 10.1523/JNEUROSCI.2735-08.2008

Oertel, D., Wu, S. H., Garb, M. W., and Dizack, C. (1990). Morphology and physiology of cells in slice preparations of the posteroventral cochlear nucleus of mice. *J. Comp. Neurol.* 295, 136–154. doi: 10.1002/cne.902950112

Pecka, M., Brand, A., Behrend, O., and Grothe, B. (2008). Interaural time difference processing in the mammalian medial superior olive: the role of glycinergic inhibition. *J. Neurosci.* 28, 6914–6925. doi: 10.1523/JNEUROSCI.1660-08.2008

Pouille, F., and Scanziani, M. (2001). Enforcement of temporal fidelity in pyramidal cells by somatic feed-forward inhibition. *Science* 293, 1159–1163. doi: 10.1126/science.1060342

Recio-Spinoso, A. (2012). Enhancement and distortion in the temporal representation of sounds in the ventral cochlear nucleus of chinchillas and cats. *PLoS ONE* 7:e44286. doi: 10.1371/journal.pone.0044286

Rhode, W. S. (2008). Response patterns to sound associated with labeled globular/bushy cells in cat. *Neuroscience* 154, 87–98. doi: 10.1016/j.neuroscience.2008.03.013

Roberts, M. T., Seeman, S. C., and Golding, N. L. (2013). A mechanistic understanding of the role of feedforward inhibition in the Mammalian sound localization circuitry. *Neuron* 78, 923–935. doi: 10.1016/j.neuron.2013.04.022

Roberts, M. T., and Trussell, L. O. (2010). Molecular layer inhibitory interneurons provide feedforward and lateral inhibition in the dorsal cochlear nucleus. *J. Neurophysiol.* 104, 2462–2473. doi: 10.1152/jn.00312.2010

Scott, L. L., Mathews, P. J., and Golding, N. L. (2005). Posthearing developmental refinement of temporal processing in principal neurons of the medial superior olive. *J. Neurosci.* 25, 7887–7895. doi: 10.1523/JNEUROSCI.1016-05.2005

Seidl, A. H. (2013). Regulation of conduction time along axons. *Neuroscience* doi: 10.1016/j.neuroscience.2013.06.047 [Epub ahead of print].

Seidl, A. H., Rubel, E. W., and Barría, A. (2014). Differential conduction velocity regulation in ipsilateral and contralateral collaterals innervating brainstem coincidence detector neurons. *J. Neurosci.* 34, 4914–4919. doi: 10.1523/JNEUROSCI.5460-13.2014

Seidl, A. H., Rubel, E. W., and Harris, D. M. (2010). Mechanisms for adjusting interaural time differences to achieve binaural coincidence detection. *J. Neurosci.* 30, 70–80. doi: 10.1523/JNEUROSCI.3464-09.2010

Smith, P. H., Joris, P. X., Carney, L. H., and Yin, T. C. (1991). Projections of physiologically characterized globular bushy cell axons from the cochlear nucleus of the cat. *J. Comp. Neurol.* 304, 387–407. doi: 10.1002/cne.903040305

Spangler, K. M., Warr, W. B., and Henkel, C. K. (1985). The projections of principal cells of the medial nucleus of the trapezoid body in the cat. *J. Comp. Neurol.* 238, 249–262. doi: 10.1002/cne.902380302

Spirou, G. A., and Berrebi, A. S. (1996). Organization of ventrolateral periolivary cells of the cat superior olive as revealed by PEP-19 immunocytochemistry and Nissl stain. *J. Comp. Neurol.* 368, 100–120. doi: 10.1002/(SICI)1096-9861(19960422)368:1<100::AID-CNE7>3.0.CO;2-7

Spirou, G. A., and Berrebi, A. S. (1997). Glycine immunoreactivity in the lateral nucleus of the trapezoid body of the cat. *J. Comp. Neurol.* 383, 473–488. doi: 10.1002/(SICI)1096-9861(19970714)383:4<473::AID-CNE6>3.0.CO;2-#

Spirou, G. A., Brownell, W. E., and Zidanic, M. (1990). Recordings from cat trapezoid body and HRP labeling of globular bushy cell axons. *J. Neurophysiol.* 63, 1169–1190.

Spirou, G. A., Rowland, K. C., and Berrebi, A. S. (1998). Ultrastructure of neurons and large synaptic terminals in the lateral nucleus of the trapezoid body of the cat. *J. Comp. Neurol.* 398, 257–272. doi: 10.1002/(SICI)1096-9861(19980824)398:2<257::AID-CNE7>3.0.CO;2-#

Spitzer, M. W., and Semple, M. N. (1995). Neurons sensitive to interaural phase disparity in gerbil superior olive: diverse monaural and temporal response properties. *J. Neurophysiol.* 73, 1668–1690.

Stotler, W. A. (1953). An experimental study of the cells and connections of the superior olivary complex of the cat. *J. Comp. Neurol.* 98, 401–431. doi: 10.1002/cne.900980303

Taschenberger, H., and von Gersdorff, H. (2000). Fine-tuning an auditory synapse for speed and fidelity: developmental changes in presynaptic waveform, EPSC kinetics, and synaptic plasticity. *J. Neurosci.* 20, 9162–9173.

Thompson, A. M., and Schofield, B. R. (2000). Afferent projections of the superior olivary complex. *Microsc. Res. Tech.* 51, 330–354. doi: 10.1002/1097-0029(20001115)51:4<330::AID-JEMT4>3.0.CO;2-X

Tolbert, L. P., Morest, D. K., and Yurgelun-Todd, D. A. (1982). The neuronal architecture of the anteroventral cochlear nucleus of the cat in the region of the cochlear nerve root: horseradish peroxidase labelling of identified cell types. *Neuroscience* 7, 3031–3052. doi: 10.1016/0306-4522(82)90228-7

Tsuchitani, C. (1977). Functional organization of lateral cell groups of cat superior olivary complex. *J. Neurophysiol.* 40, 296–318.

van der Heijden, M., Lorteije, J. A. M., Plauška, A., Roberts, M. T., Golding, N. L., and Borst, J. G. G. (2013). Directional hearing by linear summation of binaural inputs at the medial superior olive. *Neuron* 78, 936–948. doi: 10.1016/j.neuron.2013.04.028

Wang, L. Y., Gan, L., Forsythe, I. D., and Kaczmarek, L. K. (1998). Contribution of the Kv3.1 potassium channel to high-frequency firing in mouse auditory neurones. *J. Physiol.* 509(Pt 1), 183–194. doi: 10.1111/j.1469-7793.1998.183bo.x

Wu, S. H., and Kelly, J. B. (1995). In vitro brain slice studies of the rat's dorsal nucleus of the lateral lemniscus. I. Membrane and synaptic response properties. *J. Neurophysiol.* 73, 780–793.

Yang, Y.-M., Aitoubah, J., Lauer, A. M., Nuriya, M., Takamiya, K., Jia, Z., et al. (2011). GluA4 is indispensable for driving fast neurotransmission across a high-fidelity central synapse. *J. Physiol.* 589, 4209–4227. doi: 10.1113/jphysiol.2011.208066

Yin, T. C., and Chan, J. C. (1990). Interaural time sensitivity in medial superior olive of cat. *J. Neurophysiol.* 64, 465–488.

Zhang, S., and Oertel, D. (1993a). Cartwheel and superficial stellate cells of the dorsal cochlear nucleus of mice: intracellular recordings in slices. *J. Neurophysiol.* 69, 1384–1397.

Zhang, S., and Oertel, D. (1993b). Tuberculoventral cells of the dorsal cochlear nucleus of mice: intracellular recordings in slices. *J. Neurophysiol.* 69, 1409–1421.

6

Developmental expression of inhibitory synaptic long-term potentiation in the lateral superior olive

Vibhakar C. Kotak[1] and Dan H. Sanes[1,2]*

[1] Center for Neural Science, New York University, New York, NY, USA
[2] Department of Biology, New York University, New York, NY, USA

Correspondence:
Dan H. Sanes, Center for Neural Science, 4 Washington Place, New York University, New York, NY, 10003, USA
e-mail: dhs1@nyu.edu

Principal neurons of the lateral superior olivary nucleus (LSO) respond selectively to interaural level differences (ILD). To perform this computation, LSO neurons integrate excitatory synaptic drive from the ipsilateral ear with inhibitory synaptic drive from the contralateral ear via the medial nucleus of the trapezoid body (MNTB). Previous research demonstrated that inhibitory terminals from the MNTB to the LSO are eliminated during development. Furthermore, MNTB synapses display an activity- and age-dependent long-term depression (iLTD) that may contribute to inhibitory synapse elimination. However, inhibitory synapses that are stabilized become stronger. Here, we asked whether MNTB synapses displayed activity-dependent strengthening. Whole-cell recordings were obtained from LSO neurons in a gerbil brain slice before and after hearing onset. The inhibitory MNTB afferents were stimulated at a low rate, similar to spontaneous discharge rates observed *in vivo*. The MNTB-evoked inhibitory responses were strengthened by 40–300% when synaptic activity was coupled with postsynaptic membrane depolarization, exogenous glutamate application, or activation of ipsilateral excitatory synaptic inputs. This inhibitory long-term potentiation (iLTP) was associated with increased spontaneous inhibitory postsynaptic current (IPSC) amplitude and frequency. One hour after iLTP induction, IPSCs could not be de-potentiated by the MNTB stimulation pattern that induces iLTD in control slices. iLTP could only be induced after hearing onset (>P12), and was blocked in the presence of a $GABA_B$ receptor antagonist. Together, these results suggest a developmental period during which the induction of iLTP depends on the conjoint activation of $GABA_B$ receptors and postsynaptic depolarization. We propose that iLTP may support stabilization of un-pruned MNTB connections and contribute to the emergence of ILD processing in the mature LSO.

Keywords: GABA, glycine, $GABA_B$, synaptic potentiation, plasticity, LSO

INTRODUCTION

The encoding of sound localization cues, such as interaural level (ILD) and time differences (ITD), begins in the ventral auditory brain stem. For ILD coding, the discharge rate of lateral superior olivary (LSO) neurons is proportional to the integration of ipsilateral excitatory drive arising from the cochlear nucleus and contralateral inhibitory drive from the medial nucleus of the trapezoid body (MNTB) (Boudreau and Tsutchitani, 1968; Caird and Klinke, 1983; Harnischfeger et al., 1985; Tollin, 2003; Sterenborg et al., 2010). The inhibitory MNTB afferents form a tonotopic projection in the LSO that is aligned precisely with the ipsilateral excitatory projection in the adult (Sanes and Rubel, 1988). Furthermore, this precision evolves as inhibitory synapses are eliminated during postnatal development (Sanes and Siverls, 1991; Sanes and Friauf, 2000; Kim and Kandler, 2003; Kandler, 2004; Kandler and Gillespie, 2005; Kandler et al., 2009). A similar elimination of inhibitory MNTB terminals occurs at the medial superior olivary nucleus, which encodes ITD (Kapfer et al., 2002), although one study did not find a significant developmental change in amplitude (Walcher et al., 2011). It is, therefore, plausible that that the establishment of properly aligned excitatory and inhibitory maps involves the dynamic addition and elimination of inhibitory synapses. One mechanism that could participate in synapse elimination, inhibitory long-term depression (iLTD), has been described previously for MNTB synapses (Kotak and Sanes, 2000, 2002; Kotak et al., 2001; Chang et al., 2003). As inhibitory synapses are eliminated and the remaining contacts are strengthened in the rat LSO, there is a 12-fold increase in inhibitory conductance (Kim and Kandler, 2003). Here, we describe a mechanism that could account for this strengthening.

A vast literature on excitatory long-term potentiation (LTP) and depression (LTD) in the hippocampus and neocortex supports their involvement in adult learning, memory and neurodevelopmental disorders (see Bear and Malenka, 1994; Bliss et al., 2013). Many studies have also shown that inhibitory synapses can be strengthened or weakened in an activity-dependent manner. However, the functional consequence of such

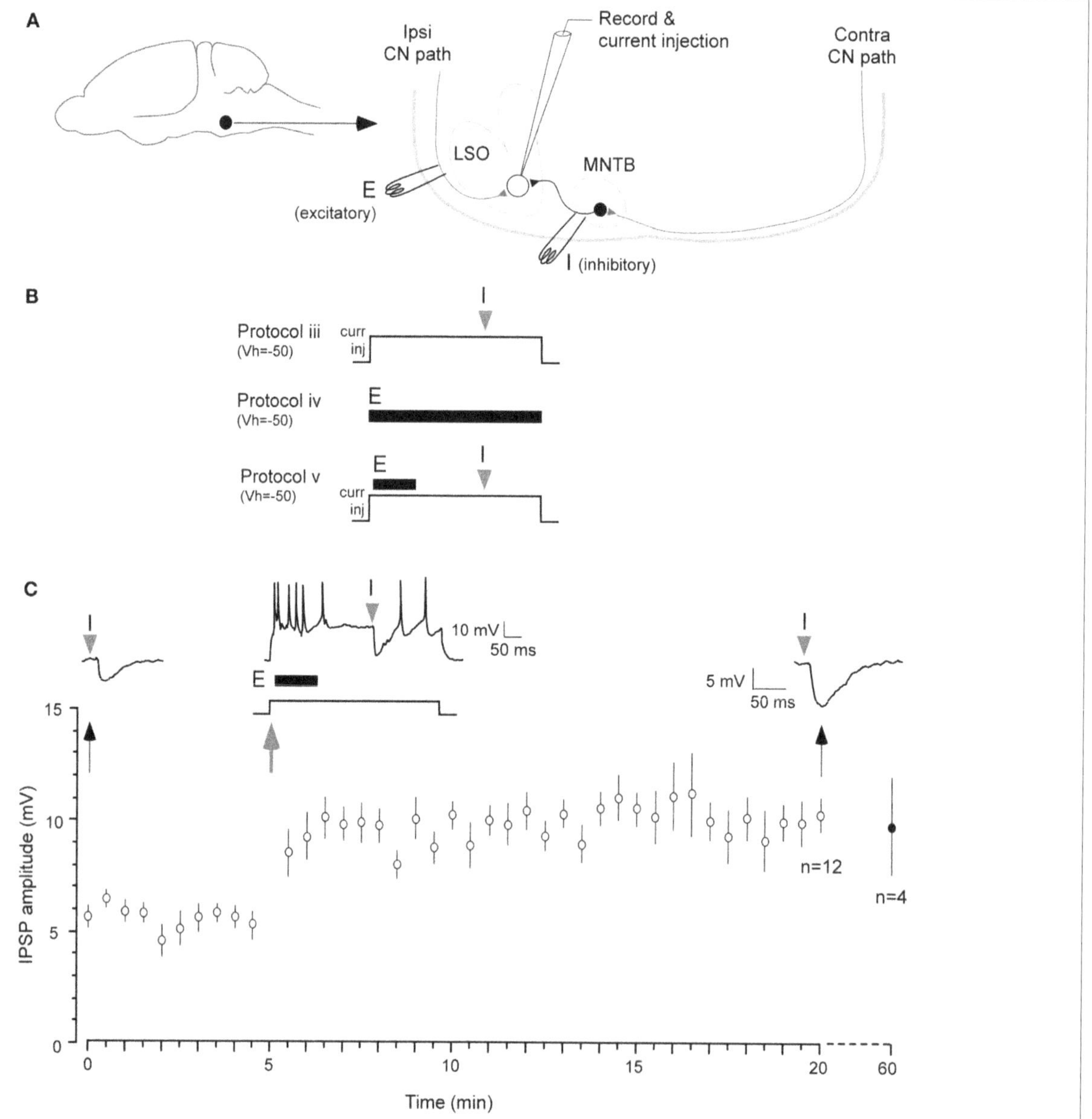

FIGURE 1 | Iaqnduction of inhibitory LTP in P12–15 day neurons. (A) A schematic of the LSO circuit in brain slice preparation. Filled circle and arrow indicate auditory brainstem. E: ipsilateral excitatory pathway from cochlear nucleus (CN), I: MTNB pathway activated by contralateral CN. **(B)** Three of the stimulus protocols are shown (see Results for details). Only Protocol v was effective in inducing iLTP, as shown in **(C)**. **(C)** A pre-conditioning MNTB-evoked IPSP evoked by MNTB stimulus (I). Such IPSPs were obtained at 0.033 Hz for 5 min at $V_{HOLD} = -50$ mV (baseline). A single suprathreshold depolarization (500 ms, +5–10 pA) injection was used to trigger neuronal firing by up to 50 Hz. The ipsilateral excitatory afferents were then stimulated at 100 Hz 10 ms after the onset of 500 ms depolarization (10 pulses, dark bar under the trace, E). MNTB evoked IPSP was timed at 300 ms after the injection of the 500 ms depolarizing pulse (gray arrowhead). The 0.033 Hz acquisition of IPSP was continued through the recording session. IPSPs displayed a significant enhancement in amplitude for at least 20 min (top right trace 20 min after). Bottom panel shows summary data (mean ± s.e.m.). In 4 neurons, recordings were continued for an additional 40 min, and the increased amplitude IPSPs persisted. IPSP means (Y axis) are sub-maximum amplitude and not normalized.

inhibitory synapse plasticity and the underlying biochemical and molecular factors are not well understood. Inhibitory plasticity, including GABAergic LTP and LTD, may contribute to memory formation or motor learning (Morishita and Sastry, 1996; Aizenman et al., 1998; Ouardouz and Sastry, 2000). Glycinergic LTP at the goldfish Mauthner neuron may dampen the escape response (Oda et al., 1995, 1998), and GABAergic LTP in the visual cortex may alter visual coding properties (Komatsu and Iwakiri, 1993; Komatsu, 1994, 1996; Komatsu and Yoshimura, 2000). Since MNTB-mediated iLTD gradually wanes following hearing onset (Kotak and Sanes, 2000), it is possible that iLTP emerges during this time. Our results demonstrated that even very low levels of inhibitory afferent activity, when coupled with excitatory transmission, can trigger iLTP after hearing onset.

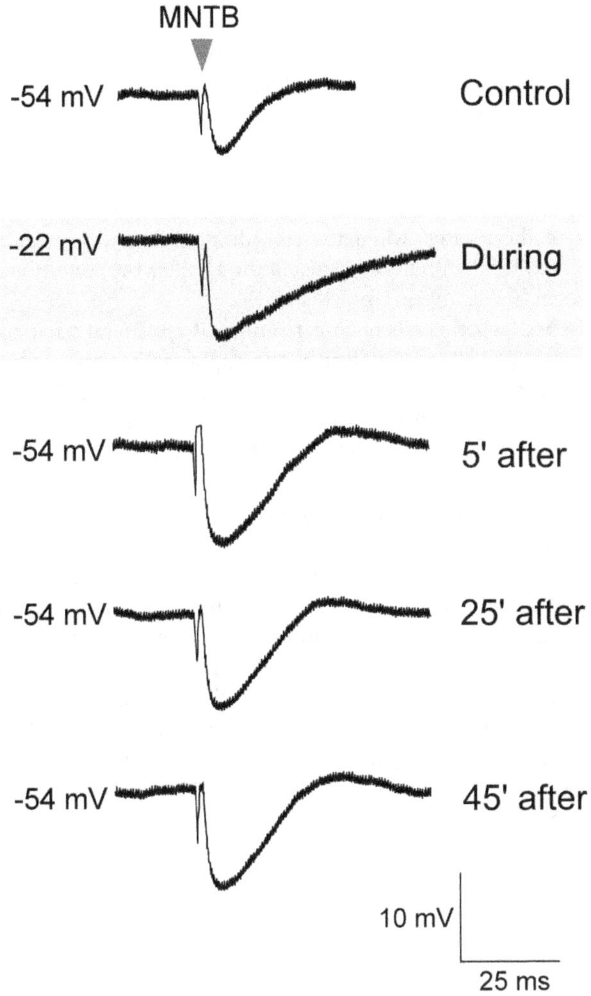

FIGURE 2 | Glutamate exposure potentiated MNTB-evoked IPSPs. Control MNTB-evoked IPSPs were recorded at 0.033 Hz. An initial response is shown in the top trace. While continuing with this stimulation, glutamate (10 mM) was bath perfused (45 s), and the neuron became depolarized (gray panel), and discharged intensely (not shown). After the cell had completely repolarized to its original resting potential, the IPSP amplitudes were significantly larger. Baseline IPSPs (pre glutamate) and those acquired during glutamate exposure and then at 5, 25, and 45 min after the cell had repolarized are shown.

Thus, early binaural cues may be critical in consolidating the functional maturation of LSO inhibitory synapses.

MATERIALS AND METHODS

All protocols were reviewed and approved by the New York University Institutional Animal Care and Use Committee. Gerbil pups *(Meriones unguiculatus)* aged postnatal (P) days 7–15, were used to generate 300 μm transverse brain slices containing the MNTB-LSO circuit (Sanes, 1993). The artificial cerebrospinal fluid (ACSF) contained (in mM): 125 NaCl, 4 KCl, 1.2 KH_2PO_4, 1.3 $MgSO_4$, 24 $NaHCO_3$, 15 glucose, 2.4 $CaCl_2$, and 0.4 L-ascorbic acid (pH = 7.3 when bubbled with 95% O_2/5% CO_2). ACSF was continuously superfused in the recordingchamber at 3 ml per min at 32 ± 1°C. Whole-cell current clamp or voltage or recordings were obtained from LSO neurons (Warner PC-501A) and 200 μs current pulses were delivered directly to the MNTB via bipolar stimulating electrodes to elicit IPSPs or IPSCs, respectively (Kotak et al., 1998). Ipsilateral excitatory afferents were stimulated by a separate bipolar stimulating electrodes at specific frequencies (Results) (**Figure 1**). Recording electrodes were fabricated from borosylicate glass microcapillaries (1.5 mm OD), and when filled with internal solution the resistance was 5–15 MΩ. For current clamp recordings, the internal patch solution contained (in mM): 127.5 mM potassium gluconate, 0.6 EGTA, 10 HEPES, 2 $MgCl_2$ 5 KCl, 2 ATP, and 0.3 GTP. For both internal solutions, the pH of was adjusted to 7.2 with KOH. For voltage clamp recordings, the internal solution was similar to current clamp solution (follows) except potassium gluconate was replaced by an equimolar concentration of cesium gluconate to block voltage-dependent potassium channels, and QX-314 (5 mM) was added to block voltage-dependent sodium channels. The pH was adjusted to 7.2 with CsOH. Further, kynurenic acid (4 mM) was added to the ACSF to block ionotropic glutamate receptors (Moore et al., 1998). Access resistance was balanced throughout the recordings and ranged between 10 and 40 MΩ.

All data were collected using a Macintosh G4 platform running a Mac OS X compatible custom IGOR (WaveMetrics, v3.5) macro called SLICE. The data were analyzed off-line using a second IGOR macro called SLICE ANALYSIS (Kotak et al., 2001). Custom algorithms were used to measure the amplitude and frequency of sIPSCs (Kotak et al., 2005). Data values are presented as mean and standard error of the mean (SEM). Initial IPSP/IPSC amplitudes were compared vs. IPSC amplitudes at the end of the recording session with a non-parametric test (Wilcoxon; Kotak and Sanes, 2000). All statistical analyses were performed using the SAS-based statistical software (JMP v5.0).

RESULTS

The data in this paper were collected from 60 principal neurons from 42 animals located in the high frequency medial limb of the LSO, each from a separate brain slice. We first asked whether iLTP could be induced under normal physiological conditions in a brain slice preparation without any intracellular or pharmacological manipulations. These current clamp recordings were similar to those employed for the induction of iLTD as described previously (Kotak and Sanes, 2000) except the stimulation rates and postsynaptic depolarization was different.

CURRENT CLAMP RECORDINGS

First, to determine whether IPSPs recorded in current clamp without glutamate receptor antagonists exhibited any change in strength, we attempted the following protocols. The stimulus to evoked IPSPs was first calibrated to evoke an IPSP at 50% of its maximum amplitude. This enabled us to observe the possible expression of either potentiation or depression. To do this, MNTB was stimulated in incremental intensity (200 μs, 5 μA increments) until maximum amplitude IPSP was obtained. We then selected the stimulus intensity that evoked an approximately 50% maximum amplitude (200 μs, ~80–90 μA).

Protocol i: IPSPs were recorded at a rate of 0.033 Hz for approximately 1 h. Under this condition, no change in amplitude was observed (initial IPSP amplitude: 7.4 ± 0.8 mV vs. IPSP amplitude at 60 min: 6.3 ± 0.7 mV; $t = 2.1$, $p > 0.05$; $n = 7$). *Protocol ii*: Our next step was to test MNTB stimulation rates of 0.1 or 5 Hz. These rates were dissimilar to the rate that produced iLTD (1 Hz, 15 min) in our previous study. Under these conditions, no significant change in IPSP amplitude was observed for up to 10 min (not shown). *Protocol iii*: LSO neurons were held slightly more depolarized (at −50 mV) than their resting membrane potential (ranged between −51 and −55 mV) by injection of a small DC current (+5–10 pA). This provided a steady membrane potential baseline against which inhibitory strength could be recorded. In addition, a suprathreshold depolarization (500 ms) was used to increase neuronal firing by up to 50 Hz, a firing rate that may elevate intracellular calcium to support induction of iLTP. Furthermore, a single MNTB-evoked IPSP was timed to occur 300 ms after the onset of postsynaptic depolarization. This regimen was ineffective in triggering iLTP ($n = 4$, not shown). *Protocol iv*: To test whether glutamatergic transmission was sufficient to induce iLTP, ipsilateral excitatory afferents were stimulated at 20 Hz (10 pulses) while cells were held at −50 mV. This protocol did not induce a significant change in IPSP amplitude ($n = 4$, not shown). Since each of these protocols was ineffective, we predicted that the induction of iLTP would require a greater level of postsynaptic glutamate receptor activation.

The protocol that proved to be effective, involved a combination of the above manipulations. *Protocol v*: Cells were held at −50 mV and a single 500 ms postsynaptic depolarization to induce up to 50 Hz firing was elicited with current injection. An increased level of ipsilateral excitatory afferent stimulation (100 Hz, 10 pulses) was timed to occur 10 ms after the onset of this depolarization. Lastly, MNTB stimulation was timed to occur 300 ms after the onset of the 500 ms postsynaptic depolarization (**Figure 1**, top panel). Under these conditions, IPSPs were potentiated for 20 min or longer (**Figure 1C**; initial IPSP amplitude: 5.9 ± 0.3 mV, IPSP amplitude 20 min after conditioning: 10.1 ± 0.6 mV; Wilcoxon test, $X^2 = 3.9$, $p = 0.001$, $n = 7$). In 4 of these cases, when the recording session was extended, increased IPSP amplitude persisted for 1 h after the conditioning protocol (9.7 ± 1.95 mV).

To test whether such co-activation of ipsilateral excitatory afferents could have involved postsynaptic activation of glutamate receptors to induce iLTP, in separate experiments, glutamate was bath applied (10 mM, 45 s) in the absence of ipsilateral afferent stimulation (Kotak and Sanes, 1995). Thus, this protocol was designed to bypass the possible co-recruitment of ipsilaterally evoked inhibition (Kotak and Sanes, 1997). Sub-maximum IPSPs were first elicited for 10 min to establish a baseline, before the application of glutamate. Glutamate treatment depolarized the LSO neurons from none to by up to 20 mV, and increased the discharge rate of recorded neurons from none up to 50 Hz. The MNTB stimulation was maintained during this depolarization for 30 min and MNTB stimulation continued after the cells had returned to the starting V_{REST}. As shown in **Figure 2**, when IPSPs were recorded after complete recovery of the membrane potential, we observed significantly enhanced IPSP amplitudes (IPSP pre-glutamate treatment: 8.4 ± 0.12 mV vs. IPSP 30 min after the recovery of membrane potential, 12.6 ± 0.2 mV; Wilcoxon test, $X^2 = 3.8$, $p < 0.05$, $n = 3$).

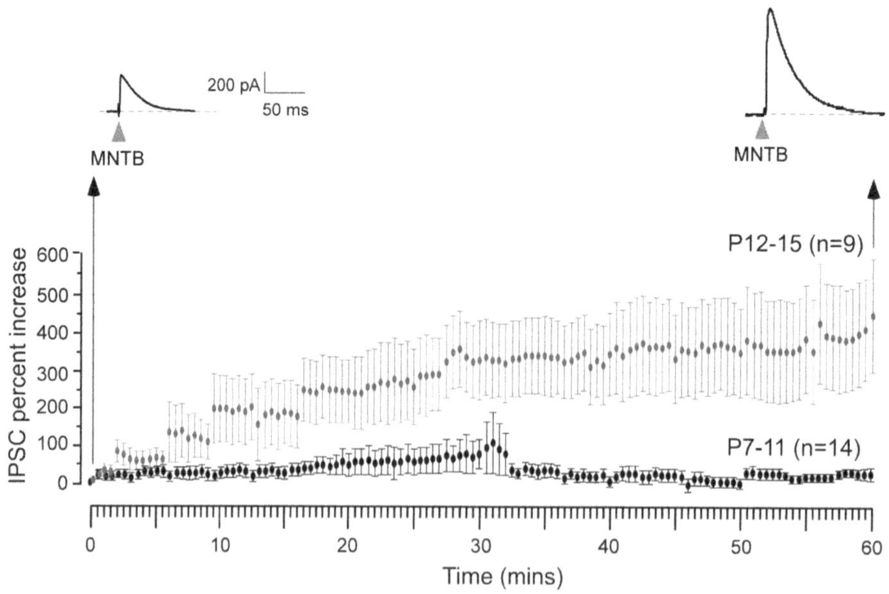

FIGURE 3 | Expression of iLTP is age-dependent. MNTB was continuously stimulated at 0.033 Hz for 1 h while voltage clamp recordings were obtained from the LSO neurons in the presence of ionotropic glutamate receptor antagonist kynuranic acid at $V_{HOLD} = 0$ mV. Under these circumstances, IPSCs were recorded as outward currents. An IPSC recorded 1 h after this stimulation protocol shows a dramatic enhancement in its amplitude (top right trace) when compared to the initial IPSC (top left trace). Long-term potentiation of IPSCs was observed for neurons recorded at P12–15 (gray symbols), but not at P7–11 (black symbols).

VOLTAGE CLAMP RECORDINGS

We then asked whether iLTP could be induced by stimulation of the MNTB afferents under voltage clamp conditions ($V_{HOLD} = 0$ mV, ionotropic glutamate receptors blocked, thus in an absence of ipsilateral afferent stimulation) identical to the recording conditions employed for experiments in which iLTD was induced (Kotak and Sanes, 2000). For iLTD induction, we had used low frequency stimulation paradigm (LFS, 1 Hz for 15 min) that led to long-term inhibitory depression for at least an hour. We could also induce and perturb iLTD in current clamp conditions using similar LFS regimen (Kotak et al., 2001). In pilot voltage clamp recordings when the MNTB was stimulated at a very low rate (0.033 Hz) to monitor baseline inhibitory strength we observed a small increase in IPSC amplitude. Therefore, we chose to carry out a full set of experiments using 0.033 Hz. Continuous stimulation of the MNTB at 0.033 Hz produced a gradual increase in IPSC amplitude, and this enhancement became progressively larger during the recording session. As shown in **Figure 3**, neurons from P12–15 animals displayed a ~400% increase in IPSC amplitude over the course of 1 hr, as compared to the initial baseline values (initial IPSC: 156 ± 26 pA vs. IPSC at 10 min of stimulation: 224 ± 74 pA, Wilcoxon test, $X^2 = 5$, $p = 0.02$; initial IPSC: 156 ± 26 pA vs. IPSC at 30 min of stimulation: 472 ± 90, $X^2 = 7.7$, $p = 0.005$; initial IPSC: 156 ± 26 pA vs. IPSC at 60 min of stimulation: 495 ± 94, $X^2 = 8.7$, $p = 0.003$; $n = 9$). When an identical stimulation protocol was employed on neurons from P7 to 11 animals, no significant change in IPSC amplitude was observed for up to 60 min (**Figure 3**). (Initial IPSC: 220 ± 68 pA vs. IPSC at 10 min of stimulation: 194 ± 54 pA, IPSC at 30 min of stimulation: 227 ± 58 pA, IPSC at 60 min of stimulation: 198 ± 67 pA, Wilcoxon test, $p > 0.05$ for each comparison; $n = 14$).

For controls, we have previously shown that the baseline of evoked IPSPs or IPSCs were stable through the entire 90 min recording session (see Figure 2 in Kotak and Sanes, 2000; Kotak et al., 2001). In the current study, whereas stimulation at 0.033 Hz produced robust iLTP after hearing onset, identical recording conditions and stimulation rates did not lead to any change in baseline sIPSCs before hearing onset (see **Figure 3**). Therefore, we did not perform additional controls. Voltage clamp recordings, similar to conditions in our previous iLTD studies (Kotak and Sanes, 2000; Chang et al., 2003), cells were held depolarized at 0 mV and 4 mM kynurenic acid was added to the ACSF (pH 7.3 after bubbling with O_2/CO_2) to block ionotropic AMPA and NMDA receptors. Spontaneous IPSCs (sIPSC) too were recorded as outward currents before and after the stimulation protocol at $V_{HOLD} = 0$ mV. The very low frequency stimulation paradigm (0.033 Hz) was then applied continuously through the recording session (1 h) both to induce plasticity as well as acquire IPSCs.

To assess whether there was any alteration in the presynaptic release properties following the conditioning protocol, spontaneous IPSC (sIPSC) amplitude and frequency were monitored at early (initial 10 min) and late (60 min) periods of the iLTP expression. As shown in **Figure 4**, these data indicate that iLTP was accompanied by a large increase in both the frequency and amplitude of spontaneous IPSCs (sIPSC amplitude before LTP: 6.3 ± 1.8 pA vs. sIPSC amplitude 60 min afterLTP: 61 ± 19.5 pA; Wilcoxon test, $X^2 = 7.8$, $p < 0.001$; sIPSC frequency before

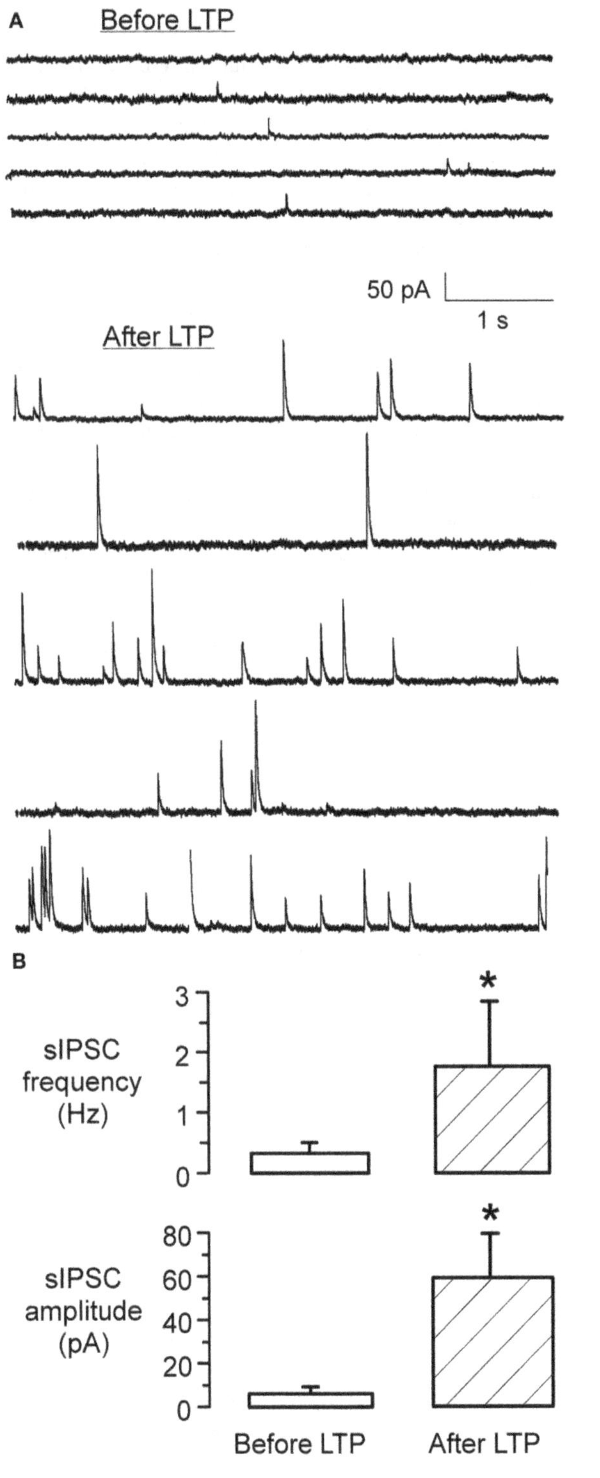

FIGURE 4 | iLTP is associated with increased sIPSC frequency and amplitude. (A) sIPSCs recorded in an LSO neuron before the induction of iLTP (top) displayed a low frequency and small amplitudes. In contrast, sIPSCs recorded from the same neuron after the induction of iLTP, during the last 5 min of the recording session, displayed a dramatic increase in frequency and amplitude (bottom). **(B)** Bar graph shows the significant increase in sIPSC frequency 1 h following the induction of LTP ($p < 0.001$) (top). Similarly, there was a dramatic increase in the mean amplitude of sIPSCs ($p = 0.01$) (bottom).

LTP: 0.28 ± 0.14 Hz vs. sIPSC frequency 60 min after LTP: 1.76 ± 1.2 Hz; Wilcoxon test, $X^2 = 6.9, p = 0.01$). Further, 1 h after iLTP induction, MNTB-evoked IPSCs could not be de-potentiated using an MNTB afferent stimulation pattern (LFS, 1 Hz, 15 min) previously shown to induce iLTD in naive slices (Kotak and Sanes, 2000). There was no significant difference between the IPSC amplitude at 60 min after LTP induction (541 ± 178 pA), as compared to the amplitude after an additional 15 min of 1 Hz/15 min stimulation (531 ± 163 pA; Wilcoxon test, $X^2 = 1.6$, $p > 0.1$; $n = 3$).

Our previous study showed that iLTD in the LSO requires the activation of $GABA_B$ receptors (Kotak et al., 2001). Therefore, we tested whether inhibitory LTP was also dependent on $GABA_B$ receptor activation using a specific $GABA_B$ receptor antagonist (SCH-50911) during induction of inhibitory LTP in P12–15 neurons. The MNTB was stimulated at the frequency that induced iLTP (0.033 Hz) in voltage clamp condition (Vh = 0 mV) while the slice was continuously exposed to 10 μM SCH-50911 ($n = 4$). As shown in **Figure 5**, the mean IPSC amplitude over an hour period did not display a significant change (initial IPSC: 260 ± 68 pA; IPSC at 60 min: 295 ± 56 pA, Wilcoxon test, $X^2 = 0.7, p = 0.8, n = 4$). Thus, inhibitory LTP was blocked by the SCH compound.

DISCUSSION

The major finding of this study is that inhibitory MNTB synapses onto the LSO display an activity-dependent long-term potentiation (iLTP) following hearing onset (P12) but not prior to that. This contrasts with the induction of an equally robust iLTD before hearing onset (Kotak and Sanes, 2000). We do not imply that transition from no iLTD to iLTP occurs suddenly or precisely at hearing onset; rather, such plasticity mechanisms may develop gradually and may even become more pronounced during the several weeks thereafter as sound coding properties associated with ILD are consolidated in the LSO. We had proposed that iLTD before hearing onset may underlie the elimination of redundant inhibitory synapses in LSO and MSO (Sanes and Siverls, 1991; Sanes and Takàcs, 1993; Kotak and Sanes, 2000; Kapfer et al., 2002; Kim and Kandler, 2003). Even as the numbers of inhibitory boutons per axon are decreased (Sanes and Takàcs, 1993), the strength of individual existing connections becomes much stronger as revealed by the increase in the amplitude of inhibitory events (Sanes, 1993; Kim and Kandler, 2003). Therefore, we propose that the emergence of iLTP may be one form of plasticity to support inhibitory synapse stabilization and strengthening *in vivo*.

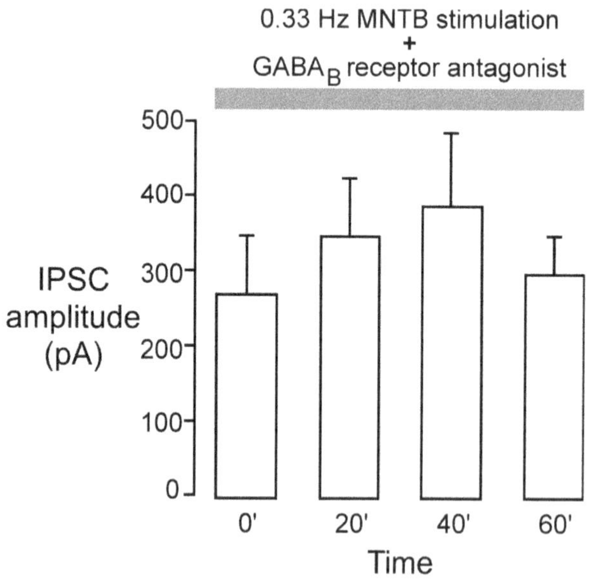

FIGURE 5 | $GABA_B$ receptor blockade perturbs inhibitory iLTP. MNTB was continuously stimulated at 0.033 Hz for 1 h while voltage clamp recordings were obtained from P12 to 15 LSO neurons in the presence of an ionotropic glutamate receptor antagonist (V_{HOLD} = 0 mV). The $GABA_B$ receptor blocker, SCH-50911 (10 μM), was present throughout the recordings. Under these conditions, IPSC amplitudes did not show any significant change toward potentiation. Each bar represents the mean current (±s.e.m.) calculated at the beginning of the experiment, and at 20, 40, and 60 min.

When coupled with MNTB stimulation, either postsynaptic depolarization alone, or activation of ipsilateral excitatory afferents alone, was not sufficient to induce iLTP under current clamp conditions. We propose two mechanisms that could mediate iLTP in an intact developing animal. First, sufficient postsynaptic depolarization could result from the synergistic activity of developing excitatory terminals and/or the co-release of glutamate from the MNTB terminals themselves (Gillespie and Kandler, 2005; Case and Gillespie, 2011; Alamilla and Gillespie, 2013). Second, it is possible that very low levels of glutamatergic afferent activity can activate postsynaptic metabotropic glutamate receptors, which trigger prolonged depolarizations and calcium entry by low levels of synaptic activity (Kotak and Sanes, 1995; Ene et al., 2003) that may be sufficient to support iLTP. This is consistent with our observation that IPSPs could be potentiated by the direct application of glutamate that may have led to calcium influx via activation of ionotropic as well as metabotropic glutamate receptors (**Figure 2**).

Our previous results have shown that $GABA_B$ receptors are involved in the generation of iLTD (Kotak et al., 2001). Similarly, it appears that $GABA_B$ receptors are involved in iLTP. Both sets of experiments were performed in voltage clamp conditions where the internal recording solution contained QX-314, which blocks the postsynaptic $GABA_B$ receptor-gated K^+ channel (Nathan et al., 1990; Andrade, 1991). The fact we did not observe iLTP in the presence of a selective antagonist (SCH-50911) could be consistent with either pre- or postsynaptic $GABA_B$ receptor signaling (**Figure 5**). One reason for this is that blockade of the $GABA_B$ receptor-gated potassium conductance by QX-314 in the pipette solution leaves open the possibility that other second messengers are involved (Kotak et al., 2001). In addition, the increase in sIPSC frequency that occurs during iLTP (**Figure 4**) suggests that a presynaptic mechanism may accompany postsynaptic strengthening.

The adjustments of auditory neuron response properties to dynamic range, frequency, or sound location during early life may well depend on activity-dependent synaptic plasticity mechanisms (Sanes and Constantine-Paton, 1983, 1985; Knudsen et al., 1984; Joseph and Hyson, 1993; Zhang et al., 2001;

Magnusson et al., 2008). For mature LSO principal neurons to properly compute ILDs, the excitatory and inhibitory synapses must become precisely matched along the tonotopic axes during development (Moore and Caspary, 1983; Spangler et al., 1985; Cant and Casseday, 1986; Sanes and Rubel, 1988; Glendenning et al., 1991; Sanes and Siverls, 1991). Our observations raise the possibility that increased inhibitory synapse strength may permit these to stabilize during the time when specificity is achieved *in vivo*.

AUTHOR CONTRIBUTIONS

Vibhakar C. Kotak and Dan H. Sanes conceived and designed the experiments, Vibhakar C. Kotak performed the experiments and analyzed the data, and Vibhakar C. Kotak and Dan H. Sanes wrote the paper.

REFERENCES

Aizenman, C. D., Manis, P. B., and Linden, D. J. (1998). Polarity of long-term synaptic gain change is related to postsynaptic spike firing at a cerebellar inhibitory synapse. *Neuron* 21, 827–835. doi: 10.1016/S0896-6273(00)80598-X

Alamilla, J., and Gillespie, D. C. (2013). Maturation of calcium-dependent GABA, glycine, and glutamate release in the glycinergic MNTB-LSO pathway. *PLoS ONE* 8:e75688. doi: 10.1371/journal.pone.0075688

Andrade, R. (1991). Blockade of neurotransmitter-activated K conductance by QX-314 in the rat hippocampus. *Eur. J. Pharmacol.* 199, 259–262. doi: 10.1016/0014-2999(91)90467-5

Bear, M., and Malenka, R. C. (1994). Synaptic plasticity: LTP and LTD. *Curr. Opin. Neurobiol.* 4, 389–400. doi: 10.1016/0959-4388(94)90101-5

Bliss, T. V. P., Collingridge, G. L., and Morris, R. G. M. (2013). Synaptic plasticity in health and disease: introduction and overview. *Philos. Trans. R. Soc. Lond. B Biol. Sci.* 369, 20130129. doi: 10.1098/rstb.2013.0129

Boudreau, J. C., and Tsutchitani, C. (1968). Binaural interaction the cat superior olive s-segment. *J. Neurophysiol.* 31, 442–454.

Caird, D., and Klinke, R. (1983). Processing of binaural stimuli by cat superior olivary complex neurons. *Exp. Brain Res.* 52, 385–399. doi: 10.1007/BF00238032

Cant, N. B., and Casseday, J. H. (1986). Projections from the anteroventral cochlear nucleus to the lateral and medial superior olivary nuclei. *J. Comp. Neurol.* 247, 457–476. doi: 10.1002/cne.902470406

Case, D. T., and Gillespie, D. C. (2011). Pre- and postsynaptic properties of glutamatergic transmission in the immature inhibitory MNTB-LSO pathway. *J. Neurophysiol.* 106, 2570–2579. doi: 10.1152/jn.00644.2010

Chang, E. H., Kotak, V. C., and Sanes, D. H. (2003). Long-term depression of synaptic inhibition is expressed postsynaptically in the developing auditory system. *J. Neurophysiol.* 90, 1479–1488. doi: 10.1152/jn.00386.2003

Ene, F. A., Kullman, P. H., Gillespie, D. C., and Kandler, K. (2003). Glutamatergic calcium responses in the developing lateral superior olive: receptor types and their specific activation by synaptic activity patterns. *J. Neurophys.* 90, 2581–2591. doi: 10.1152/jn.00238.2003

Gillespie, D. C., and Kandler, K. (2005). Inhibitory synapses in the developing auditory system are glutamatergic. *Nat. Neurosci.* 8, 332–338. doi: 10.1038/nn1397

Glendenning, K. K., Masterton, R. B., Baker, B. N., and Wenthold, R. J. (1991). Acoustic chiasm. *III*: Nature, distribution, and sources of afferents to the lateral superior olive in the cat. *J. Comp. Neurol.* 310, 377–400. doi: 10.1002/cne.903100308

Harnischfeger, G., Neuweiler, G., and Schlegel, P. (1985). Interaural time and intensity coding in superior olivary complex and inferior colliculus of the echo locating bat *Molossus ater*. *J. Neurophysiol.* 53, 89–109.

Joseph, A. W., and Hyson, R. L. (1993). Coincidence detection by binaural neurons in the chick brain stem. *J. Neurophysiol.* 69, 1197–1211.

Kandler, K. (2004). Activity-dependent organization of inhibitory circuits: lessons from the auditory system. *Curr. Opin. Neurobiol.* 14, 96–104. doi: 10.1016/j.conb.2004.01.017

Kandler, K., Clause, A., and Jihyun, N. J. (2009). Tonotopic reorganization of developing auditory brainstem circuits. *Nat. Neurosci.* 12, 711–717. doi: 10.1038/nn.2332

Kandler, K., and Gillespie, D. C. (2005). Developmental refinement of inhibitory sound-localization circuits. *TINS* 28, 290–296. doi: 10.1016/j.tins.2005.04.007

Kapfer, C., Seidl, A. H., Schweizer, H., and Grothe, B. (2002). Experience-dependent refinement of inhibitory inputs to auditory coincidence-detector neurons. *Nat. Neurosci.* 5, 247–253. doi: 10.1038/nn810

Kim, G., and Kandler, K. (2003). Elimination and strengthening of glycinergic/GABAergic connections during tonotopic map formation. *Nat. Neurosci.* 6, 282–290. doi: 10.1038/nn1015

Knudsen, E. I., Esterly, S. D., and Knudsen, P. F. (1984). Monaural occlusion alters sound localization during a sensitive period in the barn owl. *J. Neurosci.* 4, 1001–1011.

Komatsu, Y. (1994). Age-dependent long-term potentiation of inhibitory synaptic transmission in rat visual cortex. *J. Neurosci.* 14, 6488–6499.

Komatsu, Y. (1996). $GABA_B$ receptors, monoamine receptors, and postsynaptic inositol trisphosphate-induced Ca^{2+} release are involved in the induction of long-term potentiation at visual cortical inhibitory synapses. *J. Neurosci.* 16, 6342–6352.

Komatsu, Y., and Iwakiri, M. (1993). Long-term modification of inhibitory synaptic transmission in developing visual cortex. *Neuroreport* 4, 907–910. doi: 10.1097/00001756-199307000-00017

Komatsu, Y., and Yoshimura, Y. (2000). Activity-dependent maintenance of long-term potentiation at visual cortical inhibitory synapses. *J. Neurosci.* 15, 7539–7546.

Kotak, V. C., DiMattina, C., and Sanes, D. H. (2001). GABA(B) and Trk receptor signaling mediates long-lasting inhibitory synaptic depression. *J. Neurophysiol.* 86, 536–540.

Kotak, V. C., Fujisawa, S., Lee, F. A., Karthikeyan, O., Aoki, C., and Sanes, D. H. (2005). Hearing loss raises excitability in the auditory cortex. *J. Neurosci.* 25, 3908–3918. doi: 10.1523/JNEUROSCI.5169-04.2005

Kotak, V. C., Korada, S., Schwartz, I. R., and Sanes, D. H. (1998). A developmental shift from GABAergic to glycinergic transmission in the central auditory system. *J. Neurosci.* 18, 4646–4655.

Kotak, V. C., and Sanes, D. H. (1995). Synaptically evoked prolonged depolarizations in the developing auditory system. *J. Neurophysiol.* 74, 1611–1620.

Kotak, V. C., and Sanes, D. H. (1997). Deafferentation of glutamatergic afferents weakens synaptic strength in the developing auditory system. *Eur. J. Neurosci.* 9, 2340–2347.

Kotak, V. C., and Sanes, D. H. (2000). Long-lasting inhibitory synaptic depression is age- and calcium-dependent. *J. Neurosci.* 20, 5820–5826.

Kotak, V. C., and Sanes, D. H. (2002). Postsynaptic kinase signaling underlies inhibitory synaptic plasticity in the lateral superior olive. *J. Neurobiol.* 53, 36–43. doi: 10.1002/neu.10107

Magnusson, A. K., Park, T. J., Pecka, M., Grothe, B., and Koch, U. (2008). Retrograde GABA signaling adjusts sound localization by balancing excitation and inhibition in the brainstem. *Neuron* 59, 125–137. doi: 10.1016/j.neuron.2008.05.011

Moore, D. R., Kotak, V. C., and Sanes, D. H. (1998). Commissural and lemniscal synaptic input to the gerbil inferior colliculus. *J. Neurophysiol.* 80, 2229–2236.

Moore, M. J., and Caspary, D. M. (1983). Strychnine blocks binaural inhibition in lateral superior olivary neurons. *J. Neurosci.* 3, 237–242.

Morishita, W., and Sastry, B. R. (1996). Postsynaptic mechanisms underlying long-term depression of GABAergic transmission in neurons of the deep cerebellar nuclei. *J. Neurophysiol.* 76, 59–68.

Nathan, T., Jensen, M. S., and Lambert, J. D. (1990). The slow inhibitory postsynaptic potential in rat hippocampal CA1 neurones is blocked by intracellular injection of QX-314. *Neurosci. Lett.* 110, 309–313. doi: 10.1016/0304-3940(90)90865-7

Oda, Y., Charpier, S., Murayama, Y., Suma, C., and Korn, H. (1995). Long-term potentiation of glycinergic inhibitory synaptic transmission. *J. Neurophysiol.* 74, 1056–1074.

Oda, Y., Kawasaki, K., Morita, M., Korn, H., and Matsui, H. (1998). Inhibitory long-term potentiation underlies auditory conditioning of goldfish escape behavior. *Nature* 394, 182–185. doi: 10.1038/28172

Ouardouz, M., and Sastry, B. R. (2000). Mechanisms underlying LTP of inhibitory synaptic transmission int he deep cerebellar nuclei. *J. Neurophysiol.* 84, 1414–1421.

Sanes, D. H. (1993). The development of synaptic function and integration in the central auditory system. *J. Neurosci.* 13, 2627–2637.

Sanes, D. H., and Constantine-Paton, M. (1983). Altered activity patterns during development reduce neural tuning. *Science* 221, 1183–1185. doi: 10.1126/science.6612332

Sanes, D. H., and Constantine-Paton, M. (1985). The development of stimulus following the cochlear nerve and inferior colliculus of the mouse. *Brain Res.* 354, 255–267. doi: 10.1016/0165-3806(85)90177-4

Sanes, D. H., and Friauf, E. (2000). Development and influence of inhibition in the lateral superior olivary nucleus. *Hear. Res.* 147, 46–58. doi: 10.1016/S0378-5955(00)00119-2

Sanes, D. H., and Rubel, E. W. (1988). The ontogeny of inhibition and excitation in the gerbil lateral superior olive. *J. Neurosci.* 8, 682–700.

Sanes, D. H., and Siverls, V. (1991). Development and specificity of inhibitory terminal arborizations in the central nervous system. *J. Neurobiol.* 22, 837–854. doi: 10.1002/neu.480220805

Sanes, D. H., and Takàcs, C. (1993). Activity-dependent refinement of inhibitory connections. *Eur. J. Neurosci.* 5, 570–574. doi: 10.1111/j.1460-9568.1993.tb00522.x

Spangler, K. M., Warr, W. B., and Henkel, C. K. (1985). The projections of principal cells of the medial nucleus of the trapezoid body in the cat. *J. Comp. Neurol.* 238, 249–262. doi: 10.1002/cne.902380302

Sterenborg, J. C., Pilati, N., Sheridan, C. J., Uchitel, O. D., Forsythe, I. D., and Barnes-Davies, M. (2010). Lateral olivocochlear (LOC) Neurons of the mouse LSO receive excitatory and inhibitory synaptic inputswith slower kinetics than LSO principal neurons. *Hear. Res.* 270, 119–126. doi: 10.1016/j.heares.2010.08.013

Tollin, D. J. (2003). The lateral superior olive: a functional role in sound source localization. *Neuroscientist* 9, 127–143. doi: 10.1177/1073858403252228

Walcher, J., Hassfurth, B., Grothe, B., and Koch, U. (2011). Comparative posthearing development of inhibitory inputs to the lateral superior olive in gerbils and mice. *J. Neurophysiol.* 106, 1443–1453. doi: 10.1152/jn.01087.2010

Zhang, L., Bao, S., and Merzenich, M. M. (2001). Persistent and specific influences of early acoustic environments on primary auditory cortex. *Nat. Neurosci.* 4, 1123–1130. doi: 10.1038/nn745

7

Interplay between low threshold voltage-gated K^+ channels and synaptic inhibition in neurons of the chicken nucleus laminaris along its frequency axis

William R. Hamlet[1,2], Yu-Wei Liu[1], Zheng-Quan Tang[1†] and Yong Lu[1,2] *

[1] Department of Anatomy and Neurobiology, College of Medicine, Northeast Ohio Medical University, Rootstown, OH, USA
[2] School of Biomedical Sciences, Kent State University, Kent, OH, USA

***Correspondence:**
Yong Lu, Department of Anatomy and Neurobiology, College of Medicine, Northeast Ohio Medical University, Rootstown, OH, USA
e-mail: ylu@neomed.edu

†Present address:
Zheng-Quan Tang, Oregon Hearing Research Center and Vollum Institute, Oregon Health & Science University, Portland, OR, USA

Central auditory neurons that localize sound in horizontal space have specialized intrinsic and synaptic cellular mechanisms to tightly control the threshold and timing for action potential generation. However, the critical interplay between intrinsic voltage-gated conductances and extrinsic synaptic conductances in determining neuronal output are not well understood. In chicken, neurons in the nucleus laminaris (NL) encode sound location using interaural time difference (ITD) as a cue. Along the tonotopic axis of NL, there exist robust differences among low, middle, and high frequency (LF, MF, and HF, respectively) neurons in a variety of neuronal properties such as low threshold voltage-gated K^+ (LTK) channels and depolarizing inhibition. This establishes NL as an ideal model to examine the interactions between LTK currents and synaptic inhibition across the tonotopic axis. Using whole-cell patch clamp recordings prepared from chicken embryos (E17–E18), we found that LTK currents were larger in MF and HF neurons than in LF neurons. Kinetic analysis revealed that LTK currents in MF neurons activated at lower voltages than in LF and HF neurons, whereas the inactivation of the currents was similar across the tonotopic axis. Surprisingly, blockade of LTK currents using dendrotoxin-I (DTX) tended to broaden the duration and increase the amplitude of the depolarizing inhibitory postsynaptic potentials (IPSPs) in NL neurons without dependence on coding frequency regions. Analyses of the effects of DTX on inhibitory postsynaptic currents led us to interpret this unexpected observation as a result of primarily postsynaptic effects of LTK currents on MF and HF neurons, and combined presynaptic and postsynaptic effects in LF neurons. Furthermore, DTX transferred subthreshold IPSPs to spikes. Taken together, the results suggest a critical role for LTK currents in regulating inhibitory synaptic strength in ITD-coding neurons at various frequencies.

Keywords: GABAergic inhibition, voltage-gated low-threshold potassium current, IPSC, IPSP, tonotopy, whole-cell patch, interaural time difference

INTRODUCTION

Neurons rely on a variety of intrinsic and synaptic neuronal properties to ensure precise coding of temporal information from sensory inputs. An extensive body of research has demonstrated the prominent roles of synaptic inhibition in auditory neurons that encode the location of sound in azimuth space using interaural time difference (ITD) as a cue (e.g., Grothe and Sanes, 1993, 1994; Funabiki et al., 1998; Brand et al., 2002; Grothe, 2003; Zhou et al., 2005; Pecka et al., 2008; Fukui et al., 2010). These neurons encode sound location by producing maximal spiking activity when bilateral excitatory inputs from the two cochleae converge, a process termed coincidence detection (Jeffress, 1948; Konishi, 2003; MacLeod and Carr, 2012). Synaptic inhibition can improve coincidence detection via shunting the impact of depolarizing postsynaptic currents on the membrane potential and thus sharpening the time window for spike generation (Brückner and Hyson, 1998; Funabiki et al., 1998; Ingham and McAlpine, 2005; Howard and Rubel, 2010; Tang et al., 2011; Roberts et al., 2013).

In most mature neurons, synaptic inhibition mediated by ionotropic $GABA_A$ and glycine receptors produces conventional hyperpolarizing inhibitory postsynaptic currents (IPSCs). In contrast, GABAergic and glycinergic IPSCs in chicken auditory brainstem neurons are depolarizing, caused by a depolarized reversal potential for Cl^- (between −45 and −35 mV) that appears to be maintained in mature animals (Hyson et al., 1995; Lu and Trussell, 2001; Monsivais and Rubel, 2001; Kuo et al., 2009; Tang et al., 2009). Of particular interest, sound-localizing neurons in the nucleus laminaris (NL) of the chick receive depolarizing inhibitory inputs originating primarily from ipsilateral superior olivary nucleus (SON) neurons and sparsely from local GABAergic neurons (von Bartheld et al., 1989; Code and Churchill, 1991; Lachica et al., 1994; Yang et al., 1999; Burger et al., 2005; Tang et al., 2011; Yamada et al., 2013). There exists a tonotopic distribution of GABAergic inhibition along the frequency axis of NL. Neurons coding low frequency (LF) sound receive small and fast phasic inhibition with minimal tonic inhibition, whereas neurons coding middle and high frequency (MF and HF, respectively) sound receive large and slow phasic inhibition with prominent tonic inhibition (Tang et al., 2011; Tang and Lu, 2012; Yamada et al., 2013). The depolarizing inhibition improves coincidence detection via both a shunting effect of the GABAergic conductance and the activation of a low threshold voltage-gated K^+ (LTK) conductance (Funabiki et al., 1998; Monsivais et al., 2000; Howard et al., 2007; Tang et al., 2011).

LTK currents are prominent in auditory brainstem neurons involved in sound localization circuitry (Manis and Marx, 1991; Forsythe and Barnes-Davies, 1993; Reyes et al., 1994; Brew and Forsythe, 1995; Rathouz and Trussell, 1998; Golding et al., 1999; Brew et al., 2003; Barnes-Davies et al., 2004). In these neurons, LTK currents minimize the impact of small and slow excitatory postsynaptic currents (EPSCs) on membrane potential, regulate the threshold for action potential generation, and suppress hyperexcitability at presynaptic terminals (Dodson et al., 2002, 2003; Svirskis et al., 2002; Scott et al., 2005; Gittelman and Tempel, 2006; Mathews et al., 2010). Ion channels containing subunits from K_{v1}, K_{v4}, and K_{v7} subfamilies underlie the LTK currents (Coetzee et al., 1999; Johnston et al., 2010). In the tonotopically organized NL (Rubel and Parks, 1975), $K_{v1.1}$and $K_{v1.2}$ subunits show stronger anatomical expression in MF and HF neurons compared to LF neurons, and physiological data also suggests stronger LTK channel activity at rest in MF and HF neurons (Kuba et al., 2005). Therefore, LTK channels are poised to strongly affect synaptic integration of depolarizing synaptic inputs, particularly in MF and HF neurons. Given the unusual depolarizing nature of the inhibitory input to NL neurons and the robust presence of LTK channels in these neurons, it is important to determine how LTK currents interact with synaptic inhibition at subthreshold and suprathreshold membrane potentials, and how this interaction differs across the tonotopic axis.

MATERIALS AND METHODS

SLICE PREPARATION AND *IN VITRO* WHOLE-CELL RECORDINGS

Brainstem slices (250–300 μm in thickness) were prepared from chick embryos E17–E18 as described previously (Tang et al., 2009). An ice-cold artificial CSF (ACSF) used for dissecting and slicing the brain tissue contained the following (in millimolar): 250 glycerol, 3 KCl, 1.2 KH_2PO_4, 20 $NaHCO_3$, 3 HEPES, 1.2 $CaCl_2$, 5 $MgCl_2$, and 10 dextrose (pH 7.4 when gassed with 95% O_2 and 5% CO_2). The procedures were approved by the Institutional Animal Care and Use Committee at Northeast Ohio Medical University, and are in accordance with National Institutes of Health policies on animal use. Slices were incubated at 34–36°C for approximately 1 h in normal ACSF containing the following (in millimolar): 130 NaCl, 26 $NaHCO_3$, 3 KCl, 3 $CaCl_2$, 1 $MgCl_2$, 1.25 NaH_2PO_4, and 10 dextrose, pH 7.4. For recording, slices were transferred to a 0.5 ml chamber mounted on an upright Olympus BX51 microscope (Japan) with a 40× water-immersion objective. The chamber was continuously superfused with ACSF (1–2 ml/min) by gravity. Recordings were performed at 34–36°C, except K_v current recordings which were performed at 22–24°C (room temperature). Patch pipettes were drawn on an Electrode Puller PP-830 (Narishige) to 1–2 μm tip diameter using borosilicate glass micropipettes (inner diameter of 0.86 mm; outer diameter of 1.60 mm) (VWR Scientific). Electrode resistance was between 3 and 5 MΩ when filled with a solution containing the following (in millimolar): 105 K-gluconate, 35 KCl, 5 EGTA, 10 HEPES, 1 $MgCl_2$, 4 ATP-Mg, and 0.3 GTP-Na, with pH of 7.2 (adjusted with KOH) and osmolarity between 280 and 290 mOsm/L. The Cl^- concentration (37 mM) in the internal solution approximated the physiological Cl^- concentration in NL neurons (Tang et al., 2009). Placement of recording electrodes was controlled by a micromanipulator NMN-25 (Narishige). The liquid junction potential was 10 mV, and data were corrected accordingly. Voltage- and current clamp experiments were performed with an AxoPatch 200B and an AxoClamp 2B amplifier, respectively (Molecular Devices). Voltage-clamp recordings were obtained at a holding potential of −60 mV. Data were low-pass filtered at 2–10 kHz and digitized with a Data Acquisition Interface ITC-18 (InstruTECH) at 20 kHz. Recording protocols were written and run using the acquisition and analysis software AxoGraph X (AxoGraph Scientific). In K_v current recordings, R_s compensation was done at approximately 75%. When Rs changed more than 25% during recording, the neuron was not included in data analysis. In current clamp experiments, bridge balance was used to compensate for the voltage drop across the electrode resistance.

All chemicals were purchased from Sigma–Aldrich except: (1*S*,2*S*)-2-[2-[[3-(1*H*-Benzimidazol-2-yl)propyl]methylamino] ethyl]-6-fluoro-1,2,3,4-tetrahydro-1-(1-methylethyl)-2-naphthal enyl methoxyacetoacetate dihydrochloride (Mibefrandil), 4-Ethylphenylamino-1,2-dimethyl-6-methylaminopyrimidinium chloride (ZD-7288), which were obtained from Tocris, and 6-imino-3-(4-methoxyphenyl)-1(6*H*)-pyridazine butanoic acid (SR95531), and 6,7-Dinitroquinoxaline-2,3-dione (DNQX) which were obtained from Abcam.

SYNAPTIC STIMULATION AND RECORDINGS OF SYNAPTIC RESPONSES

Extracellular stimulation was performed using concentric bipolar electrodes with a tip core diameter of 127 μm (World Precision Instruments). The stimulating electrodes were placed using a Micromanipulator NMN-25 (Narishige) at the lateral fiber bundle, which carries both excitatory and inhibitory fibers. Blockade of AMPA receptors with DNQX (20 μM) completely blocks EPSCs, so all synaptic recordings were done in the presence of DNQX. Square electric pulses (0.2 ms duration) were delivered through a Stimulator A320RC (World Precision Instruments). Optimal stimulation parameters were selected for each cell to give postsynaptic potentials of maximal amplitude. In experiments designed to examine the effect of LTK currents on subthreshold responses, QX-314 (5 mM) was included in the pipette solution to block Na_v channels. A comparison of K_v recordings with and without QX-314 in the pipette solution showed little to no difference in LTK current size, although QX-314 can block other K^+ conductances (Andrade, 1991; Alreja and Aghajanian, 1994).

IDENTIFICATION OF TONOTOPIC CHARACTERISTIC FREQUENCY (CF) REGION

It is not possible to define the characteristic frequency of NL neurons in an *in vitro* slice preparation. Therefore, to categorize neurons into LF, MF, and HF regions, we used an approach modified from Kuba et al. (2005), by using the rostral–caudal and medial–lateral position as an indicator of CF. Generally five slices of brainstem tissue containing relevant nuclei were collected, and the most caudal one was slice #1 and the most rostral one slice #5. Neurons in the lateral NL of slices #2 and #3 were considered LF neurons. MF neurons were considered to be present in the medial NL of slice #2 and #3 and the lateral portion of slice #4. HF neurons were found in the medial portion of slice #4 and in slice #5 (**Figure 1**). Images were taken with a Provis AX70 (Olympus) microscope using SPOT software (Diagnostic Instruments), from freshly sliced tissue. Image contrast and colorization was adjusted using Creative Suites v2.0 (Adobe). Because boundaries between the regions are subjective, we recorded from neurons clearly present in one of the three CF regions.

DATA ANALYSIS

The resting membrane potential was read from the amplifiers immediately after the whole-cell configuration was established. The input resistance was calculated from the voltage responses to a somatic current injection (50 pA). Current density was calculated by normalizing the raw current to each cell's membrane capacitance, obtained during C_m compensation prior to recording. For K_V current recordings, leak subtraction was performed using a linear fitting to $V_{command}$ −100 to −70 mV. The amount of inactivated current was calculated by subtracting the maximum current (I_{max}) evoked during the $V_{command}$ from the minimum current (I_{min}) evoked during the $V_{command}$. Current activation was measured by a single exponential function, $f(t) = A^*\exp(-t/\text{decay } \tau)$, in which t stands for time and τ for time constant. Spontaneous synaptic events were detected by a template using a function for product of exponentials, $f(t) = [1 - \exp(-t/\text{rise time})]^*\exp(-t/\text{decay } \tau)$. Due to differences in synaptic event size and shape within the NL, the values of these parameters for the template were determined based on the average of real events from individual cells. The detection threshold was three to four times the noise standard deviation, which allowed for a detection rate with the least number of false positives. Graphs were made in Igor (Wavemetrics). Means and SEMs are reported. Prior to hypothesis testing, normality and outliers were observed within each set of data to determine the appropriate statistical test. Outliers (>3× larger than the interquartile range) were dropped from the dataset. Wilks-Shapiro test was used to confirm whether sample distributions were approximately normally distributed. Violations of normality were present when $p < 0.05$. When significant violations of normality were present or where datasets contained $n_i \leq 7$, nonparametric inferential statistical tests were used. Statistical differences were determined by Analysis of Variance (ANOVA) and Kruskal–Wallis test for parametric and nonparametric samples, respectively. When significant group differences were found, a Tukey's *post hoc* test or Mann–Whitney U-test was conducted. Paired-sample t-tests were conducted for repeated-measures sample comparisons. Alpha-levels were corrected using the Holm–Bonferroni method.

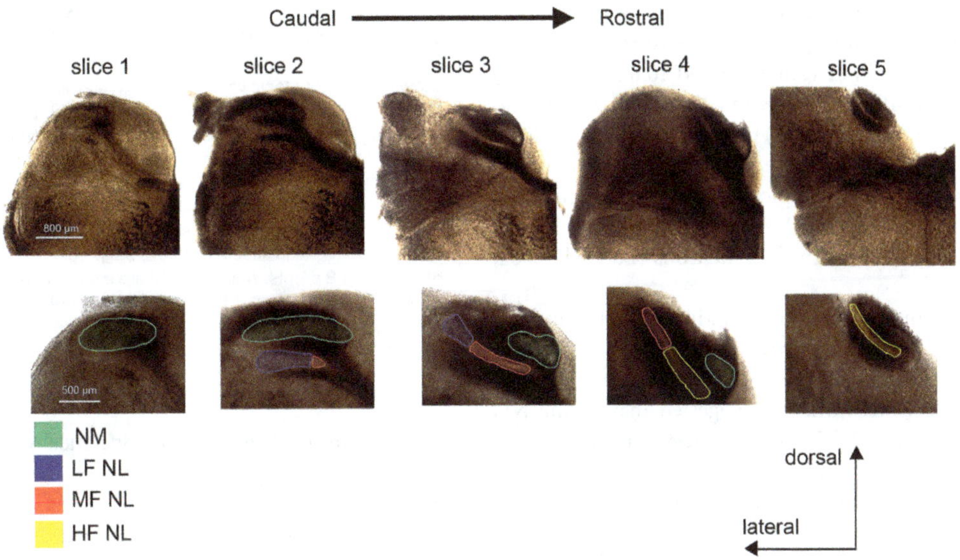

FIGURE 1 | Determination of characteristic frequency (CF) regions of nucleus laminaris (NL) in coronal brainstem slices. Typically a total of five slices (300 μm in thickness) from each animal were collected and numbered #1 through #5, in a caudal to rostral direction. Slice #1 is characterized by the nucleus magnocellularis (NM, green) without NL. The NM is present in all but slice #5. The NL appears in slice #2 and contains mostly low frequency (LF, blue) neurons, with some middle frequency (MF, red) neurons present at the most medial end. MF neurons are most prevalent in slice #3, with LF neurons at the lateral end of the nucleus. In slice #4, HF (yellow) neurons are located in the medial portion of the NL while MF neurons are found laterally. In slice #5 only HF neurons are present. The colored boundaries between CF regions are approximate.

RESULTS

Nucleus laminaris neurons were categorized into three groups based on CF region as function of position: caudolateral, caudomedial/rostrolateral, and rostromedial neurons corresponded to LF, MF, and HF groups, respectively (**Figure 1**). A total of 162 neurons were recorded, with 50, 57, and 55 cells from the LF, MF, and HF regions, respectively.

CHARACTERIZATION OF LTK CURRENTS ALONG THE FREQUENCY AXIS OF NL

In order to assess the interaction between LTK currents and synaptic inhibition, a detailed analysis of LTK currents along the frequency axis of NL was conducted. LTK currents were isolated in the presence of blockers for Na_V channels (TTX, 1 μM), low threshold Ca_V channels (Mibefrandil, 10 μM), HCN channels (ZD7288, 80 μM), AMPA receptors (DNQX, 20 μM), and $GABA_A$ receptors (Gabazine, 20 μM). LTK currents showed a striking tonotopic variation in the amplitude of the onset current (I_{Onset}, measured at 4–9 ms after the onset of the $V_{command}$) and steady state current (I_{SS}, measured at 94–99 ms) (**Figure 2**). Because K_V currents activated at −40 mV primarily represent the LTK component, with little contamination of high threshold K_V (HTK) (Brew and Forsythe, 1995; Wang et al., 1998), we analyzed and compared LTK current amplitude at −40 mV. I_{Onset} was significantly smaller in LF ($n = 15$, 0.4 ± 0.2 nA) compared to MF ($n = 19$, 1.3 ± 0.2 nA) and HF ($n = 16$, 1.1 ± 0.2 nA) neurons, and no difference was observed between MF and HF neurons ($p = 0.002$, **Figure 2D**). I_{SS} at −40 mV was also significantly smaller in LF (0.6 ± 0.2 nA) neurons than in MF (1.4 ± 0.2 nA) neurons but not HF (1.3 ± 0.2 nA) neurons ($p = 0.021$, **Figure 2H**). Due to differences in membrane area across the tonotopic axis (gradual reduction in area from LF to MF and HF regions), current density (defined as the ratio of current amplitude over cell capacitance) was compared. Both I_{Onset} and I_{SS} densities at −40 mV were significantly smaller in LF (7.6 ± 4.1 and 10.0 ± 4.5 pA/pF) neurons compared to MF (26.1 ± 3.8 and 27.1 ± 4.0 pA/pF) and HF (34.0 ± 4.0 and 38.4 ± 4.4 pA/pF) neurons (I_{Onset}: $p < 0.0001$; I_{ss}: $p < 0.0001$, **Figures 2E,I**). These results confirm anatomical data that there is a robust tonotopic variation in LTK channels in NL neurons such that MF and HF neurons have substantially higher LTK current amplitude than LF neurons (Lu et al., 2004; Kuba et al., 2005).

Coincident detecting neurons in the auditory brainstem have fast membrane time constants, partly due to a strong active LTK conductance at rest (Kuba et al., 2005; Scott et al., 2005; Mathews et al., 2010). Previous work has suggested that in the NL, MF neurons possess more LTK current at rest than LF and HF neurons (Kuba et al., 2005), however little is known about the amount of active LTK conductances at rest along the tonotopic axis. Therefore, we assessed how much LTK current was available at rest (approximately −60 mV for NL neurons; Reyes et al., 1994; Funabiki et al., 1998; Gao and Lu, 2008) by introducing a −90 mV pre-pulse (1000 ms duration) prior to the voltage commands (100 ms duration) (**Figure 3**). At −60 mV, neither I_{Onset} nor I_{SS} amplitude was significantly different across the tonotopic axis (**Figures 3D,H**). However, the onset and steady state current density of MF neurons were significantly higher than that of LF and HF neurons (**Figures 3E,I**). Specifically, a significant difference in I_{Onset} density between MF ($n = 7$, 8.9 ± 1.9 pA/pF) and HF ($n = 10$, 2.1 ± 1.7 pA/pF) emerged ($p = 0.038$) (**Figure 3E**), and I_{SS} density of MF neurons (10.9 ± 2.3 pA/pF) was higher compared to LF ($n = 8$, 3.5 ± 2.3 pA/pF) neurons ($p = 0.041$, **Figure 3I**). To some extent, LTK current was active at rest in all CF regions, with MF neurons having the largest conductance.

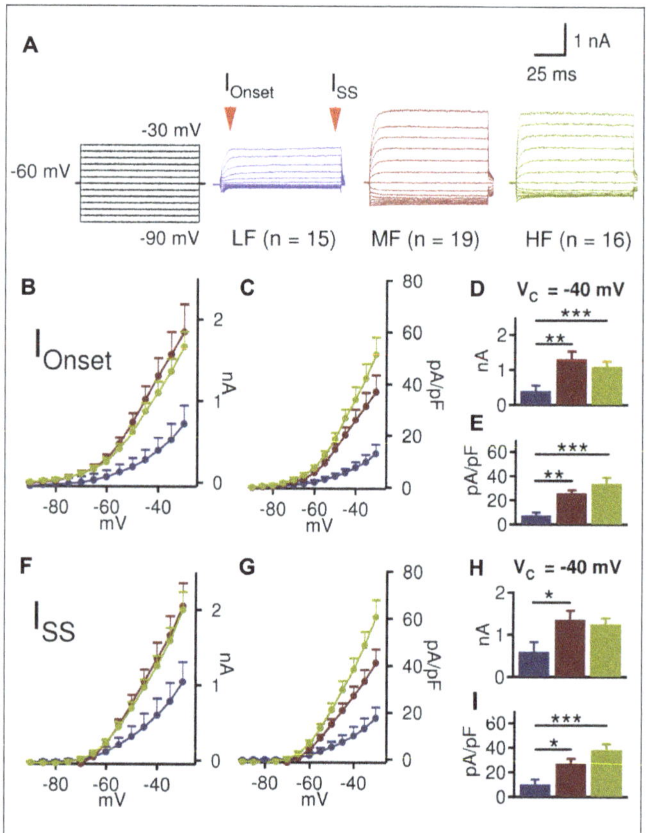

FIGURE 2 | MF and HF NL neurons have larger low threshold voltage-gated K⁺ (LTK) currents than LF neurons. (A) Sample protocol ($V_{hold} = -60$ mV; $V_{Command} = -90$ to −30 mV, 100 ms duration), and representative LTK current recordings from LF (blue, $n = 15$), MF (red, $n = 19$), and HF (yellow, $n = 16$) NL neurons. **(B,C)** Onset current (I_{Onset}) amplitude and current density in MF and HF neurons are higher than those in LF neurons. **(D)** At −40 mV, LF (0.4 ± 0.2 nA) neurons have significantly smaller I_{Onset} than MF (1.3 ± 0.2 nA) and HF (1.1 ± 0.1 nA) neurons. MF and HF neurons do not significantly differ. **(E)** I_{Onset} density at −40 mV shows similar tonotopic variations to I_{Onset} amplitude (LF: 7.6 ± 2.1 pA/pF; MF: 26.1 ± 4.1 pA/pF; and HF: 34.0 ± 4.9 pA/pF). **(F,G)** Steady state current (I_{SS}) amplitude and current density reveal similar tonotopic variations to I_{Onset}, with higher current amplitude and density in MF and HF neurons compared to LF neurons. **(H)** At −40 mV, LF (0.6 ± 0.2 nA) neurons have significantly smaller I_{SS} than MF (1.4 ± 0.2 nA) and HF (1.3 ± 0.1 nA) neurons. **(I)** I_{SS} density at −40 mV shows similar tonotopic variations to I_{SS} amplitude (LF: 10.0 ± 3.9 pA/pF; MF: 27.1 ± 4.1 pA/pF; and HF: 38.4 ± 4.8 pA/pF). Mean ± SEM are shown in this and subsequent figures. $^*p < 0.05$, $^{**}p < 0.01$, $^{***}p < 0.001$ (ANOVA, Tukey's *post hoc* analysis, unless otherwise indicated). Cells were held at −60 mV for voltage clamp experiments.

Low threshold voltage-gated K⁺ current kinetics may also vary across the tonotopic axis, which may influence how LTK currents interact with inhibitory synaptic input. Therefore we assessed LTK kinetics across the tonotopic axis by examining LTK activation and

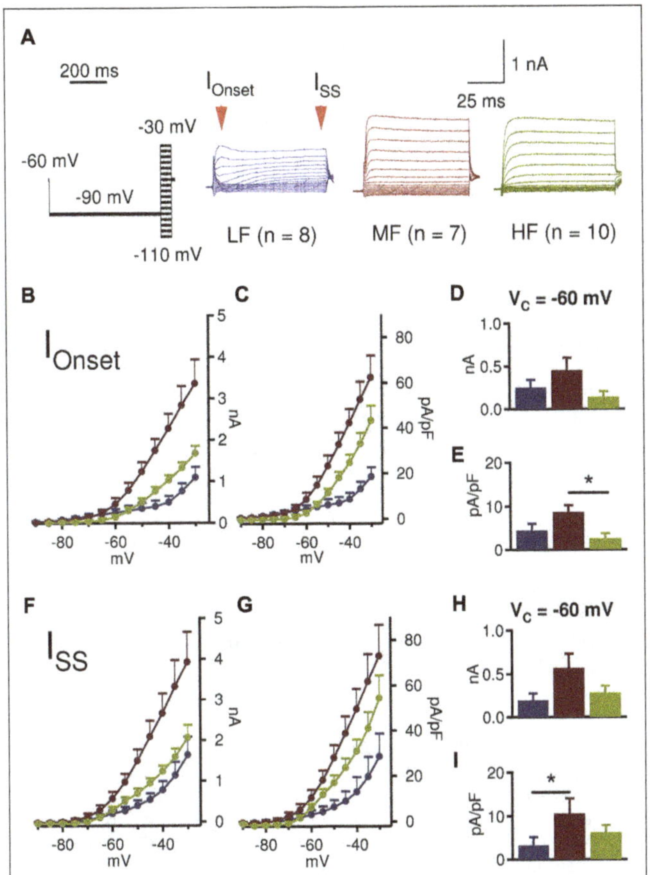

FIGURE 3 | MF neurons have higher LTK conductance active at rest. **(A)** Sample protocol ($V_{hold} = -60$ mV, $V_{prepulse} = -90$ mV, 1000 ms duration; $V_C = -110$ to -30 mV, 100 ms duration), and representative LTK current recordings from LF (blue, $n = 8$), MF (red, $n = 7$), and HF (yellow, $n = 10$) NL neurons. **(B–E)** At −60 mV, MF (0.5 ± 0.1 nA) neurons appear to have higher I_{Onset} amplitude than LF (0.3 ± 0.1 nA) and HF (0.2 ± 0.1 nA) neurons. The I_{Onset} density at −60 mV in MF (8.9 ± 1.9 pA/pF) neurons is significantly higher than in HF (2.1 ± 1.7 pA/pF) neurons, while LF neurons have intermediate current density (4.3 ± 1.9 pA/pF). **(F,G)** I_{SS} amplitude and current density reveal similar tonotopic variations to I_{Onset}. **(H)** I_{SS} amplitude at −60 mV in MF (0.6 ± 0.1 nA) neurons seems to be higher than LF (0.2 ± 0.1 nA) and HF (0.3 ± 0.1 nA) neurons. **(I)** I_{SS} density at −60 mV in MF (10.9 ± 2.3 pA/pF) neurons is significantly higher than in LF (3.5 ± 2.3 pA/pF) neurons. HF neurons have intermediate current density (5.4 ± 2.0 pA/pF). Kruskal–Wallis tests with follow-up Mann–Whitney *U*-tests. $*p < 0.05$, $**p < 0.01$, $***p < 0.001$.

steady state inactivation. For activation kinetics, we analyzed the fast membrane time constants ($\tau < 10$ ms) because they are relevant to the peak amplitude and rise time of the depolarizing synaptic conductances. To do this, we used an exponential function, $f(t) = A*\exp(-t/\text{decay } \tau)$. A fast τ was found in most MF (14/19) and HF (13/16) neurons but in less than half LF (5/14 cells) neurons (**Figure 4A**). The absence of a fast τ in many LF neurons may suggest that LF neurons lack prominent fast activating LTK currents. At −45 mV, MF (1.6 ± 0.3 ms) neurons had a significantly faster τ than LF (2.3 ± 0.3 ms) and HF (3.1 ± 0.5 ms) neurons (**Figure 4B**, $p = 0.018$). LTK inactivation was analyzed from K_V currents obtained at two voltages: −45 and −30 mV (**Figure 4C**). While at −45 mV virtually only LTK currents were activated, the current evoked at −30 mV may be contaminated by small amounts of HTK currents (Brew and Forsythe, 1995; Wang et al., 1998). In many recordings, a fast transient inward current was evoked at −45 and −30 mV, likely caused by a low threshold Ca_V current incompletely blocked by Mibefrandil (Blackmer et al., 2009). Because the fast inward current corrupted accurate measurement of I_{Onset}, we analyzed I_{SS} LTK inactivation. I_{SS} showed relatively little inactivation and similar kinetics across the tonotopic axis. Nonetheless, HF neurons had slightly less LTK channel inactivation (15–25% inactivated) compared to LF (20–30%) and MF (20–30%) neurons (**Figures 4D–F**). MF ($n = 8$, 0.45 ± 0.8 nA) had a larger amount of current inactivation compared to LF ($n = 11$, 0.14 ± 0.6 nA) and HF ($n = 11$, 0.19 ± 0.6 nA) neurons at −45 mV ($p = 0.008$, **Figure 4G**). No tonotopic differences in the amount of current inactivation were observed at −30 mV (**Figure 4H**). Taken together, these data suggest that LTK inactivation kinetics is relatively similar across the tonotopic axis, and the LTK currents are more readily activated in MF neurons.

One caveat to the LTK currents reported here is that the recordings were made at room temperature to achieve a better voltage clamp (Rathouz and Trussell, 1998). LTK currents at physiological temperature would be expected to be slightly larger in peak amplitude and show faster activation kinetics (Cao and Oertel, 2005). Another caveat is the use of embryonic neurons in this study. Although K_V currents are relatively mature by E18 (Gao and Lu, 2008), there is evidence that membrane conductances including LTK currents increase after E21 (Kuba et al., 2002). However, the effects of DTX on the firing properties of NL neurons are similar between early chick hatchlings and late embryos (Kuba et al., 2002). Despite these caveats, our data confirm and elaborate on previous research, indicating that LTK current size and kinetics vary across the tonotopic axis of NL.

CHARACTERIZATION OF IPSPS ALONG THE FREQUENCY AXIS OF NL

The driving question behind this study is how LTK currents differentially modulate depolarizing inhibitory postsynaptic potentials (IPSPs) in NL neurons. Prior work from our lab has demonstrated a robust tonotopic difference in synaptic inhibition in the NL. LF neurons show less frequent spontaneous inhibitory postsynaptic currents (sIPSCs) than MF and HF neurons, and IPSCs of LF neurons are smaller and faster (Tang et al., 2011; Tang and Lu, 2012). We sought to confirm these tonotopic variations in current clamp recordings (**Figure 5**). Evoked IPSPs were isolated by stimulating the fiber bundle lateral to the NL in the presence of AMPA receptor blocker DNQX (20 μM). To prevent action potentials from occurring on the top of IPSP, QX-314 (5 mM) was included in the intracellular recording solution. A comparison of LTK currents recorded with and without QX-314 in the pipette solution revealed little to no difference in LTK currents (data not shown). No tonotopic differences in IPSP peak amplitude and 10–90% rise time were observed (**Figures 5B,C**). However, IPSP half width was significantly different across the tonotopic axis (**Figure 5D**, $p = 0.035$). The half width of IPSPs was significantly larger in HF ($n = 13$, 97.3 ± 32.8 ms) neurons compared to LF ($n = 14$, 39.0 ± 9.6 ms) neurons, while MF ($n = 14$, 61.3 ± 13.0 ms) neurons had an intermediate value. Analysis of spontaneous IPSPs (sIPSPs) revealed that while there

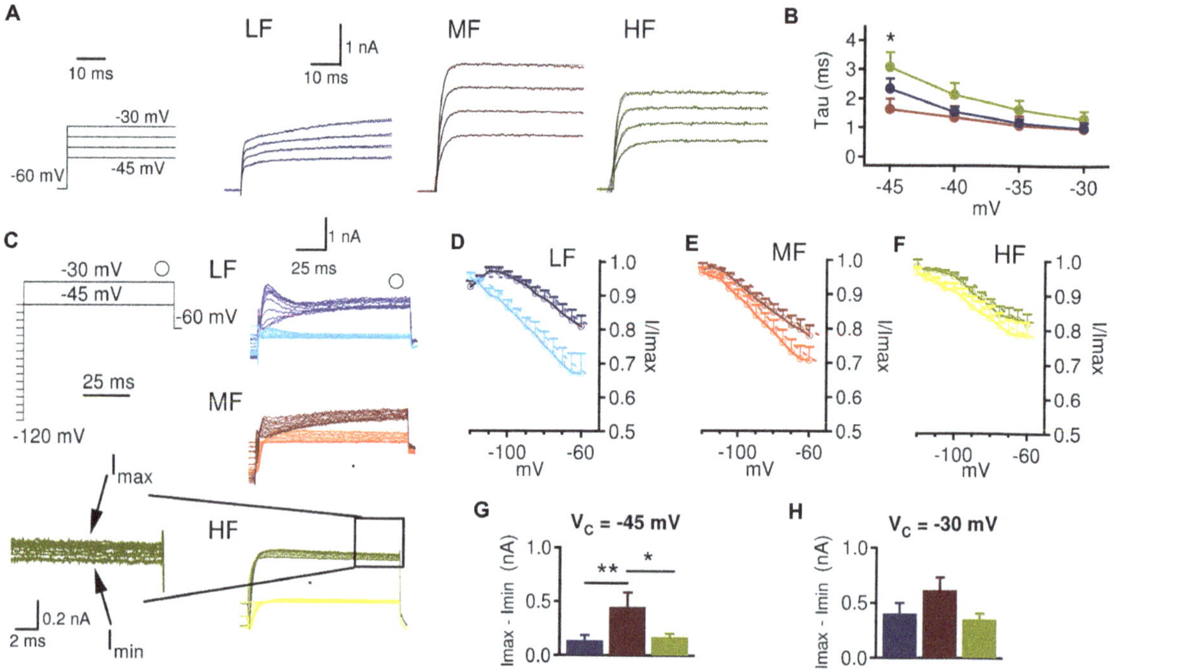

FIGURE 4 | LTK currents in MF neurons are of faster activation and stronger inactivation than in LF and HF neurons. (A) To obtain the time constant (τ) for LTK current activation, a single exponential fitting (black dashed line) was performed on the LTK currents recorded at V_C from −45 to −30 mV (V_{hold} = −60 mV). **(B)** At −45 mV, MF (1.6 ± 0.3 ms) neurons have significantly faster τ than LF (2.3 ± 0.3 ms) and HF (3.1 ± 0.5 ms) neurons. Kruskal–Wallis tests with follow-up Mann–Whitney *U*-tests. **(C)** Sample protocol used to study LTK inactivation at −45 and −30 mV following increasing voltage steps (−120 to −45 mV, 100 ms duration, and 5 mV increment). The open circle indicates where I_{SS} was measured. The traces with darker colors were obtained at −30 mV and those with lighter colors at −45 mV. Inset shows the I_{max} and I_{min} used to calculate the amount of inactivated current. **(D)** Normalized I_{SS} inactivation at −45 (n = 11, $V_{1/2}$ = −83.9 mV; k = 19.6) and −30 mV (n = 13, $V_{1/2}$ = −71.9 mV; k = 7.7) in LF neurons. **(E)** Normalized I_{SS} inactivation at −45 (n = 8, $V_{1/2}$ = −83.1 mV; k = 14.4) and −30 mV (n = 12, $V_{1/2}$ = −82.3 mV; k = 13.8) in MF neurons. **(F)** Normalized I_{SS} inactivation at −45 (n = 11, $V_{1/2}$ = −85.0 mV; k = 13.6) and −30 mV (n = 12, $V_{1/2}$ = −82.5 mV; k = 8.6) in HF neurons. **(G, H)** The raw amount of inactivated current was calculated by subtracting the maximum current from the minimum I_{SS}. MF (0.45 ± 0.8 nA) neurons had significantly more inactivated LTK current at −45 mV than LF (0.14 ± 0.6 nA) and HF (0.19 ± 0.6 nA) neurons. No differences between CF regions were observed in the amount of inactivated LTK current at −30 mV. $^*p < 0.05$, $^{**}p < 0.01$.

was no tonotopic variation in the sIPSP kinetics (half width and rise time), the frequency and peak amplitude of sIPSPs were different across the tonotopic axis (**Figures 5E–I**). The inter-event interval (IEI) of sIPSPs was significantly smaller in MF (n = 14, 120.0 ± 11.0 ms) and HF (n = 13, 120.4 ± 21.4 ms) neurons compared to LF (n = 12, 333.3 ± 58.9 ms) neurons (**Figure 5F**, p = 0.001). Peak amplitude was also significantly different across the tonotopic axis (**Figure 5G**, p = 0.003). LF neurons had smaller sIPSP amplitude (1.6 ± 0.2 mV) compared to MF (3.3 ± 0.3 mV) and HF (2.5 ± 0.2 mV). The data on sIPSP frequency and amplitude are consistent with our previous voltage clamp studies on sIPSC parameters (Tang et al., 2011; Tang and Lu, 2012). The lack of differences in sIPSP kinetics across CF regions may result from differential influences of LTK currents and other intrinsic conductances on the depolarizing inhibition.

INTERACTIONS BETWEEN LTK CURRENTS AND IPSPS ALONG THE FREQUENCY AXIS OF NL

To assess the role of LTK currents in regulating subthreshold changes in membrane potentials caused by activation of inhibitory inputs to NL neurons, we studied the effects of DTX (0.08 μM), a selective blocker for K_{v1}-subunit containing channels (Harvey, 2001), on IPSPs (**Figure 6**) and sIPSPs (**Figure 7**). DTX significantly increased the input resistance (R_{in}) in MF (n = 12, control: 51.6 ± 6.5 MΩ, DTX: 101.2 ± 16.9 MΩ, p = 0.008) and HF (n = 11, control: 68.6 ± 6.8 MΩ, DTX: 108.1 ± 12.0 MΩ, p = 0.001) neurons, but not in LF (n = 12, control: 88.4 ± 8.2 MΩ, DTX: 126.6 ± 26.5 MΩ, p = 0.054) neurons (**Figure 6B**). R_{in} was increased significantly more in MF (99.8 ± 25.6%) compared to LF (38.3 ± 13.2%) neurons (p = 0.028) (**Figure 6C**), agreeing with Kuba et al. (2005). DTX significantly increased the peak IPSP amplitude in all CF regions: LF (control: 6.7 ± 0.8 mV, DTX: 14.5 ± 2.1 mV, p = 0.004), MF (control: 7.8 ± 1.4 mV, DTX: 11.7 ± 2.1 mV, p = 0.030), and HF (control: 6.8 ± 1.1 mV, DTX: 12.5 ± 2.1 mV, p = 0.002, **Figure 6D**). DTX also increased the half width of IPSPs all CF regions: LF (control: 50.9 ± 9.6 ms, DTX: 97.6 ± 14.8 ms, p = 0.002), MF (control: 66.2 ± 13.0 ms, DTX: 179.3 ± 59.2 ms, p = 0.040) and HF (control: 79.4 ± 32.8 ms, DTX: 197.4 ± 73.6 ms, p = 0.028) neurons (**Figure 6F**). No tonotopic differences in the percent effect of DTX on IPSP peak amplitude or half width were detected (**Figures 6E,G**). The analysis of coefficient of variation (CV) of synaptic responses can be

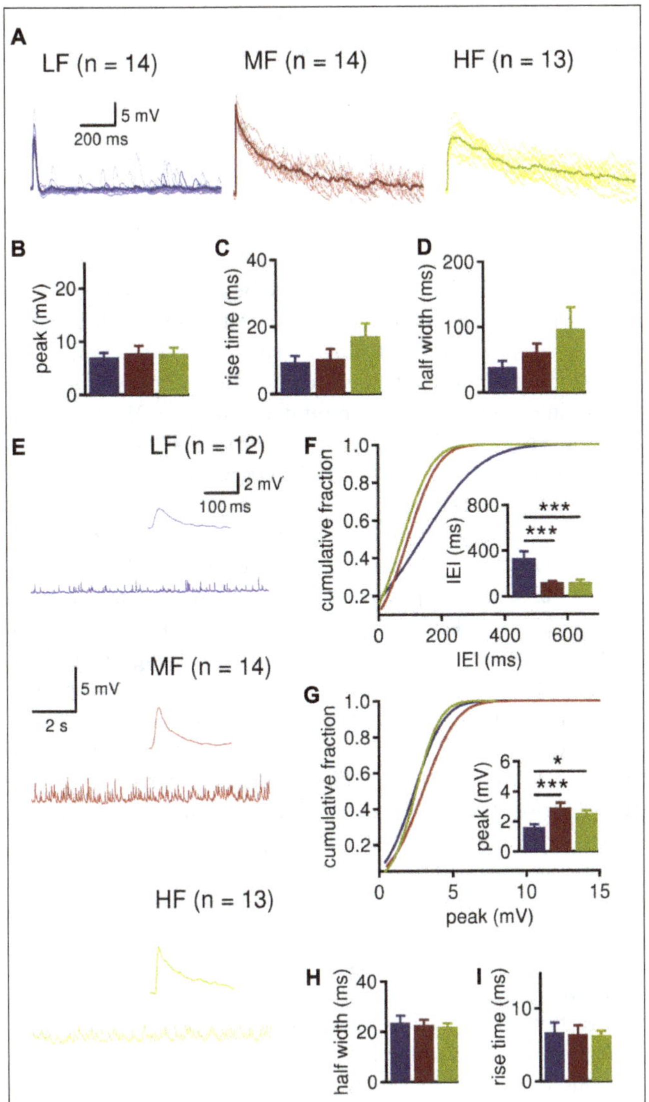

FIGURE 5 | MF and HF neurons tend to have wider IPSPs and larger sIPSPs than LF neurons. (A) Sample evoked inhibitory postsynaptic potentials (IPSP) recordings (the average traces shown as thicker lines). A square current pulse (0.2 ms) was delivered to a mixed excitatory and inhibitory fiber tract, and IPSPs were isolated in the presence of DNQX (20 μM). QX-314 (5 mM) was present in the intracellular solution to prevent action potentials in the recorded neurons. LF (blue, $n = 14$) neurons tend to have more narrow IPSPs than MF (red, $n = 14$) and HF (yellow, $n = 13$) neurons. **(B)** Peak IPSP amplitude is not significantly different in LF (7.1 ± 0.8 mV), MF (7.8 ± 1.4 mV), and HF (7.7 ± 1.1 mV) neurons. **(C)** 10–90% rise time of IPSP is not significantly different in LF (9.5 ± 1.9 ms), MF (10.4 ± 3.0 ms), and HF (17.1 ± 3.8 ms) neurons. **(D)** The half width of IPSPs is significantly larger in HF (97.3 ± 32.8 ms) neurons compared to LF (39.0 ± 9.6 ms) neurons. MF (61.3 ± 13.0 ms) neurons do not differ from LF or HF neurons. **(E)** Sample spontaneous IPSP (sIPSP) recordings from LF (blue, $n = 12$), MF (red, $n = 14$), and HF (yellow, $n = 13$) neurons, with a sample single sIPSP shown as an inset. **(F)** MF (120.0 ± 11.0 ms) and HF (120.4 ± 21.4 ms) neurons have significantly shorter inter-event intervals (IEI) than LF (333.3 ± 58.9) neurons. **(G)** LF neurons (1.6 ± 0.2 mV) have smaller sIPSP peak amplitude than MF (3.3 ± 0.3 mV) and HF (2.5 ± 0.2 mV) neurons. **(H,I)** sIPSP half width and 10–90% rise time are not different between CF regions. $^{*}p < 0.05$, $^{**}p < 0.01$, $^{***}p < 0.001$.

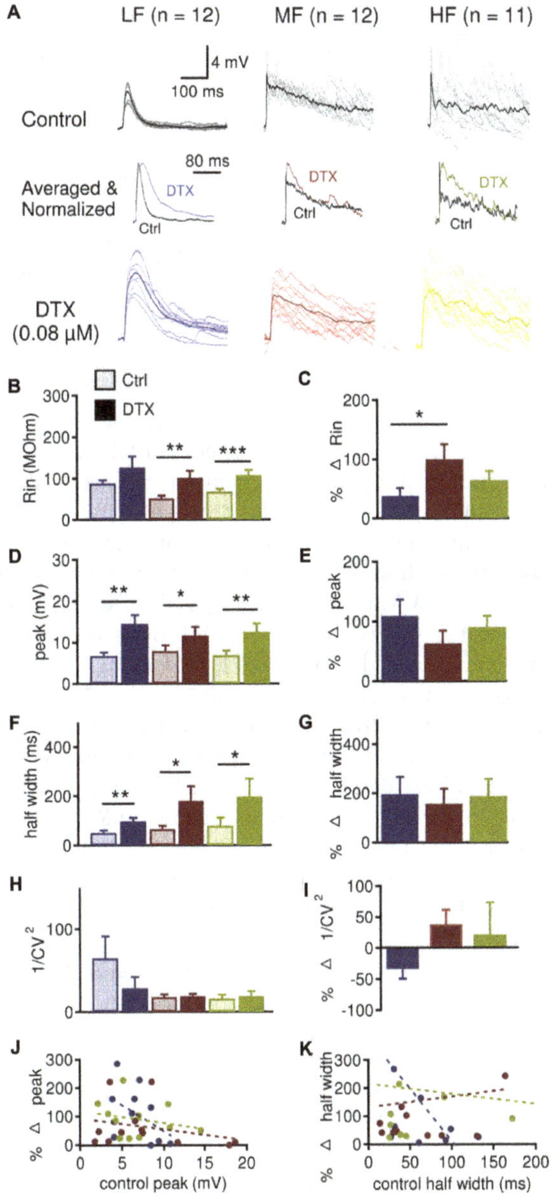

FIGURE 6 | LTK currents regulate evoked IPSP size in the NL. (A) Sample IPSP recordings before (dark traces) and after (color traces) bath application of DXT (0.08 μM), in LF ($n = 12$), MF ($n = 12$) and HF ($n = 11$) NL neurons. QX-314 (5 mM) was present in the intracellular solution. Above and below are raw (gray or light color) and averaged (black or dark color) IPSP recordings. Normalized averaged IPSP recordings before (black) and after (color) dendrotoxin I (DTX) are shown in the center. **(B)** DTX significantly increased the input resistance (R_{in}) in MF (control: 51.6 ± 6.5 MΩ, DTX: 101.2 ± 16.9 MΩ), and HF (control: 68.6 ± 6.8 MΩ, DTX: 108.1 ± 12.0 MΩ) neurons but not in LF (control: 88.4 ± 8.2 MΩ, DTX: 126.6 ± 26.5 MΩ) neurons. **(C)** R_{in} was increased significantly more in MF (99.8 ± 25.6%) compared to LF (38.3 ± 13.2%) neurons, while HF (64.2 ± 15.8%) did not differ from LF or MF neurons. **(D)** DTX significantly increased the peak IPSP amplitude in LF (control: 6.7 ± 0.8 mV, DTX: 14.5 ± 2.1 mV), MF (control 7.8 ± 1.4 mV, DTX: 11.7 ± 2.1 mV), and HF (control: 6.8 ± 1.1 mV, DTX: 12.5 ± 2.1 mV) neurons. **(E)** No tonotopic differences in the effect of DTX on peak IPSP amplitude were observed. **(F)** DTX significantly increased the half width of IPSP in LF (control: 50.9 ± 9.6 ms, DTX: 97.6 ± 14.8 ms), MF (control: 66.2 ± 13.0 ms,

(Continued)

FIGURE 6 | Continued
DTX: 179.3 ± 59.2 ms) or HF (control: 79.4 ± 32.8 ms, DTX: 197.4 ± 73.6 ms) neurons. **(G)** No tonotopic differences in the effect of DTX on IPSP half width. **(H)** $1/CV^2$ was not significantly changed in LF, MF, or HF neurons after DTX application. **(I)** Percent change in $1/CV^2$ was not significantly different across the tonotopic axis. **(J)** Peak IPSP amplitude plotted against the percent change in peak amplitude after DTX reveals that neurons with smaller IPSP peak amplitudes showed a greater change in IPSP peak amplitude after DTX treatment. The change appeared to be larger in LF ($r^2 = 0.215$, $p = 0.076$) neurons than MF ($r^2 = 0.067$) and HF ($r^2 = 0.061$) neurons. **(K)** IPSP half width plotted against the percent change in half width after DTX reveals that neurons with smaller IPSP half width showed a greater change in IPSP half width after DTX treatment. The change appeared to be larger in LF ($r^2 = 0.347$, $p = 0.022$) neurons than MF ($r^2 = 0.009$) and HF ($r^2 = 0.010$) neurons. $^*p < 0.05$, $^{**}p < 0.01$, $^{***}p < 0.001$.

used as one indicator of whether changes in IPSP size and shape is due to pre- or postsynaptic mechanism (Scheuss et al., 2002; Clements, 2003). No significant differences in $1/CV^2$ were found between control and DTX conditions, nor among CF regions (**Figures 6H–I**). However, LF (64.9 ± 26.1) neurons had significantly larger $1/CV^2$ in control conditions than MF (18.0 ± 3.2) and HF (16.1 ± 4.6) neurons ($p = 0.041$, not shown in figure) and LF neurons tended to show a reduction in $1/CV^2$ after DTX application (control: 64.9 ± 26.1; DTX: 28.7 ± 13.5; $p = 0.069$). LF neurons also showed a correlation between control IPSP peak amplitude and half width with their respective percent changes (amplitude: $r^2 = 0.215$, $p = 0.076$; half width: $r^2 = 0.347$, $p = 0.022$) after DTX application (**Figures 6J,K**). These data demonstrate that LTK currents regulate the size and shape of IPSPs in NL neurons across the entire frequency axis and suggest the possibility of a presynaptic component of this effect in LF neurons.

These findings were somewhat surprising because MF and HF neurons had stronger LTK current amplitude and density than LF neurons (**Figures 2** and **3**), and therefore MF and HF neurons were expected to show a greater change in IPSP parameters than LF neurons. One potential explanation for this apparent discrepancy is that presynaptic LTK currents regulate the inhibitory inputs to LF neurons to a greater extent than in MF and HF neurons. Analysis of the effects of DTX on sIPSP supported this hypothesis (**Figure 7**). DTX significantly decreased IEI in LF ($n = 11$, control: 347.2 ± 63.1 ms, DTX: 192.3 ± 30.2 ms, $p = 0.011$) but not in MF ($n = 13$, control: 119.4 ± 12.8 ms, DTX: 124.7 ± 15.1 ms, $p = 0.646$) and HF ($n = 10$, control: 129.4 ± 24.8 ms, DTX: 164.5 ± 57.2 ms, $p = 0.374$) neurons (**Figure 7B**). The percent decrease in IEI was significantly different in LF (−35.3 ± 10.4%) neurons compared to MF (8.1 ± 9.8%) and HF (15.5 ± 14.4%) neurons ($p = 0.017$, **Figure 7C**). There was a significant increase in sIPSP peak amplitude after DTX treatment in LF (control: 1.5 ± 0.2 mV, DTX: 2.1 ± 0.4 mV, $p = 0.010$) and HF (control: 2.5 ± 0.2 mV, DTX: 3.2 ± 0.4 mV, $p = 0.018$) neurons but not in MF neurons (**Figure 7D**). DTX increased in sIPSP half width in HF (control: 21.9 ± 1.7 ms, DTX: 28.6 ± 2.8 ms, $p = 0.038$) but not LF and MF neurons (**Figure 7G**). In spite of robust tonotopic differences in postsynaptic LTK currents, there were no significant differences in the effect of DTX on percent changes in peak amplitude or half width of sIPSP among LF, MF and HF neurons (**Figures 7E,G**), and LTK currents appear to regulate the sIPSP frequency in LF neurons, suggesting that presynaptic LTK currents regulate inhibitory synapses.

LTK CURRENTS ON IPSCS: ACTION LOCI OF DTX

To better understand the presynaptic versus postsynaptic roles of LTK currents in regulating synaptic inhibition, we studied the effects of DTX on IPSCs recorded under voltage clamp ($V_h = -60$ mV). Ideally, under voltage clamp, changes in IPSCs observed after DTX application should be attributable to blockade of presynaptic LTK channels because postsynaptic LTK channels are not activated. Evoked IPSCs were subject to LTK modulation (**Figure 8**). DTX tended to increase the peak amplitude, decay time constant, and amount of charge (Q) in LF neurons ($n = 10$; peak amplitude: control: −429.8 ± 72.6 pA, DTX: −656.4 ± 112.7 pA, $p = 0.031$; decay time constant: control 55.4 ± 10.7 ms, DTX: 113.5 ± 23.7 ms, $p = 0.071$; Q: control: 12.7 ± 2.4 pC, DTX: 30.7 ± 7.3 pC, $p = 0.012$), and in MF neurons ($n = 8$; peak amplitude: control: −357.1 ± 83.3 pA, DTX: −662.5 ± 172.7 pA, $p = 0.018$; decay time constant: control: 101.9 ± 25.3 ms, DTX: 170.5 ± 29.3 ms, $p = 0.063$; Q: control: 31.0 ± 13.0 pC, DTX: 76.4 ± 22.5 pC, $p = 0.012$) (**Figures 8D,F,H**). HF neurons ($n = 9$) did not show increases in peak amplitude, decay time constant, and amount of charge, but showed a significant increase in 10–90% rise time (control 5.8 ± 3.3 ms, DTX: 10.5 ± 3.1 ms, $p = 0.045$) (**Figure 8B**). The percent change in 10–90% rise time, peak, decay time constant, and amount of charge did not differ across the tonotopic axis (**Figures 8C,E,G,I**). These data suggest that presynaptic LTK may, to some extent, regulate IPSCs in all CF regions but more prominently in LF neurons.

To further confirm and define the role of presynaptic LTK currents, we studied the effect of DTX on spontaneous IPSCs (sIPSCs; **Figure 9**). Cumulative probability of sIPSC IEI revealed that DTX decreased IEI predominantly in LF ($n = 12$, −53.1 ± 8.3%) neurons compared to MF ($n = 11$, −22.7 ± 4.2%) and HF ($n = 13$, −19.8 ± 6.4%) neurons (**Figures 9B–E**, $p = 0.002$). sIPSC peak amplitude also similarly increased after DTX application in LF (46.6 ± 17.7%), MF (33.7 ± 18.2%), and HF (26.1 ± 12.2%) neurons (**Figures 9F–I**). sIPSC decay time constant was significantly increased in LF (control: 6.0 ± 0.4 ms, DTX: 8.0 ± 0.7 ms, $p = 0.022$) but not in MF (control: 9.1 ± 1.5 ms, DTX: 9.3 ± 1.2 ms, $p = 0.829$) or HF (control: 9.7 ± 0.8 ms, DTX: 10.9 ± 1.4 ms, $p = 0.193$) neurons (**Figure 9J**). The amount of charge transferred per sIPSC (Q) increased after DTX application in LF (control: 0.5 ± 0.1 pC, DTX: 0.8 ± 0.1 pC, $p = 0.011$) and HF (control: 0.9 ± 0.1 pC, DTX: 1.2 ± 0.2 pC, $p = 0.040$), but not in MF (control: 1.1 ± 0.2 pC, DTX: 1.4 ± 0.3 pC, $p = 0.078$) neurons (**Figure 9L**). No differences in the percent change in peak amplitude, decay time constant, and charge were observed between LF, MF, and HF neurons (**Figures 9I,K,M**). These data support the notion that LTK currents have a presynaptic role in modulating IPSC size and shape in NL neurons especially in LF neurons. The discrepancy in the effects of DTX on sIPSCs versus evoked IPSCs in MF neurons might be caused by relatively weak influences of LTK currents on the spontaneous release of GABA in MF neurons.

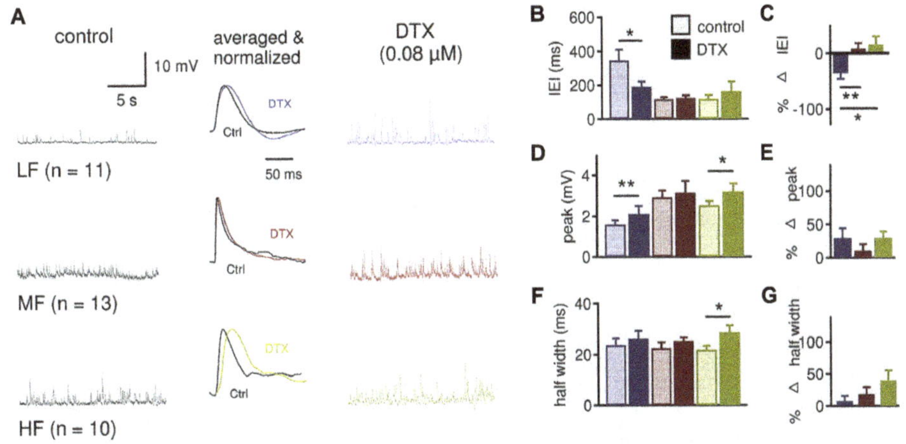

FIGURE 7 | LTK currents strongly regulate sIPSP frequency in LF neurons and sIPSP shape in HF neurons. (A) Sample sIPSP recordings before (dark traces) and after (color traces) bath application of DTX (0.08 μM) in LF ($n = 11$), MF ($n = 13$) and HF ($n = 10$) NL neurons. See **Figure 6A** for legend. **(B)** The IEI significantly decreased in LF (control: 347.2 ± 63.1 ms, DTX: 192.3 ± 30.2 ms) but not MF (control: 120.0 ± 11.0 ms, DTX: 119.4 ± 12.8 ms) and HF (control: 129.4 ± 24.8 ms, DTX: 164.5 ± 57.2 ms) neurons after DTX. **(C)** The percent decrease in IEI of sIPSPs is significantly greater in LF (−35.3 ± 10.4%) neurons compared to MF (8.1 ± 9.8%) and HF (15.5 ± 14.4%) neurons. **(D)** There is a significant increase in sIPSP peak amplitude after DTX treatment in LF (control: 1.5 ± 0.2 mV, DTX: 2.1 ± 0.4 mV) and HF (control: 2.5 ± 0.2 mV, DTX: 3.2 ± 0.4 mV) neurons but not in MF (control: 3.0 ± 0.3 mV, DTX: 3.1 ± 0.6 mV) neurons. **(E)** The percent change in sIPSP peak amplitude was not different across the tonotopic axis. **(F)** DTX increased the sIPSP half width in HF (control: 21.9 ± 1.7 ms, DTX: 28.6 ± 2.8 ms) but not in LF (control: 23.7 ± 2.7 ms, DTX: 26.3 ± 3.0 ms) and MF (control: 22.5 ± 2.1 ms, DTX: 25.2 ± 1.5 ms) neurons. **(G)** Although HF neurons show a substantial increase in sIPSP half width, the percent change in sIPSP half width is not significantly different across the tonotopic axis ($p = 0.075$). $^*p < 0.05$, $^{**}p < 0.01$, $^{***}p < 0.001$.

LTK CURRENTS ON EXCITABILITY OF NL NEURONS

Finally, we assessed the role of LTK currents in regulating neuronal excitability in NL. Specifically, we tested whether the presence of LTK currents prevented GABA-induced action potentials in NL neurons, as suggested in NM neurons (Monsivais et al., 2000; Howard et al., 2007). We thus investigated such interactions in NL neurons using current clamp recordings (**Figure 10**). We first confirmed the effects of DTX (0.1 μM) on the intrinsic firing properties of NL neurons in MF and HF regions. Under control conditions, NL cells fired one action potential in response to prolonged suprathreshold current injections followed by a plateau of subthreshold membrane potential (**Figure 10A**), a characteristic hallmark of time-coding neurons in the central auditory system. DTX produced a small depolarization (2 mV) in RMP, substantially lowered the threshold current, and changed the phasic firing pattern to a tonic mode (**Figures 10B,C**), consistent with previous findings in auditory brainstem neurons where K_{V1}-containing channels are highly expressed (e.g., Brew and Forsythe, 1995; Gittelman and Tempel, 2006). Furthermore, spontaneous action potentials, which were absent under control conditions, appeared prior to the onset and after the termination of the current injections. Because ionotropic glutamate receptors were blocked throughout these experiments, the spontaneous spikes occurred on the top of depolarizing IPSPs. Under control condition, sIPSP varied widely in amplitude, with maximal membrane depolarization of up to several millivolt without spike activity (**Figure 10D**). DTX increased the amplitude of sIPSP and transformed some into spikes (**Figures 10E,F**, $n = 9$). To further study the effects of DTX on evoked IPSP and GABA-induced spikes, train stimulations at different frequencies were applied to evoke GABA responses. At 50 and 100 Hz, IPSPs summated temporally, forming a sustained membrane depolarization of about 15 mV. GABA-induced spikes were seen occasionally (**Figure 10G**). Under DTX, more spikes were seen at all three frequencies tested, and bursts of spikes occurred at the beginning of the simulation. Significant increase in AP probability was detected for the stimulations at frequency of 10 and 50 Hz (**Figures 10H,I**, $n = 9$). These data confirm that LTK currents prevent GABA-induced excitation, providing a critical role for LTK currents in maintaining synaptic inhibition in NL.

DISCUSSION

This study sought to determine the interplay between intrinsic LTK currents and extrinsic synaptic inhibition in NL neurons across the tonotopic axis. We characterized the LTK currents in LF, MF, and HF neurons, and then demonstrated a tonotopic relationship between LTK currents and inhibitory synaptic input. Interestingly, the data suggest that while MF and HF neurons possess larger postsynaptic LTK currents than LF neurons, robust presynaptic LTK currents in LF neurons may compensate for the relatively lower postsynaptic LTK counterpart, leading to equally strong LTK influences on synaptic inhibition across different frequency-coding regions. In addition to shaping inhibitory inputs, LTK currents also prevent GABAergic-driven excitation and therefore are critical for the maintenance of inhibition in NL.

Postsynaptic LTK currents in NL neurons exhibit tonotopic variation in amplitude and kinetics along the tonotopic axis of NL. LTK currents were substantially higher in MF and HF neurons compared to LF neurons. The presence of a tonotopic gradient of K_V currents, with stronger current expression with increasing CF, has been shown in peripheral (Pantelias et al., 2001) and a variety

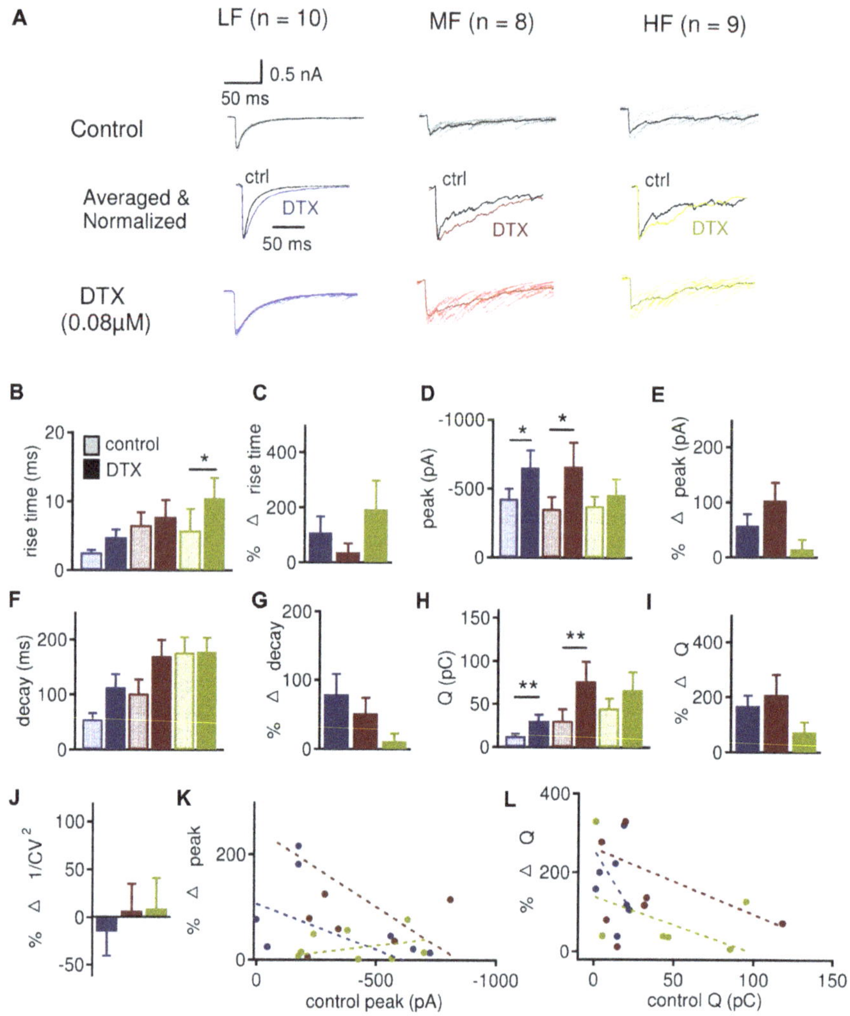

FIGURE 8 | DTX preferentially regulates IPSC frequency and shape in LF and MF neurons. (A) Sample evoked IPSC recordings before (dark traces) and after (color traces) bath application of DXT (0.08 μM) in LF (n = 10), MF (n = 8), and HF (n = 9) NL neurons. See **Figure 6A** for legend. **(B,C)** DTX increases the 10–90% rise time in HF (control: 5.8 ± 3.3 ms, DTX: 10.5 ± 3.1 ms) neurons, but not in LF (control: 2.6 ± 0.4 ms, DTX: 4.8 ± 1.2 ms) and MF (control: 6.1 ± 1.9 ms, DTX: 6.6 ± 2.4 ms) neurons, without significant differences in percent changes across tonotopic axis. **(D)** DTX increased the IPSC peak amplitude in LF (control: −429.8 ± 72.6 pA, DTX: −656.4 ± 112.7 pA) and MF (control: −357.1 ± 83.3 pA, DTX: −662.5 ± 172.7 pA) but not in HF (control: −379.9 ± 66.6 pA, DTX: −460.4 ± 113.4 pA) neurons. **(E)** Percent change in IPSC peak amplitude is not significantly different between LF (58.5 ± 20.6%), MF (103.8 ± 32.5%), and HF (15.2 ± 17.4%) neurons. **(F)** No change in the decay time constant was observed in LF (control: 55.4 ± 10.7 ms, DTX: 113.5 ± 23.7 ms), MF (control: 101.9 ± 25.3 ms, DTX: 170.5 ± 29.3 ms) or HF (control: 158.8 ± 27.3 ms, DTX: 178.7 ± 25.1 ms) neurons. **(G)** Percent change in IPSC decay time constant is not significantly different across CF regions. **(H)** DTX increases the amount of charge per IPSC (Q) in LF (control: 12.7 ± 2.4 pC, DTX: 30.7 ± 7.3 pC) and MF (control: 31.0 ± 13.0 pC, DTX: 76.4 ± 22.5 pC) neurons but not in HF (control: 45.6 ± 10.8 pC, DTX: 66.6 ± 20.9 pC) neurons. **(I)** The percent change in Q is not different between CF regions. **(J)** No significant differences are observed between CF regions in $1/CV^2$ after DTX treatment. **(K,L)** Control peak amplitude and total area plotted against the percent change in peak amplitude and total area, respectively, after DTX reveals that there was little to no correlation between control and percent change after DTX in all CF regions: LF (peak amplitude: r^2 = 0.076; area: r^2 = 0.156), MF (amplitude: r^2 = 0.140; area: r^2 = 0.088), and HF (amplitude: r^2 = 0.060; area: r^2 = 0.190). $^*p < 0.05$, $^{**}p < 0.01$.

of central auditory structures (Li et al., 2001; Fukui and Ohmori, 2004; Brew and Forsythe, 2005; Kuba et al., 2005). In NL, the LTK currents seem to be most specialized in MF neurons. One important measure of the LTK channels in timing coding neurons in the auditory system is the amount of active current at rest. It is well known that active LTK conductances at rest contribute to making the membrane leaky, and result in a narrow time window for converging excitatory inputs to drive the cells to spike (Golding et al., 1999; Scott et al., 2005). Although all NL neurons possessed active LTK conductance at rest, MF neurons had a higher LTK current density at rest than LF and HF neurons (**Figures 3** and **6**), consistent with the observation of specialized fast membrane time constants and fast synaptic inputs in MF neurons (Kuba et al., 2005). Furthermore, in terms of

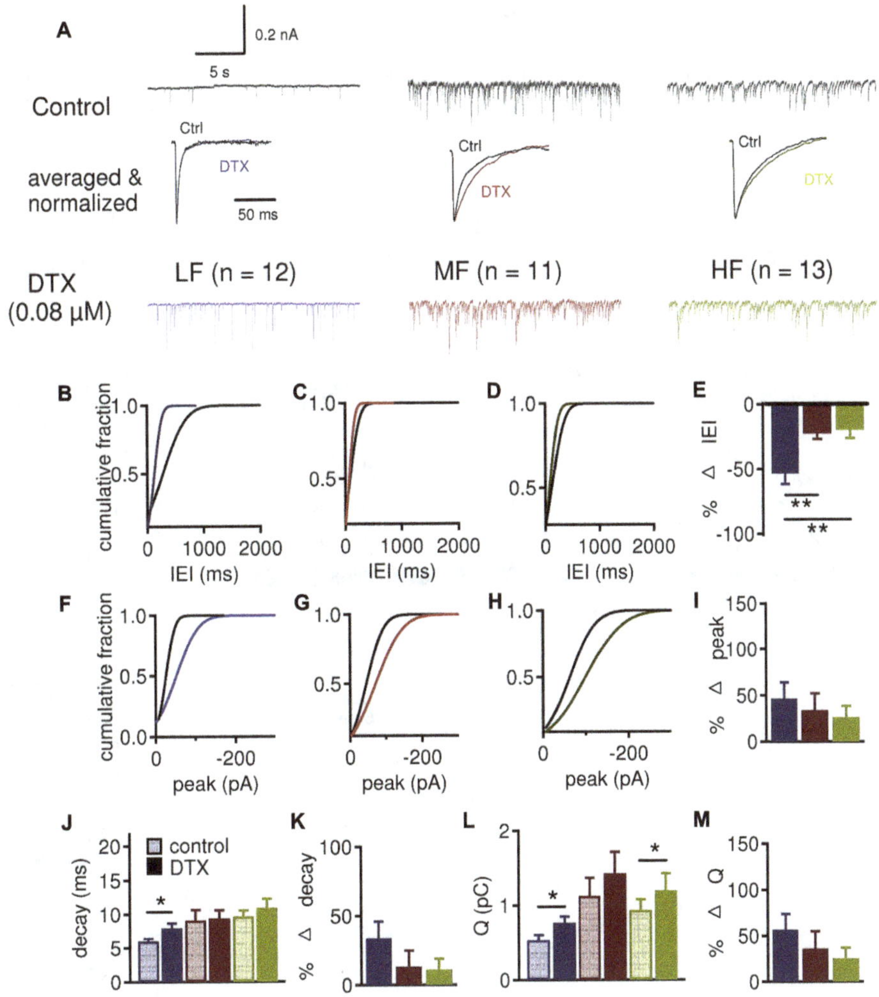

FIGURE 9 | LTK currents strongly regulate the frequency of sIPSCs in LF neurons. (A) Sample sIPSC recordings before (dark traces) and after (color traces) bath application of DXT (0.08 μM) in LF (blue, $n = 12$), MF (red, $n = 11$) and HF (yellow, $n = 13$) NL neurons. See **Figure 6A** for legend. **(B–D)** Cumulative fraction of IEI in LF **(B)**, MF **(C)**, and HF **(D)** neurons before (black) and after (color) DTX. **(E)** Percent change in IEI is significantly larger in LF (−53.1 ± 8.3%) neurons compared to MF (−22.7 ± 4.2%) and HF (−19.8 ± 6.4%) neurons. No differences were observed between MF and HF neurons. **(F–H)** Cumulative fraction of sIPSC IEI in LF **(F)**, MF **(G)**, and HF **(H)** neurons before (black) and after (color) DTX. **(I)** No significant differences in percent change in sIPSC peak after DTX treatment between LF (46.6 ± 17.7%), MF (33.7 ± 18.2%), and HF (26.1 ± 12.2%) neurons. **(J)** The sIPSC decay time constant is significantly increased in LF (control: 6.0 ± 0.4 ms, DTX: 8.0 ± 0.7 ms) but not in MF (control: 9.1 ± 1.5 ms, DTX: 9.3 ± 1.2 ms) or HF (control: 9.7 ± 0.8 ms, DTX: 10.9 ± 1.4 ms) neurons. **(K)** No significant differences in percent change in the sIPSC decay time constant were observed between LF, MF, and HF neurons after DTX treatment. **(L)** The amount of charge transferred per sIPSC (Q) is significantly increased in LF (control: 0.5 ± 0.1 pC, DTX: 0.8 ± 0.1 pC) and HF (control: 0.9 ± 0.1 pC, DTX: 1.2 ± 0.2 pC) but not in MF (control: 1.1 ± 0.2 pC, DTX: 1.4 ± 0.3 pC) neurons. **(M)** No significant differences in percent change in sIPSC area after DTX treatment across CF regions. $^*p < 0.05$, $^{**}p < 0.01$.

activation kinetics of LTK currents, MF neurons had the fastest τ at −45 mV compared to LF and HF neurons. The activation kinetics of LTK currents in MF neurons indeed were similarly fast compared to those found in NM neurons (Rathouz and Trussell, 1998), with τ ranging from 2 to 1 ms at membrane potentials between −45 and −30 mV. These data reaffirm that MF neurons have a more active LTK conductance at low membrane potentials. There were, however, no significant differences in inactivation kinetics of LTK currents across the tonotopic axis. A relatively small portion (∼20%) of steady state LTK currents in NL neurons inactivate at −45 to −30 mV, similar to NM neurons (Rathouz and Trussell, 1998).

One potential caveat in these experiments would be errors in current measurement due to poor space clamping, particularly in LF neurons, which are known to have longer dendrites than MF and HF neurons. While long dendrites can introduce space clamp errors, the number of dendritic bifurcations and the diameter of primary dendrites can also dramatically influence space clamp. Specifically, thin primary dendrites with numerous bifurcations will also introduce relatively large space clamp errors. Furthermore, the membrane resistance is also a major factor in determining the degree of space clamp errors (Bar-Yehuda and Korngreen, 2008; Poleg-Polsky and Diamond, 2011). Space clamp errors are unlikely to account for the differences in LTK amplitude

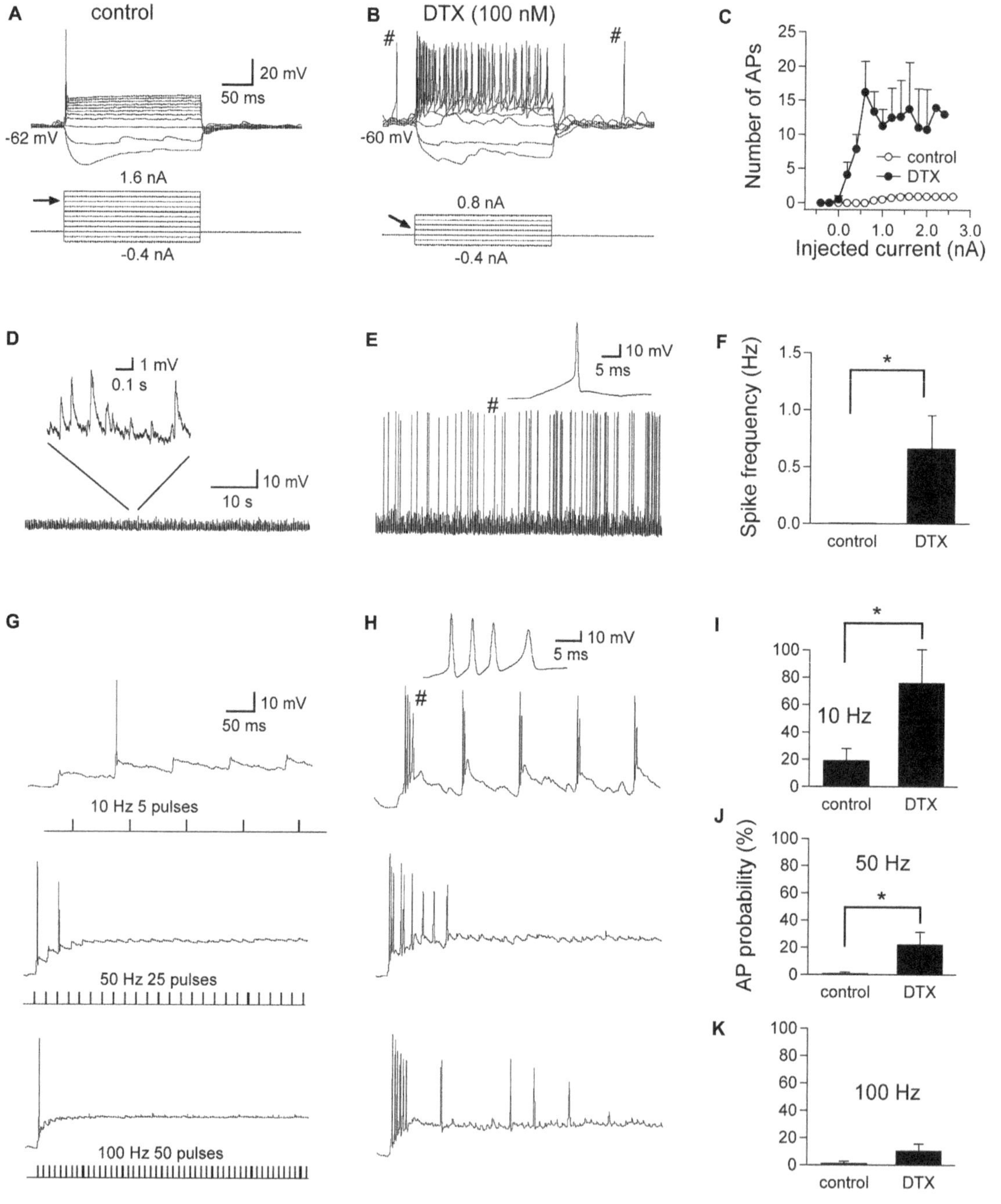

FIGURE 10 | Regulation of GABA responses in NL neurons by LTK channels. (A) Under control conditions, the cell fires one single action potential (AP) in response to prolonged suprathreshold current injections (threshold current indicated by the arrow, 1.2 nA in this case). **(B)** DTX slightly depolarizes the RMP, substantially lowers the threshold current to 0.2 nA, and changed the phasic firing pattern to a tonic mode. **(C)** Pooled data show a dramatic increase in the number of APs in response to DTX application ($n = 9$). Furthermore, spontaneous APs, which are absent under control condition, appear prior to and after the current injections (indicated by #). Because ionotropic glutamate receptors were blocked throughout the experiments, these two spontaneous spikes likely occurred on top of two depolarizing IPSPs. **(D)** Chart recordings show sIPSP with amplitude of up to several millivolts, without spike activity. **(E)** DTX increased the amplitude of sIPSP and transforms some into spikes (one spike indicated by # is shown at an enlarged time scale). **(F)** Spike frequency was significantly higher after DTX application than in control conditions ($n = 9$). **(G,H)** Train stimulations at different frequencies were applied to evoke GABA responses. At 50 and 100 Hz, IPSPs summate, forming a sustained membrane depolarization of about 15 mV. GABA-induced spikes were seen occasionally. Under DTX, more spikes were seen at all three frequencies tested, and bursts of spikes are noted (a burst of four APs shown at an enlarged time scale). **(I–K)** Significant increase in AP probability was detected for the stimulations at frequency of 10 and 50 Hz but not 100 Hz ($n = 9$). $^*p < 0.05$.

across the tonotopic axis, because the dendritic gradient in the NL is such that LF neurons have longer, thicker primary dendrites with relatively few bifurcations. With increasing CF, dendritic length and diameter decrease, while the number of primary dendrites and bifurcations increase (Smith and Rubel, 1979). Additionally, MF neurons have lower R_{in} than LF and HF neurons (Kuba et al., 2005). Therefore, given the tonotopic differences in R_{in}, dendritic length, width and branching, we expect that space clamp errors did not contribute to the significant differences in LTK currents across the tonotopic axis.

Given the tonotopic arrangement of LTK currents in NL, we expected to find more robust change in IPSP shape and size in MF and HF neurons than in LF neurons after application of K_{v1} channel blocker DTX. To the contrary, the effect of DTX was about equally evident in all CF regions. We found increases in IPSP and sIPSP peak amplitude and half width after DTX treatment in most CF regions. Although MF neurons have more LTK currents active at rest, there were no significant differences in the percent changes caused by DTX in the size and shape of IPSP and sIPSP between LF, MF, and HF neurons. The concurrent increase in sIPSP frequency (reduction in sIPSP IEI) in LF but not MF and HF neurons suggests that presynaptic LTK currents may have contributed to the changes in IPSP amplitude in LF neurons. We tested this hypothesis by conducting voltage clamp experiments, which should minimize the influence of postsynaptic LTK currents and therefore allow us to assess to what extent presynaptic LTK currents contributed to DTX-induced changes in the size and shape of the synaptic inhibitory responses. Our data were suggestive of a tonotopic arrangement of presynaptic LTK currents in NL, which is supported by the observation that DTX induced an increase in sIPSC frequency preferentially in LF neurons. Furthermore, DTX caused significant changes in the peak, decay, and amount of charge (Q) of IPSCs and sIPSCs in LF neurons, reflecting a combined effect of both presynaptic and postsynaptic LTK currents on the synaptic inhibition in LF neurons. Fewer parameters of IPSC were affected by DTX in MF neurons, and the effects of DTX on IPSCs in HF neurons were even less significant. These results suggest that presynaptic LTK currents are more prevalent in LF than in MF and HF neurons. A recent study (Yamada et al., 2013) demonstrates that local GABAergic neurons project primarily to LF neurons. It remains to be determined whether these GABAergic terminals express stronger LTK channels than those that originate from the SON.

Presynaptic mechanisms can be confirmed with analysis of variability ($1/CV^2$) of peak amplitude of evoked synaptic responses and paired pulse ratio (PPR; del Castillo and Katz, 1954; Oleskevich et al., 2000; Scheuss et al., 2002). PPR paradigm, however, is not effective in studying synaptic inhibition of NL neurons due to dramatic fluctuations in IPSC peak amplitude under control conditions (Kuo et al., 2009; Tang et al., 2013). Analyses of $1/CV^2$ of IPSPs (**Figures 6H,I**) and IPSCs (**Figure 8J**) did not show significant differences in the percent change of $1/CV^2$ caused by DTX between CF regions. However, DTX tended to substantially reduce $1/CV^2$ in LF neurons while slightly increasing $1/CV^2$ in MF and HF neurons (**Figures 6** and **8**), suggesting that presynaptic LTK currents preferentially influence inhibitory synaptic input in LF neurons. We speculate that there may be a tonotopic arrangement of presynaptic LTK currents opposing the postsynaptic arrangement of LTK currents. In other words, postsynaptic LTK currents are largest in HF neurons while presynaptic LTK currents are largest in LF neurons. To support this hypothesis, further research will need to demonstrate the presence of LTK-subfamily channels (e.g.; K_{v1}, K_{v4}, K_{v7}) on inhibitory synapses in the NL.

The presence of presynaptic LTK channels on inhibitory terminals of LF neurons provides an intriguing possibility for interplay between these two neuronal properties that may be critical for forming fast inhibition in LF neurons. The fast kinetics of IPSCs in LF NL neurons can be attributed to both a presynaptic release profile with strong synchronization (Tang and Lu, 2012) and a postsynaptic enrichment of the fast $\alpha 1$-$GABA_A$ receptor subunit (Yamada et al., 2013). MF and HF neurons display stronger asynchronous release of GABA than LF neurons (Tang and Lu, 2012), which is consistent with the results of the current study (**Figures 5, 6,** and **8**). We propose that in addition to these mechanisms, presynaptic LTK currents also contribute to accelerating IPSCs in LF neurons. In fact, K_{v1}-containing channels have been shown to regulate presynaptic spiking activity in a variety of structures, including the cerebellum, hippocampus, and motor nerve (Trussell and Roberts, 2008). After DTX application, a fair amount of asynchronous events emerged in LF neurons, whereas qualitatively there was not an obvious change in MF and HF neurons (**Figures 6** and **8**), supporting a role of presynaptic LTK channels in LF neurons. This suggests that LF neurons may utilize similar mechanisms including intrinsic voltage-gated conductances and fast synaptic inhibition to code ITD as observed in mammalian medial superior olive neurons (Grothe and Sanes, 1993, 1994; Brand et al., 2002; Dodson et al., 2002, 2003; Grothe, 2003; Roberts et al., 2013). While presynaptic LTK currents may regulate fast phasic inhibition in LF neurons, postsynaptic LTK currents prevent GABA-induced excitation. In NM neurons, GABA-driven excitation is prevalent in E14 chicks, but decreases during development and becomes predominantly inhibitory at E18. The decrease in GABA-induced excitation coincides with the increase in LTK currents (Howard et al., 2007). The same principle may apply to the maturation of GABAergic inhibition in NL neurons. The LTK currents are thus critical not only in switching the sign of GABA inputs from excitation to inhibition but also maintenance of synaptic inhibition in coincidence detector neurons. The interactions between these two critical neuronal properties along the tonotopic axis help create optimal ITD coding strategies dependent upon the frequency of the auditory inputs.

AUTHOR CONTRIBUTIONS

Yong Lu conceived and supervised the study; William R. Hamlet and Yong Lu designed the experiments; William R. Hamlet, Yu-Wei Liu, Zheng-Quan Tang, and Yong Lu performed the research and analyzed data; William R. Hamlet and Yong Lu wrote the paper.

ACKNOWLEDGMENTS

We thank Rebecca Curry, Jennifer Gay, and Zahra Ghasemahmad for helpful discussion and comments, and thank Patrick Cullen for advice on statistical analysis. This work was supported by National Institute on Deafness and other Communication Disorders Grant R01DC008984 (Yong Lu).

REFERENCES

Alreja, M., and Aghajanian, G. K. (1994). QX-314 blocks the potassium but not the sodium-dependent component of the opiate response in locus coeruleus neurons. *Brain Res.* 639, 320–324. doi: 10.1016/0006-8993(94)91746-9

Andrade, R. (1991). Blockade of neurotransmitter-activated K+ conductance by QX-314 in the rat hippocampus. *Eur. J. Pharmacol.* 199, 259–262. doi: 10.1016/0014-2999(91)90467-5

Bar-Yehuda, D., and Korngreen, A. (2008). Space clamp problems when voltage-clamping neurons expressing voltage-gated conductances. *J. Neurophysiol.* 99, 1127–1136. doi: 10.1152/jn.01232.2007

Barnes-Davies, M., Barker, M. C., Osmani, F., and Forsythe, I. D. (2004). Kv1 currents mediate a gradient of principal neuron excitability across the tonotopic axis in the rat lateral superior olive. *Eur. J. Neurosci.*19, 325–333. doi: 10.1111/j.0953-816X.2003.03133.x

Blackmer, T., Kou, S. P., Bender, K. J., Apostolides, P. F., and Trussell, L. O. (2009). Dendritic calcium channels and their activation by synaptic signals in auditory coincidence detector neurons. *J. Neurophysiol.* 102, 1218–1226. doi: 10.1152/jn.90513.2008

Brand, A., Behrend, O., Marquardt, T., McAlpine, D., and Grothe, B. (2002). Precise inhibition is essential for microsecond interaural time difference coding. *Nature* 417, 543–547. doi: 10.1038/417543a

Brew, H. M., and Forsythe, I. D. (1995). Two voltage-dependent K+ conductances with complementary functions in postsynaptic integration at a central auditory synapse. *J. Neurosci.* 15, 8011–8022.

Brew, H. M., and Forsythe, I. D. (2005). Systematic variation of potassium current amplitudes across the tonotopic axis of the rat medial nucleus of the trapezoid body. *Hear. Res.* 206, 116–132. doi: 10.1016/j.heares.2004.12.012

Brew, H. M., Hallows, J. L., and Tempel, B. L. (2003). Hyperexcitability and reduced low threshold potassium currents in auditory neurons of mice lacking the channel subunit Kv1.1. *J. Physiol.* 548, 1–20. doi: 10.1113/jphysiol.2002.035568

Brückner, S., and Hyson, R. L. (1998). Effect of GABA on the processing of interaural time differences in nucleus laminaris neurons in the chick. *Eur. J. Neurosci.* 10, 3438–3450, doi: 10.1046/j.1460-9568.1998.00353.x

Burger, R. M., Cramer, K. S., Pfeiffer, J. D., and Rubel, E. W. (2005). Avian superior olivary nucleus provides divergent inhibitory input to parallel auditory pathways. *J. Comp. Neurol.* 481, 6–18. doi: 10.1002/cne.20334

Cao, X. J., and Oertel, D. (2005). Temperature affects voltage-sensitive conductances differentially in Octopus cells in the mammalian cochlear nucleus. *J. Neurophysiol.* 94, 821–832. doi: 10.1152/jn.01049.2004

Clements, J. D. (2003). Variance–mean analysis: a simple and reliable approach for investigating synaptic transmission and modulation. *J. Neurosci. Methods* 130, 115–125. doi: 10.1016/j.jneumeth.2003.09.019

Code, R. A., and Churchill, L. (1991). GABAA receptors in auditory brainstem nuclei of the chick during development and after cochlea removal. *Hear. Res.* 54, 281–295. doi: 10.1016/0378-5955(91)90122-P

Coetzee, W. A., Amarillo, Y., Chiu, J., Chow, A., Lau, D., McCormack, T., et al. (1999). Molecular diversity of K^+ channels. *Ann. N. Y. Acad. Sci.* 868, 233–285. doi: 10.1111/j.1749-6632.1999.tb11293.x

del Castillo, J., and Katz, B. (1954). Statistical factors involved in neuromuscular facilitation and depression. *J. Physiol.* 124, 574–585.

Dodson, P. D., Barker, M. C., and Forsythe, I. D. (2002). Two heteromeric Kv1 potassium channels differentially regulate action potential firing. *J. Neurosci.* 22, 6953–6961.

Dodson, P. D., Billups, B., Rusznák, Z., Szûcs, G., Barker, M. C., and Forsythe, I. D. (2003). Presynaptic rat Kv1.2 channels suppress synaptic terminal hyperexcitability following action potential invasion. *J. Physiol.* 550, 27–33. doi: 10.1113/jphysiol.2003.046250

Forsythe, I. D., and Barnes-Davies, M. (1993). The binaural auditory pathway: membrane currents limiting multiple action potential generation in the rat medial nucleus of the trapezoid body. *Proc. Biol. Sci.* 251, 143–150. doi: 10.1098/rspb.1993.0021

Fukui, I., Burger, R. M., Ohmori, H., and Rubel, E. W. (2010). GABAergic inhibition sharpens the frequency tuning and enhances phase locking in chicken nucleus magnocellularis neurons. *J. Neurosci.* 30, 12075–12083. doi: 10.1523/JNEUROSCI.1484-10.2010

Fukui, I., and Ohmori, H. (2004). Tonotopic gradients of membrane and synaptic properties for neurons of the chicken nucleus magnocellularis. *J. Neurosci.* 24, 7514–7523. doi: 10.1523/JNEUROSCI.0566-04.2004

Funabiki, K., Koyano, K., and Ohmori, H. (1998). The role of GABAergic inputs for coincidence detection in the neurons of nucleus laminaris of the chick. *J. Physiol.* 508, 851–869. doi: 10.1111/j.1469-7793.1998.851bp.x

Gao, H., and Lu, Y. (2008). Early development of intrinsic and synaptic properties of chicken nucleus laminaris neurons. *Neuroscience* 153, 131–143. doi: 10.1016/j.neuroscience.2008.01.059

Gittelman, J. X., and Tempel, B. L. (2006). Kv1.1-containing channels are critical for temporal precision during spike initiation. *J. Neurophysiol.* 96, 1203–1214. doi: 10.1152/jn.00092.2005

Golding, N. L., Ferragamo, M. J., and Oertel, D. (1999). Role of intrinsic conductances underlying responses to transients in octopus cells of the cochlear nucleus. *J. Neurosci.* 19, 2897–2905.

Grothe, B., and Sanes, D. H. (1993). Bilateral inhibition by glycinergic afferents in the medial superior olive. *J. Neurophysiol.* 69, 1192–1196.

Grothe, B., and Sanes, D. H. (1994). Synaptic inhibition influences the temporal coding properties of medial superior olivary neurons: an in vitro study. *J. Neurosci.* 14, 1701–1709.

Grothe, B. (2003). New roles for synaptic inhibition in sound localization. *Nat. Rev. Neurosci.* 4, 540–550. doi: 10.1038/nrn1136

Harvey, A. L. (2001). Twenty years of dendrotoxins. *Toxicon.* 39, 15–26. doi: 10.1016/S0041-0101(00)00162-8

Howard, M. A., Burger, M. A., and Rubel E. W. (2007). A developmental switch to GABAergic inhibition dependent on increase in Kv1-type K^+ currents. *J. Neurosci.* 27, 2112–2123. doi: 10.1523/JNEUROSCI.5266-06.2007

Howard, M. A., and Rubel, E. W. (2010). Dynamic spike thresholds during synaptic integration preserve and enhance temporal response properties in the avian cochlear nucleus. *J. Neurosci.* 30, 12063–12074. doi: 10.1523/JNEUROSCI.1840-10.2010

Hyson, R. L., Reyes, A. D., and Rubel, E. W. (1995). A depolarizing inhibitory response to GABA in brainstem auditory neurons of the chick. *Brain Res.* 677, 117–126. doi: 10.1016/0006-8993(95)00130-I

Ingham, N. J., and McAlpine, D. (2005). GABAergic inhibition controls neural gain in inferior colliculus neurons sensitive to interaural time differences. *J. Neurosci.* 25, 6187–6198. doi: 10.1523/JNEUROSCI.0146-05.2005

Jeffress, L. A. (1948). A place theory of sound localization. *J. Comp. Physiol. Psychol.* 41, 35–39. doi: 10.1037/h0061495

Johnston, J., Forsythe, I. D., and Kopp-Scheinpflug, C. (2010). Going native: voltage-gated potassium channels controlling neuronal excitability. *J. Physiol.* 588, 3187–3200. doi: 10.1113/jphysiol.2010.191973

Konishi, M. (2003). Coding of auditory space. *Annu. Rev. Neurosci.* 26, 31–55. doi: 10.1146/annurev.neuro.26.041002.131123

Kuba, H., Koyano, K., and Ohmori, H. (2002). Development of membrane conductance improves coincidence detection in the nucleus laminaris of the chicken. *J. Physiol.* 540, 529–542. doi: 10.1113/jphysiol.2001.013365

Kuba, H., Yamada, R., Fukui, I., and Ohmori, H. (2005). Tonotopic specialization of auditory coincidence detection in nucleus laminaris of the chick. *J. Neurosci.* 25, 1924–1934. doi: 10.1523/JNEUROSCI.4428-04.2005

Kuo, S. P., Bradley, L. A., and Trussell, L. O. (2009). Heterogeneous kinetics and pharmacology of synaptic inhibition in the chick auditory brainstem. *J. Neurosci.* 29, 9625–9634. doi: 10.1523/JNEUROSCI.0103-09.2009

Lachica, E. A., Rübsamen, R., and Rubel, E. W. (1994). GABAergic terminals in nucleus magnocellularis and laminaris originate from the superior olivary nucleus. *J. Comp. Neurol.* 348, 403–418. doi: 10.1002/cne.903480307

Li, W., Kaczmarek, L. K., and Perney, T. M. (2001). Localization of two high-threshold potassium channel subunits in the rat central auditory system. *J. Comp. Neurol.* 437, 196–218. doi: 10.1002/cne.1279

Lu, T., and Trussell, L. O. (2001). Mixed excitatory and inhibitory GABA-mediated transmission in chick cochlear nucleus. *J. Physiol.* 535, 125–131. doi: 10.1111/j.1469-7793.2001.t01-1-00125.x

Lu, Y., Monsivais, P., Tempel, B. L., and Rubel, E. W. (2004). Activity-dependent regulation of the potassium channel subunits Kv1.1 and Kv3.1. *J. Comp. Neurol.* 470, 93–106. doi: 10.1002/cne.11037

MacLeod, K. M., and Carr, C. E. (2012). "Synaptic mechanisms of coincidence detection," in *Synaptic Mechanisms in the Auditory System*, eds L. O. Trussell, A. N. Popper, and R. R. Fay (New York: Springer Press), 135–164. doi: 10.1007/978-1-4419-9517-9_6

Manis, P. B., and Marx, S. O. (1991). Outward currents in isolated ventral cochlear nucleus neurons. *J. Neurosci.* 11, 2865–2880.

Mathews, P. J., Jercog, P. E., Rinzel, J., Scott, L. L., and Golding, N. L. (2010). Control of submillisecond synaptic timing in binaural coincidence detectors by Kv1 channels. *Nat. Neurosci.* 13, 601–609. doi: 10.1038/nn.2530

Monsivais, P., and Rubel, E. W. (2001). Accommodation enhances depolarizing inhibition in central neurons. *J. Neurosci.* 21, 7823–7830.

Monsivais, P., Yang, L., and Rubel, E. W. (2000). GABAergic inhibition in nucleus magnocellularis: implications for phase locking in the avian auditory brainstem. *J. Neurosci.* 20, 2954–2963.

Oleskevich, S., Clements, J., and Walmsley, B. (2000). Release probability modulates short-term plasticity at a rat giant terminal. *J. Physiol.* 524, 513–523. doi: 10.1111/j.1469-7793.2000.00513.x

Pantelias, A. A., Monsivais, P., and Rubel, E. W. (2001). Tonotopic map of potassium currents in chick auditory hair cells using an intact basilar papilla. *Hear. Res.* 156, 81–94. doi: 10.1016/S0378-5955(01)00269-6

Pecka, M., Brand, A., Behrend, O., and Grothe, B. (2008). Interaural time difference processing in the mammalian medial superior olive: the role of glycinergic inhibition. *J. Neurosci.* 28, 6914–6925. doi: 10.1523/JNEUROSCI.1660-08.2008

Poleg-Polsky, A., and Diamond, J. S. (2011). Imperfect space clamp permits electrotonic interactions between inhibitory and excitatory synaptic conductances, distorting voltage clamp recordings. *PLoS ONE* 6:e19463. doi: 10.1371/journal.pone.0019463

Rathouz, M., and Trussell, L. (1998). Characterization of outward currents in neurons of the avian nucleus magnocellularis. *J. Neurophysiol.* 80, 2824–2835.

Reyes, A. D., Rubel, E. W., and Spain, W. J. (1994). Membrane properties underlying the firing of neurons in the avian cochlear nucleus. *J. Neurosci.* 14, 5352–5364.

Roberts, M. T., Seeman, S. C., and Golding, N. L. (2013). A mechanistic understanding of the role of feedforward inhibition in the mammalian sound localization circuitry. *Neuron* 78, 923–935. doi: 10.1016/j.neuron.2013.04.022

Rubel, E. W., and Parks, T. N. (1975). Organization and development of brain stem auditory nuclei of the chicken: tonotopic organization of *N. magnocellularis* and *N. laminaris*. *J. Comp. Neurol.* 164, 411–433. doi: 10.1002/cne.901640403

Scheuss, V., Schneggenburger, R., and Neher, E. (2002). Separation of presynaptic and postsynaptic contributions to depression by covariance analysis of successive EPSCs at the calyx of held synapse. *J. Neurosci.* 22, 728–739.

Scott, L. L., Mathews, P. J., and Golding, N. L. (2005). Posthearing developmental refinement of temporal processing in principal neurons of the medial superior olive. *J. Neurosci.* 25, 7887–7895. doi: 10.1523/JNEUROSCI.1016-05.2005

Smith, D. J., and Rubel, E. W. (1979). Organization and development of brain stem auditory nuclei of the chicken: dendritic gradients in nucleus laminaris. *J. Comp. Neurol.* 186, 213–239. doi: 10.1002/cne.901860207

Svirskis, G., Kotak, V., Sanes, D. H., and Rinzel, J. (2002). Enhancement of signal-to-noise ratio and phase locking for small inputs by a low threshold outward current in auditory neurons. *J. Neurosci.* 22, 11019–11025.

Tang, Z.-Q., and Lu, Y. (2012). Two GABAA responses with distinct kinetics in a sound localization circuit. *J. Physiol.* 590, 3787–3805. doi: 10.1113/jphysiol.2012.230136

Tang, Z.-Q., Dinh, E. H., Shi, W., and Lu, Y. (2011). Ambient GABA-activated tonic inhibition sharpens auditory coincidence detection via a depolarizing shunting mechanism. *J. Neurosci.* 31, 6121–6131. doi: 10.1523/JNEUROSCI.4733-10.2011

Tang, Z.-Q., Gao, H., and Lu, Y. (2009). Control of a depolarizing GABAergic input in an auditory coincidence detection circuit. *J. Neurophysiol.* 102, 1672–1683. doi: 10.1152/jn.00419.2009

Tang, Z.-Q., Liu, Y.-W., Shi, W., Dinh, E. H., Hamlet, W. R., Curry, R. J., et al. (2013). Activation of synaptic group II metabotropic glutamate receptors induces long-term depression at GABAergic synapses in CNS neurons. *J. Neurosci.* 33, 15964–15977. doi: 10.1523/JNEUROSCI.0202-13.2013

Trussell, L. O., and Roberts, M. T. (2008). "The role of potassium channels in the regulation of neurotransmitter release," in *Molecular Mechanisms of Neurotransmitter Release*, ed. Z.-W. Wang (New York: Humana Press), 171–185.

von Bartheld, C. S., Code, R. A., and Rubel, E. W. (1989). GABAergic neurons in brainstem auditory nuclei of the chick: distribution, morphology, and connectivity. *J. Comp. Neurol.* 287, 470–483. doi: 10.1002/cne.902870406

Wang, L. Y., Gan, L., Forsythe, I. D., and Kaczmarek, L. K. (1998). Contribution of the Kv3.1 potassium channel to high frequency firing in mouse auditory brainstem neurones. *J. Physiol.* 509, 183–194. doi: 10.1111/j.1469-7793.1998.183bo.x

Yamada, R., Okuda, H., Kuba, H., Nishino, E., Ishii, T. M., and Ohmori, H. (2013). The cooperation of sustained and phasic-inhibition increased the contrast of ITD-tuning in low-frequency neurons of the chick nucleus laminaris. *J. Neurosci.* 33, 3927–3938. doi: 10.1523/JNEUROSCI.2377-12.2013

Yang, L., Monsivais, P., and Rubel, E. W. (1999). The superior olivary nucleus and its influence on nucleus laminaris: a source of inhibitory feedback for coincidence detection in the avian auditory brainstem. *J. Neurosci.* 19, 2313–2325.

Zhou, Y., Carney, L. H., and Colburn, H. S. (2005). A model for interaural time difference sensitivity in the medial superior olive: interaction of excitatory and inhibitory synaptic inputs, channel dynamics, and cellular morphology. *J. Neurosci.* 25, 3046–3058. doi: 10.1523/JNEUROSCI.3064-04.2005

8

Linear coding of complex sound spectra by discharge rate in neurons of the medial nucleus of the trapezoid body (MNTB) and its inputs

Kanthaiah Koka and Daniel J. Tollin*

Department of Physiology and Biophysics, University of Colorado School of Medicine, Aurora, CO, USA

***Correspondence:**
Daniel J. Tollin, Department of Physiology and Biophysics, University of Colorado School of Medicine, RC1-N, Stop 8307, 12800 E. 19th Avenue, Aurora, CO 80045, USA
e-mail: daniel.tollin@ucdenver.edu

The interaural level difference (ILD) cue to sound location is first encoded in the lateral superior olive (LSO). ILD sensitivity results because the LSO receives excitatory input from the ipsilateral cochlear nucleus and inhibitory input indirectly from the contralateral cochlear nucleus via glycinergic neurons of the ipsilateral medial nucleus of the trapezoid body (MNTB). It is hypothesized that in order for LSO neurons to encode ILDs, the sound spectra at both ears must be accurately encoded via spike rate by their afferents. This spectral-coding hypothesis has not been directly tested in MNTB, likely because MNTB neurons have been mostly described and studied recently in regards to their abilities to encode temporal aspects of sounds, not spectral. Here, we test the hypothesis that MNTB neurons and their inputs from the cochlear nucleus and auditory nerve code sound spectra via discharge rate. The Random Spectral Shape (RSS) method was used to estimate how the levels of 100-ms duration spectrally stationary stimuli were weighted, both linearly and non-linearly, across a wide band of frequencies. In general, MNTB neurons, and their globular bushy cell inputs, were found to be well-modeled by a linear weighting of spectra demonstrating that the pathways through the MNTB can accurately encode sound spectra including those resulting from the acoustical cues to sound location provided by head-related directional transfer functions (DTFs). Together with the anatomical and biophysical specializations for timing in the MNTB-LSO complex, these mechanisms may allow ILDs to be computed for complex stimuli with rapid spectrotemporally-modulated envelopes such as speech and animal vocalizations and moving sound sources.

Keywords: calyx of held, medial nucleus of the trapezoid body, lateral superior olive, spectrotemporal receptive field, sound localization, temporal processing

INTRODUCTION

The interaural level difference (ILD) cue to sound location requires neural encoding of the shapes and magnitudes of sound spectra. ILDs result from frequency- and direction-dependent modifications of sound by the head and pinnae and are defined as the difference in spectra of the signals at the two ears (Tollin and Koka, 2009a,b). In the mammalian brainstem, the superior olivary complex contains a circuit comprising the ipsilateral medial nucleus of the trapezoid body (MNTB) and the lateral superior olive (LSO) that is essential for ILD encoding (Tollin, 2003). LSO neurons receive excitatory input from spherical bushy cells (SBCs) of the ipsilateral cochlear nucleus (CN) and inhibitory input from the contralateral ear via the MNTB; the MNTB receives excitatory input from globular bushy cells (GBCs) of the contralateral CN. SBCs and GBCs receive excitatory inputs from the auditory nerve. These inputs confer upon single LSO neurons the ability to compute a neural correlate of ILDs (Boudreau and Tsuchitani, 1968).

Although there is consensus that the LSO initially encodes ILDs and that the inhibitory input to the LSO from the MNTB is essential, the mechanisms are still not well understood. The accurate and precise encoding of ILD observed in LSO neurons (e.g., Tollin et al., 2008) would seem to imply that the neurons comprising the ascending inputs to LSO must be accurately encoding sound spectra at the two ears. However, this hypothesis has not been explicitly tested. One reason for this may be that the MNTB and bushy cells are mostly described, and thus studied, in regards to their exquisite abilities to encode *temporal* aspects of sounds (Wu and Kelly, 1993; Taschenberger and Von Gersdorff, 2000; Futai et al., 2001; Joshi et al., 2004; Lorteije et al., 2009) but not spectral. The exquisite temporal processing capabilities of MNTB result from several specializations. First, the input from GBCs onto MNTB neurons forms the largest, most secure synapses in the CNS, the calyx of Held (Jean-Baptiste and Morest, 1975; McLaughlin et al., 2008). Each MNTB neuron receives only a single calyx, which can envelop up to half the soma surface, and large pre-synaptic terminals that produce large post-synaptic currents (Banks and Smith, 1992; Smith et al., 1998), facts that have made this synapse a model for synaptic transmission (Forsythe, 1994; Borst et al., 1995; Schneggenburger and Forsythe, 2006). MNTB neurons have short membrane time constants, receptors with fast kinetics, and specialized ion channels that together with specializations in the calyx result in large, rapid EPSPs that excite MNTB neurons with nearly invariant synaptic delays (Wu and Kelly, 1991; Banks and Smith, 1992; von Gersdorff and Borst, 2002; Trussell, 2002; although see Tolnai et al., 2009) making them indeed well suited to preserve temporal information that is important for the encoding of the binaural cues to sound location (Joris and Yin, 1998; Tollin and Yin, 2005).

Despite these extraordinary specializations for temporal fidelity, we hypothesize that MNTB neurons must also accurately code the shapes of the sound spectra at the ears over short time intervals in order to account for the abilities of LSO neurons to encode the frequency-dependent acoustic ILDs (Tollin and Yin, 2002a,b; Tollin et al., 2008; Tsai et al., 2010) and for animals such as cats to use these ILD cues to accurately and precisely localize high-frequency sound sources (Tollin et al., 2005, 2013; Moore et al., 2008; Gai et al., 2013; Ruhland et al., 2013). Here, a systems identification method, the Random Spectral Shape (RSS) technique (Yu and Young, 2000), was used to test the hypothesis that MNTB neurons and their inputs, the GBCs and auditory nerve fibers, encode stationary sound spectra linearly via their discharge rate. The RSS technique estimates the spectral weighting function that describes how spectra are linearly and non-linearly weighted to produce a discharge rate. Both GBC and MNTB neurons were well modeled by a linear weighting of sound spectra, consistent with previous reports in auditory nerve and other CN neurons (Yu and Young, 2000, 2013; Young and Calhoun, 2005). Together with the anatomical and biophysical specializations for timing in the neural circuits comprising the GBC, MNTB, and LSO, the mechanisms that produce accurate linear coding of spectral levels in these neurons may allow ILD cues to be coded for complex biologically-relevant stimuli with rapid spectrotemporally-modulated envelopes such as speech and animal vocalizations and moving sound sources.

MATERIALS AND METHODS

ANIMALS, APPARATUS, AND EXPERIMENTAL PROCEDURES

All surgical and experimental procedures complied with the guidelines of the University of Colorado Anschutz Medical Campus Animal Care and Use Committee and the National Institutes of Health. Methods are based on those described in Tollin et al. (2008) and Tsai et al. (2010). Adult cats with clean external ears were initially anesthetized with ketamine hydrochloride (20 mg/kg) along with acepromazine (0.1 mg/kg). Atropine sulfate (0.05 mg/kg) was also given to reduce mucous secretions, and a tracheal cannula was inserted. Supplemental doses of sodium pentobarbital (3–5 mg/kg) were administered intravenously into the femoral vein as needed to maintain areflexia. Heart rate was continuously monitored as was core body temperature (with a rectal probe), the latter maintained with a heating pad at 37°C (Model TC 100, CWE, Inc., Ardmore, PA). Blood-oxygen levels, respiratory rate, and end-tidal CO_2 were measured continuously via a capnograph (Surgivet V90040, Waukesha, WI) and mean arterial blood pressure (femoral artery) was monitored with a pressure transducer (Harvard Apparatus research blood pressure transducer, Holliston, MA). Both pinnae were cut transversely, removed, and tight-fitting custom built hollow earpieces were fitted tightly into the external auditory meati. Polyethylene tubing (Intramedic, PE-90, 30 cm, 0.9 mm ID) was glued into a small hole made in each bulla to maintain normal middle ear pressure.

The trapezoid body and the MNTB was approached ventrally by drilling small holes into the basioccipital bone. Parylene-coated tungsten microelectrodes (1–2 MΩ, Microprobe, Clarksburg, MD) were advanced ventromedially to dorsolaterally at an angle of 26–30° into the brainstem by a microdrive (Kopf Model 662, Tujunga, CA) affixed to a micromanipulator that could be remotely advanced from outside the double-walled sound-attenuating chamber (Industrial Acoustics, Bronx, NY). Electrical activity was amplified (ISO-80, WPI, Sarasota, FL) and filtered (300–3000 Hz; Stanford Research Systems SRS 560, Sunnyvale, CA). Unit responses were discriminated with a BAK amplitude-time window discriminator (Model DDIS-1, Mount Airy, MD) and spike times were stored at a precision of 1 μs via a Tucker-Davis Technologies (TDT, Alachua, FL) RV8.

Stimuli: general

All stimuli were generated digitally at 24-bit resolution and converted to analog at a nominal rate of 100 kHz by a TDT RX-6. Overall stimulus level to each ear was independently controlled in 1 dB steps using a pair of TDT PA-5s. The conditioned output of the D/A converter was sent to an acoustic assembly (one for each ear) comprising a TDT EC1 electrostatic speaker, a calibrated probe-tube microphone (Bruel and Kjaer Type 4182, Norcross, GA), and a hollow earpiece that was fit tightly into the cut end of the auditory meatus and sealed with petroleum jelly. The hollow earpiece accommodated the small probe-tube microphone by which the sound delivery system to each ear was calibrated for tones between 50 Hz and 40 kHz in 50–100 Hz steps. The calibration data was used to compute 256 tap Finite Impulse Response digital filters that equalized the responses of the acoustical system and typically yielded flat frequency responses within ±2 dB for frequencies less than 35 kHz (Koka et al., 2010).

Tone bursts of varying frequency were used as search stimuli. Once a single unit was isolated, the characteristic frequency (CF), spontaneous activity, and threshold were measured using an automated threshold tracking routine or by measuring a frequency-intensity response area (±2 octaves around the CF with 1/8 octave frequency increments and ~0–80 dB SPL in 5 dB increments). The sharpness of the tuning curves was measured as the Q_{10} (CF/bandwidth at 10 dB above threshold). Rate-level functions were measured by presenting 200 repetitions of a 50-ms tone pip at CF (5-ms rise-fall times) every 100 ms from which the resulting PST histograms (PSTHs) were examined on-line. For some neurons, the sensitivity to ILDs was examined by holding the sound level presented to the contralateral, excitatory ear constant at ~20 dB above the contralateral-ear only threshold level and varying the stimulus level to the ipsilateral ear ±25 dB about the contralateral ear sound level (i.e., ILDs varied between ±25 dB). Discharge rate vs. sound level functions were also measured for 100-ms duration flat-spectrum broadband noise by presenting 20 repetitions of the noise at each stimulus level tested.

MNTB and GBC neuron classification

When recording extracellularly with metal electrodes, care must be taken in positively categorizing neurons as MNTB due to the presence of the large numbers of fibers of the trapezoid body passing directly through the MNTB; many of these fibers respond to sound stimuli similar to MNTB neurons (Smith et al., 1991, 1993). Here, the criteria of Smith et al. (1998) were used to classify MNTB principal cells based on their extracellular responses. Neurons were classified as MNTB based on three properties: (1) responses only to stimuli presented to the contralateral ear (Guinan et al., 1972a,b; Smith et al., 1998); (2) the presence of a prepotential in the action potential waveform (Guinan and Li, 1990); and (3) a primary-like (PL) or a primary-like with notch (PLN) PSTH to short tone burst stimuli (Smith et al., 1998). GBC-like responses were obtained from fiber recordings in the trapezoid body. GBCs fibers were also classified according to Smith et al. (1991, 1998) by monaural-only responses, PLN or onset-L (OnL; Rhode, 2008) PSTHs to short tone stimuli, the lack of a pre-potential in the extracellular waveform, and a more ventral recording depth than MNTB. This is a conservative characterization of GBCs from electrophysiological responses because some morphologically-identified GBCs can have primary-like PSTHs to tones at some stimulus levels (Rhode, 2008).

Histology

In many experiments, electrolytic DC lesions ($5\,\mu A \times 10\,s$) were made to differentiate electrode tracks, mark locations of interest, and assist in estimating tissue shrinkage after histological processing. At the conclusion of each experiment, the brain was fixed in formalin or 4% buffered paraformaldehyde by immersion or perfusion through the heart. The fixed tissue was cut into 50-μm frozen sections and stained with cresyl violet so that electrode tracks and lesions made during the recordings could be seen.

RSS method and spectral weight function model

The RSS technique is a systems identification method (Yu and Young, 2000, 2013; Young and Calhoun, 2005; Bandyopadhyay et al., 2007; Reiss et al., 2007) to determine how neurons linearly and non-linearly weight sound spectra to increase or decrease their discharge rate. For this paper, 264 different pseudorandom RSS noises were created, each consisting of the sum of 512 random-phase tones spaced logarithmatically in frequency at 1/64-octave spacing and covering the range from 0.17 to 40 kHz. The random phase of the tones eliminates the formation of an onset transient after the summation of the tones. The tones were grouped into 64 frequency bins each containing 8 tones, so that each bin spanned 1/8 octave. Relative to the mean overall spectral level of each stimulus (i.e., a flat-spectrum broadband noise where all bins are set to a gain of 0 dB), the amplitude of the tones in each of the 64 bins, $S(f)$ in dB, were chosen randomly from a normal distribution that had a mean and standard deviation of 0 and 10 dB, respectively, so that all 8 components in a single bin have the same amplitude. Of the 264 RSS stimuli 4 had a flat spectrum, $S(f) = 0$ dB for all f, while the remaining 260 stimuli had spectral patterns as just described. **Figure 1** shows the amplitude spectra in terms of the gain in dB re: the reference level for three of the stimuli among 264 stimuli, including one with a flat spectrum.

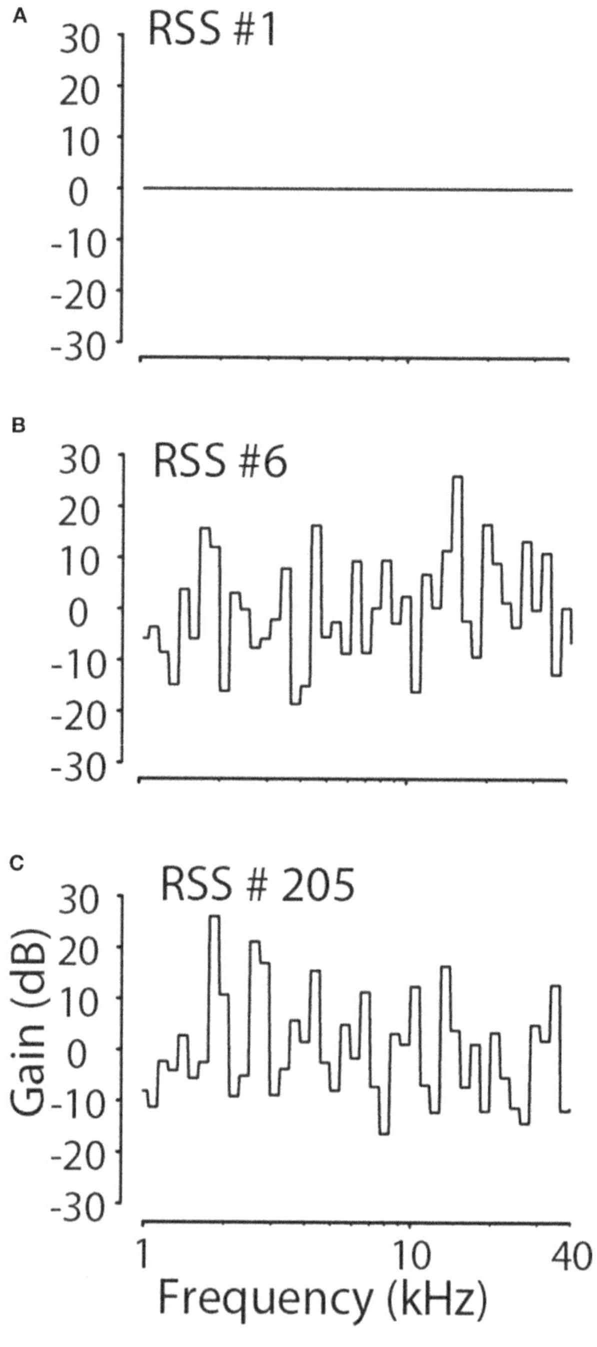

FIGURE 1 | Examples of three of 264 RSS stimulus spectra. The RSS stimuli had spectral contrasts chosen from a normal distribution with a standard deviation of 10 dB. Four of 264 stimuli had flat spectra **(A)**, while the remaining stimuli had spectra resembling those in **(B,C)**.

Across the 264 stimuli, the amplitudes in each frequency bin were specifically constructed to be uncorrelated with the amplitudes in all other bins. This constraint allows the use of linear least squares techniques (Press et al., 1986) to compute the spectral weights from the rate responses to the ensemble of RSS stimuli.

Moreover, the zero mean and uncorrelated spectral levels in the different frequency bins allows the computation of both first order and second order weighting functions separately. In order for this to occur, as described by Reiss et al. (2007), the ensemble of RSS stimuli were ordered into successive plus-minus pairs such that the spectral levels of the first stimulus of the pair $S_i(f)$ were simply inverted in the second stimulus $S_{i+1}(f)$ [i.e., $S_{i+1}(f) = -S_i(f)$]. These plus-minus pairs of stimulus were used to separate the estimation of the even and the odd order terms in the model presented below. The full description and validation of this technique can be found in Reiss et al. (2007).

The ensemble of 264 RSS stimuli was presented at 4–10 overall levels spanning ~20 dB below to ~40 dB above the threshold level for the flat spectrum noise alone. The threshold was estimated to within ±2.5 dB from the rate-level function for one of the flat-spectrum RSS stimuli. In all cases, the RSS stimuli were 100 ms in duration and were gated on and off with 10-ms linear ramps.

The weight function model is based on the following equation for average discharge rate r of a neuron computed over the 100-ms duration of the stimulus:

$$r = R_0 + \sum_{j=1} w_j S(f_i) + \sum_{j=1}\sum_{k=j} w_{jk} S(f_i) S(f_k) \quad (1a)$$

which can be re-written in matrix form in the following way:

$$r = R_0 + \mathrm{w}^T \mathrm{s} + \mathrm{s}^T \mathrm{M} \mathrm{s} \quad (1b)$$

where s is a vector containing the dB values of each stimulus at different frequencies [i.e., $S(f_i)$], w is a vector containing the first order, or linear, weights (i.e., w_j) of the neuron [in units of spikes/(s·dB)], M is a matrix of second order, or non-linear, weights (i.e., w_{jk}) of the neuron [units of spikes/(s·dB^2)] and T indicates transposition. The matrix of second order weights measures the contribution to the response of the neuron to quadratic terms like the energy-squared at a particular frequency [e.g., w_{jj} for $S^2(f_j)$] or the product of the energy at two different frequencies. Finally R_0 is a constant, which is the rate response to the flat spectrum stimulus with all frequency bins set to 0 dB level. For all the calculations, dB levels were not always corrected for the speaker calibration; however, because the headphone calibrations are locally flat (re: the spectral receptive field of a given neuron), correcting for the calibration had negligible effects on the data (see also Young and Calhoun, 2005).

For each neuron the model parameters for Equation (1) were estimated using the discharge rates in responses to single presentations of each of the 264 RSS stimuli, which thus results in 264 equations as expressed by Equation (1). The variable R_0 was estimated directly as part of Equation (1b). The first- and second-order model weights, w and M Equation (1b), were estimated by the method of normal equations (e.g., Press et al., 1986) by minimizing the chi-square error:

$$\chi^2(w, M) = \sum_j \frac{\left[r_j - \hat{r}_j(s_j, w, M)\right]^2}{\sigma_j^2} \quad (2)$$

Here r_j are the empirical rates measured in the experiment and $r_j(\mathrm{s}_j,\mathrm{w},\mathrm{M})$ are the rates predicted by the model in Equation (1) for the stimulus s_j and the first and second-order weights w and M, respectively, and σ_j^2 is the variance of the rate response r_j. We did not attempt to estimate directly σ_j^2 (the variance of the rates computed over multiple repetitions of the same stimulus) in all neurons due to the limited recording time for each neuron. Instead, we assumed that the response counts (i.e., r_j/T, where $T = 100$ ms, the duration of the stimuli used here) were Poisson distributed such that the variance of the count was equal to the mean count. Also, to avoid having the denominator in Equation (2) go to zero, σ_j^2 was not allowed to have a value <0.1. Using Equations (1) and (2), the model weights were computed using the weighted least squares technique (Press et al., 1986) in MATLAB (v7.1, The Mathworks, Inc., Natick, MA), where the diagonal of the weight matrix is equal to σ_j^2.

As one check of the applicability of the Poisson variance assumption, in 8 neurons the response variance σ_j^2 was estimated from a power-law fit of the response variance vs. the mean response computed from the flat-spectrum stimulus rate-level function where multiple presentations of the same stimuli were presented (see Tollin et al., 2008). From the power-law fitted function, given an arbitrary discharge rate, the corresponding rate variance could be accurately predicted. Using this empirically-determined response variance instead of the Poisson variance assumption did not materially change the weight functions (e.g., see **Figures 3A1,B1**) or the predicted responses to arbitrary stimuli not used in the fitting of the model parameters (see below).

Computational estimation of the first- and second-order weights was simplified due to the design of the plus-minus RSS stimulus pairs as mentioned earlier. Following from Reiss et al. (2007), let r^+ and r^- be the rates in response to a plus-minus stimulus pair s^+ and s^- (i.e., where $s^+ = -s^-$). From Equation (1):

$$\frac{r^+ + r^-}{2} = R_0 + \mathrm{s}^{+T}\mathrm{M}\mathrm{s}^+ \text{ and } \frac{r^+ - r^-}{2} = \mathrm{s}^{+T}\mathrm{w} \quad (3)$$

Here, the estimation of the second-order weight matrix M is based on $(r^+ + r^-)/2$ and the first order weight vector w based on $(r^+ - r^-)/2$. As before, R_0 is estimated either from the responses to the flat spectrum RSS stimuli or as part of the parameters in Equation (2). For each neuron and overall sound level we used that R_0 which maximized the fraction of explained variance (*fv*, see next section). We adopted this procedure because the R_0 measured from only four presentations of the flat-spectrum stimuli did not always maximize *fv*; more than four presentations of the flat spectrum stimuli apparently need to be measured to get a more accurate estimate of R_0. Because the estimates of different orders of weights are not necessarily orthogonal (see Reiss et al., 2007), if the neuron were to actually be influenced by third (or higher) order weights, this would appear as an error in the estimation of the lower-order weights. Estimating the first and second order weights separately in the way described above reduces this error by keeping the error from un-estimated odd-order components from affecting even-order estimates and vice versa.

The standard deviations (SDs) of the spectral weights were estimated using standard statistical bootstrapping techniques (Efron and Tibshirani, 1993). This was done because neural responses to multiple repetitions of stimuli were not collected in all neurons. The SDs of the weights were computed in the following way. A set of 200 RSS stimulus/response pairs were chosen at random with replacement from the 200 RSS stimuli estimation set (see next section) and the spectral weight functions computed using Equation (1b). This process of selecting stimulus/response pairs with replacement and computing the spectral weights was repeated at least 200 times. From the resulting 200 spectral weight functions the mean and SD of each the weights were calculated.

Prediction of responses to arbitrary stimuli: quality of the model fit

A rigorous test of the spectral weight model Equation (1a) was the ability to predict the rate responses to arbitrary stimuli that were not used in the fitting process. To this end, the 264 RSS stimuli were divided in to two groups: (1) an estimation set of the rate responses to 200 RSS stimuli [1–100 from positive-spectra half and 1–100 from negative-spectra half, see Equation (3)] and (2) a prediction set consisting of the responses to the remaining 64 RSS stimuli (101–132 from positive half and 101–132 from negative half). The set of 200 RSS stimuli was used to estimate the spectral weights using Equation (1b). These weights were then used to predict the responses to the 64 stimuli also using Equation (1b). The quality of the model was quantified by an adaptation of the fraction of unexplained variance (Hays, 1988) which has been defined by Young and Calhoun (2005) as:

$$fv = 1 - \frac{\sum (r_j - \hat{r}_j)^2}{\sum (r_j - \bar{r})^2} \quad (4)$$

Here, for the *i*th RSS stimulus, r_j the empirical rate, $\hat{r}_j$ is the rate predicted by the model, and $\bar{r}$ is the mean rate computed over all RSS stimuli. *fv* values vary from a maximum of 1 (perfect fit) and decrease with poorer predictions; *fv* can take values <0 when the fit is particularly poor. The *fv* was also used to assist in the determination of the numbers of first- and second-order model parameters for the spectral weight functions. The numbers of spectral weights were systematically added to the model beginning with the weight at BF, along with the corresponding number of second-order weights. More weights were added until the *fv* for prediction was maximized. The frequency range of the weights was typically within one octave below and one-half octave above BF. Choosing weights in this way helps to avoid over fitting the model. The correlation coefficients were also quantified for the predictions along with the *fv* values and compared.

Rationale for using the random spectral shape technique

For neurons in the auditory system with complex receptive fields, researchers often characterize the so-called spectrotemporal receptive field (STRF; Aertsen et al., 1981; Eggermont, 1993; Kowalski et al., 1996; deCharms et al., 1998; Theunissen et al., 2000; Schnupp et al., 2001; Escabi and Schreiner, 2002). The STRF estimates the average power spectrum of the stimulus as a function of time (e.g., the spectrogram) preceding an action potential elicited from a neuron. Here, it is assumed that the STRFs for MNTB neurons are spectrally and temporally separable, which is a good assumption for neurons peripheral to the inferior colliculus (Qiu et al., 2003; Lewis and van Dijk, 2004; Lesica and Grothe, 2008; Versnel et al., 2009). When any separable STRF is averaged over time, the temporal component in any particular frequency bin reduces to a constant. The resultant STRF summation, then, gives rise to precisely the RSS weight function as given in Equation (1) (Young et al., 2005). Moreover, for stimulus sets for which the spectra are stationary (i.e., fixed throughout the stimulus duration), such as the RSS stimuli used here, any residual spectral-temporal interactions may be minimized (Young et al., 2005). While temporal interactions probably do play an important role in establishing the ultimate responsiveness of MNTB neurons (see Kopp-Scheinpflug et al., 2008), we wanted to test here the specific hypothesis that the neurons of the MNTB accurately encode stationary spectral characteristics of the stimuli via discharge rate. Toward this specific goal, the RSS technique (Yu and Young, 2000) represents an efficient method.

Responses to acoustic directional transfer function-filtered broadband noise stimuli

As an additional test of the weight function model, a behaviorally-relevant set of acoustical stimuli was used. Here, the first- and second-order weights of the estimated spectral weight models for each neuron tested were used to predict the responses to 100-ms duration flat-spectrum broadband noise filtered by directional transfer functions (DTFs) from 325 to 627 locations in the front and rear hemispheres. Acoustic DTFs contain the sound source location dependent features of the head related transfer functions (HRTF) (Koka et al., 2011). The acoustic DTFs were measured in each animal in this paper immediately prior to the physiological studies. The methods for measuring the DTFs and the associated acoustical cues to location computed from them are described in detail in Tollin and Koka (2009a,b). Spatial plotting of the DTF-stimuli and the neural responses to them was done using Aitov projections. These spatial plots are shown in this paper for just the frontal hemisphere from elevations −45° to +90° and azimuths −90° (contralateral to MNTB being studied) to +90°. This area consists of 325 DTF filtered stimuli. The fraction of variance *fv* was quantified for the predicted rate responses for DTF stimuli. Two-dimensional smoothing was done on empirical responses along with responses predicted from either first order alone or first order and second order together for plotting purposes only. The spatial correlation coefficients were calculated and compared along with the *fv* values. The spatial correlation coefficients explain how well the model can predict the general two-dimensional shape of the neural spatial receptive fields.

RESULTS

Results are based on recordings of 103 MNTB and 51 GBC neurons collected from 22 subjects. All 103 MNTB neurons exhibited a complex "pre-potential" that preceded the action potential by ~0.5–0.7 ms and all responded only to stimuli presented to the contralateral ear. **Figure 2A** shows examples of the complex waveforms of the extracellularly-recorded action potentials from five neurons. The diversity in waveform shapes is consistent with other reported recordings in cat MNTB (e.g., Guinan

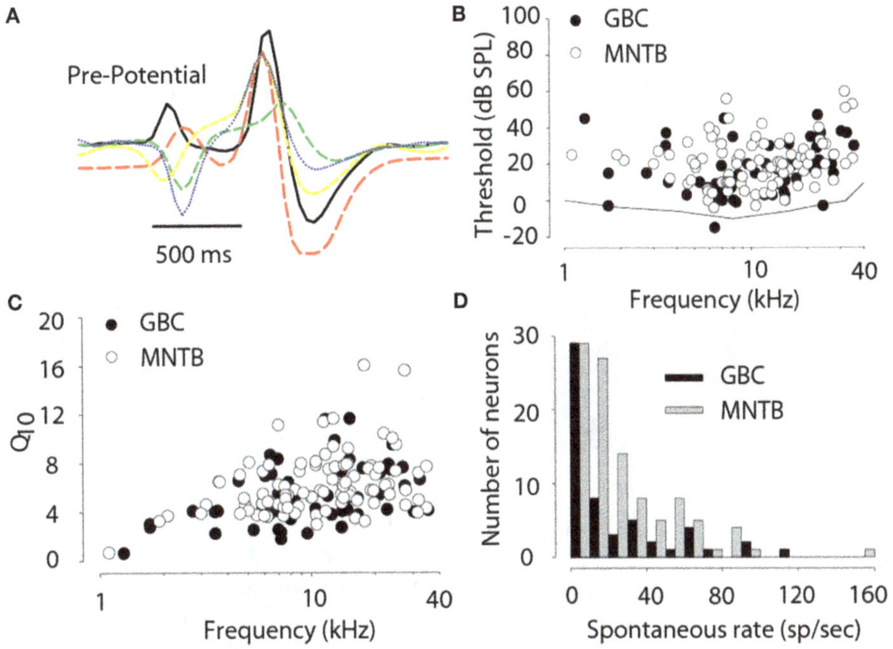

FIGURE 2 | (A) Examples of extracellular voltage waveforms illustrating the pre-potential component in 5 MNTB neurons. **(B)** Threshold SPL for tones as a function of the characteristic frequency of each neuron. Behavioral audiogram for cat from Heffner and Heffner (1985) (solid line). **(C)** Frequency tuning bandwidth, Q_{10} (characteristic frequency divided by the bandwidth 10 dB above threshold), as a function of characteristic frequency. **(D)** Histogram of spontaneous activity. Data in **(B–D)** are based on 103 MNTB and 51 GBC neurons.

and Li, 1990; Joris and Yin, 1998; Smith et al., 1998). Electrode tracks were able to be reconstructed from the histology in 8 cats, allowing the verification of 44/103 neurons in the MNTB. The location of neurons as a function of their CF was in agreement with prior studies (Guinan et al., 1972a; Sommer et al., 1993; Smith et al., 1998; Tollin and Yin, 2005) with high-CF neurons located medioventral and lower-CF neurons located dorsolateral in the nucleus. Histology was either not available or the electrode tracks could not be reconstructed to localize the remaining neurons. These remaining neurons are included here because they all had properties consistent with MNTB neurons in the cat: complex "pre-potential" wave shape (e.g., **Figure 2A**), responsive to contralateral ear stimulation only, gave PL or PLN response type, and where two or more MNTB neurons were recorded in the same electrode penetration there was systematically increasing progression of CF with electrode depth. Thirty eight MNTB neurons were studied extensively with 8 bin/oct RSS stimuli. Finally, 14 of these 38 neurons were studied with virtual acoustic space stimuli consisting of broadband noise appropriately filtered by a set of DTFs. Responses from 51 putative GBC fibers were recorded, 21 of which were studied with RSS stimuli.

BASIC ACOUSTICAL RESPONSE PROPERTIES

Several basic acoustic response properties were measured for all 103 MNTB neurons and 51 GBC fibers. **Figure 2B** shows the threshold SPL as a function of CFs for all neurons and also the cat audiogram (Heffner and Heffner, 1985). The CFs ranged from 0.32 to 35 kHz (mean $CF = 12.4 \pm 8$ kHz, median = 10.6 kHz) and 1.3–35.5 kHz (12.7 ± 8.44 kHz; 10.5 kHz) and thresholds ranged from -4 to 60 dB SPL (mean threshold = 20.5 ± 12.8, median = 20 dB) and −15 to 47 dB SPL (16.5 ± 14.0, 15.0) for MNTB and GBC, respectively. In MNTB the Q_{10} (**Figure 2C**) ranged from 0.5 to 16 and was highly dependent on CF with low Q_{10} of ~1–2 for CFs of <1 kHz increasing to ~8 for high CFs. The Q_{10} (**Figure 2C**) in GBCs ranged similarly across CF from 0.64 to 11.6. MNTB neurons exhibited a high degree of spontaneous activity (**Figure 2D**) ranging from 0 to 150 spikes/s (mean spontaneous activity = 25.5 ± 25.9 spikes/s; median = 17.5 spikes/s) while GBC fibers ranged from 0 to 40 spikes/s (23.6 ± 25.1; 13.0). In 20/20 (100%) MNTB neurons tested (CFs spanning 1.9–35 kHz) exhibited no sensitivity to ILDs (i.e., the responses were not affected by stimuli at the ipsilateral ear). Finally, the spontaneous activity and thresholds were not significantly different, as assessed by an independent-samples *t*-test [$t_{(152)} < 1.8, p > 0.05$ for both tests] between the GBC and MNTB neurons consistent with GBC providing MNTB with its afferent excitatory input via the calyx of Held; however MNTB neurons tended to have significantly, albeit slightly, narrower frequency selectivity than GBCs as assessed from Q_{10} (**Figure 2C**) [$t_{(152)} = 2.0, p = 0.03$].

GENERAL PROPERTIES OF THE SPECTRAL WEIGHT FUNCTIONS

For all MNTB and GBC neurons, the first order weight functions, e.g., Equation (1a) showed an excitatory area (positive weights) near the neuron CF. The frequency bin corresponding to the largest spectral weight will be called the best frequency (BF). **Figures 3A1,B1** (black symbols) show the first order weights for one MNTB neuron ($BF = 15.4$ kHz) taken at −5 and 15 dB

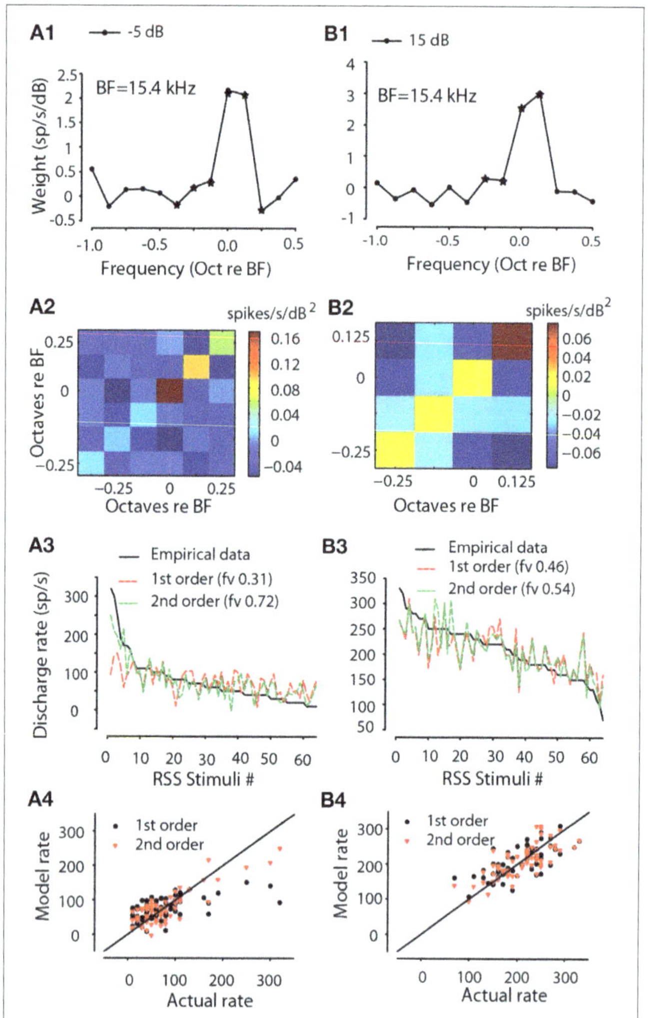

FIGURE 3 | Encoding of sound spectra by MNTB neuron via RSS method. First order (linear) spectral weight functions for one neuron (*CF* = 15.4 kHz) at two levels re: threshold (**A1** −5 dB, **B1** 15 dB). Second-order weights for the same two levels **(A2,B2)**. Empirical discharge rates plotted rank-ordered vs. RSS stimuli (black line) along with the predicted rates using the estimated first-order (red line) and full-order (green line) spectral weight models for the same two levels **(A3,B3)**. The fraction of explained variance, *fv*, is indicated for each model. Scatter plot of modeled rate vs. empirical rate for first-order (black) and full-order (red) models for the same two levels **(A4,B4)**. Solid line is line of equality.

sound levels above the flat-spectrum noise threshold, respectively. At both sound levels, the peak weight was at BF with smaller weights at adjacent higher and lower frequencies. Standard deviations of the weights (not shown) were estimated using statistical resampling techniques (Efron and Tibshirani 86). Weights ±1 SD away from 0 were considered significant and were subsequently used for predictions (see below); significant weights are indicated by a star symbol in **Figures 3A1,B1**. The second order weights (**Figures 3A2,B2**) were positive (red) at the BF and along the diagonal (i.e., same frequency bins on the x and y axes) but negative (blue) at the adjacent off diagonal frequencies. In general, the second order weights were about an order of magnitude smaller than the first order weights.

TESTING THE VALIDITY OF THE SPECTRAL WEIGHT FUNCTION MODEL

The weight functions (Equation 1 and **Figures 3A1,B1**) are designed to quantify the transformation of spectral levels into discharge rate and indicates the frequency range over which these transformations occur (i.e., spectral selectivity). But how accurate and valid is this model for GBC and MNTB neurons? The validity of the spectral weight model and the RSS technique in general was tested by using the fitted weights and Equation (1) to make predictions of rate responses to arbitrary RSS (and DTF-filtered stimuli, see below) stimuli that were not used for the fitting. Model quality was quantified by the fraction of explained variance, *fv* [see Equation (4), Methods]. *fv* values vary from a maximum of 1 (perfect fit) and decrease with poorer predictions; *fv* can take values <0 when the fit is particularly poor.

As an example of this procedure, **Figures 3A3,B3** show the empirical responses to the 64 RSS stimuli comprising the prediction set, plus the predicted rates for the first-order model (R_0 and first order weights, red) and the full-order model that also includes the second order terms, e.g., Equation (1a). For this neuron as well as all others, addition of the second order terms (e.g., **Figures 3A3,B3**) improved the quality of the fit as assessed by the *fv* value. For the 15 dB stimulus level (**Figure 3B3**), addition of the second order terms improved the prediction quality from *fv* of 0.46 to 0.54. For the −5 dB stimulus level (**Figure 3A3**), addition of the second order terms improved the prediction more substantially from *fv* of 0.31 to 0.72. The *fv* metric is approximately equal to the coefficient of determination (R^2; Hays, 1988; see also Young and Calhoun, 2005); the calculated R^2 from the data can, in some instances (e.g., poor estimation of the R_0 parameter), be larger than the corresponding *fv* value. Thus, for the example in **Figure 3A3** the full model explains *at least* 72% of the variance in the discharge rates. Note that since $fv = \sim R^2$, an *fv* of 0.72 corresponds to *R* of 0.85. *fv* is a stricter test of the model than correlation coefficient because it is sensitive to deviations of predictions from a slope of 1.0 and a y-intercept of 0.0, whereas correlation coefficient (and thus, R^2) is not. Finally, **Figures 3A4,B4** show scatter plots of the predicted rates (model rates) as a function of the empirical rates. Note that the data cluster along the line of equality (slope = 1.0) indicating that the spectral weight function model, e.g., Equation (1a) predicts accurately (at least within the unexplained error due to nearly-Poisson response variability) the discharge rate of this MNTB neuron to arbitrary RSS stimuli that were not used to estimate the parameters of the model.

For all GBC and MNTBs neurons and at all sound levels tested for each neuron, the validity of the spectral weight model was assessed by the accuracy of the rate predictions, as illustrated for the one neuron in **Figure 3**. **Figure 4** plots histograms of the first- and second-order prediction qualities, *fv*, for all MNTB (**Figures 4A,B**) and GBC (**Figures 4D,E**) neurons and all sound levels tested. Across the 38 MNTB neurons ($n = 109$ sound levels), the median *fv* was 0.40 [interquartile (IQ) range 0.29–0.54] for the linear first-order model predictions and increased significantly (Wilcoxon signed-ranks test, $Z = 7.48, p < 0.0001$) to 0.55 (IQ range 0.37–0.7) for the full-order model. **Figure 4D** plots the *fv* for the GBC neurons over all sound levels tested. Across the 21 GBC neurons ($n = 76$ sound levels) the median *fv* was

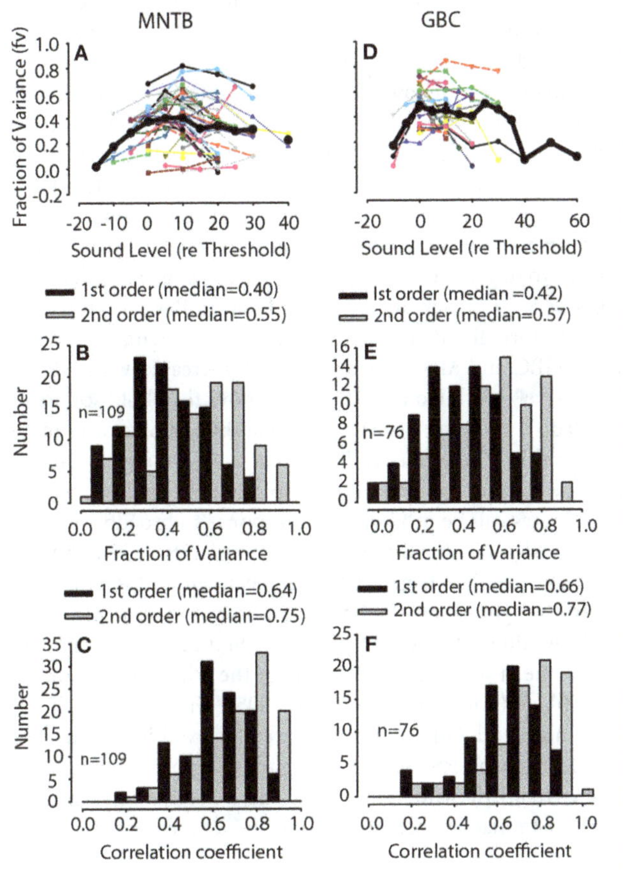

FIGURE 4 | Predictive validation of the spectral weight function model. Fraction of variance, *fv*, as a function of RSS stimulus level for MNTB **(A)** and GBC **(D)** neurons; thin lines indicate data for individual neurons and thick black lines the across-neurons mean. Histogram of the maximum fraction of explained variance Equation (4), *fv*, in 42 MNTB neurons (109 total RSS levels) **(B)** and 21 GBC neurons (76 total RSS levels) **(E)** for both the first-order linear model (black) and the full-order model (gray) containing the second-order non-linear terms. The *fv* were computed by predicting the discharge rates to arbitrary RSS stimuli that were not used in the estimation of the spectral weight models. The across-neuron median *fv* for each model is indicated. Histograms of the correlation coefficient, r, relating the predicted spike rate to the empirical rate (e.g., **Figure 3B4**) are shown in **(C,F)** for MNTB and GBC neurons, respectively.

0.42 (IQ range 0.3–0.56) for the linear first-order model predictions and increased significantly (Wilcoxon signed-ranks test, $Z = 7.57$, $p < 0.0001$) to 0.57 (IQ range 0.39–0.68) for the full-order model. In most MNTB and GBC neurons, the linear model alone explained at least 40-90% of the variance ($R \sim 0.63$–0.95).

Although the median *fv* values plotted in **Figure 4** may appear low (given the 1.0 maximum value for *fv*), the values underestimate model performance when considering the variance (nearly Poisson) of the empirical discharge rate data. Given just a single repetition and short duration (100 ms) of each RSS stimulus used here, the large response variance will ensure that the *fv* will *always* be less than 1.0; that is, a sizeable fraction of the responses are random and thus not predictable at all by the model. This can be appreciated somewhat by observing the vertical scatter of the responses in **Figures 3A4,B4**. The error in *fv* due to random effects obscures the actual capabilities of the spectral weighting model, and thus the functional implications of the model for neural processing. There are a variety of ways of correcting for the effects of finite data sampling on such predictions (see David and Gallant, 2005). Here we used the technique described in Young and Calhoun (2005, p. 4448) to correct the *fv* values for such unexplained variance (assuming Poisson variability). After correction, the maximum *fv* we could theoretically obtain with our empirical data was in the range of ~0.5–0.7, which is comparable to that computed by Young and Calhoun (2005) for auditory nerve fibers stimulated with similar RSS stimulus sets. For the examples in **Figures 3A4,B4**, the estimated maximum *fv* values using the correction method were 0.746 and 0.521, respectively, which were comparable to the empirical *fv* values for the full-order model predictions of 0.73 and 0.47, respectively. In other words, assuming the variance correction above, across the population of neurons (**Figures 4B,E**) the linear model can generally explain most of the variance in the rate responses of MNTB and GBC neurons to arbitrary RSS stimuli. That the second-order terms only marginally, but still significantly, increased the prediction accuracy suggests that a simple linear weighting is a good model for how MNTB and GBC neurons encode sound spectra. Similar results are reported below for predictions of rate responses to noise stimuli filtered through DTFs.

As another objective measure of model performance that is less susceptible to random errors in rate predictions, **Figures 4C,F** plot histograms of the first- and second-order prediction qualities, *correlation coefficient* (r), for all MNTB and GBC neurons, respectively, and all sound levels tested. Across the 38 MNTB neurons ($n = 109$ sound levels), the median r was 0.64 (IQ range 0.54–0.75) for the linear first-order model predictions and increased significantly (Wilcoxon signed-ranks test, $Z = 8.23$, $p < 0.0001$) to 0.75 (IQ range 0.67–0.84) for the full-order model. Across the 21 GBC neurons ($n = 76$ sound levels), the median r was 0.66 (IQ range 0.56–0.76) for the linear first-order model predictions and increased significantly (Wilcoxon signed-ranks test, $Z = 7.55$, $p = 0.003$) to 0.77 (IQ range 0.66–0.85) for the full-order model.

MNTB neurons receive a single large calyceal input from the GBCs. To test the hypothesis that MNTB inherit their spectral coding capabilities from GBCs we compared the distributions of *fv* and correlation coefficients plotted in **Figure 4**. There were no significant differences in *fv* (i.e., **Figures 4B,E**) between MNTB and GBC neurons for either the first order (Mann-Whitney $U = 4412$, $p = 0.45$) or full order models (Mann-Whitney $U = 4375$, $p = 0.52$). Similarly, there were no significant differences between correlation coefficients (e.g., **Figures 4C,F**) between MNTB and GBC neurons for either the first order (Mann-Whitney $U = 4439$, $p = 0.41$) or full order models (Mann-Whitney $U = 4367$, $p = 0.53$). These results support the hypothesis that the spectral coding capabilities of GBCs are largely recapitulated in MNTB.

FUNCTIONAL PROPERTIES OF FIRST ORDER SPECTRAL WEIGHT FUNCTIONS AND THEIR DEPENDENCE ON STIMULUS LEVEL

The validation of the spectral weight model via accurate predictions to arbitrary stimuli suggests that the properties of the weight functions may have functional meaning (although see Materials and Methods for caveats). The first order (linear) weight functions were examined in one way by averaging weights across all neurons after grouping them into three ranges of BFs: 1–3, 3–10, and 10–30 kHz. **Figure 5** shows that the weight functions were quite similar across all neurons in the respective BF groupings when computed at reference sound levels 5–15 dB above threshold. The weight functions in **Figure 5** were aligned on the peak of the weight functions (i.e., BF). The gray lines are for individual neurons and the across-neuron average is shown with black lines. The lower frequency BF neurons generally had lower overall weights and the significant weights spanned a larger range of frequencies than those for the mid- to high-BF neurons.

Because the general shapes of the first-order spectral weight functions were quite similar across both MNTB and GBC neurons computed over similar BF ranges, shown in **Figures 5A,B**, respectively, the functions could then be adequately summarized across neurons and nuclei by two main parameters: maximum weight at BF and the bandwidth of the weight function at half the maximal weight. The bandwidth at half-height (see **Figure 7C**) gives an estimate of the frequency selectivity of the neuron and the maximum weight at BF indicates the strength by which the neuron transforms spectral levels into discharge rate. Across-neuron average first-order spectral weight functions from auditory nerve fibers from the study of Young and Calhoun (2005) are also plotted in **Figure 5C** for comparison; note that the plotted weights for the auditory nerve fibers are smaller (by approximately a factor of 2) than those for the MNTB and GBC neurons because weights were estimated for twice as many frequency bins (i.e., 1/16 bins/octave) as the weights for the MNTB and GBC neurons (1/8 bins/oct).

As an example of how the spectral weights depended on overall sound level, for each MNTB (**Figure 6A**), GBC (**Figure 6B**) and auditory nerve (Figure 6C, from Young and Calhoun, 2005) neuron the maximum spectral weight was plotted as a function of the sound level at which it was measured. To summarize across neurons, each of the functions for the individual neurons was normalized to its maximum weight and then averaged across neurons (**Figures 6A–C**, black lines, right ordinates). Based on the across-neuron normalized average, the spectral weights of auditory nerve, GBC and MNTB neurons at BF increased with reference sound level, saturated at ~10–15 dB above threshold sound level (i.e., 0 dB), and then decreased with additional increases in level beyond this. These data indicate that across this population of neurons comprising the inhibitory pathway to the LSO, their discharge rates can be modulated in response to broadband stimuli over at least a 60–70 dB range of stimulus levels (−20 to 50 dB re: threshold). While the general level dependence of the maximum spectral weight was similar from auditory nerve to MNTB, the absolute value of the weights were not. **Figure 6D** plots the across neuron mean spectral weight at BF for the population of auditory nerve fibers (Young and Calhoun, 2005), GBC and MNTB neurons. In general, GBC and MNTB weights exhibited both similar dependencies on RSS sound level and their absolute magnitudes were virtually the same. Both GBC and MNTB weights, however, were substantially larger by a factor of 1.5-2 (even after accounting

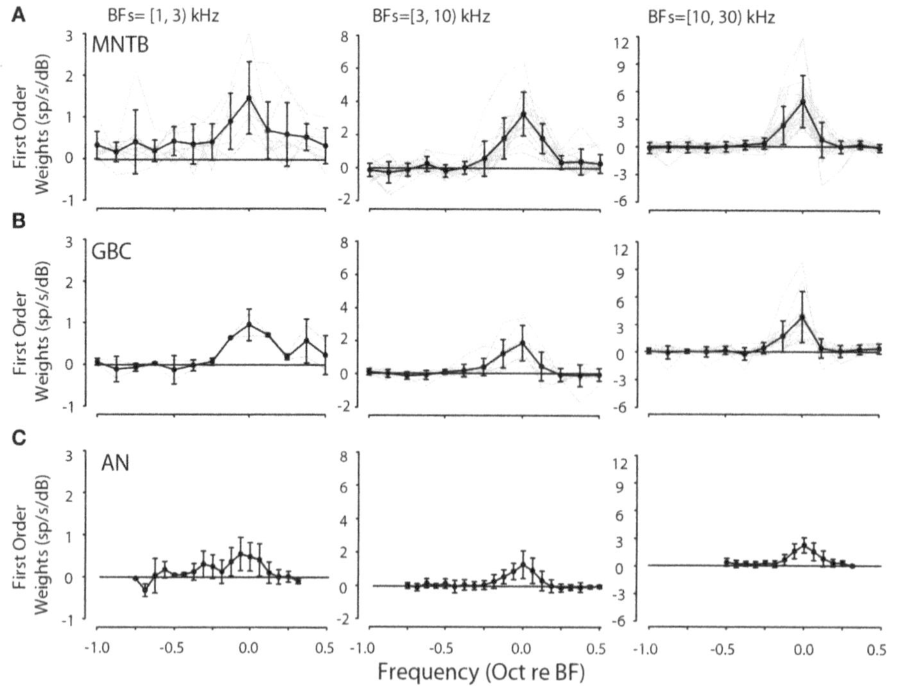

FIGURE 5 | First-order linear weight functions for all 42 MNTB (A) and 21 GBC (B) neurons studied binned according to BF (BF ranges in upper left of each panel). Weight functions were taken from spectral levels in the range of 5–15 dB. Weight function for auditory nerve fibers (AN, **C**) are replotted from Young and Calhoun (2005). In each panel, the light gray lines indicate weight functions for individual neurons while the solid line with symbols and error bars indicate the across-neuron mean weight function ±1 standard deviation. Generally, the weight functions in each range of BFs were similar in terms of shape and magnitude.

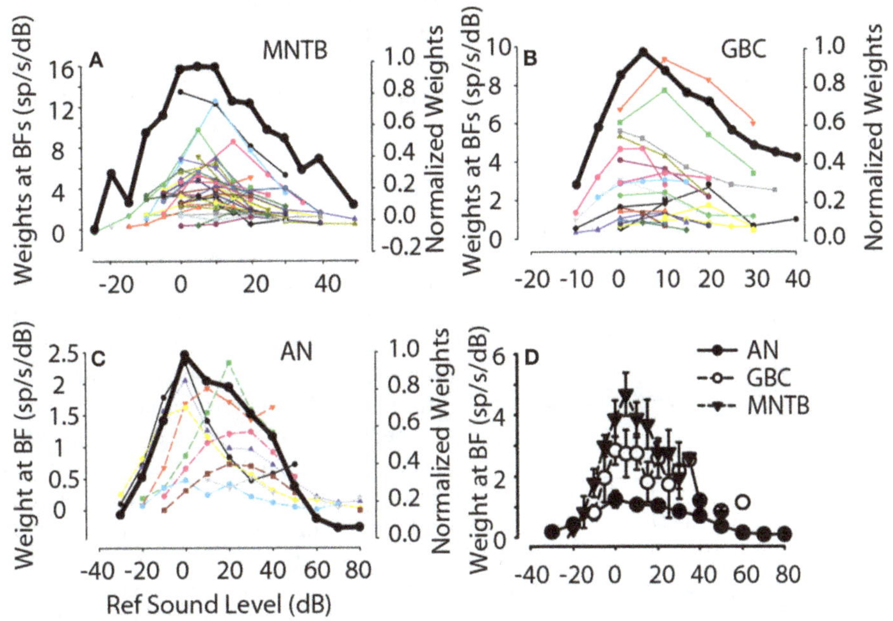

FIGURE 6 | Dependence of first-order weights at BF on overall sound level. For all MNTB **(A)**, GBC **(B)**, and ANF **(C)** neurons studied (individual lines and symbols), the first-order weight at BF (left-hand ordinate) is plotted as a function of sound level (re: threshold for flat-spectrum stimulus, **Figure 1A**). In general, for each neuron the first-order weights were small for low and high sound levels and peaked for moderate sound levels. To summarize this trend, the solid black line shows the across-neuron mean first-order weight as a function of sound level; data for individual neurons was first normalized by the maximum weight before averaging across neurons. **(D)** Summarizes the across-neuron first-order weights at BF in AN, GBC, and MNTB neurons.

for the differences in the weights for auditory nerve fibers discussed in the prior paragraph). That is, for every 1 dB increase in stimulation at BF, MNTB and GBCs produce nearly twice as many additional spikes as auditory nerve fibers.

In addition to characterizing the spectral weights at BF, the BF estimated from the weight function for MNTB neurons was positively correlated with the CF estimated from pure tones (i.e., the frequency at which a neuron just responds at the lowest sound level) and shown in **Figure 7A**; the linear regression of the data indicated a strong correlation ($R = 0.992$, $p < 0.0001$) with a relationship of the form $BF_{RSS} = 1.0 \times CF_{tones} + 0.18$. Thus, as an additional validation of the RSS technique, the properties of the spectral weight functions can yield accurate measurements of traditional metrics for frequency selectivity, BF and Q_{10}. Bandwidths as computed above can be converted to Q_{10} using the approximation of Young and Calhoun (2005) $Q_{10} = 1/[\ln(2) \times \textit{octave halfwidth}]$, where *octave halfwidth* was computed from the formulae earlier in this section. **Figure 7B** shows the Q_{10} estimated from the first-order weight functions for MNTB neurons compared with Q_{10} measured with tones. The linear regression of the Q_{10}estimated from the first-order spectral weight functions (for all neurons measured at each stimulus level tested) as a function of the empirical Q_{10} measured with pure tones was significant ($R = 0.85$, $P < 0.0001$, $n = 144$) with a relationship of the form $Q_{10\,RSS} = 0.9 \times Q_{10\,tones} + 1.0$.

LEVEL TOLERANCE OF SPECTRAL CODING

In addition to the spectral weight dependence on stimulus level, **Figures 7C,D** shows how the bandwidth of spectral tuning depended on stimulus level for GBC and MNTB neurons. First, **Figure 7C** shows an example of how the bandwidth of the weighting function at half the maximum weight was calculated for one MNTB neuron. Generally for stimulus levels above 0 dB, the weights at BF were positive and followed the general trends with overall stimulus level as that shown in **Figure 6**. The neuron in **Figure 7C** also showed significant off-BF inhibition/suppression (i.e., negative spectral weights) on the high-frequency side for high stimulus levels. By plotting normalized spectral weight functions (i.e., each weight function normalized by its maximum weight), the neuron in **Figure 7C** also revealed that the bandwidth was not affected much by changing the sound level over a range of 40 dB, 30 dB of which are shown (−15 to 15 dB re: threshold). Following Young and Calhoun (2005), for each neuron and for each sound level tested, the bandwidth corresponding to half the maximal spectral weight was computed on an octave scale using the formula $log(F_{upper}/F_{lower})/log(2)$. **Figures 7D,E** show the general stimulus level independence of the half-maximum weight bandwidth for all high-BF (>3 kHz) MNTB and GBC neurons, respectively. As stimulus levels increased, the spectral selectivity remained generally constant. The across-neuron mean bandwidths (**Figures 7D,E**, thick black lines) were constant in the range of ~0.2–0.225 octaves over at least a ~60 dB range of sound levels for both GBC and MNTB neurons. The observed bandwidths for four low-BF MNTB neurons (BF < 2 kHz, not shown in **Figure 7D**) were quite broad relative to the higher-BF neurons, with widths in the range of 1.0–1.2 octaves.

Figure 7F shows the across neuron mean bandwidths for auditory nerve fibers (Young and Calhoun, 2005), GBC and MNTB neurons. While the auditory nerve fiber bandwidths

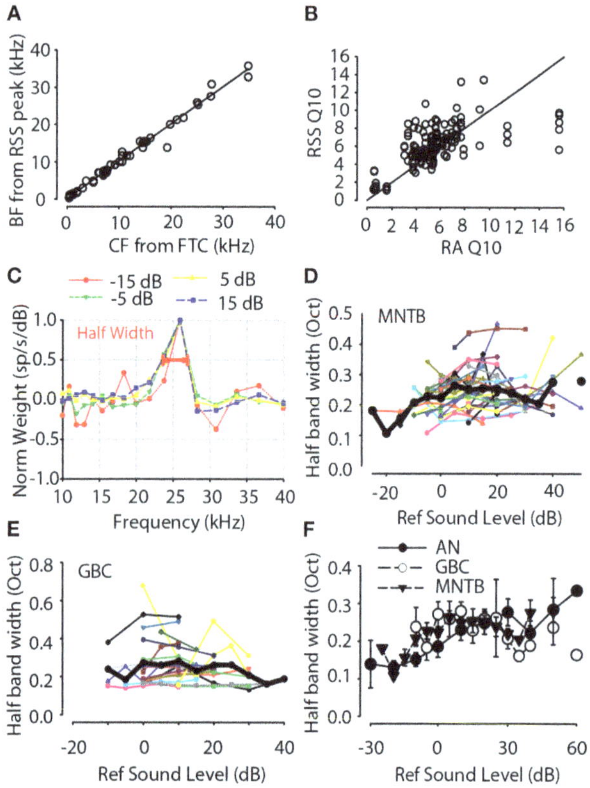

FIGURE 7 | (A) BF estimated from the RSS weight function as a function of the CF measured from pure tone frequency-intensity response area. **(B)** Frequency tuning estimated from the RSS weight functions (RSS Q_{10}, see text for equation) for all neurons and all levels tested as a function of Q_{10} measured from pure tone frequency-intensity response area (RA Q_{10}). **(C)** First-order weight function for one neuron ($BF = 25.9$ kHz) computed over a range of sound levels (−15 to 15 dB). The weight function for each sound level has been normalized by the maximum weight at BF at each particular sound level. For higher sound levels (> −15 dB), the normalized weight function shapes were similar. The bandwidth of the weight functions was computed at one-half the maximum weight at BF (see bar at normalized weight of 0.5). Significant off-BF inhibition (negative weights) can be seen at higher levels (error bars not shown for clarity). **(D)** Half-height bandwidth for 38 high-BF (>3 kHz) MNTB neurons as a function of sound level re: threshold. Lines and points show data for individual neurons while the solid black line shows the across-neuron mean. **(E)** Same as in **(D)**, but for GBC neurons. **(F)** Across-neuron mean spectral selectivity of GBC and MNTB neurons was quite consistent, or level-tolerant, across a wide range levels while the selectivity of AN neurons tended to widen. AN data replotted from Young and Calhoun (2005).

generally increased with increasing sound level (see also Young and Calhoun, 2005), the bandwidths for GBC and MNTB neurons remained quite constant, and similar, suggesting that the spectral selectivity of the inhibitory pathway through GBC and MNTB to LSO is invariant to sound level. Over a range of 50 dB (from −10 to 40 dB re: threshold) the high BF (>2 kHz) GBC and MNTB neurons had median bandwidths of 0.21 (IQ range = 0.17–0.27) and 0.23 (IQ range = 0.19–0.26), respectively, which were not significantly different than each other (Mann-Whitney $U = 3572$, $p = 0.34$). These data are consistent with the hypothesis that MNTB neurons inherit most of their level tolerance for spectral coding from the GBCs.

PREDICTION OF RATE RESPONSES FOR DTF-FILTERED BROADBAND NOISE STIMULI

A primary function of the neural circuit comprising the LSO is the computation of the ILD cues for sound localization (Tollin, 2003). The inhibitory pathway to the LSO including the auditory nerve, GBC and MNTB should thus accurately encode sound spectra. Therefore, as an additional test of the biological relevance and also generalizability of the spectral weight model, in 14 MNTB neurons, we also collected responses to 100-ms duration noise that was filtered by the DTFs measured in each animal prior to the physiological experiments (see Tollin and Koka, 2009a,b for methods). The DTFs covered 627 locations in the frontal hemisphere, which contain spectral notch cues. These DTF-filtered stimuli provide a more ecologically-relevant set of test stimuli because they contain the spectral components necessary for sound localization based on ILDs. Responses to DTF stimuli were predicted for each neuron using the spectral weighting functions estimated with the RSS stimuli. Compared to the RSS spectra (e.g., **Figure 1**), the DTF spectra are much smoother, except perhaps at frequencies corresponding to the spectral notches; an example DTF spectrum is shown in **Figure 11A**. In order predict the responses using the spectral weight functions, first the energy in the DTF spectra was resampled into frequency bins corresponding exactly to those bins (8 bins/oct) used in the RSS stimulus set. These DTF spectra were also corrected for speaker calibration (either directly via the *in situ* speaker calibration filter, or *post-hoc*) and then reexpressed in terms of dB level relative to the reference stimulus level. Both the DTF and RSS stimuli were presented at different reference sound levels in steps of 5 or 10 dB. For each DTF stimuli set, the spectral weight function model used for prediction was taken from the RSS data set that was measured with a reference level nearest (within 5–10 dB) the mean DTF sound level computed at the neuron BF. This method is adapted from that used by Young and Calhoun (2005).

Figure 8 shows an example for one MNTB neuron ($CF = 10$ kHz). **Figure 8A** shows the spatial plot of the acoustical gain of the head and pinnae of the DTF at a frequency bin corresponding to the CF (10 kHz) of the neuron (positive gain indicates amplification by the head and pinnae, negative gain indicates attenuation). The acoustic gain was maximal (~15 dB) for sounds ipsilateral to the ear being measured, and the gain was reduced systematically for sound source locations away from this point (see Tollin and Koka, 2009a for detailed analyses of acoustical gains of head and pinnae in the cat). **Figure 8B** shows the first order weight function at sound level 20 dB above threshold and **Figure 8C** shows the second order terms. The first order terms with star symbol are the weights which optimized the *fv* (see Methods). The spatial distribution of empirical responses to DTF-filtered stimuli presented at 20 dB re: threshold and the first and full-order model predictions are shown graphically in **Figures 8D–F**. The distribution of empirical responses (**Figure 8D**) roughly matches the distribution of acoustical gain corresponding to the neuron BF, as might be expected. The spatial distributions of responses predicted by the linear- (**Figure 8E**) and full-order (**Figure 8F**) spectral weight models are similar to the empirical rate distributions (**Figure 8D**) in terms of the areas of space over which the neuron responded. The *fv* values for

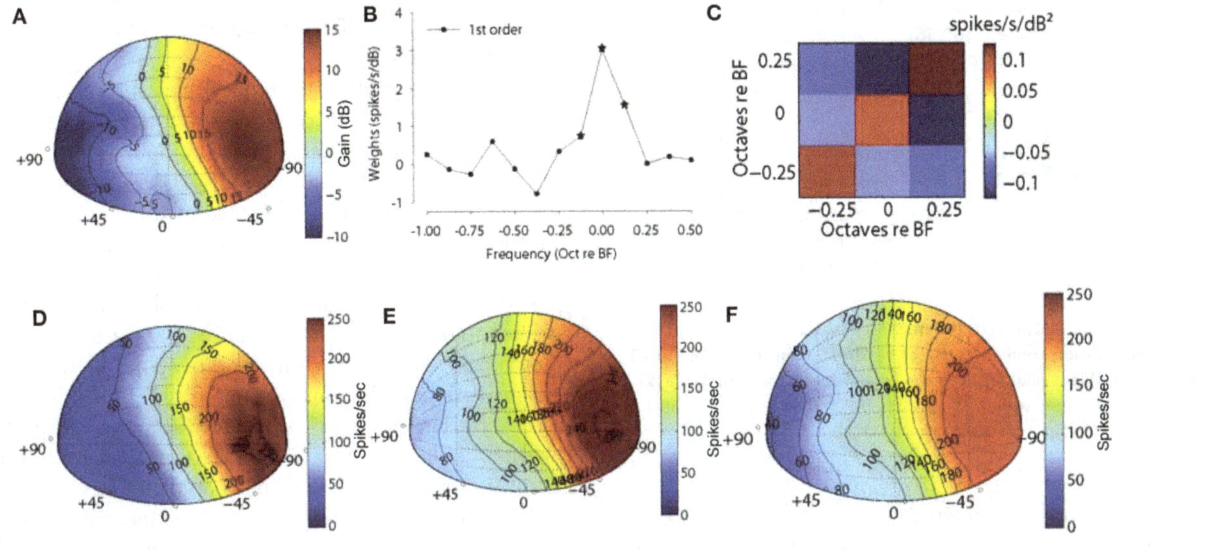

FIGURE 8 | Discharge rate predictions to broadband noise filtered through acoustical head related directional transfer functions (DTFs). **(A)** Spatial plot of the spectral levels (dB) for DTF filtered broadband noise stimuli corresponding to the CF of one neuron (10 kHz). **(B,C)** show the first- and second-order weights, respectively, used for predicting rate responses to DTF stimuli. **(D)** Spatial plot of empirical discharge rates for the 325 (out of 627) front-hemisphere DTF stimuli and predicted rates with first-order **(E)** and full-order **(F)** spectral weight models.

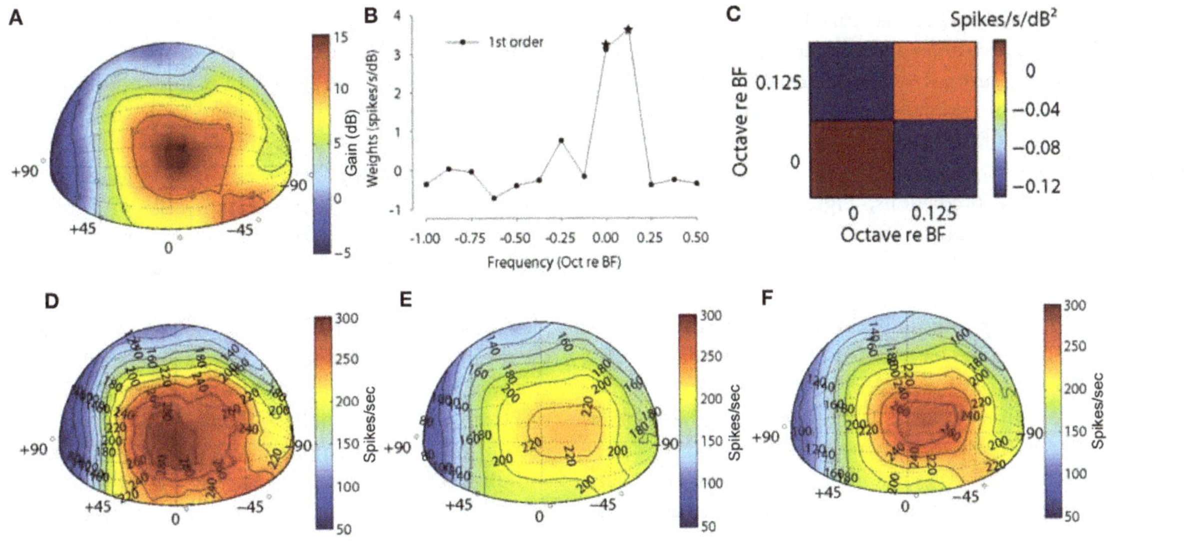

FIGURE 9 | Discharge rate predictions to broadband noise filtered through acoustical head related directional transfer functions (DTFs). Same as in **Figure 8** but for a MNTB neuron with a CF of 15.4 kHz.

prediction for this neuron were 0.62 and 0.71 and spatial correlation coefficients were 0.98 and 0.99 for the first-order and all order models, respectively. In general, even the first-order linear model produces predictions of the spatial receptive field structure nearly perfectly.

Figure 9 shows an example for another MNTB neuron ($CF =$ 15.4 kHz). **Figure 9A** shows the spatial plot of the acoustical gain of the head and pinnae of the DTF at a frequency bin corresponding to the CF (15.4 kHz) of the neuron (positive gain indicates amplification by the head and pinnae, negative gain indicates attenuation). The acoustic gain was maximal (~15 dB) for sounds immediately in front, and the gain was reduced systematically for sound source locations away from this point. As such, the spatial distribution of acoustical gain is somewhat more complex than that in the example in **Figure 8**. **Figure 9B** shows the first order weight function at sound level 15 dB above threshold and 9C shows the second order terms. The first order terms with star symbol are the weights which optimized the *fv*. The spatial distribution of empirical responses to DTF-filtered stimuli presented at 15 dB re: threshold and the first and full-order

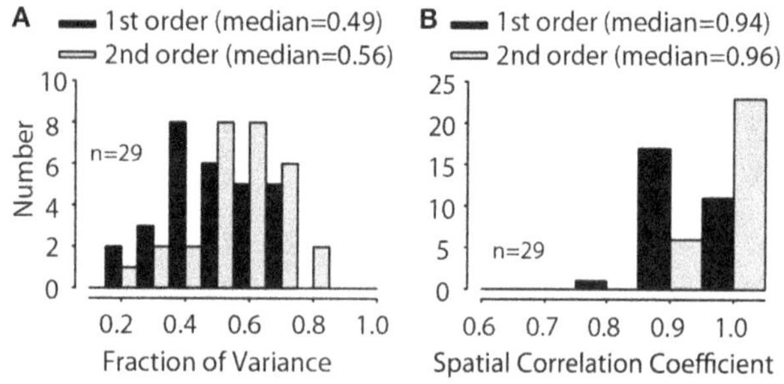

FIGURE 10 | Distributions of the fraction of variance, *fv* (A), and the spatial correlation coefficient (B) for 14 MNTB neurons (tested at 29 overall stimulus levels) for both the first-order linear model (black) and the full-order model (gray). The across-neuron median *fv* and spatial correlation coefficient for each model is indicated.

model predictions are shown graphically in **Figures 9D–F**. The distribution of empirical responses (**Figure 9D**) roughly matches the distribution of acoustical gain corresponding to the neuron BF, as might be expected. The spatial distributions of responses predicted by the linear- (**Figure 9E**) and full-order (**Figure 9F**) spectral weight models are similar to the empirical rate distributions (**Figure 9D**) in terms of the areas of space over which the neuron responded. The *fv* values for prediction for this neuron were 0.72 and 0.78 and the spatial correlation coefficients were 0.96 and 0.97 for the first-order and all order models, respectively. As with the example neuron shown in **Figure 8**, a linear weighting of the stimulus spectrum provided by the DTFs producted predictions of the structure of the neuron's spatial receptive field nearly perfectly.

To summarize the predictions, **Figure 10A** shows the histogram of the quality of fit *fv* values for the 14 MNTB neurons studied at different sound levels ($n = 29$ levels). The *fv* values from the full-order weight function model (median = 0.56, IQ range 0.47–0.67) were significantly (Wilcoxon signed-ranks test, $Z = 4.7, p < 0.0001$) different from the *fv* values (median = 0.49, IQ range 0.39–0.61) from first-order model. Over all, the *fv* values from the prediction of these DTF-filtered stimuli accounted for ~60% of the variance in the empirical data, and they were generally better than the *fv* values for RSS data sets. Given just a single repetition and short duration (100 ms) of each DTF-filtered stimulus used here, the large response variance will ensure that the *fv* will always be less than 1.0; that is, some fraction of the responses are random and thus not predictable at all by the model. When *fv* is corrected (as described above) for this, the linear spectral weight model can account for virtually all of the variance in the empirical rates in response to DTF-filtered stimuli. **Figure 10B** shows the histogram of spatial correlation coefficients for the quality of predictions. The spatial correlation coefficient shows how well the models can predict the actual shape of the acoustics via discharge rate. The spatial correlation coefficients values from the full-order weight function model (median = 0.97, IQ range 0.95–0.98) were significantly (Wilcoxon signed-ranks test, $Z = 4.62$, $p < 0.0001$) different from the *fv* values (median = 0.94, IQ range 0.93–0.96) from first-order model.

THE SPECTRAL MODULATION SELECTIVITY OF MNTB NEURONS IS SUFFICIENT TO ENCODE THE MODULATION SPECTRA OF THE CUES TO SOUND LOCATION

The MNTB is hypothesized to play an essential role in the encoding of the ILD cues to sound location as it provides the direct inhibitory input necessary for the computation of ILD by LSO (Tollin and Yin, 2002a,b; Tollin, 2003). Acoustically, ILDs are defined as the binaural difference in the sound spectra at the two ears. Examination of the ILD cues to location in a variety of mammalian species (Koka et al., 2008, 2011; Greene et al., 2014), including the cat (Tollin and Koka, 2009b) have demonstrated that large ILDs are produced in part due to the spectral notch cues induced by diffraction of sound by the pinnae. The results here have demonstrated that MNTB neurons are capable of accurately encoding via spike rate the monaural spectral information contained in DTF-filtered stimuli (**Figures 8–10**). This result implies that the spectral modulation resolving capacities of MNTB neurons must encompass the spectral modulations, or spectral-envelope frequency, of the ensemble of DTFs.

In order to test this hypothesis, following the method described by Macpherson and Middlebrooks (2003, p. 437) we computed the distributions of spectral modulations of the DTFs used for this study as well as the ensemble of RSS stimuli themselves. We then compared these distributions to the spectral modulation selectivity of the MNTB neurons as computed from the spectral weighting functions. **Figure 11A** shows the DTF for a midline (0°, 0°) sound source and the red line in **Figure 11B** shows the spectral modulation for this sound in terms of spectral ripple (or spectral envelope) depth (in dB) as a function of spectral ripple frequency (in ripples/octave) for this location. The DTFs of cats for frontal hemisphere locations contain pronounced features such as spectral peaks and deep notches for frequencies above ~8 kHz (Rice et al., 1992; Tollin and Koka, 2009a). The resulting DTF ripple spectrum for the (0°, 0°) source shows two prominent ripples >10 dB over the range of 0.25–1 ripples/octave. Across all source locations in the frontal hemisphere the mean DTF ripple depth was >5 dB for ripples/octave < ~1.5 and was lower for ripples/octave higher than 2. The modulation spectrum of the ensemble of RSS stimuli used in this study was flat up to around 4 ripples/octave, demonstrating that the RSS stimuli were sufficient to probe the spectral modulation coding capability of the neurons at least over this range of modulation.

The RSS spectral weighting functions can be used to estimate the spectral resolving power of neurons based on rate responses. The high spatial correlation coefficients between predicted and empirical spike rates for DTF-filtered stimuli imply that MNTB neurons can accurately encode the spectral envelopes contained in these stimuli. To more directly examine whether MNTB neurons have sufficient spectral resolving power to encode the modulation spectra of directional information contained in the DTFs (**Figure 11B**) we decomposed the spectral weighting functions for MNTB neurons with BFs > 3 kHz as a function of ripples/octave. The results shown in **Figure 11C** reveal that MNTB neurons prefer low ripple densities, as indicated by higher spectral weights (spikes/s/dB), indicating that they prefer broad spectral features, similar to those produced by the distributions of DTFs. Thus, the spectral modulation sensitivities of the population of MNTB

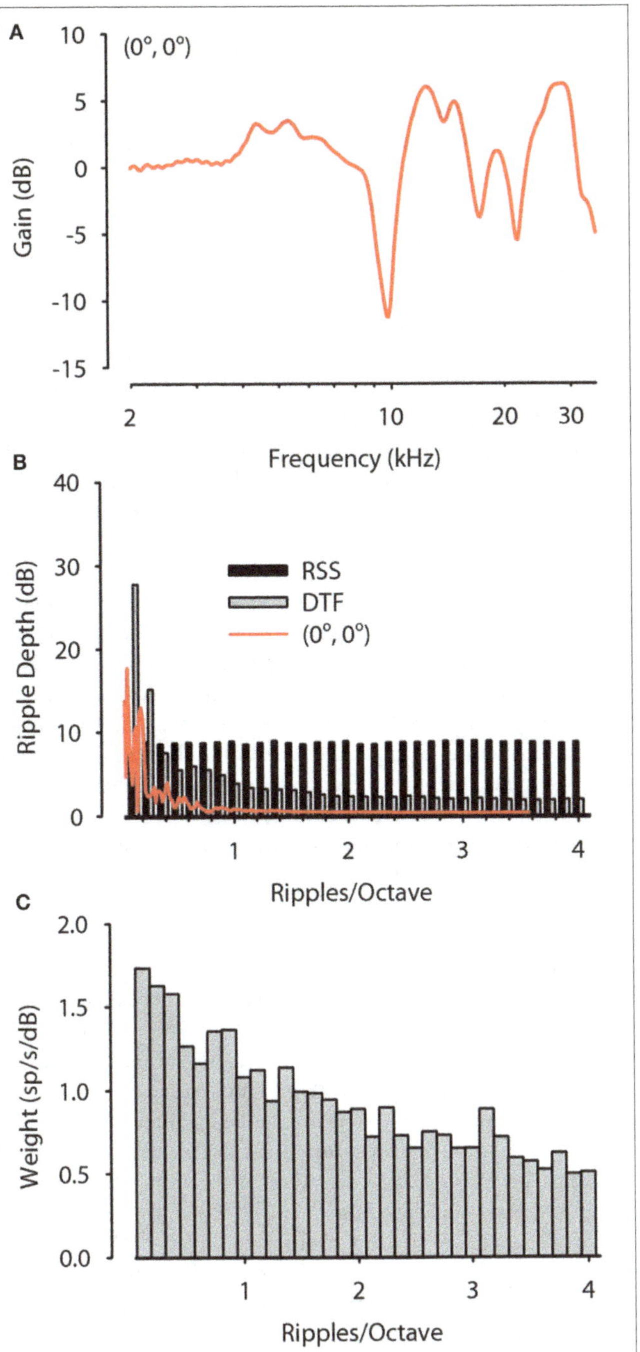

FIGURE 11 | Spectral modulation selectivity of MNTB neurons are sufficient to encode the spectral modulations contained in spatial head related transfer functions. (A) The directional transfer function (DTF) for a sound source located at (0°, 0°). **(B)** Spectral modulation distribution of the DTF in **(A)**, the ensemble of RSS stimuli, and the ensemble of DTFs used in this study plotted as mean ripple depth (dB) as a function of ripples/octave. DTFs have large ripple depth at low ripples/octave while RSS have constant mean ripple depth up to at least 4 ripples/octave. **(C)** Spectral modulation selectivity of the population of MNTB neurons in terms of spectral weighting (spikes/s/dB) as a function of ripples/octave. MNTB neurons preferentially resolve low spectral modulations consistent with those provided by the DTFs.

neurons studied here are sufficient to encode the biologically-relevent spectral modulations contained in the directional information conveyed by the DTFs. This ability is essential in order for MNTB neurons to transmit information about stimulus spectrum via rate to the LSO for accurate encoding of the ILD cues to location.

DISCUSSION

The classical function of the MNTB is to provide inhibitory input to the LSO necessary for encoding the ILD cue to location (Yin, 2002; Tollin, 2003). However, based largely on *in vitro* studies, MNTB neurons have recently been described and intensely studied in terms of their abilities to encode *temporal* information (Taschenberger and Von Gersdorff, 2000; Trussell, 2002; Schneggenburger and Forsythe, 2006). In addition to the input to ipsilateral LSO, the MNTB sends glycinergic projections to the MSO, the superior paraolivary nucleus, and the ventral nucleus of the lateral lemniscus (Spangler et al., 1985; Banks and Smith, 1992; Sommer et al., 1993; Smith et al., 1998). The projection of MNTB to MSO is considered to be an important mechanism for the encoding of ITDs by the MSO in small mammals (Brand et al., 2002; Pecka et al., 2008). The hypothesized function of these projections is to provide temporally-precise inhibition. Here, however, we reexamined the traditional hypothesis that MNTB neurons provide the inhibitory input to the LSO required for ILD encoding and thus encode the shapes of sound spectra via discharge rate.

THE MNTB AS A SPECTRAL ANALYZER

The ability of receptive field models to generate response predictions to arbitrary stimuli is essential to establishing functional properties based on the model parameters (see Methods). The spectral weight models here produced predictions that supported the hypothesis that MNTB neurons and their inputs, the GBCs, encode stationary spectra via discharge rate. Both GBC and MNTB neurons were well modeled by a linear weighting of spectra, consistent with auditory nerve (Young and Calhoun, 2005; Reiss et al., 2007) and other CN neurons (Yu and Young, 2000; Yu, 2003). The non-linear terms reflected the need to model the curvature of the discharge rate-level function near threshold and at high sound levels. Addition of the non-linear terms marginally, but significantly, increased the predictive capacity of the model. Given the predictive validation of the model and because we also accounted for possible non-linear aspects, the properties of the weight functions, like bandwidth, sideband suppression/inhibition (hereafter referred to as inhibition), BF and the magnitudes of the weights have functional meaning. See Christianson et al. (2008) for the importance of non-linearities for predictive validation.

MNTB neurons were able to accurately encode via rate the complex spectral shapes of the DTFs produced by the directional filtering of sounds by the head and pinnae. A comparison of the spectral modulation spectra of cat DTFs (**Figure 11B**) and the spectral resolution of MNTB neurons as assessed from the RSS-derived spectral weight functions (**Figure 11C**) revealed that there was sufficient spectral resolution of MNTB neurons to adequately encode the spectral modulations contained in the DTFs of cats.

Hence, the MNTB is capable of providing via rate response the full range of spectral information necessary to localize sound based on ILD or spectral shape cues in the frontal hemisphere.

LEVEL TOLERANCE FOR SPECTRAL CODING IN THE NEURAL CIRCUIT FOR INTERAURAL LEVEL DIFFERENCE CUE COMPUTATION

The spectral-tuning bandwidths of GBC and MNTB neurons were similar and remarkably stable over a wide range of intensities (**Figures 7D,E**), or level tolerant. Level tolerance may emerge from or be sustained by on- and/or off-BF inhibition. Spectral coding by auditory nerve fibers has been shown to be not as level tolerant as that seen here and in other areas of the auditory system (Young and Calhoun, 2005; Yu and Young, 2013). We hypothesize that level tolerance may be required for encoding of the spectral levels of stimuli via discharge rate necessary for level-tolerant ILD coding (see Tsai et al., 2010). Level-tolerant frequency selectivity has many hypothesized computational attributes, including the capability to create a more accurate neural representation of spectra (Suga, 1977; Sadagopan and Wang, 2008), computation of ILDs (Tsai et al., 2010) and the use of spectral cues for sound localization over a wide range of sound levels (Tollin et al., 2005, 2013; Gai et al., 2013). In the context of the GBC-MNTB-LSO circuit, level-tolerance may function to preclude confounds between sound level and the bandwidth of neural spectral selectivity. This is necessary because the ILD cue in cats can vary by as much as ±40 dB (Tollin and Koka, 2009b). Thus, the capabilities of individual afferents to LSO, including the GBC and MNTB, to maintain consistent spectral coding over a 40 dB range or more is essential. Similar invariance, but to varying degrees, has been reported in AN (Young and Calhoun, 2005), CN (Yu and Young, 2000), inferior colliculus (Yu and Young, 2013), and auditory cortex (Suga and Tsuzuki, 1985; Ehret and Schreiner, 1997; Sutter, 2000; Barbour and Wang, 2003; Sadagopan and Wang, 2008). Here we demonstrate that spectral coding was relatively more invariant to level in GBC and MNTB neurons than in AN fibers (**Figure 7F**), which suggests that some degree of invariance is produced at the level of the cochlear nucleus and/or MNTB itself.

One potential mechanism for level tolerance may be on- or off-BF inhibition to GBC and/or MNTB neurons. The BF and frequency selectivity estimated from the weight functions were highly correlated with measures using tones, CF and Q_{10}. The broadband and stationary nature of the RSS stimuli also allowed for revelation of properties not easily observable with tones. For example, 49% of high-BF (>3 kHz) MNTB neurons showed significant off-BF inhibition. The lack of observable off-BF effects in other neurons does not preclude on-BF or other inhibitory effects. Because similar forms of inhibition (or suppression) are observed in auditory nerve (Sachs and Kiang, 1968) and GBCs (Caspary et al., 1994; Kopp-Scheinpflug et al., 2002) that provide input to MNTB, it cannot be determined here whether this off-BF inhibition was created and/or enhanced directly at the MNTB.

It is known, however, that MNTB neurons do indeed receive direct inhibitory inputs (Adams and Mugnaini, 1990) from a variety of sources including the ventral nucleus of the trapezoid body (Kuwabara et al., 1991; Albrecht et al., 2014), dorsomedial periolivary nucleus (Kuwabara et al., 1991; Schofield, 1994) and intrinsic collaterals from neighboring MNTB neurons (Bledsoe et al., 1988; Kuwabara and Zook, 1991). These sources are comprised of neurons containing GABA and glycine (Helfert et al., 1989). *In vitro* studies have demonstrated that glycine, and GABA, can influence MNTB responses directly (Banks and Smith, 1992; Wu and Kelly, 1995; Turecek and Trussell, 2001; Awatramani et al., 2004, 2005; Lu et al., 2008). Glycine also acts presynaptically to enhance glutamate release by the calyx onto MNTB neurons (Turecek and Trussell, 2001). A possible function of inhibition has been suggested by *in vivo* studies where sideband inhibition in the frequency-intensity response areas has been demonstrated (Kopp-Scheinpflug et al., 2003; Tolnai et al., 2008a,b). Kopp-Scheinpflug et al. (2008) reported 10/19 (53%) neurons had off-BF inhibition, comparable to the 49% observed here. Tolnai et al. (2008a,b) also reported some high-CF MNTB neurons with off-BF inhibition. Tsuchitani (1997) did not report any suppression of spontaneous activity by off-BF tones in 40 MNTB neurons in cat.

By independently analyzing the acoustically-evoked prepotentials and action potentials of the complex waveforms (e.g., **Figure 2A**), Kopp-Scheinpflug et al. (2003) suggested that off-BF inhibition was enhanced by some mechanism acting at MNTB neurons directly (although see McLaughlin et al., 2008). Kopp-Scheinpflug et al. (2008) subjected MNTB neurons to acoustic stimulation before, during, and after iontophoretic application of the glycine receptor antagonist strychnine. Strychnine was found to enhance or reduce discharge rates. Rate reductions were most common for spontaneous activity and for sound-evoked responses throughout the excitatory response areas, with the largest reductions occurring for frequencies near CF. Outside the excitatory area, strychnine often caused rate increases, consistent with the hypothesis that blockage of glycine action reduced the strength of putative on/off-BF inhibition. Frequency selectivity in these latter neurons decreased (i.e., poorer selectivity). Comparable results have been observed in CN (Caspary et al., 1994; Kopp-Scheinpflug et al., 2002). Thus, one function of direct glycinergic inhibition to MNTB may be to increase frequency selectivity. There is evidence from prior studies that MNTB neurons may be more sharply tuned than the GBCs that provide the input (Kopp-Scheinpflug et al., 2003) and the ipsilateral excitatory responses of LSO neurons to which MNTB projects (Tsuchitani, 1997). Consistent with these findings our results here also revealed a slight, but significant, increase in frequency selectivity (**Figure 2C**) in MNTB neurons over GBCs when assessed with tones; however, there was no difference in frequency selectivity between MNTB and GBC when assessed with the broadband RSS-derived spectral weight functions (**Figure 7F**). The later result, along with the striking similarities between GBCs and MNTB neurons in terms of the characteristics of the spectral weight functions, and the similar rates of spontaneous activity are consistent with the hypothesis that MNTB neurons largely inherit their spectral coding capabilities from GBCs via the calyx of Held.

Given the anatomical and *in vitro* evidence for inhibitory inputs to MNTB, it was surprising that we and others find only a portion of neurons exhibiting off-BF inhibition. The spectral coding properties of MNTB and their GBC inputs were found here to be remarkably similar, consistent with the large calyceal input. Perhaps inhibition is on-BF and thus matched to the excitatory RF. Such mechanisms have been demonstrated in whole-cell studies by Wehr and Zador (2003) in auditory cortex and Gittleman et al. (2009) in inferior colliculus. Alternatively, there may be temporal interactions of excitation and inhibition that cannot be revealed by extracellular recordings (e.g., Xie et al., 2007). Perhaps the spectrally stationary stimuli used here are not sufficient to evoke underlying inhibitory mechanisms in some neurons.

A SOLUTION TO THE TEMPORAL "CORRESPONDENCE PROBLEM" FOR ILD COMPUTATION—THE MNTB ENCODES SOUND SPECTRA WITH HIGH TEMPORAL PRECISION

As mentioned in the Introduction, the MNTB and bushy cells have recently been mostly described, and studied, in regards to their exquisite abilities to encode *temporal* aspects of sounds, not spectral. Indeed the inhibitory inputs to MNTB may play important roles in temporal processing that would not be revealed in the present study. It has been suggested that enhanced temporal precision allows transient or complex stimuli with slowly varying envelopes to be more precisely encoded in MNTB than their afferents (Joris and Yin, 1998; Kopp-Scheinpflug et al., 2003, 2008; Tollin and Yin, 2005). Inhibition may thus help to extract and represent spectrotemporally modulated envelopes of natural sounds, like speech, animal vocalizations, or transients like rustling leaves and snapping twigs. To compute the ILD cue to location in these kinds of signals at the LSO requires care (see Tollin, 2003). As suggested by Joris and Yin (1998) and Tollin (2003), there is a time correspondence problem for ILD computation not unlike the classical spatial correspondence problem for stereoscopic vision (Julesz, 1971). The anatomical and biophysical specializations in the GBC-MNTB-LSO circuit may minimize the relative timing delays and the jitter in synaptic delays so that ILD can be computed at corresponding points in frequency and *time* (Joris and Yin, 1998; Tollin, 2003).

The precise spectrotemporal encoding of sound by LSO afferents is well-matched by correspondingly short integration times of LSO neurons. Contralateral stimulus-evoked IPSPs recorded in LSO neurons have relatively long durations (3.2–8.1 ms), nearly twice the duration of ipsilaterally-evoked EPSPs (1.5–4.2 ms) (Sanes, 1990). Functionally, however, contralateral inhibition suppresses ipsilaterally-evoked discharges of LSO neurons for only ~1.0–2.0 ms (Sanes, 1990; Wu and Kelly, 1992; Joris and Yin, 1995; Park et al., 1996; Irvine et al., 2001). The integration time for the comparison of afferent inputs by LSO neurons is sufficiently short so that the ILD is only computed over brief, temporally corresponding portions of the sounds at each ear, thus solving the temporal correspondence problem for ILD computation. Integration times of 1–2 ms would presumably allow ongoing ILD computation for envelope fluctuations up to ~1 kHz before synaptic inputs would be temporally integrated. Some LSO neurons can track ILDs in binaural amplitude-modulated stimuli at rates up to 800 Hz (Joris and Yin, 1995). Such short integration times in the MNTB-LSO spectral processing pathway are wholly consistent with spectral integration times of 1–5 ms estimated from human and animal psychophysical sound localization studies (Hofman and van Opstal, 1998; Tollin and Henning, 1999; Martin and McAnally, 2008; Gai et al., 2013). In order to reconcile the exquisite temporal and spectral coding capabilities of MNTB and their GBC inputs, we propose that together with the anatomical and biophysical specializations for timing in the GBC-MNTB-LSO complex, the linear spectral coding mechanisms demonstrated here may ultimately function synergistically to allow ILDs to be computed for biologically-relevant complex stimuli with rapid spectrotemporally-modulated envelopes such as speech and animal vocalizations and moving sound sources.

ACKNOWLEDGMENTS

This work was supported by National Institutes of Deafness and Other Communicative Disorders Grant DC-006865 and DC-011555. We would like to acknowledge Dr. Eric Young for providing software and suggestions that greatly assisted us in the early parts of these experiments. We thank Dr. Michael Hall for preparing custom hardware (supported by NIH grant P30 NS041854).

REFERENCES

Adams, J. C., and Mugnaini, E. (1990). Immunocytochemical evidence for inhibitory and disinhibitory circuits in the superior olive. *Hear. Res.* 49, 281–298. doi: 10.1016/0378-5955(90)90109-3

Aertsen, A. M., Olders, J. H., and Johannesma, P. I. (1981). Spectro-temporal receptive fields of auditory neurons in the grassfrog. III. Analysis of the stimulus-event relation for natural stimuli. *Biol. Cybern.* 39, 195–209. doi: 10.1007/BF00342772

Albrecht, O., Dondzillo, A., Mayer, F., Thompson, J. A., and Klug, A. (2014). Inhibitory projections from the ventral nucleus of the trapezoid body to the medial nucleus of the trapezoid body in the mouse. *Front. Neural Circuits* 8:83. doi: 10.3389/fncir.2014.00083

Awatramani, G. B., Turecek, R., and Trussell, L. O. (2004). Inhibitory control at a synaptic relay. *J. Neurosci.* 24, 2643–2647. doi: 10.1523/JNEUROSCI.5144-03.2004

Awatramani, G. B., Turecek, R., and Trussell, L. O. (2005). Staggered development of GABAergic and glycinergic transmission in the MNTB. *J. Neurophysiol.* 93, 819–828. doi: 10.1152/jn.00798.2004

Bandyopadhyay, S., Reiss, L. A. J., and Young, E. D. (2007). Receptive field for dorsal cochlear nucleus neurons at multiple sound levels. *J. Neurophysiol.* 98, 3505–3515. doi: 10.1152/jn.00539.2007

Banks, M. I., and Smith, P. H. (1992). Intracellular recordings from neurobiotin-labeled cells in brain slices of the rat medial nucleus of the trapezoid body. *J. Neurosci.* 12, 2819–2837.

Barbour, D. L., and Wang, X. (2003). Auditory cortical responses elicited in awake primates by random spectral stimuli. *J. Neurosci.* 23, 7194–7206. doi: 10.1126/science.1080425

Bledsoe, S. C., Pandya, P., Altschuler, R. A., and Helfert, R. H. (1988). Axonol projections of PHA-labeled neurons in the medial nucleus of the trapezoid body. *Soc. Neurosci. Abst.* 14, 491.

Borst, J. G. G., Helmchen, F., and Sakmann, B. (1995). Pre- and postsynaptic whole-cell recordings in the medial nucleus of the trapezoid body of the rat. *J. Physiol. (Lond.)* 489, 825–840.

Boudreau, J. C., and Tsuchitani, C. (1968). Binaural interaction in the cat superior olive S-segment. *J. Neurophysiol.* 31, 442–454.

Brand, A., Behrend, O., Marquardt, T., McAlpine, D., and Grothe, B. (2002). Precise inhibition is essential for microsecond interaural time difference coding. *Nature* 417, 543–547. doi: 10.1038/417543a

Caspary, D. M., Backoff, P. M., Finlayson, P. G., and Palombi, P. S. (1994). Inhibitory inputs modulate discharge rate within frequency receptive fields of anteroventral cochlear nucleus neurons. *J. Neurophysiol.* 72, 2124–2133.

Christianson, G. B., Sahani, M., and Linden, J. (2008). The consequences of response nonlinearities for interpretation of spectrotemporal receptive fields. *J. Neurosci.* 28, 446–455. doi: 10.1523/JNEUROSCI.1775-07.2007

David, S. V., and Gallant, J. L. (2005). Predicting neuronal responses during natural vision. *Netw. Comput. Neural Syst.* 16, 239–260. doi: 10.1080/09548980500464030

deCharms, R. C., Blake, D. T., and Merzenich, M. M. (1998). Optimizing sound features for cortical neurons. *Science* 280, 1439–1443. doi: 10.1126/science.280.5368.1439

Efron, B., and Tibshirani, R. J. (1993). *An Introduction to the Bootstrap*. New York, NY: Chapman and Hall.

Eggermont, J. J. (1993). Wiener and volterra analyses applied to the auditory system. *Hear. Res.* 66, 177–201. doi: 10.1016/0378-5955(93)90139-R

Ehret, G., and Schreiner, C. E. (1997). Frequency resolution and spectral integration (critical band analysis) in single units of the cat primary auditory cortex. *J. Comp. Physiol. A.* 181, 635–650. doi: 10.1007/s003590050146

Escabi, M. A., and Schreiner, C. E. (2002). Nonlinear spectrotemporal sound analysis by neurons in the auditory midbrain. *J. Neurosci.* 15, 4114–4131.

Forsythe, I. D. (1994). Direct patch recording from identified presynaptic terminals mediating glutamatergic EPSCs in the rat CNS, *in vitro*. *J. Physiol. (Lond.)* 479, 381–387.

Futai, K., Okada, M., Matsuyama, K., and Takahashi, T. (2001). High-fidelity transmission acquired via a developmental decrease in NMDA receptor expression at an auditory synapse. *J. Neurosci.* 21, 3342–3349.

Gai, Y., Ruhland, J. L., Yin, T. C. T., and Tollin, D. J. (2013). Behavioral and modeling studies of sound localization in cats: effects of stimulus level and duration. *J. Neurophysiol.* 110, 607–620. doi: 10.1152/jn.01019.2012

Gittleman, J. X., Li, N., and Pollak, G. D. (2009). Mechanisms underlying directional selectivity for frequency-modulated sweeps in the inferior colliculus revealed by *in vivo* whole-cell recordings. *J. Neurosci.* 29, 13030–13041. doi: 10.1523/JNEUROSCI.2477-09.2009

Greene, N. T., Anbuhl, K. L., Williams, W., and Tollin, D. J. (2014). The acoustical cues to sound location in the guinea pig (Cavia porcellus). *Hear. Res.* 316, 1–15. doi: 10.1016/j.heares.2014.07.004

Guinan, J. J. Jr., Guinan, S. S., and Norris, B. E. (1972a). Single auditory units in the superior olivary complex. I: responses to sounds and classifications based on physiological properties. *Int. J. Neurosci.* 4, 101–120. doi: 10.3109/00207457209147165

Guinan, J. J. Jr., and Li, R. Y. (1990). Signal processing in brainstem auditory neurons which receive giant endings (calyces of Held) in the medial nucleus of the trapezoid body of the cat. *Hear. Res.* 49, 321–334. doi: 10.1016/0378-5955(90)90111-2

Guinan, J. J. Jr., Norris, B. E., and Guinan, S. S. (1972b). Single auditory units in the superior olivary complex. II: location of unit categories and tonotopic organization. *Int. J. Neurosci.* 4, 147–166. doi: 10.3109/00207457209164756

Hays, W. L. (1988). *Statistics*. Fort Worth, TX: Holt, Rinehart, and Winston.

Heffner, R. S., and Heffner, H. E. (1985). Hearing range of the domestic cat. *Hear. Res.* 19, 85–88. doi: 10.1016/0378-5955(85)90100-5

Helfert, R. H., Bonneau, J. M., Wenthold, R. J., and Altschuler, R. A. (1989). GABA and glycine immunoreactivity in the guinea pig superior olivary complex. *Brain Res.* 501, 269–286. doi: 10.1016/0006-8993(89)90644-6

Hofman, P. M., and van Opstal, A. J. (1998). Spectro-temporal factors in two-dimensional human sound localization. *J. Acoust. Soc. Am.* 103, 2634–2648. doi: 10.1121/1.422784

Irvine, D. R., Park, V. N., and McCormick, L. (2001). Mechanisms underlying the sensitivity of neurons in the lateral superior olive to interaural intensity differences. *J. Neurophysiol.* 86, 2647–2666.

Jean-Baptiste, M., and Morest, D. K. (1975). Transneuronalchanges of synaptic endings and nuclear chromatin in the trapezoidbody following cochlear ablation in cats. *J. Comp. Neurol.* 162, 111–134 doi: 10.1002/cne.901620107

Joris, P. X., and Yin, T. C. T. (1995). Envelope coding in the lateral superior olive. I. Sensitivity to interaural time differences. *J. Neurophysiol.* 73, 1043–1062.

Joris, P. X., and Yin, T. C. T. (1998). Envelope coding in the lateral superior olive. III. Comparison with afferent pathways. *J. Neurophysiol.* 79, 253–269.

Joshi, I., Shokralla, S., Titis, P., and Wang, L. Y. (2004). The role of AMPA receptor gating in the development of high-fidelity neurotransmission at the calyx of Held synapse. *J. Neurosci.* 24, 183–196. doi: 10.1523/JNEUROSCI.1074-03.2004

Julesz, B. (1971). *Foundations of Cyclopean Perception*. Chicago: The University of Chicago Press.

Koka, K., Holland, N. J., Lupo, J. E., Jenkins, H. A., and Tollin, D. J. (2010). Electrocochleographic and mechanical assessment of round window stimulation with an active middle ear prosthesis. *Hear. Res.* 263, 128–137. doi: 10.1016/j.heares.2009.08.009

Koka, K., Jones, H., Thornton, J. L., and Tollin, D. J. (2011). Sound pressure transformations by the head and pinnae of the adult Chinchilla (Chinchilla lanigera). *Hear. Res.* 272, 135–147. doi: 10.1016/j.heares.2010.10.007

Koka, K., Read, H. L., and Tollin, D. J. (2008). The acoustical cues to sound location in the rat: measurements of directional transfer functions. *J. Acoust. Soc. Am.* 123, 4297–4309. doi: 10.1121/1.2916587

Kopp-Scheinpflug, C., Dehmel, S., Dorrscheidt, G. J., and Rubsamen, R. (2002). Interaction of excitation and inhibition in anteroventral cochlear nucleus neurons that receive large endbulb synaptic endings. *J. Neurosci.* 22, 11004–11018.

Kopp-Scheinpflug, C., Dehmel, S., Tolnai, S., Dietz, B., Milenkovic, I., and Rubsamen, R. (2008). Glycine-mediated changes of onset reliability at a mammalian central synapse. *Neuroscience* 157, 432–445. doi: 10.1016/j.neuroscience.2008.08.068

Kopp-Scheinpflug, C., Lippe, W. R., Dorrscheidt, G. J., and Rubsamen, R. (2003). The medial nucleus of the trapezoid body in the gerbil is more than a relay: comparison of pre- and postsynaptic activity. *J. Assoc. Res. Otolaryngol.* 4, 1–23. doi: 10.1007/s10162-002-2010-5

Kowalski, N., Depireux, D. A., and Shamma, S. A. (1996). Analysis of dynamic spectra in ferret primary auditory cortex. I. Characteristics of single-unit responses to moving ripple spectra. *J. Neurophysiol.* 76, 3503–3523.

Kuwabara, N., DiCaprio, R. A., and Zook, J. M. (1991). Afferents to the medial nucleus of the trapezoid body and their collateral projections. *J. Comp. Neurol.* 314, 684–706. doi: 10.1002/cne.903140405

Kuwabara, N., and Zook, J. M. (1991). Classification of the principal cells of the medial nucleus of the trapezoid body. *J. Comp. Neurol.* 314, 707–720. doi: 10.1002/cne.903140406

Lesica, N. A., and Grothe, B. (2008). Dynamic spectrotemporal feature selectivity in the auditory midbrain. *J. Neurosci.* 28, 5412–5421. doi: 10.1523/JNEUROSCI.0073-08.2008

Lewis, E. R., and van Dijk, P. (2004). New variations on the derivation of spectro-temporal receptive fields for primary auditory afferent axons. *Hear. Res.* 189, 120–136. doi: 10.1016/S0378-5955(03)00406-4

Lorteije, J. A. M., Rusu, S. I., Kushmerick, C., and Borst, J. G. (2009). Reliability and precision of the mouse calyx of Held synapse. *J. Neurosci.* 29, 13770–13784. doi: 10.1523/JNEUROSCI.3285-09.2009

Lu, T., Rubio, M. E., and Trussell, L. O. (2008). Glycinergic transmission shaped by the corelease of GABA in a mammalian auditory synapse. *Neuron* 57, 524–535. doi: 10.1016/j.neuron.2007.12.010

Macpherson, E. A., and Middlebrooks, J. C. (2003). Vertical-plane sound localization probed with ripple-spectrum noise. *J. Acoust. Soc. Am.* 114, 430–445. doi: 10.1121/1.1582174

Martin, R. L., and McAnally, K. I. (2008). Spectral integration time of the auditory localization system. *Hear. Res.* 238, 118–123. doi: 10.1016/j.heares.2007.08.006

McLaughlin, M., van der Heihden, M., and Joris, P. X. (2008). How secure is *in vivo* synaptic transmission at the calyx of Held? *J. Neurosci.* 28, 10206–10219. doi: 10.1523/JNEUROSCI.2735-08.2008

Moore, J., Tollin, D. J., and Yin, T. C. T. (2008). Can measures of sound localization acuity be related to the precision of absolute location estimates? *Hear. Res.* 238, 94–109. doi: 10.1016/j.heares.2007.11.006

Park, T. J., Grothe, B., Pollak, G. D., Schuller, G., and Koch, U. (1996). Neural delays shape selectivity to interaural intensity differences in the lateral superior olive. *J. Neurosci.* 16, 6554–6566.

Pecka, M., Brand, A., Behrend, O., and Grothe, B. (2008). Interaural time difference processing in the mammalian medial superior olive: the role of glycinergic inhibition. *J. Neurosci.* 28, 6914–6925. doi: 10.1523/JNEUROSCI.1660-08.2008

Press, W. H., Flannery, B. P., Teukolsky, S. A., and Vetterling, W. T. (1986). *Numerical Recipes: The Art of Scientific Computing*. Cambridge: Cambridge University Press.

Qiu, A., Schreiner, C. E., and Escabí, M. A. (2003). Gabor analysis of auditory midbrain receptive fields: spectro-temporal and binaural composition. *J. Neurophysiol.* 90, 456–476. doi: 10.1152/jn.00851.2002

Reiss, L. A. J., Bandyopadhyay, S., and Young, E. D. (2007). Effects of stimuls spectral contrast on receptive fields of dorsal cochlear nucleus neruons. *J. Neurophysiol.* 98, 2133–2143. doi: 10.1152/jn.01239.2006

Rhode, W. S. (2008). Response patterns to sound associated with labeled globular/bushy cells in cat. *Neuroscience* 154, 87–98. doi: 10.1016/j.neuroscience.2008.03.013

Rice, J. J., May, B. J., Spirou, G. A., and Young, E. D. (1992). Pinna-based spectral cues for sound localization in cat. *Hear. Res.* 58, 132–152. doi: 10.1016/0378-5955(92)90123-5

Ruhland, J. L., Yin, T. C. T., and Tollin, D. J. (2013). Gaze shifts of the cat to auditory and visual stimuli. *J. Assoc. Res. Otolaryngol.* 14, 731–755. doi: 10.1007/s10162-013-0401-4

Sachs, M. B., and Kiang, N. Y. (1968). Two-tone inhibition in auditory-nerve fibers. *J. Acoust. Soc. Am.* 43, 1120–1128. doi: 10.1121/1.1910947

Sadagopan, S., and Wang, X. (2008). Level invariant representation of sounds by populations of neurons in primary auditory cortex. *J. Neurosci.* 28, 3415–3426. doi: 10.1523/JNEUROSCI.2743-07.2008

Sanes, D. H. (1990). An *in vitro* analysis of sound localization mechanisms in the gerbil lateral superior olive. *J. Neurosci.* 10, 3494–3506.

Schneggenburger, R., and Forsythe, I. D. (2006). The calyx of Held. *Cell Tissue Res.* 326, 311–337. doi: 10.1007/s00441-006-0272-7

Schnupp, J. W. H., Mrsic-Flogel, T. D., and King, A. J. (2001). Linear processing of spatial cues in primary auditory cortex. *Nature* 414, 200–204. doi: 10.1038/35102568

Schofield, B. R. (1994). Superior peraolivary nucleus in the pigmented guinea pig: separate classes of neurons project to the inferior colliculus and cochlear nucleus. *J. Comp. Neurol.* 312, 68–76. doi: 10.1002/cne.903120106

Smith, P. H., Joris, P. X., Carney, L. H., and Yin, T. C. T. (1991). Projections of physiologically characterized globular bushy cells from the cochlear nucleus of the cat. *J. Comp. Neurol.* 304, 387–407. doi: 10.1002/cne.903040305

Smith, P. H., Joris, P. X., and Yin, T. C. T. (1993). Projections of physiologically characterized spherical bushy cell axons from the cochlear nucleus of the cat: evidence for delay lines to the medial superior olive. *J. Comp. Neurol.* 331, 245–260. doi: 10.1002/cne.903310208

Smith, P. H., Joris, P. X., and Yin, T. C. T. (1998). Anatomy and physiology of principal cells of the medial nucleus of the trapezoid body (MNTB) of the cat. *J. Neurophysiol.* 79, 3127–3142.

Sommer, I., Lingenhohl, K., and Friauf, E. (1993). Principal cells of the rat medial nucleus of the trapezoid body: an intracellular *in vivo* study of their physiology and morphology. *Exp. Brain Res.* 95, 223–239. doi: 10.1007/BF00229781

Spangler, K. M., Warr, W. B., and Henkel, C. K. (1985). The projections of principal cells of the medial nucleus of the trapezoid body in the cat. *J. Comp. Neurol.* 238, 249–262. doi: 10.1002/cne.902380302

Suga, N. (1977). Amplitude spectrum representation in the doppler-shifed-CF processing area of the auditory cortex of the mustached bat. *Science* 196, 64–67. doi: 10.1126/science.190681

Suga, N., and Tsuzuki, K. (1985). Inhibition and level-tolerant frequency tuning in the auditory cortex of the mustached bat. *J. Neurophysiol.* 53, 1109–1145.

Sutter, M. L. (2000). Shapes and level tolerances of frequency tuning curves in primary auditory cortex: quantitative measures and population codes. *J. Neurophysiol.* 84, 1012–1025.

Taschenberger, H., and Von Gersdorff, H. (2000). Fine-tuning an auditory synapse for speed and fidelity: developmental changes in presynaptic waveform, EPSC kinetics, and synaptic plasticity. *J. Neurosci.* 20, 9162–9173.

Theunissen, F. E., Sen, K., and Doupe, A. J. (2000). Spectral-temporal receptive fields of nonlinear auditory neurons obtained using natural sounds. *J. Neurosci.* 20, 2315–2331.

Tollin, D. J. (2003). The lateral superior olive: a functional role in sound source localization. *Neuroscientist* 9, 127–143. doi: 10.1177/1073858403252228

Tollin, D. J., and Henning, G. B. (1999). Some aspects of the lateralization of echoed sound in man. II. The role of stimulus spectrum. *J. Acoust. Soc. Am.* 105, 838–849. doi: 10.1121/1.426273

Tollin, D. J., and Koka, K. (2009a). Postnatal development of sound pressure transformations by the head and pinnae of the cat: monaural characteristics. *J. Acoust. Soc. Am.* 125, 980–994. doi: 10.1121/1.3058630

Tollin, D. J., and Koka, K. (2009b). Postnatal development of sound pressure transformations by the head and pinnae of the cat: binaural characteristics. *J. Acoust. Soc. Am.* 126, 3125–3136. doi: 10.1121/1.3257234

Tollin, D. J., Koka, K., and Tsai, J. J. (2008). Interaural level difference discrimination thresholds for single neurons in the lateral superior olive. *J. Neurosci.* 28, 4848–4860. doi: 10.1523/JNEUROSCI.5421-07.2008

Tollin, D. J., Populin, L. C., Moore, J., Ruhland, J. L., and Yin, T. C. (2005). Sound localization performance in the cat: the effect of restraining the head. *J. Neurophysiol.* 93, 1223–1234. doi: 10.1152/jn.00747.2004

Tollin, D. J., Ruhland, J. L., and Yin, T. C. (2013). The role of spectral composition of sounds on the localization of sound sources by cats. *J. Neurophysiol.* 109, 1658–1668. doi: 10.1152/jn.00358.2012

Tollin, D. J., and Yin, T. C. (2002a). The coding of spatial location by single units in the lateral superior olive of the cat. I. Spatial receptive fields in azimuth. *J. Neurosci.* 22, 1454–1467.

Tollin, D. J., and Yin, T. C. (2002b). The coding of spatial location by single units in the lateral superior olive of the cat. I. The determinants of spatial receptive fields in azimuth. *J. Neurosci.* 22, 1468–1479.

Tollin, D. J., and Yin, T. C. T. (2005). Interaural phase and level difference sensitivity in low-frequency neurons in the lateral superior olive. *J. Neurosci.* 25, 10648–10657. doi: 10.1523/JNEUROSCI.1609-05.2005

Tolnai, S., Englitz, B., Kopp-Scheinpflug, C., Dehmel, S., Jost, J., and Rubsamen, R. (2008b). Dynamic coupling of excitatory and inhibitory responses in the medial nucleus of the trapezoid body. *Eur. J. Neurosci.* 27, 3191–3204. doi: 10.1111/j.1460-9568.2008.06292.x

Tolnai, S., Englitz, B., Scholbach, J., Jost, J., and Rubsamen, R. (2009). Spike transmission delay at the Calyx of Held *in vivo*: rate dependence, phenomenological modeling, and relevance for sound localization. *J. Neurophysiol.* 102, 1206–1217. doi: 10.1152/jn.00275.2009

Tolnai, S., Hernandez, O., Englitz, B., Rubsamen, R., and Malmierca, M. S. (2008a). The medial nucleus of the trapezoid body in rat: spectral and temporal properties vary with anatomical location of the units. *Eur. J. Neurosci.* 27, 2587–2598. doi: 10.1111/j.1460-9568.2008.06228.x

Trussell, L. O. (2002). "Cellular mechanisms for information coding in auditory brainstem nuclei," in *Integrative Functions in the Mammalian Auditory Pathway*, eds D. Oertel, A. N. Popper, and R. R. Fay (New York, NY: Springer-Verlag), 72–98.

Tsai, J. J., Koka, K., and Tollin, D. J. (2010). Roving overall sound intensity to the two ears impacts interaural level difference discrimination thresholds by single neurons in the lateral superior olive. *J. Neurophysiol.* 103, 875–886. doi: 10.1152/jn.00911.2009

Tsuchitani, C. (1997). Input from the medial nucleus of trapezoid body to an interaural level detector. *Hear. Res.* 105, 211–224. doi: 10.1016/S0378-5955(96)00212-2

Turecek, R., and Trussell, L. O. (2001). Presynaptic glycine receptors enhance transmitter release at a mammalian central synapse. *Nature* 411, 587–590. doi: 10.1038/35079084

Versnel, H., Zwiers, M. P., and van Opstal, J. A. (2009). Spectrotemporal response properties of inferior colliculus neurons in alert monkey. *J. Neurosci.* 29, 9725–9739. doi: 10.1523/JNEUROSCI.5459-08.2009

von Gersdorff, H., and Borst, J. G. G. (2002). Short-term plasticity at the calyx of Held. *Nat. Rev. Neurosci.* 3, 53–64. doi: 10.1038/nrn705

Wehr, M., and Zador, A. M. (2003). Balanced inhibition underlies tuning and sharpens spike timing in auditory cortex. *Nature* 426, 442–446. doi: 10.1038/nature02116

Wu, S. H., and Kelly, J. B. (1991). Physiological properties of neurons in the mouse superior olive: membrane characteristics and postsynaptic responses studied *in vitro*. *J. Neurophysiol.* 65, 230–246.

Wu, S. H., and Kelly, J. B. (1992). Synaptic pharmacology of the superior olivary complex studied in mouse brain slice. *J. Neurosci.* 12, 3084–3097.

Wu, S. H., and Kelly, J. B. (1993). Response of neurons in the lateral superior olive and medial nucleus of the trapezoid body to repetitive stimulation: intracellular and extracellular recordings from mouse brain slice. *Hear. Res.* 68, 189–201. doi: 10.1016/0378-5955(93)90123-I

Wu, S. H., and Kelly, J. B. (1995). Inhibition in the superior olivary complex: pharmacological evidence from mouse brain slice. *J. Neurophysiol.* 73, 256–269.

Xie, R., Gittleman, J. X., and Pollak, G. D. (2007). Rethinking tuning: *in vivo* whole-cell recordings of the inferior colliculus in awake bats. *J. Neurosci.* 27, 9469–9481. doi: 10.1523/JNEUROSCI.2865-07.2007

Yin, T. C. T. (2002). "Neural mechanisms of encoding binaural localization cues in the auditory brainstem," in *Integrative Functions in the Mammalian Auditory*

Pathway, eds D. Oertel, A. N. Popper, and R. R. Fay (New York, NY: Springer), 99–159.

Young, E. D., and Calhoun, B. M. (2005). Nonlinear modeling of auditory-nerve rate responses to wideband stimuli. *J. Neurophysiol.* 94, 4441–4454. doi: 10.1152/jn.00261.2005

Young, E. D., Yu, J. J., and Reiss, L. A. (2005). Non-linearities and the representation of auditory spectra. *Int. Rev. Neurobiol.* 70, 135–168. doi: 10.1016/S0074-7742(05)70005-2

Yu, J. J. (2003). *Spectral Information Encoding in the Cochlear Nucleus and Inferior Colliculus: A Study Based on the Random Spectral Shape Method.* Ph.D. thesis, Baltimore, MD: Johns Hopkins University.

Yu, J. J., and Young, E. D. (2000). Linear and nonlinear pathways of spectral information transmission in the cochlear nucleus. *Proc. Natl. Acad. Sci. U.S.A.* 97, 11780–11786. doi: 10.1073/pnas.97.22.11780

Yu, J. J., and Young, E. D. (2013). Frequency response areas in the inferior colliculus: nonlinearity and binaural interaction. *Front. Neural Circuits* 7:90. doi: 10.3389/fncir.2013.00090

9

Neuronal specializations for the processing of interaural difference cues in the chick

Harunori Ohmori*

Department of Physiology and Neurobiology, Faculty of Medicine, Kyoto University, Kyoto, Japan

****Correspondence:***
Harunori Ohmori, Department of Physiology and Neurobiology, Faculty of Medicine, Kyoto University, Bldg. C, Kyoto 606-8501, Japan
e-mail: ohmori@nbiol.med.kyoto-u.ac.jp

Sound information is encoded as a series of spikes of the auditory nerve fibers (ANFs), and then transmitted to the brainstem auditory nuclei. Features such as timing and level are extracted from ANFs activity and further processed as the interaural time difference (ITD) and the interaural level difference (ILD), respectively. These two interaural difference cues are used for sound source localization by behaving animals. Both cues depend on the head size of animals and are extremely small, requiring specialized neural properties in order to process these cues with precision. Moreover, the sound level and timing cues are not processed independently from one another. Neurons in the nucleus angularis (NA) are specialized for coding sound level information in birds and the ILD is processed in the posterior part of the dorsal lateral lemniscus nucleus (LLDp). Processing of ILD is affected by the phase difference of binaural sound. Temporal features of sound are encoded in the pathway starting in nucleus magnocellularis (NM), and ITD is processed in the nucleus laminaris (NL). In this pathway a variety of specializations are found in synapse morphology, neuronal excitability, distribution of ion channels and receptors along the tonotopic axis, which reduces spike timing fluctuation in the ANFs-NM synapse, and imparts precise and stable ITD processing to the NL. Moreover, the contrast of ITD processing in NL is enhanced over a wide range of sound level through the activity of GABAergic inhibitory systems from both the superior olivary nucleus (SON) and local inhibitory neurons that follow monosynaptic to NM activity.

Keywords: brainstem auditory nucleus, interaural difference cues, SON, tonic inhibition, phasic inhibition

INTRODUCTION

The auditory nervous system is highly sensitive to changes in acoustic signals both in the frequency and the level (Dooling et al., 2000; Klump, 2000). Activity of ANFs codes the sound timing as the phase-locked-firing and the level as the firing-rate. Anatomically separate, and physiologically distinct pathways process these two auditory features (Oertel, 1999; Carr and Code, 2000). Anatomical separation is particularly distinct in the avian auditory system (**Figure 1**), where the pathway starting from NM carries the temporal information, and ITD is processed in NL. The pathway starting from NA carries the intensity information and ILD is processed in LLDp (Sullivan and Konishi, 1984; Takahashi et al., 1984). These two interaural differences inherent in auditory signals are used as cues for sound source localization (Moiseff, 1989). ITDs are generally used for processing low frequency sounds, while ILD is a cue used for high frequencies (Rayleigh, 1907).

Sharpening of ITD selectivity by GABAergic inputs has been demonstrated in higher auditory nuclei such as the inferior colliculus of the barn owl (Fujita and Konishi, 1991). In mammals, neurons in medial superior olive receive glycinergic inhibitory innervation from the medial and the lateral nucleus of the trapezoid body (Kuwabara and Zook, 1992; Grothe and Sanes, 1994). We are therefore interested in the presence and the roles of such inhibitory innervations in the ITD processing of NL. GABAergic innervations in NL are mostly from neurons in SON and some from the GABA positive interneurons located near NM and NL (Code et al., 1989; von Bartheld et al., 1989; Yamada et al., 2013). SON receives excitatory inputs from ipsilateral NA and NL, and inhibitory inputs from the contralateral SON, and makes projections to the ipsilateral NL, NM, NA and to the contralateral SON (**Figure 1**; Lachica et al., 1994; Yang et al., 1999; Monsivais et al., 2000; Burger et al., 2005).

In this review article I will first discuss the possible interplay between ILD and ITD, then I will detail the specializations found in the timing processing pathway, and the role of inhibition to make the ITD tuning tolerant to the sound level.

ILD PROCESSING IS AFFECTED BY INTERAURAL PHASE DIFFERENCE

Timing and level information is processed in separate neuronal pathways originating in the cochlear nuclei but ultimately merge in the midbrain, mesencephalicus lateralis dorsalis (avian homolog of the inferior colliculus; Pena and Konishi, 2001; Konishi, 2003). However, they are not processed in total separation even at lower levels. They influence one another at multiple steps of encoding and processing. Sound level affects processing of ITD under certain conditions (Viete et al., 1997; Dasika et al., 2005; Nishino et al., 2008), and sound timing affects processing of ILD (Sato et al., 2010; in mammals see Finlayson and

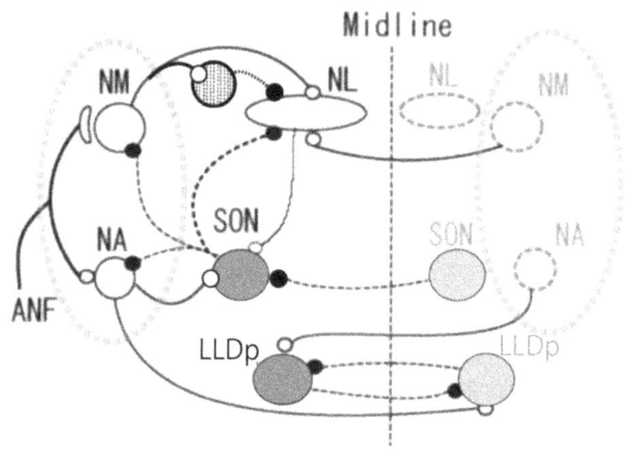

FIGURE 1 | Schema of avian auditory brainstem nuclei. Symbols indicate as follows: large open circles (excitatory neurons), large gray circles (inhibitory neurons), small open circles and solid lines (excitatory inputs) small filled circles and dashed lines (inhibitory inputs), and circle filled with dots (local inhibitory neurons). The local inhibitory neurons receive monosynaptic excitatory input from the ipsilateral NM. ANF, auditory nerve fiber; NM, nucleus magnocellularis; NA, nucleus angularis; NL, nucleus laminaris; SON, superior olivary nucleus; LLDp, posterior part of dorsal lateral lemniscus nucleus.

Caspary, 1991; Joris and Yin, 1995; Tollin and Yin, 2005). ILD is processed in the avian LLDp. LLDp neurons are excited by contralateral sound and inhibited by ipsilateral sound, reflecting excitation by the contralateral NA and inhibition from the ipsilateral NA through the contralateral LLDp as it is detailed in the barn owl (**Figure 1**; Manley et al., 1988; Mogdans and Knudsen, 1994).

Neural activity in NA and LLDp is changed with sound location, and is affected by the interaural phase difference (IPD). IPD modulates the activity of NA neurons in the chick through the acoustic interaction across the interaural canal that connects the middle ear cavities of two sides (Hyson et al., 1994; see also Christensen-Dalsgaard et al., 2011). The activity of NA neurons is suppressed by strong contralateral tones when binaural stimuli were presented in-phase, but activity increased monotonically with sound level when dichotic tones were at 180° out-of-phase (**Figure 2A**; Sato et al., 2010). Consequently, IPD dependence of firing activity of the NA neuron affects the ILD processing of the LLDp units of the chick (**Figure 2B**). However, in the barn owl, because of a sharp attenuation of the acoustic coupling across the interaural canal at frequencies above 3 kHz, the acoustic binaural interaction is negligible (Moiseff and Konishi, 1981).

The firing rate of LLDp units increases with increasing contralateral sound level, and decreases with increasing ipsilateral sound level. Moreover, the strength of inhibition by ipsilateral sound level varied among LLDp units, and a group of LLDp neurons was inhibited strongly by the ipsilateral sound (**Figures 2B,C**). IPD affected the rate-ILD function of LLDp neurons, and LLDp neurons that were inhibited strongly enhanced the selectivity toward the contralateral ear through the modulation of rate-ILD function (**Figures 2C,D**). The ratio of slopes of rate-ILD relationship between the contralateral dominant sound and the ipsilateral dominant sound across 0 ILD indicates the direction selectivity of LLDp units. This IPD effect on ILD processing in LLDp neurons may compensate for the small ILD cue available to the animal (Sato et al., 2010). The balance of excitation and inhibition changes with sound location, and in the barn owl LLDp, it is reported that the reliability of the response to spectrotemporal feature of LLDp neuron is enhanced by temporally delayed inhibition of LLDp neurons through gain modulation of the input-output function of the neuron (Steinberg et al., 2013).

SYNAPTIC SPECIALIZATIONS IN NM

Neurons in NM do not have appreciable dendrites, and ANFs make synapses on the cell soma. ANFs form enfolding end-bulbs of Held around the cell body in the high and middle characteristic frequency (CF) neuron but not in low CF neurons. Accordingly the EPSCs recorded in the high-middle CF NM neurons are large and generated in all-or-none manner with a small number of amplitude steps when the intensity of electrical stimulation applied to the ANFs bundle is changed, while the EPSCs recorded in the low CF neurons are small and the size gradually increases depended on the intensity of electrical stimulus (Fukui and Ohmori, 2004). NM neurons express low-voltage-activated Kv1.1 channels with a gradient along the tonotopic axis. High CF neurons have stronger Kv1.1 channel expression and conductance, resulting in more negative resting membrane potential and higher spike threshold. Blocking these channels by dendrotoxin depolarizes the resting membrane potential and reduces the spike threshold (Fukui and Ohmori, 2004). Dendrotoxin is known to block low-voltage-activated K^+ channels of Kv1.1, Kv1.2, and Kv1.6 subtypes (Hopkins et al., 1994; Harvey, 2001). Synaptic transmission during on-going stimuli is robust in the high-middle CF synapse but is depressed quickly in low CF synapses (Oline and Burger, 2014). A large readily releasable pool size in the high-middle CF terminals could maintain the reliable transmission. This may function to maintain the suprathreshold EPSCs in high CF neurons while enabling summation to enhance phase-locking in low CF neurons as it is discussed below.

NM neurons are specialized to encode temporal information of sound from ANFs activity. The low frequency sound information is strongly phase-locked, however it is actually encoded with a large timing jitter in ANFs. This timing fluctuation is reduced during transmission from ANFs to NM neurons (Fukui and Ohmori, 2004; Fukui et al., 2006; see Joris et al., 1994). Here, the mechanism is explained by the temporal integration of small EPSPs. Because the low frequency NM neuron is innervated by a large number of small bouton shaped synapses, single EPSPs are so small that multiple EPSPs are required to summate in order to reach spike threshold (Fukui and Ohmori, 2004; Kuba and Ohmori, 2009). Therefore, only those synaptic inputs arriving within a limited time window could contribute to NM spike; NM activity becomes more precisely phase-locked than ANF activity. However, the integration makes the depolarization of the NM neuron slow, which increases the level of inactivation of Na^+ channels. Axon initial segment (AIS), the site of action potential initiation, is extended longer in the axon of low CF NM neurons than the high-middle CF NM neurons. Clustering of a large number of Na^+ channels at the AIS would allow sufficient

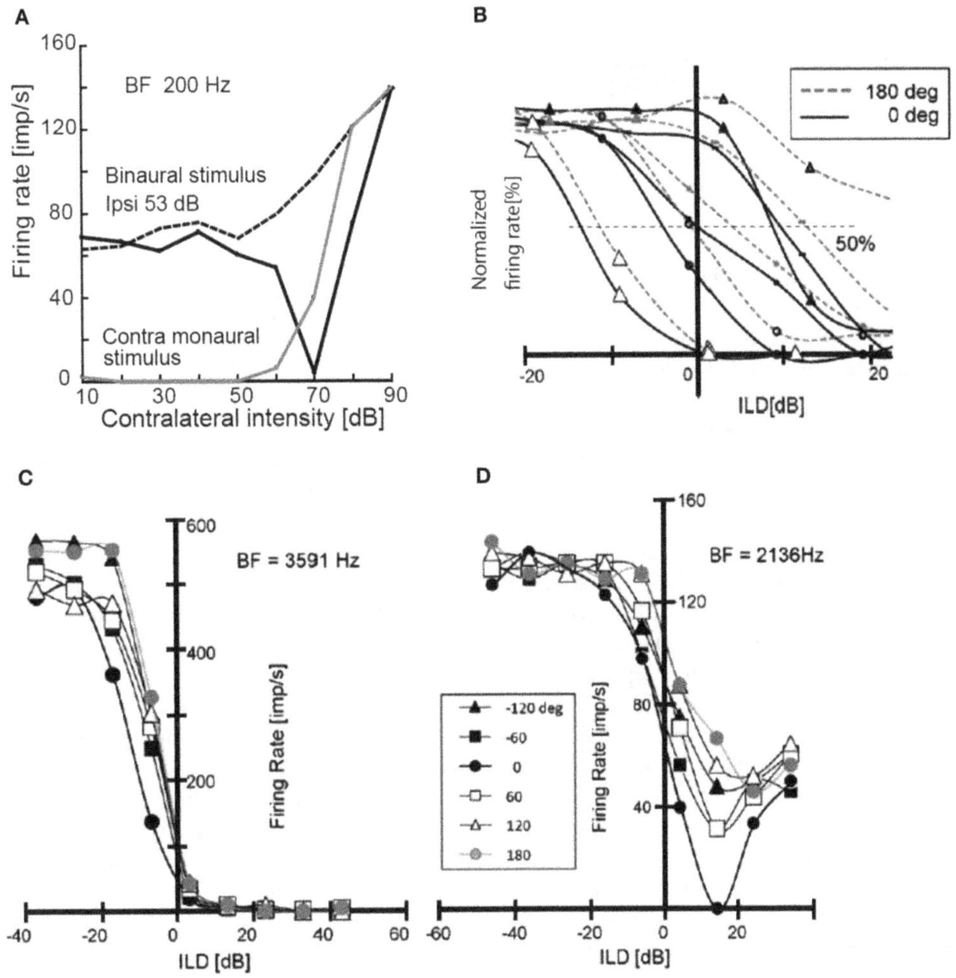

FIGURE 2 | Responses of NA unit and LLDp units to binaural stimuli. **(A)** Response of NA units to contralateral tone of 200 Hz. Binaural stimulus was applied in-phase (solid black line) or 180° out of phase (dotted line) with a constant ipsilateral tone of 53 dB; 20 dB above the threshold. Responses induced by contralateral monaural stimulus are included (solid gray line). **(B)** Rate-ILD relationship of LLDp units. ILD was defined as ipsi-contra SPL [dB]. Different symbols indicate different cells. Solid lines are for in-phase and broken lines are for 180° out-of-phase relationships. **(C,D)** IPD modulation of rate-ILD relationship of LLDp units with strong ipsilateral inhibition **(C)** with weak ipsilateral inhibition **(D)**. The inset indicates IPDs applied to both **(C,D)**. The slope of rate-ILD relationship across zero ILD is affected by IPD in **(C)** but not in **(D)**. Reproduced with permission from Sato et al. (2010).

current to generate action potentials even under a certain level of inactivation (Kuba and Ohmori, 2009). On the other hand, high frequency neurons are innervated by a small number of end-bulb shaped large terminal of ANF. Large EPSCs are generated and timing information is transmitted more precisely to high frequency NM neurons (Fukui and Ohmori, 2004; Fukui et al., 2006; Oline and Burger, 2014).

SPECIALIZATIONS OF ITD ENCODING IN THE NL

Somas of NL neurons have bipolar tufted dendrites and an axon emerges from the cell body. Dentrite morphology changes systematically along the tonotopic axis. Dendrites are short, relatively unbranched, occur in large numbers in high CF NL cells. The number of dendrites decreases in the middle-CF neurons but they become thicker and longer. Only a few primary dendrites extend away from the soma in the low-CF neurons, and they have extensive branching (Smith and Rubel, 1979; Kuba et al., 2005; Sanchez et al., 2010).

ITD depends on head size, and in most birds, the physiological maximum ITD is smaller than 100 μs. Considering the maximum firing rate of most neurons is less than or equal to 1 kHz, this maximum available ITD cue is extremely small; thus the auditory system needs specialization to process ITDs accurately.

During embryonic development, NMDA receptor currents increase in the NM-NL synapse, however it decreases dramatically before hatching. AMPA receptor currents increase during the embryonic development, particularly in the high CF NL cells. The EPSC kinetics becomes faster with development and rectifies in all CF regions, suggesting the exclusion of GluR2 receptor subunits from the synapse (Sanchez et al., 2010). Kinetics and amplitude of EPSCs are symmetrical in single NL neurons between inputs of two sides (Lu, 2009). Moreover, tonotopic gradients are matched between the EPSC time course and the feature of postsynaptic band-pass filtering in single NL neurons (Slee et al., 2010). These are consistent with the faster EPSC and mEPSC kinetics in NL neurons after hatching (Kuba et al., 2005).

LOW-VOLTAGE-ACTIVATED K^+ CHANNELS ENHANCE COINCIDENCE DETECTION, AND MAKE ITD DETECTION MOST SENSITIVE FOR MID-FREQUENCY SOUND

The best sensitivity to ITD or the smallest error of sound source localization was observed in the mid-audible frequency range in the avian species (Klump, 2000). Consistent with this observation, we found that the coincidence detection of bilateral NM spikes was most accurate in the middle-CF NL neurons. In brainstem slice experiments of the post-hatch chicks conducted at body temperature, 40°C, the time window of coincidence detection was 1700, 300, and 600 μs, for the low, middle and high CF neurons, respectively; the time window is defined as the time separation of bilateral stimuli applied to projection fibers from NM, which generates spikes in more than 50% trials (Kuba et al., 2003). Moreover, we found that the time course of EPSP measured as the half amplitude width have a significant positive correlation with the time window of coincidence detection (**Figure 3**); therefore, NL neuron with fast EPSPs has temporally sharp coincidence detection. The time course of EPSC is progressively faster toward high CF neurons. However, the time course of EPSP is fastest in mid-CF neurons, which is almost the same or sometimes faster than the time course of EPSC recorded in the same neuron (Kuba et al., 2005). The falling phase of the EPSP was accelerated due to strong activation of low-voltage-activated K^+ channels caused by EPSPs. Application of dendrotoxin prolonged the falling phase of EPSP. The expression of Kv1.2 channels is confirmed immunohistochemically in the NL, and the density of immuno-reactivity is the highest in the mid-CF region, where the time window for the coincidence detection is most precise (Kuba et al., 2005). These findings are consistent with the idea that Kv1.2 channels accelerate EPSP time course in the middle-CF NL neurons.

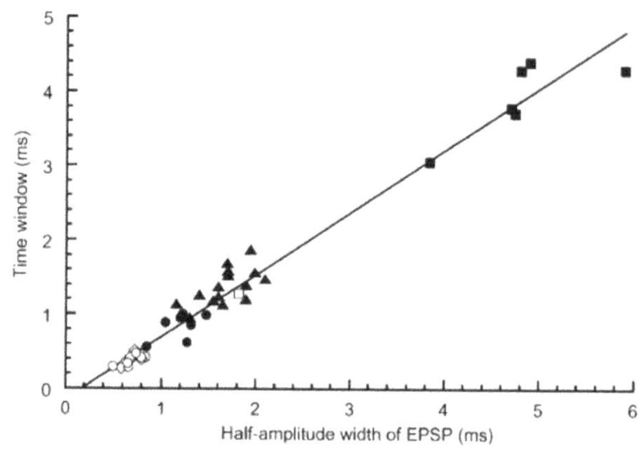

FIGURE 3 | Correlation between the time window for coincidence detection and the width of EPSP measured in the NL neurons. Time windows were plotted against the half amplitude width of EPSP recorded at −62 mV. Different symbols indicate different experimental conditions: ■, embryo recorded at 20–25°C ($n = 6$); □, embryo 40°C ($n = 1$); ▲, chick 20–25°C ($n = 15$); ●, chick 30°C ($n = 7$); ○, chick 40°C ($n = 8$); ◇, chick 40°C without bicuculline using low-Cl internal solution ($n = 5$). Reproduced with permission from Kuba et al. (2003).

Na^+ CHANNEL DISTRIBUTION IN AIS MAKES SPIKE-GENERATION STABLE IN WIDE FREQUENCY RANGES

We have been puzzled for a long time by the observation that the spikes and Na^+ currents were small in the high and middle CF NL neurons than those of low CF NL neurons (Kuba et al., 2003, 2005, 2006). By immuno-histochemical observations we found that the AIS is extended in length and located close to the cell soma in low CF NL neurons while short and located distant in the high CF NL neurons. The significance of this Na^+ channel distribution is interpreted by a computer simulation using a NEURON model under an assumption that NL neurons receive excitatory synaptic inputs at the frequency that closely matches with their CF; namely the frequency of synaptic inputs is high in the high CF NL neurons and low in the low CF NL neurons. Simulations demonstrated that the depolarization of the cell soma is greater in high CF NL neurons than the low CF NL neurons during sound inputs. This depolarization would inactivate Na^+ channels and prevent spike generation if the AIS, thus Na^+ channel, is located close to the cell soma. By displacing the AIS to a distance where the level of steady depolarization is small because of the electro-tonic property of the axon, the level of Na^+ channel inactivation should be reduced; however the reduced level of membrane depolarization may also reduce the activation level of Na^+ channels at a distance. Consequently, the balance of activation and inactivation of Na^+ channels is achieved, and the spike generation is optimized by controlling the spatial distribution of Na^+ channels for each NL neuron depending on its CF. This is likely the underlying mechanism for the stable processing of ITD in each NL neuron (Kuba et al., 2006; see also Ashida et al., 2007).

HCN CHANNELS MODIFY THE COINCIDENCE DETECTION

Hyperpolarization-activated cyclic nucleotide-gated (HCN) channels have a reversal potential around −30 mV, are activated by membrane hyperpolarization, and the voltage-sensitivity is modulated by cyclic nucleotides. Channel gating is shifted in the positive direction when the cytosolic concentration of cyclic nucleotides is high, and the sensitivity to cyclic nucleotide is greater in HCN2 than in HCN1 channel subtype (Pape, 1996; Santoro and Tibbs, 1999; Biel et al., 2009). In the chicken NL, both HCN1 and HCN2 channels are expressed along the tonotopic axis with a gradient (Yamada et al., 2005). Expression of HCN1 is graded extensively toward the low CF region of the nucleus, while the expression of HCN2 is less graded across the nucleus. The membrane depolarization of NL neurons was confirmed when the level of cyclic AMP was raised either by incubation of slices with 8-Br-cAMP or by photo-illumination of the cell that was loaded with a caged compound of cyclic AMP through the patch electrode, which likely reflected an increased level of activation of HCN channels (Yamada et al., 2005). The membrane depolarization improved the coincidence detection by accelerating the time course of EPSPs, presumably because of the activation of low-voltage-activated K^+ channels. The relatively high density of HCN2 channels over HCN1 channels in the high CF NL neurons made the high CF neurons more sensitive to the level of cyclic AMP (Yamada et al., 2005). Accordingly, by incubation of slices prepared from the high CF NL region with nor-adrenaline for a few minutes, the coincidence detection became more precise. Nor-adrenaline is a neurotransmitter released from sympathetic nerve terminals and is expected to activate G-protein-coupled receptors and increase cyclic AMP concentration in the target neurons (Gilman, 1987). These results raise the possibility that coincidence detection is under sympathetic control. HCN channel activity could be coupled with the improved sound source localization capability of the barn owl observed when owls were exposed to a sound stimulus of long duration (Knudsen and Konishi, 1979). Listening to a sound of long duration may increase the tension that likely mobilizes the sympathetic activity. Expression pattern of HCN channel subunits in the owl has not yet been examined.

METABOTROPIC GLUTAMATE RECEPTORS (mGluRs) ENHANCE THE LOW FREQUENCY COINCIDENCE DETECTION

The fast time course of EPSPs is critical to enhance the coincidence detection; however the sharpness of coincidence detection depends also on the size of EPSPs (Kuba et al., 2002). The size was not only affected by the short term synaptic plasticity, but was affected through the presynaptic mGluR activity as well (Okuda et al., 2013). A non-specific agonist of mGluRs (t-ACPD) reduced the amplitude of EPSCs, which reduced the depression of EPSCs during a stimulus train, while the paired pulse ratio and the coefficient of variation of EPSC amplitude were increased. In contrast, the amplitude of spontaneous EPSCs was not affected, but the frequency was reduced. Thus, the effects of t-ACPD were presynaptic and t-ACPD likely reduced the release of neurotransmitter from the NM terminal. Both group-II (DCG-IV) and group-III (L-AP4) specific agonists reduced EPSC amplitude by presynaptic mechanisms, and the effects were greater in low CF NL neurons. The reduced EPSP amplitude in DCG-IV improved the coincidence detection. A specific antagonist of group-II mGluRs (LY341495) increased the amplitude of both EPSCs and EPSPs, and enhanced depression during the stimulus train, which indicated a constitutive activation of mGluRs in the NL even though experiments were conducted in slice preparations. We have detected expression of group-II mGluRs immuno-histochemically, and the expression level was increased after hatching. The expression was greater toward the low CF NL region. These observations indicate that the presynaptic mGluRs may operate as a self-regulatory mechanism to optimize the size of EPSP and have roles in sharpening the coincidence detection, particularly during the on-going sound stimulus.

INHIBITORY SYNAPSES IN THE NL

Because of the relatively high intracellular concentration of Cl^-, GABA was depolarizing in brainstem auditory neurons (Hyson et al., 1995). GABA-induced depolarization could exceed the spike threshold and could be excitatory; however GABA application reduced input impedance and was primarily inhibitory. Therefore, sustained GABA effects are critical in improving the temporal processing of sounds (Funabiki et al., 1998; Tang et al., 2011). Moreover, GABAergic inhibitory synapse was affected by $GABA_B$ receptors and mGluRs in NL of embryonic age (E19-E21, Tang et al., 2009). These $GABA_B$ and mGluRs are cooperative and may improve the coincidence detection in NL neurons.

SUSTAINED GABAergic INHIBITION IMPROVES ITD PROCESSING

Firing rates of ITD processing neurons alternates periodically as ITD changes during a tonal stimulation, and the period of the ITD tuning curve was determined by the CF of the neuron (Goldberg and Brown, 1969; Carr and Konishi, 1990; Yin and Chan, 1990). The sound pressure level affected the contrast between the peak and trough firing rates (Pena et al., 1996). Loud sound was expected to increase the firing rate both at the peak and the trough of ITD tuning curve, and to reduce the peak-trough contrast (or ITD sensitivity, Dasika et al., 2005). However, the peak-trough contrast was actually maintained rather than reduced at high sound pressure level in *in vivo* recordings from the barn owl (Pena et al., 1996). Pena and colleagues proposed that inhibition from SON controls the ITD tuning in NL, making it tolerant to sound pressure level.

By recording single unit activity in NL *in vivo,* ITD tuning was found dependent both on the sound frequency and the sound pressure level (Nishino et al., 2008). The peak-trough contrast in mid-to-high CF NL units (higher than 1 kHz) was maximal at intermediate sound pressure levels. The peak-trough contrast was practically lost when a very loud sound was applied because of the increased firing rate both at the peak and the trough of ITD tuning curve (90 dB or louder sound). In low CF NL units (lower than 1 kHz), neural activity was temporally suppressed after a loud sound. The peak-trough contrast became larger as the sound became louder. This is because the trough-firing rate decreased with the sound pressure level, even to the level lower

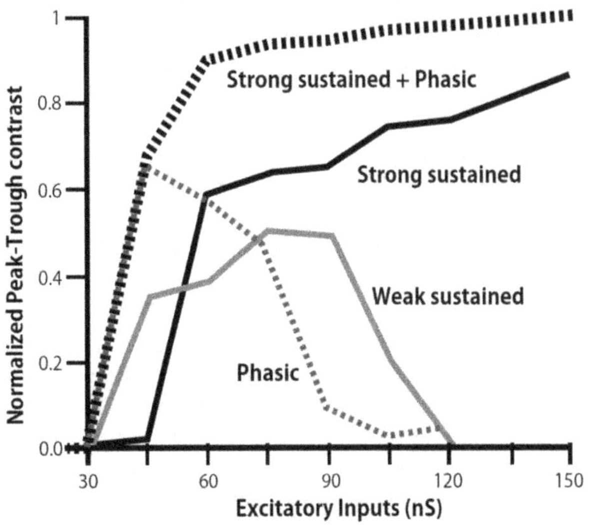

FIGURE 4 | Modulation of peak-trough contrast of ITD tuning curve of low-CF NL neurons by inhibition. Peak-trough contrasts of ITD tuning curve are calculated by including the sustained inhibition of weak (gray line), strong (black line), and phasic inhibition (dotted gray line) separately, and by including both the strong sustained and the phasic inhibition (dotted black line). Modified from Yamada et al. (2013).

than the spontaneous firing rate. These observations are consistent with the sustained SON inhibition of low CF NL neurons. Consistently after electrical lesioning of the ipsilateral SON the contrast of ITD tuning in the low CF NL neuron collapsed at loud sound (Nishino et al., 2008), and the tolerance of ITD tuning to the sound pressure level became similar to that of the mid-to-high CF NL units. The sound pressure level dependence of ITD processing of the mid-to-high CF NL neurons was not virtually affected by lesioning of the SON. SON receives sound pressure level information through NA (**Figure 1**), and GABAergic projection from SON to NL is robust in the low CF region of NL but becomes less prominent toward the high CF region. The density of the SON projection along the tonotopy is correlated with the magnitude of the response to SON lesions across the tonotopic axis in NL (Nishino et al., 2008). We conclude, accordingly, that the dense inhibitory projection from SON to NL makes the ITD tuning tolerant to the sound pressure level in NL (Nishino et al., 2008).

PHASIC INHIBITION BY LOCAL GABAergic NEURONS IMPROVES ITD PROCESSING WHEN THE EXCITATORY INPUT LEVEL IS LOW

We further found a phasic IPSC in the low CF NL neurons in slice preparations, which followed the ipsilateral NM inputs with a short time delay and small timing jitter; thus the phasic IPSC likely follows monosynaptically the ipsilateral NM activity (Yamada et al., 2013). GABA-positive small neurons are distributed in and near the NL (Carr et al., 1989; von Bartheld et al., 1989). When photoactivated by a caged glutamate compound these neurons generated IPSC in NL neurons suggesting that these GABAergic neurons are interneurons that mediate the phasic inhibition. These IPSCs in the low CF NL region have fast decay kinetics that is attributable to α1 subunit of the $GABA_A$ receptor (Goldstein et al., 2002; Eyre et al., 2012), the expression of which is dominated in the low-CF region of the NL. The fast decay kinetics is consistent with the faster kinetics of GABAergic IPSC in the low CF NL neuron observed by Tang and Lu (2012). Simulations using a NEURON model demonstrated that phasic IPSCs increase the contrast of ITD-tuning when the sound pressure level is low. Furthermore, the simulation demonstrated that the cooperation of phasic and sustained inhibitions effectively increases the contrast of ITD-tuning over a wide range of excitatory input levels (**Figure 4**; Yamada et al., 2013).

CONCLUSIONS

Interaural difference cues are small, particularly for animals endowed with small heads. This review has focused on works conducted on the chick, which provide profound insights into the mechanisms that contribute to the accuracy of ITD processing. Further, these studies reveal how ITD tuning is maintained over a wide range of sound pressure level in birds. The morphological specializations complement the roles of ionic channels in the ITD tuning. The distribution of ionic channels and receptors including the inhibitory synapses in the NL is critically arranged to optimize the ITD processing, and in turn, sound source localization. Moreover, timing and level cues of sounds are used cooperatively in both mammals and birds to improve the processing of small interaural difference cues.

ACKNOWLEDGMENTS

I thank helpful comments from anonymous reviewers greatly, and Dr. R.M. Burger for editing and kind comments on the manuscript. I appreciate all colleagues of the Department of Physiology and Neurobiology Kyoto University for their exquisite works summarized in this review. Those works were supported by grant-in-aid (12053233, 17023027, 20220008) from MEXT and JSPS.

REFERENCES

Ashida, G., Abe, K., Funabiki, K., and Konishi, M. (2007). Passive soma facilitates submillisecond coincidence detection in the owl's auditory system. *J. Neurophysiol.* 97, 2267–2282. doi: 10.1152/jn.00399.2006

Biel, M., Wahl-Schott, C., Michalakis, S., and Zong, X. (2009). Hyperpolarization-activated cation channels: from genes to function. *Physiol. Rev.* 89, 847–885. doi: 10.1152/physrev.00029.2008

Burger, R. M., Cramer, K. S., Pfeiffer, J. D., and Rubel, E. W. (2005). Avian superior olivary nucleus provides divergent inhibitory input to parallel auditory pathways. *J. Comp. Neurol.* 481, 6–18. doi: 10.1002/cne.20334

Carr, C. E., and Code, R. A. (2000). "The central auditory system of reptiles and birds," in *Comparative Hearing: Birds and Reptiles*, eds R. J. Dooling, R. R. Fay, and A. N. Popper (New York, NY: Springer), 197–248. doi: 10.1007/978-1-4612-1182-2_5

Carr, C. E., Fujita, I., and Konishi, M. (1989). Distribution of GABAergic neurons and terminals in the auditory system of the barn Owl. *J. Comp. Neurol.* 286, 190–207. doi: 10.1002/cne.902860205

Carr, C. E., and Konishi, M. (1990). A circuit for detection of interaural time differences in the brain stem of the barn owl. *J. Neurosci.* 10, 3227–3246.

Code, R. A., Burd, G. D., and Rubel, E. W. (1989). Development of GABA immunoreactivity in brainstem auditory nuclei of the chick ontogeny of gradients in terminal staining. *J. Comp. Neurol.* 284, 504–518. doi: 10.1002/cne.902840403

Dasika, V. K., White, J. A., Carney, L. H., and Colburn, H. S. (2005). Effects of inhibitory feedback in a network model of avian brain stem. *J. Neurophysiol.* 94, 400–414. doi: 10.1152/jn.01065.2004

Dooling, R. J., Bernard, L., and Dent, M. L. (2000). "Hearing in birds and reptiles," in *Comparative Hearing: Birds and Reptiles*, eds R. J. Dooling, R. R. Fay, and A. N. Popper (New York, NY: Springer), 308–359. doi: 10.1007/978-1-4612-1182-2_7

Eyre, M. D., Renzi, M., Farrant, M., and Nusser, Z. (2012). Setting the time course of inhibitory synaptic currents by mixing multiple GABAA receptor subunit isoforms. *J. Neurosci.* 32, 5853–5867. doi: 10.1523/JNEUROSCI.6495-11.2012

Finlayson, P. G., and Caspary, D. M. (1991). Low-frequency neurons in the lateral superior olive exhibit phase-sensitive binaural inhibition. *J. Neurophysiol.* 65, 598–605.

Fujita, I., and Konishi, M. (1991). The Role of GABAergic inhibition in processing of interaural time difference in the owl's auditory system. *J. Neurosci.* 11, 722–739.

Fukui, I., and Ohmori, H. (2004). Tonotopic gradients of membrane and synaptic properties for neurons of the chicken nucleus magnocellularis. *J. Neurosci.* 24, 7514–7523. doi: 10.1523/JNEUROSCI.0566-04.2004

Fukui, I., Sato, T., and Ohmori, H. (2006). Improvement of phase information at low sound frequency in nucleus magnocellularis of the chicken. *J. Neurophysiol.* 96, 633–641. doi: 10.1152/jn.00916.2005

Funabiki, K., Koyano, K., and Ohmori, H. (1998). The role of GABAergic inputs for coincidence detection in the neurones of nucleus laminaris of the chick. *J. Physiol.* 508, 851–869. doi: 10.1111/j.1469-7793.1998.851bp.x

Gilman, A. G. (1987). G proteins: transducers of receptor-generated signals. *Annu. Rev. Biochem.* 56, 615–649. doi: 10.1146/annurev.bi.56.070187.003151

Goldberg, J. M., and Brown, P. B. (1969). Response of binaural neurons of dog superior olivary complex to dichotic tonal stimuli: some physiological mechanisms of sound localization. *J. Neurophysiol.* 32, 613–636.

Goldstein, P. A., Elsen, F. P., Ying, S. W., Ferguson, C., Homanics, G. E., and Harrison, N. L. (2002). Prolongation of hippocampal miniature inhibitory postsynaptic currents in mice lacking GABAA receptor alpha1 subunit. *J. Neurophysiol.* 88, 3208–3217. doi: 10.1152/jn.00885.2001

Grothe, B., and Sanes, D. H. (1994). Synaptic inhibition influences the temporal coding properties of medial superior olivary neurons: an *in vitro* study. *J. Neurosci.* 14, 1701–1709.

Harvey, A. L. (2001). Twenty years of dendrotoxins. *Toxicon* 39, 15–26. doi: 10.1016/S0041-0101(00)00162-8

Hopkins, W. F., Allen, M. L., Houamed, K. M., and Tempel, B. L. (1994). Properties of voltage-gated K currents expressed in Xenopus oocytes by mKv1.1, mKv1.2 and their heteromultimers as revealed by mutagenesis of the dendrotoxin-binding site in mKv1.1. *Pflugers Arch.* 428, 382–390. doi: 10.1007/BF00724522

Hyson, R. L., Overholt, E. M., and Lippe, W. R. (1994). Cochlear microphonic measurements of interaural time differences in the chick. *Hear. Res.* 81, 109–118. doi: 10.1016/0378-5955(94)90158-9

Hyson, R. L., Reyes, A. D., and Rubel, E. W. (1995). A depolarizing inhibitory response to GABA in brainstem auditory neurons of the chick. *Brain Res.* 677, 117–126. doi: 10.1016/0006-8993(95)00130-I

Joris, P. X., Carney, L. H., Smith, P. H., and Yin, T. C. T. (1994). Enhancement of neural synchronization in the anteroventral cochlear nucleus. I. Responses to tones at the characteristic frequency. *J. Neurophysiol.* 71, 1022–1036.

Joris, P. X., and Yin, T. C. T. (1995). Envelope coding in the lateral superior olive. I. sensitivity to interaural time differences. *J. Neurophysiol.* 73, 1043–1062.

Klump, G. (2000). "Sound localization in birds," in *Comparative Hearing: Birds and Reptiles*, eds R. J. Dooling, R. R. Fay, and A. N. Popper (New York, NYSpringer), 249–307.

Knudsen, E. I., and Konishi, M. (1979). Mechanisms of sound localization in the barn owl (Tyto alba). *J. Comp. Physiol.* 133, 13–12. doi: 10.1007/BF00663106

Konishi, M. (2003). Coding of auditory space. *Annu. Rev. Neurosci.* 26, 31–55. doi: 10.1146/annurev.neuro.26.041002.131123

Kuba, H., Ishii, T. M., and Ohmori, H. (2006). Axonal site of spike initiation enhances auditory coincidence detection. *Nature* 444, 1069–1072. doi: 10.1038/nature05347

Kuba, H., Koyano, K., and Ohmori, H. (2002). Synaptic depression improves coincidence detection in the nucleus laminaris in brainstem slices of the chick embryo. *Eur. J. Neurosci.* 15, 984–990. doi: 10.1046/j.1460-9568.2002.01933.x

Kuba, H., and Ohmori, H. (2009). Roles of axonal sodium channels in precise auditory time coding at nucleus magnocellularis of the chick. *J. Physiol.* 587, 87–100. doi: 10.1113/jphysiol.2008.162651

Kuba, H., Yamada, R., Fukui, I., and Ohmori, H. (2005). Tonotopic specialization of auditory coincidence detection in nucleus laminaris of the chick. *J. Neurosci.* 25, 1924–1934. doi: 10.1523/JNEUROSCI.4428-04.2005

Kuba, H., Yamada, R., and Ohmori, H. (2003). Evaluation of the limiting acuity of coincidence detection in nucleus laminaris of the chicken. *J. Physiol.* 552, 611–620. doi: 10.1113/jphysiol.2003.041574

Kuwabara, N., and Zook, J. M. (1992). Projections to the medial superior olive from the medial and lateral nuclei of the trapezoid body in rodents and bats. *J. Comp. Neurol.* 324, 522–538. doi: 10.1002/cne.903240406

Lachica, E. A., Buebsamem, R., and Rubel, E. W. (1994). GABAergic terminals in nucleus magnocellularis and laminaris originate from the superior olivary nucleus. *J. Comp. Neurol.* 348, 403–418. doi: 10.1002/cne.903480307

Lu, Y. (2009). Regulation of glutamatergic and GABAergic neurotransmission in the chick nucleus laminaris: role of N-type calcium channels. *Neuroscience* 164, 1009–1019. doi: 10.1016/j.neuroscience.2009.09.013

Manley, G. A., Koppl, C., and Konishi, M. (1988). A neural map of interaural intensity differences in the brain stem of the barn owl. *J. Neurosci.* 8, 2665–2676.

Mogdans, J., and Knudsen, E. I. (1994). Representation of interaural level difference in the VLVp, the first site of binaural comparison in the barn owl's auditory system. *Hear. Res.* 74, 148–164. doi: 10.1016/0378-5955(94)90183-X

Moiseff, A. (1989). Binaural disparity cues available to the barn owl for sound localization. *J. Comp. Physiol. A* 164, 629–636. doi: 10.1007/BF00614505

Moiseff, A., and Konishi, M. (1981). Neuronal and behavioral sensitivity to binaural time differences in the owl. *J. Neurosci.* 1, 40–48.

Monsivais, P., Yang, L., and Rubel, E. W. (2000). GABAergic inhibition in nucleus magnocellularis: implications for phase locking in the avian auditory brainstem. *J. Neurosci.* 20, 2954–2963.

Nishino, E., Yamada, R., Kuba, H., Hioki, H., Furuta, T., Kaneko, T., et al.,(2008). Sound-intensity-dependent compensation for the small interaural time difference cue for sound source localization. *J. Neurosci.* 28, 7153–7164. doi: 10.1523/JNEUROSCI.4398-07.2008

Oertel, D. (1999). The role of timing in the brainstem auditory nuclei of vertebrates. *Ann. Rev. Physiol.* 61, 497–519. doi: 10.1146/annurev.physiol.61.1.497

Okuda, H., Yamada, R., Kuba, H., and Ohmori, H. (2013). Activation of metabotropic glutamate receptors improves the accuracy of coincidence detection by presynaptic mechanisms in the nucleus laminaris of the chick. *J. Physiol.* 591, 365–378. doi: 10.1113/jphysiol.2012.244350

Oline, S. N., and Burger, R. M. (2014). Short-term synaptic depression is topographically distributed in the cochlear nucleus of the chicken. *J. Neurosci.* 34, 1314–1324. doi: 10.1523/JNEUROSCI.3073-13.2014

Pape, H. C. (1996). Queer current and pacemaker: the hyperpolarization-activated cation current in neurons. *Annu. Rev. Physiol.* 58, 299–327. doi: 10.1146/annurev.ph.58.030196.001503

Pena, J. L., and Konishi, M. (2001). Auditory spatial receptive fields created by multiplication. *Science* 292, 249–252. doi: 10.1126/science.1059201

Pena, J. L., Viete, S., Albeck, Y., and Konishi, M. (1996). Tolerance to sound intensity of binaural coincidence detection in the nucleus laminaris of the owl. *J. Neurosci.* 16, 7046–7054.

Rayleigh, L. (1907). On our perception of sound direction. *Philos. Mag.* 13, 214–232. doi: 10.1080/14786440709463595

Sanchez, J. T., Wang, Y., Rubel, E. W., and Barria, A. (2010). Development of glutamatergic synaptic transmission in binaural auditory neurons. *J. Neurophysiol.* 104, 1771–1789. doi: 10.1152/jn.00468.2010

Santoro, B., and Tibbs, G. R. (1999). The HCN gene family: molecular basis of the hyperpolarization-activated pacemaker channels. *Ann. N. Y. Acad. Sci.* 868, 741–764. doi: 10.1111/j.1749-6632.1999.tb11353.x

Sato, T., Fukui, I., and Ohmori, H. (2010). Interaural phase difference modulates the neural activity in the nucleus angularis and improves the processing of level difference cue in the lateral lemniscal nucleus in the chicken. *Neurosci. Res.* 66, 198–212. doi: 10.1016/j.neures.2009.11.001

Slee, J. S., Higgs, M. H., Fairhall, A. L., and Spain, W. J. (2010). Tonotopic tuning in a sound localization circuit. *J. Neurophysiol.* 103, 2857–2875. doi: 10.1152/jn.00678.2009

Smith, D., and Rubel, E. W. (1979). Organization and development of brain stem auditory nuclei of the chicken: dendritic gradients in nucleus laminaris. *J. Comp. Neurol.* 186, 213–240. doi: 10.1002/cne.901860207

Steinberg, L. J., Fischer, B. J., and Pena, J. L. (2013). Binaural gain modulation of spectrotemporal tuning in the interaural level difference-coding pathway. *J. Neurosci.* 33, 11089–11099. doi: 10.1523/JNEUROSCI.4941-12.2013

Christensen-Dalsgaard, J., Tang, Y., and Carr, C. E. (2011). Binaural processing by the gecko auditory periphery. *J. Neurophysiol.* 105, 1992–2004. doi: 10.1152/jn.00004.2011

Tang, Z. Q., Dinh, E. H., Shi, W., and Lu, Y. (2011). Ambient GABA-activated tonic inhibition sharpens auditory coincidence detection via a depolarizing shunting mechanism. *J. Neurosci.* 31, 6121–6131. doi: 10.1523/JNEUROSCI.4733-10.2011

Tang, Z. Q., Gao, H., and Lu, Y. (2009). Control of a depolarizing GABAergic input in an auditory coincidence detection circuit. *J. Neurophysiol.* 102, 1672–1683. doi: 10.1152/jn.00419.2009

Tang, Z. Q., and Lu, Y. (2012). Two GABAA responses with distinct kinetics in a sound localization circuit. *J. Physiol.* 590, 3787–3805. doi: 10.1113/jphysiol.2012.230136

Takahashi, T., Moiseff, A., and Konishi, M. (1984). Time and intensity cues are processed independently in the auditory system of the owl. *J. Neurosci.* 4, 1781–1786.

Tollin, D. J., and Yin, T. C. T. (2005). Interaural phase and level difference sensitivity in low frequency neurons in the lateral superior olive. *J. Neurosci.* 25, 10648–10657. doi: 10.1523/JNEUROSCI.1609-05.2005

Viete, S., Pena, J. L., and Konishi, M. (1997). Effects of iteraural intensity difference on the processing of interaural time difference in the owl's nucleus laminaris. *J. Neurosci.* 17, 1815–1824.

von Bartheld, C. S., Code, R. A., and Rubel, E. W. (1989). GABAergic neurons in brainstem auditory nuclei of the chick distribution, morphology, and connectivity. *J. Comp. Neurol.* 287, 470–483. doi: 10.1002/cne.902870406

Sullivan, W. E., and Konishi, M. (1984). Segregation of stimulus phase and intensity coding in the cochlear nucleus of the barn owl. *J. Neurosci.* 4, 1787–1799.

Yamada, R., Kuba, H., Ishii, T. M., and Ohmori, H. (2005). Hyperpolarization-activated cyclic nucleotide-gated cation channels regulate auditory coincidence detection in nucleus laminaris of the chick. *J. Neurosci.* 25, 8867–8877. doi: 10.1523/JNEUROSCI.2541-05.2005

Yamada, R., Okuda, H., Kuba, H., Nishino, E., Ishii, T. M., and Ohmori, H. (2013). The cooperation of sustained and phasic inhibitions increases the contrast of ITD-tuning in low-frequency neurons of the chick nucleus laminaris. *J. Neurosci.* 33, 3927–3938. doi: 10.1523/JNEUROSCI.2377-12.2013

Yang, L., Monsivais, P., and Rubel, E. W. (1999). The superior olivary nucleus and its influence on nucleus laminaris: a source of inhibitory feedback for coincidence detection in the avian auditory brainstem. *J. Neurosci.* 19, 2313–2325.

Yin, T. C. T., and Chan, J. C. K. (1990). Interaural time sensitivity in medial superior olive of cat. *J. Neurophysiol.* 64, 465–488.

10

Inhibitory projections from the ventral nucleus of the trapezoid body to the medial nucleus of the trapezoid body in the mouse

Otto Albrecht[1], Anna Dondzillo[1], Florian Mayer[1], John A. Thompson[2] and Achim Klug[1]*

[1] Department of Physiology and Biophysics, School of Medicine, University of Colorado, Aurora, CO, USA
[2] Department of Neurosurgery, School of Medicine, University of Colorado, Aurora, CO, USA

***Correspondence:**
Achim Klug, Department of Physiology and Biophysics, School of Medicine, University of Colorado, 12800 E 19th Ave., MS 8307, Aurora, CO 80045, USA
e-mail: achim.klug@ucdenver.edu

Neurons in the medial nucleus of the trapezoid body (MNTB) receive prominent excitatory input through the calyx of Held, a giant synapse that produces large and fast excitatory currents. MNTB neurons also receive inhibitory glycinergic inputs that are also large and fast, and match the calyceal excitation in terms of synaptic strength. GABAergic inputs provide additional inhibition to MNTB neurons. Inhibitory inputs to MNTB modify spiking of MNTB neurons both *in-vitro* and *in-vivo*, underscoring their importance. Surprisingly, the origin of the inhibitory inputs to MNTB has not been shown conclusively. We performed retrograde tracing, anterograde tracing, immunohistochemical experiments, and electrophysiological recordings to address this question. The results support the ventral nucleus of the trapezoid body (VNTB) as at least one major source of glycinergic input to MNTB. VNTB fibers enter the ipsilateral MNTB, travel along MNTB principal neurons and produce several bouton-like presynaptic terminals. Further, the contribution of GABA to the total inhibition declines during development, resulting in only a very minor fraction of GABAergic inhibition in adulthood, which is matched in time by a reduction in expression of a GABA synthetic enzyme in VNTB principal neurons.

Keywords: VNTB, MNTB, glycinergic, auditory, calyx of held, trapezoid body, inhibition

INTRODUCTION

The medial nucleus of the trapezoid body (MNTB) is an auditory brainstem nucleus located in the ventro-medial aspect of the brainstem. It consists of about 3000–5000 principal neurons (Rodríguez-Contreras et al., 2006; Kulesza, 2008) that receive neural excitation from globular bushy cells located in the contralateral antero-ventral cochlear nucleus (AVCN; Held, 1893; Morest, 1968). Almost all excitatory input to MNTB neurons is conveyed via the giant calyx of Held synapse (Held, 1893; Guinan and Li, 1990). Evidence also exists for additional non-calyceal inputs from an unknown source (Banks and Smith, 1992; Hamann et al., 2003). Each MNTB neuron receives excitatory input from exactly one calyx (Rodríguez-Contreras et al., 2006), which produces large and fast excitatory currents (Forsythe, 1994; Taschenberger and von Gersdorff, 2000). The results of many studies have provided a good understanding of the excitatory input (von Gersdorff and Borst, 2002; Schneggenburger and Forsythe, 2006; Borst and van Hoeve, 2012).

Much less attention has been paid to inhibitory inputs to MNTB neurons. The inhibitory inputs comprise both GABAergic and glycinergic components, although the contribution of GABA declines during development, resulting in little GABAergic inhibition in the adult (Awatramani et al., 2005). However, at all stages, glycinergic inhibition to MNTB is large and fast, and able to follow rapid stimulus trains (~several 100 Hz; Awatramani et al., 2004). The synaptic conductance of the inhibitory input matches the extremely large synaptic conductance produced by the calyceal excitatory input, and is able to suppress MNTB spiking when activated (Awatramani et al., 2004). Even after prolonged stimulation, the inhibitory input continues to produce large, fast, and phasic synaptic currents (Florian Mayer, unpublished data). *In-vivo*, neural inhibition to MNTB shapes its response to sound (Green and Sanes, 2005; Kopp-Scheinpflug et al., 2008; Tolnai et al., 2008). Further, blocking glycinergic inhibition *in-vivo* reveals that some inhibitory inputs shape responses at or near the neurons' best excitatory frequencies, while others act off best frequency (Kopp-Scheinpflug et al., 2008).

Despite the importance of glycinergic inhibition for information processing in the MNTB, there are gaps in our knowledge about the origin of the inhibitory inputs. Evidence exists for both the ventral nucleus of the trapezoid body (VNTB) (Kuwabara et al., 1991; Thompson and Schofield, 2000) and MNTB itself (Guinan and Li, 1990; Kuwabara and Zook, 1991) as putative sources.

Our goal was to determine the source(s) of glycinergic inhibition to MNTB. We used a transgenic mouse line in which glycinergic neurons express green fluorescent protein (GlyT2-GFP mouse; Zeilhofer et al., 2005), and performed retrograde and anterograde tracing studies, immunohistochemistry, and electrophysiology. Our findings suggest that the VNTB is one area that sends substantial glycinergic inputs to MNTB. VNTB fibers travel along MNTB principal neurons and produce several bouton-like presynaptic terminals. The developmental shift in GABAergic contribution is matched by reduced detection of the GABAergic marker, GAD67, in VNTB principal neurons.

METHODS

All experimental procedures complied with all applicable laws and NIH guidelines and were approved by the University of Colorado IACUC. All experiments were conducted in a transgenic GlyT2-GFP mouse line, in which glycinergic neurons are labeled with enhanced green fluorescent protein [eGFP; Poyatos et al., 1997; Zeilhofer et al., 2005; JAX registry code: Tg(Slc6a5-EGFP)1Uze].

RETROGRADE TRACING

GlyT2-GFP mice aged p14 to p138 were anesthetized with pentobarbital (120 mg/kg bodyweight) and perfused transcardially with ice-cold phosphate buffered saline (PBS; NaCl: 137 mM, KCl: 2.7 mM, KH_2PO_4: 1.76 mM, Na_2HPO_4: 10 mM; all chemicals from Sigma-Aldrich). After exsanguination and perfusion, the animals were decapitated and the brain removed. Brain explants were cut along the caudal border (line "A" in **Figure 1**) of two ventral prominent "bulbs" containing the VNTB (black dotted lines in **Figure 1**), exposing the caudal end of the MNTB in the coronal cutting plane (white line "A" in **Figure 1**). Brainstem explants were placed in oxygenated (95% O_2, 5% CO_2) dissecting solution (NaCl: 125 mM, KCl: 2.5 mM, $MgCl_2$: 1 mM, $CaCl_2$: 0.1 mM, glucose: 25 mM, NaH_2PO_4: 1.25 mM, $NaHCO_3$: 25 mM, ascorbic acid: 0.4 mM, myo-inositol: 3 mM, pyruvic acid: 2 mM). Injection pipettes were pulled from borosilicate glass (Harvard Apparatus; GC150F-10) using a Zeitz DMZ Universal Puller (Zeitz Instruments, Germany) and filled with PBS containing 1.0 mg/ml solution of cholera toxin subunit-b conjugated to Alexa 555 ($n = 11$) (Molecular Probes; C-34776) (Conte et al., 2008, 2009), or dextran tetramethylrhodamine 555 ($n = 7$) (TMR; 3000 mW; 1%-dilution in 0.9% saline; Molecular Probes; D-7162). Pipette resistances varied from 2.5 to 3.5 MOhm.

Tracer injection locations were confirmed visually by inspecting the exposed caudal end of the explant (for further anatomical reference, see Franklin and Paxinos (2008); Franklin and Paxinos, Plate 78, Bregma ~ −5.7 mm). Based on this, the injection site was within the area marked as "Tz" (nucleus of the trapezoid body = MNTB). Electrodes were inserted into the tissue block in a perpendicular direction, as indicated by the red arrow labeled A' (**Figure 1**).

The injections consisted of 2–10 pressure pulses (15 psi, 50 ms), directed perpendicularly at the MNTB in the coronal plane of the brainstem. Single pressure pulses were administered at intervals of 10–15 s to allow for the dye to spread. For the TMR injections, additional electrical stimulation was performed to enhance the dye uptake through electroporation (Burger et al., 2005; Ford et al., 2009) After the injections, brainstems were incubated in oxygenated artificial cerebrospinal fluid (ACSF; NaCl: 125 mM, KCl: 2.5 mM, $MgCl_2$: 1 mM, $CaCl_2$: 2 mM, glucose: 25 mM, NaH_2PO_4: 1.25 mM, $NaHCO_3$: 25 mM, ascorbic acid: 0.4 mM, myo-inositol: 3 mM, pyruvic acid: 2 mM) for 1–4 h. Subsequently, the brainstems were post fixed in 4% paraformaldehyde (PFA) overnight. On the next day the

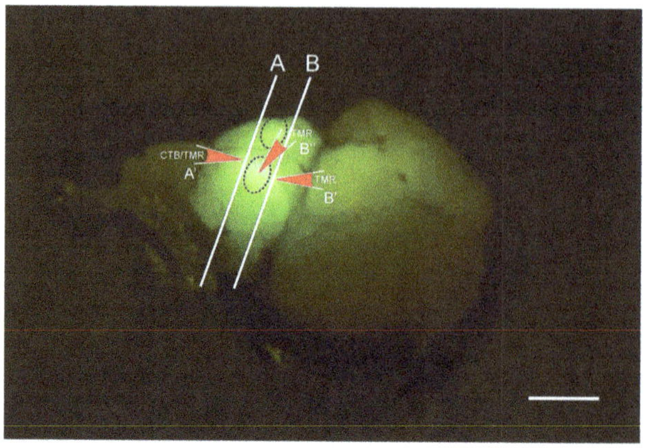

FIGURE 1 | Photo of a brain stem explant of a young (p2) GlyT2-GFP mouse showing the "bulbs" on the ventral surface of the explant (dashed oval lines). The image was taken through a yellow filter while the brain explant was illuminated with a 405 nm laser. With this type of lighting, the bulbs light up brightly and can easily be distinguished, presumably because they contain the VNTB with GFP positive neurons close to the brain surface, and presumably because other major sources of GlyT2-GFP label, such as the MNTB, are located close by. The locations of the two different coronal cutting planes for retrograde and anterograde injections are shown by lines A and B, respectively, and the injection sites and their directionality are depicted by the red arrows A', B', and B." Scale bar: 1 mm.

brainstems were washed three times in PBS (5 min for each washing step), covered in 4% agar and then cut into 50–80 μm thick slices on a Leica VT1000S vibratome. Each slice was mounted using Fluromount-G (Southern Biotech; Cat.-No: 0100-01) and coverslipped. A subset of brains ($n = 7$) were additionally labeled with fluorescent blue Nissl (1:100 dilution; Invitrogen; N21479).

ANTEROGRADE TRACING

The preparation was similar as for retrograde tracing, except that explanted brains were either not cut, or cut rostral to MNTB (Line "B" in **Figure 1**; compare with Bregma −4.6 mm; Franklin and Paxinos, 2008). TMR was injected directly from the ventral side of the brainstem into one of the prominent bulbs containing the VNTB (oval structures in **Figure 1**, injection site and direction is labeled by red arrow B") or into the exposed rostral end of VNTB (red arrow B', **Figure 1**). This location corresponded to Bregma ~ −4.6 mm;(Franklin and Paxinos, 2008), Plate 69 [labeled "MVPO" (medioventral periolivary nucleus) = VNTB].

In addition to the pressure pulses, a series of square voltage steps (8 TTL pulses, 8 Volts, 50 ms duration, 50 ms interpulse interval) were applied (Burger et al., 2005; Ford et al., 2009). The stimulus train was usually repeated 10–20 times after each pressure injection pulse to enhance the dye uptake via electroporation. The stimulus train was programmed in MC Stimulus software and used to control a STG-1002 stimulator (both Multi Channel Systems, Germany). The output of the stimulator was connected to a stimulation isolation unit (Iso-Flex, A.M.P.I., Israel), which was used to amplify the voltage steps to 55 V. Following the injection and stimulation, brainstem explants were treated as for retrograde tracer injections (incubation, fixation, and wash cycles). Then, brainstems were cut into sections of

200–500 μm, and cleared (Clear^{T2}, Kuwajima et al., 2013). After the last incubation step, slices were mounted with custom-made spacers, coverslipped with the same clearing solution that was used to incubate the sections [a mix of 50% formamide and 20% poly(ethanyl glycol), 8000 mW], and imaged.

IMMUNOHISTOCHEMISTRY

For immunostaining of the brain tissue against GAD67 (glutamic acid decarboxylase-67 kDa) GlyT2-GFP mice aged p14 (6 animals), p59 (3 animals), and p70 (2 animals) were perfused transcardially with PBS and 4% PFA. For the antibody labeling against GlyT2, five adult mice (two wild type animals aged p51 and 3 GlyT2-GFP mice, aged p59, p60, and p61) were sacrificed. Their brainstems were taken out and post fixed in 4% PFA for 2 h. After being washed in PBS (3 × 5 min), the brainstems were covered in 4% agarose and cut into 40 μm thick slices. These slices were washed 3 × 10 min in PBS and incubated in AB media [0.1 M phosphate buffer (PB; KH_2PO_4: 50 mM, Na_2HPO_4: 150 mM], 150 mM NaCl, 3 mM Triton-X, 1% bovine serum albumin; 1% normal goat serum) containing unlabeled Fab fragments of goat anti-mouse IgG (Jackson ImmunoResearch) overnight to enhance the specificity of the primary antibody in mouse tissue (in the case of the GlyT2 labeling, the Fab fragments were left out). After this blocking step the slices were kept in the primary antibody solution for 2 days at 4°C. The primary antibodies were a purified mouse monoclonal IgG2a against GAD67 (Millipore; MAB5406; RRID: AB_2278725) and a guinea pig polyclonal antibody raised against a rat GlyT2 C-terminal region (Millipore; AB1773; RRID: AB_90953). Specificity of both antibodies has been shown previously (Ito et al., 2007; Dufour et al., 2010). Following the incubation in the primary antibody solution, the slices were washed 3 × 10 min in PBS and incubated in secondary antibody solution for 2 h. The secondary antibodies were acquired from Invitrogen (goat anti-mouse IgG conjugated with Alexa 568; A11031; RRID: AB_144696 and goat anti-guinea pig IgG conjugated with Alexa 568; A11075; RRID: AB_141954). After another three washing steps in PBS, the slices were briefly washed in PB, mounted on glass slides using Fluromount-G (SouthernBiotech, Cat.-No.: 0100-01) and coverslipped.

IMAGING

The retrograde and anterograde tracer-injected brainstem slices were imaged on three different systems: 3I Vivo (Denver, USA) equipped with a 20×/N.A. 1.0 DIC water objective (1.0 mm working distance) and Slidebook 5.5 imaging software, Olympus Fluoview with 10×/N.A. 0.4, 20× oil /N.A. 0.8 and 60× oil /N.A. 1.4 objectives using Fluoview imaging software and Olympus FV1000 FCS/RICS with 10×/N.A. 0.4, 20×/N.A. 0.75 and 60× water /N.A. 1.2. Immunolabeled brain slices were imaged with the Olympus Fluoview system only. Images were background-corrected either online using the respective imaging software or *post-hoc* in ImageJ.

IMAGE ANALYSIS

VNTB delineation

We used the GlyT2-GFP signal (i.e., the glycinergic subpopulation of VNTB cells) to delineate the borders of the VNTB (white dotted line in **Figure 2A**). With this method, the VNTB typically consists of small, stellate or slightly elongated (spindle-like) GlyT2-GFP positive cells, and extends along the ventral border of a coronal brainstem section of the superior olivary complex (SOC). This delineation is consistent with Kuwabara et al. (1991) in terms of VNTB cell shapes, and is consistent with Helfert et al. (1989) in terms of the presence of glycinergic neurons in this nucleus. We defined the medio-lateral extent of VNTB between the lateral border of the ipsilateral MNTB and approximately the medial border of the ipsilateral LSO, consistent with Franklin and Paxinos (2008) and Ollo and Schwartz (1979). In the mouse, the superior paraolivary nucleus (SPN) is located directly above VNTB, marking its dorsal border. SPN was determined by its few and large glycinergic cells (Helfert et al., 1989; Saint Marie and Baker, 1990) and a dense web of glycinergic inputs appearing as a solid green area in our GlyT2-GFP mouse line. Directly lateral to the VNTB lies the lateral nucleus of the trapezoid body (LNTB, red dotted line in **Figure 2A**), a "comma-shaped" nucleus wrapping around the ventro-lateral border of the LSO. LNTB contains a similar number of glycinergic neurons as the VNTB, but some of them are larger, and rounder, and show brighter fluorescence (**Figure 2**). We typically observed a distinct non-fluorescent gap between the VNTB and the LNTB; the gap was more prominent in more posterior sections (**Figure 2C**). Based on these criteria, we were able to distinguish between the two nuclei.

Co-localization analysis

For the co-localization analysis of the GABAergic marker GAD67 in glycinergic (GFP+) VNTB neurons we chose the automatic co-localization algorithm developed by Li et al. (2004) that is implemented as one of ImageJ's plugins (Just Another Co-Localization Plugin; JACoP). Glycinergic (GFP+) VNTB neurons were marked and cropped out of the stack (in x, y, and z directions) using ImageJ's region of interest (ROI) manager and then analyzed with JACoP. This analysis algorithm is based on a user selecting a square area containing one glycinergic VNTB neuron from a single image of a confocal stack, and determining the brightness of GAD67 label within this analysis area. The result is subsequently correlated with the GFP signal intensity in the same area on a pixel-by-pixel basis. The amount of co-variation of signal intensities in both channels is formulated as the ICQ (intensity correlation quotient), with higher ICQ values indicating a higher degree of co-localization. The co-localization color map (after Jaskolski et al., 2005) was used to look for co-localization hot spots in young and adult animals. The statistical analysis was done in MS Excel and Sigmastat.

Semi-automated injection site quantification

Epifluorescent images of brain slices (80 μm thick) containing injected MNTB were collected using an Olympus BX 41 microscope (obj. × 10, N.A. 0.3) with TRITC (for tracer fluorescence) and DAPI (Nissl fluorescence) filter cubes. Image dimensions were 2048 × 2048 pixels with a pixel size of 0.742 μm (x and y) and a 12 bit depth converted to 8 bit for Matlab analysis. The exposure time for the TRITC channel was selected based on the brain section closest to the epicenter of the injection (brightest area) and was kept constant for all images per brain. The collected

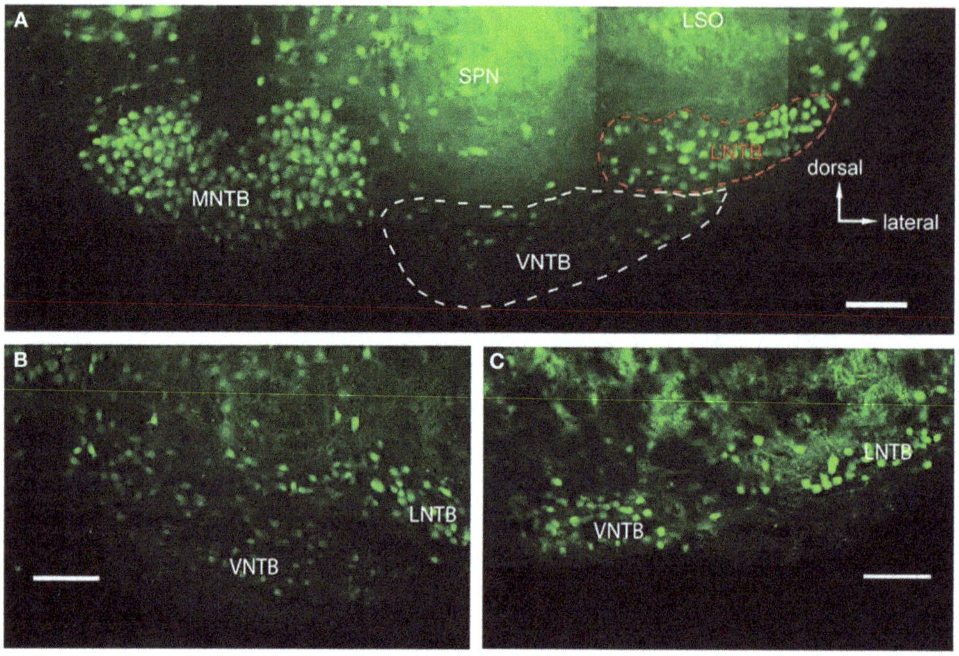

FIGURE 2 | Glycinergic auditory nuclei in a brainstem of a p14 GlyT2-GFP mouse. (A) Maximum projection of 10 tiled confocal stacks through a 200 μm brain section cleared prior to imaging using the Clear^{T2}-protocol. Five major nuclei with glycine label can be seen: the medial nucleus of the trapezoid body (MNTB), the ventral and lateral nuclei of the trapezoid body (VNTB and LNTB, outlined with white and red dashed lines, respectively), the SPN, and the ventral, high-frequency region of the lateral superior olive (LSO). **(B,C)** Closeup of the VNTB/LNTB area, showing the anatomical features used to discriminate between the VNTB and the LNTB. The image in **(B)** represents a more posterior location than **(A)** and **(C)** is located even more posterior than the ones in **(A,B)**. Note the increasing gap between the two nuclei void of glycinergic cells. Scale bars: 100 μm.

images were then used for a quantification of the injection site by a custom written routine in Matlab 2013a using base Matlab and the Image Processing Toolbox (Mathworks, Natick, MA). The quantification procedure performed in a custom Matlab GUI consisted of the following steps: (a) the experimenter traced a ROI around the MNTB in the Nissl channel (**Figure 5B**); (b) then the background of the injection signal was objectively averaged in the TRITC channel by selecting three different regions (each sample box in **Figure 5B** was comprised of an area of 1% of the total number of pixels) within the image to capture the distribution of the background signal; (c) calculation of the threshold (see below); (d) counting and displaying all pixels above the threshold located within the MNTB ROI (pink dots in **Figure 5B**). The calculation of the threshold and the number of pixels above threshold was objective and fully automated. This procedure was repeated for each section, resulting in at least 70% of the entire MNTB in the antero-posterior direction being analyzed. Additionally, to estimate the potential amount of injection outside the boundary of the MNTB ROI, a dynamically expanding box ROI was implemented. Initially the box was set to an area 25% greater than the MNTB ROI area and centered on the MNTB ROI. To ensure that the accurate estimation of area of tracer spillover was captured, an algorithm was implemented to detect whether 10% of the total pixels within any side (which varied in length, but were always 1 pixel wide) of the box ROI exceeded threshold. The algorithm would independently expand the sides of the box until all sides contained pixel populations that fell below 10% of threshold. When the parameters of the algorithm were satisfied, the area of pixels that exceeded threshold outside the MNTB and inside the box was calculated to objectively quantify the area of injection tracer spillover.

Data obtained from the custom Matlab GUI were the surface area of the MNTB and the surface area of the injection within the MNTB (in pixels) and were recalculated into volumes. We represent injection accuracy in volume percentages. Threshold was defined as a mean calculated from the MNTB ROI and the three squares selected in the TRITC channel of an image plus two standard deviations (SD), (Threshold = mean + 2*SD). All pixels above the threshold within the MNTB ROI were counted as labeled.

If the variability in pixel intensity was high such that the threshold equation resulted in intensities higher than 255, we implemented an upper boundary on the threshold. The second threshold was defined as the maximum intensity minus two standard deviations as calculated from the equation [$\text{Threshold}_{(\text{upper})} = 255 - 2^*\text{SD}$].

The Matlab script for this custom programmed GUI is available for download at the following URL: https://github.com/neuropil/DyeDist).

ELECTROPHYSIOLOGY

Slice preparation

Slices of brainstem were prepared from mice of either sex ranging in age from p14 to p70. Animals were anesthetized by isoflurane inhalation (IsoFlo, Abbott Laboratories, USA) and decapitated. The brainstem was dissected out and cut into slices of 180 μm with a vibratome (VT1000S, Leica, Wetzlar, Germany) under ice-cold dissection ringer (125 mM NaCl, 2.5 mM KCl, 1 mM $MgCl_2$, 0.1 mM $CaCl_2$, 25 mM glucose, 1.25 mM NaH_2PO_4, 25 mM $NaHCO_3$, 0.4 mM ascorbic acid, 3 mM myo-inositol, 2 mM pyruvic acid; all chemicals from Sigma–Aldrich, MO) bubbled for at least 15 min with 5% CO_2–95% O_2. Slices were transferred to an incubation chamber containing ACSF (125 mM NaCl, 2.5 mM KCl, 1 mM $MgCl_2$, 2 mM $CaCl_2$, 25 mM glucose, 1.25 mM NaH_2PO_4, 25 mM $NaHCO_3$, 0.4 mM ascorbic acid, 3 mM myo-inositol, 2 mM pyruvic acid; all chemicals from Sigma–Aldrich) and bubbled with 5% CO_2–95% O_2. Slices were incubated for 1 h at 37°C, after which the chamber was brought to room temperature. Recordings were obtained within 4–5 h of slicing.

Whole cell recordings

After incubation, slices were transferred to the recording chamber and continuously perfused with heated and oxygenated ACSF at 2–3 ml/min through a gravity-fed perfusion system. All recordings were performed at 35.5–37°C, controlled by a microcomputer thermometer with a thermo coupling wire that was attached to the 40× water immersion objective (BAT-7001H, Physitemp Instruments, USA). This configuration allowed for measurement of the ACSF temperature within 1–2 mm of the recording site. MNTB neurons were viewed and identified through a Zeiss Axioskop 2 FS plus microscope equipped with Dodt optics and a 40× water-immersion objective (Zeiss, Oberkochen, Germany). Whole cell recordings were performed with an EPC 10 double amplifier (HEKA Instruments, Lambrecht/Pfalz, Germany). Signals were filtered at 5–10 kHz and subsequently digitized at 30–50 kHz using Patchmaster Version 2.40 software (HEKA). Patch pipettes (2.4–3.2 MOhm) were pulled from 1.5-mm borosilicate glass (Harvard Instruments, Kent, UK) using a DMZ Universal Puller (Zeitz Instruments, Munich, Germany) and filled with high-chloride internal solution (130 mM CsCl, 10 mM EGTA, 1 mM $MgCl_2$, 10 mM HEPES, 2 mM ATP, 0.3 mM GTP, 10 mM phosphocreatine, and 1 mM $CaCl_2$, pH adjusted to 7.3 with CsOH 295–300 mOsm; all chemicals from Sigma–Aldrich). The series resistance was compensated to values between 1.8 and 8 MOhm with a lag time of 10 μs.

5 mM QX-314 (Alomone Labs, Jerusalem, Israel) was added to the internal solution to eliminate postsynaptic sodium currents. Glutamatergic currents were blocked by addition of 40 μM DNQX and 50 μM D-AP-V (both from Tocris Bioscience, Bristol, UK) to the ACSF. In some recordings GABAergic currents were blocked by 20 μM SR 95531 (Tocris Bioscience). In other recordings, glycine currents were blocked by 500 nM strychnine (Sigma).

Electrical stimulation of inhibitory inputs

Inhibitory postsynaptic currents (IPSCs) were evoked by electrical stimulation in the vicinity of the MNTB principal neuron via an ACSF-filled glass pipette with tip resistance of 2–3 MOhm. The location and intensity of the stimulus were optimized to obtain the largest IPSCs. Stimuli were 100-μs-long square pulses of 1 to 90 V delivered with an STG 2004 computer-controlled four-channel stimulator (Multi Channel Systems, Reutlingen, Germany) and a stimulation isolation unit (Iso-flex, AMPI, Jerusalem, Israel). IPSCs were analyzed in IGOR Pro 6.21 (WaveMetrics), Clampfit 10.3.0.2 (Molecular Devices, Sunnyvale, CA) and Axograph X (Axograph.com).

RESULTS

GlyT2-GFP TRANSGENIC MICE REVEAL GLYCINERGIC NEURONS IN AUDITORY BRAINSTEM

The main goal of this study was to identify sources of glycinergic inhibition to principal neurons in the MNTB. In GlyT2-GFP mice, somata of glycinergic neurons are GFP+, as are axons in some cases. In auditory brainstem nuclei in a medio-ventral region of a P14 transgenic mouse, neurons of the MNTB, VNTB, LNTB, SPN, as well as a LSO subpopulation, known to be at least partially glycinergic, are GFP+ (Helfert et al., 1989; **Figure 2A**). VNTB and LNTB are recognized on the basis of their GFP expression and the GFP^- gap between them (**Figures 2B,C**).

RETROGRADE TRACER INJECTIONS INTO MNTB REVEAL THE IPSILATERAL VNTB AS A PUTATIVE SOURCE OF GLYCINERGIC INHIBITION TO MNTB

To reveal potential sources of synaptic input to MNTB, we injected retrograde tracers into the MNTB of GlyT2-GFP mice. One known input nucleus is the contralateral AVCN, the home of globular bushy cells whose axons give rise to the calyx of Held(1893; Morest, 1968). As expected, we detected the tracer in globular bushy-like cells (on basis of shape and location; Webster and Trune, 1982; Kuwabara et al., 1991; Smith et al., 1991) of the AVCN (**Figures 3A,B**). To exclude the possibility that the tracer material was located in presynaptic terminals surrounding these somata, we analyzed single confocal sections and substacks consisting of only the center portions of the cell somata. We found red label clearly inside the center somata of neurons and several

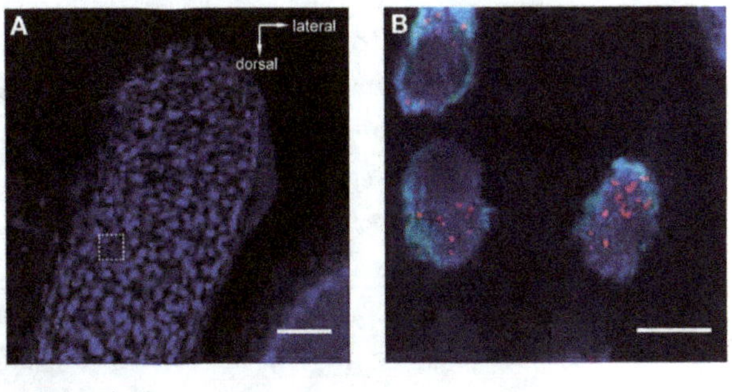

FIGURE 3 | Retrograde tracer injections into MNTB resulted in labeling of neurons in the antero-ventral cochlear nucleus (AVCN). Red = TMR, blue = Nissl. **(A)** Image of AVCN in Nissl only to highlight the globular shapes of cells in the approximate location where globular bushy cells (GCBs) are expected. The dashed square indicates the area from which the magnification in **(B)** was imaged. The image is a maximum projection of a 80 μm stack. **(B)** Maximum projection computed from a sub-stack through the mid-sections of 3 labeled GBCs (spanning a total of 9 μm). Note the punctate labeling of the cell bodies. Scale bar for **(A)**: 100 μm, for **(B)**: 10 μm; 4.6× digital zoom.

micrometers distant from the cell membranes, making it unlikely that it could represent presynaptic terminals surrounding these somata (**Figure 3B**). The results from this control experiment indicate that the tracer injection correctly targeted the MNTB suggesting successful uptake and transport to source neurons.

More importantly, we also found somata in the ipsilateral VNTB that were labeled in a similar fashion as the globular bushy cells described above (**Figure 4**). This CTB injection into the medial portion of the MNTB (**Figure 4A**) resulted in retrograde label in the VNTB, ipsilateral to the injection site (**Figures 4B–E**). These results raise the possibility that VNTB neurons send synaptic inputs to the ipsilateral MNTB, and that these inputs are glycinergic.

For all injections, we verified qualitatively the accuracy of the injection. In addition, for 7/18 cases, we performed quantitative analysis of the extent of the injection for the robust, dense labeling provided by TMR injections (**Figures 5A,B**; see Methods). The high concentration of dye and associated high levels of fluorescence makes it difficult to determine labeled presynaptic terminals in the area of the injection (but see Wang et al., 2014). Further, since intrinsic collaterals within the MNTB may exist (Guinan and Li, 1990; Kuwabara and Zook, 1991), it was not possible to distinguish between MNTB principal cells that took up the dye as a result of a "direct hit" vs. retrograde dye transport from labeled terminals to cell somata of other principal neurons. Therefore, the quantitative analysis of injection sites refers to the *apparent* injection, not the *effective* injection.

MNTB extends longitudinally along the rostro-caudal axis and thus, no single injection could evenly label tissue along this entire axis. Not surprisingly, the extent of the *apparent* tracer injection varied between 3 and 65% (average 13.8 ± 8.6%). However, when only a single section at which the tracer injection was centered was

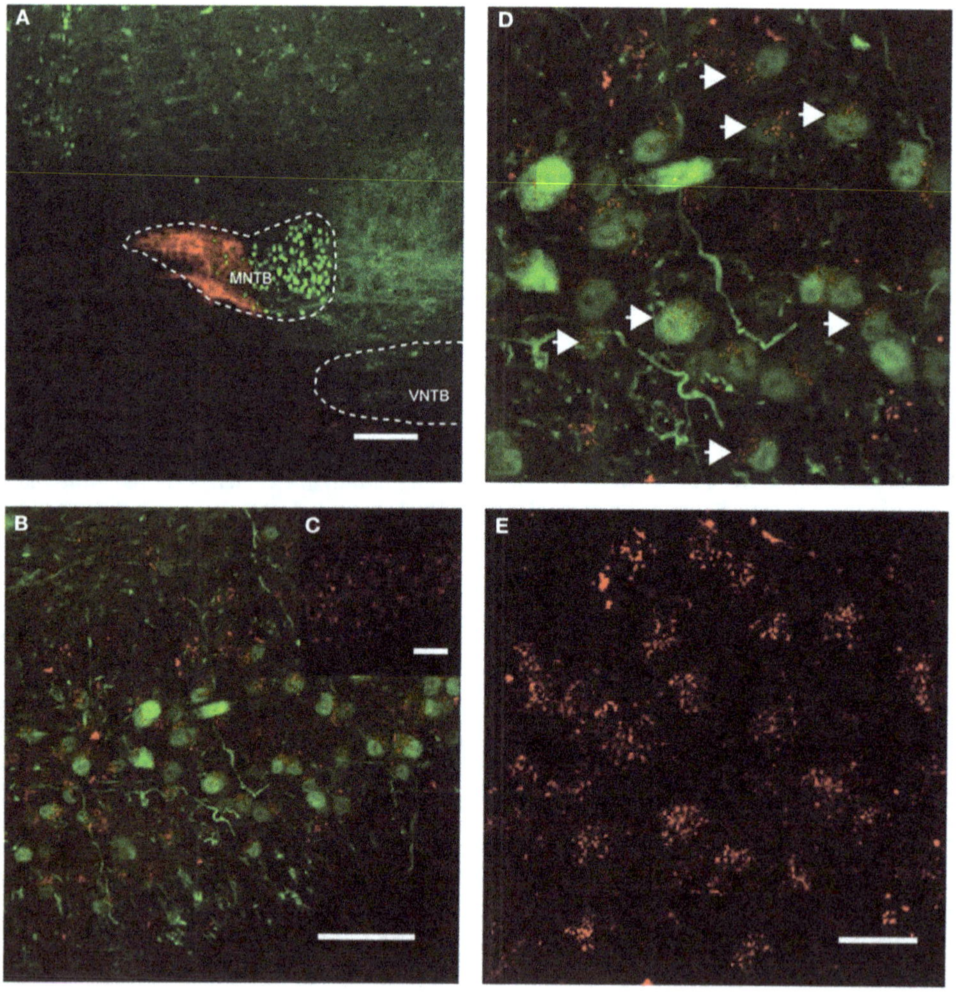

FIGURE 4 | Retrograde labeling of MNTB resulted in labeling of glycinergic neurons in the ipsilateral VNTB. The image is from a case in which CTB was injected into the MNTB of a p88 GlyT2-GFP mouse. Glycinergic neurons expressing GFP are shown in green, the tracer is shown in red. **(A)** Shows the site of injection targeting mostly the medial half of the MNTB. **(B)** Depicts the resulting label in the ipsilateral VNTB [the inset **(C)** shows the red channel for this image only]. **(D)** Is a magnification of a portion of the image shown in **(B)**, with **(E)** showing the corresponding red channel only. The white arrows in **(D)** highlight double-labeled neurons. Images are maximum projections of confocal stacks (image depth: 60 μm). Scale bar for **(A)**: 200 μm, **(B,C)**: 50 μm, for **(D,E)**: 20 μm.

analyzed, the tracer injection varied between 8 and 100% of the MNTB surface area of that section (average = 27 ± 13%). In a case where 99% of the MNTB area was injected (**Figure 5A**), a majority of neurons in the ipsilateral VNTB were labeled with the tracer substance (white arrows, **Figure 5C**).

The number of retrogradely labeled neurons in VNTB varied with the extent of the tracer injections into MNTB (**Figures 5C–E**). Overall, larger injection volumes yielded more labeled neurons in the ipsilateral VNTB.

ANTEROGRADE TRACER INJECTIONS INTO VNTB REVEAL LABELED PRESYNAPTIC TERMINALS IN THE IPSILATERAL MNTB

The results from the retrograde injections with two different dyes (CTB and TMR) presented so far suggest that glycinergic VNTB neurons might send projections to the ipsilateral MNTB. To further substantiate this concept, we performed anterograde tracer injections into the VNTB. Anterograde tracer is taken up by postsynaptic neurons and labels their axons and presynaptic terminals. In our particular case, anterograde injections into the VNTB would be expected to label glycinergic presynaptic terminals synapsing onto MNTB principal neurons.

The anterograde injections were performed into brainstem explants, similar to the retrograde injections, with two differences (**Figure 6A**): (1) The brain stem explant was cut differently and injected differently, and (2) blocks of tissue were cut into thicker sections and "cleared" before imaging (Clear^{T2} after Kuwajima et al., 2013). Clearing involves incubating the brain section in a solution that has a similar refractory index as the myelin to make it optically transparent. In cleared material, we were able to follow single projections from VNTB neurons to MNTB (**Figure 6A**). The injection site of the anterograde tracer is evident (bright saturated red spot, **Figure 6A**), as well as labeling in the ventral

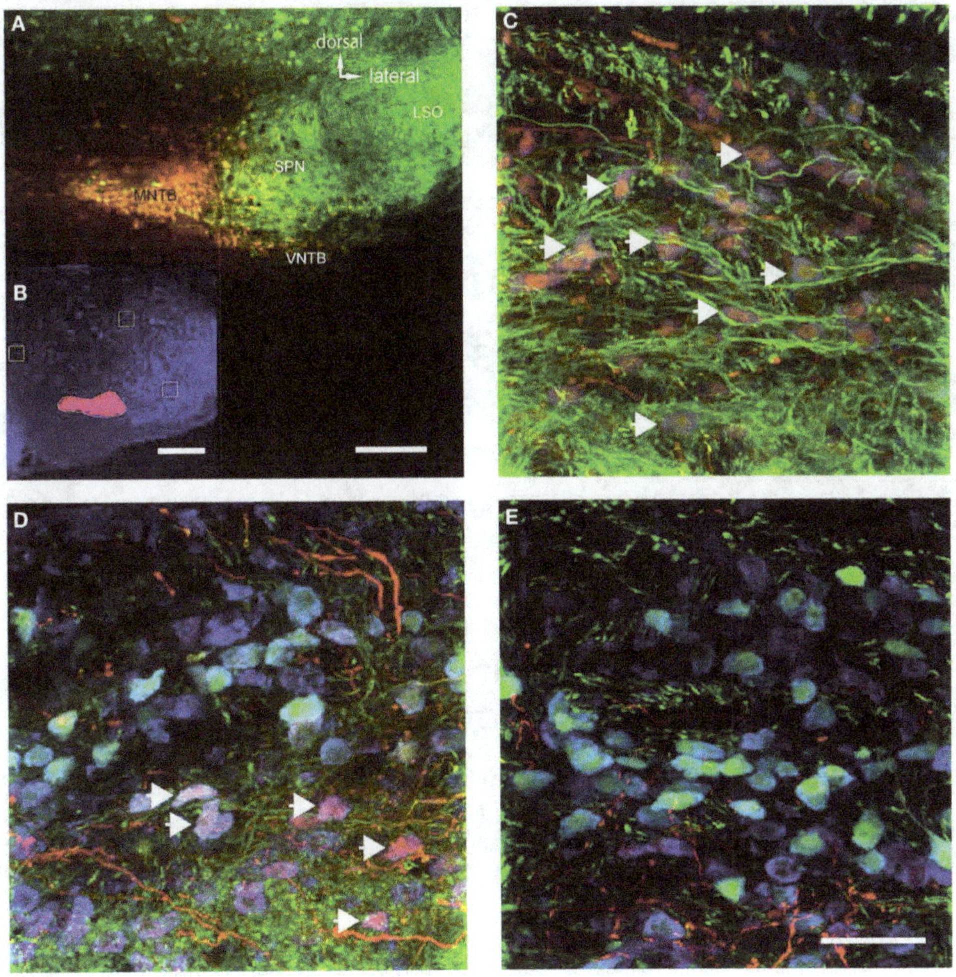

FIGURE 5 | The volume of TMR-injections into MNTB correlates with the number of labeled VNTB neurons. (A) A brain stem image showing a TMR-injected (red) MNTB. **(B)** The result of a semi-automatic analysis of the same injection with our custom-built MATLAB algorithm, illustrating the method of quantifying the apparent extent of the tracer injection. **(C)** Shows a section of VNTB from a brain where the tracer injection into the ipsilateral MNTB was extensive (65% of MNTB volume). **(D)** represents a section of VNTB from a brain where the tracer injection into the ipsilateral MNTB was moderate (5.5% of MNTB volume). **(E)** Represents a section of VNTB from a brain where the tracer injection into the ipsilateral MNTB was minimal (1.5% of MNTB volume). **(A,C–E)** are maximum projections of confocal stacks (image depth: 80 μm), **(B)** is based on an epifluorescence microscopy image taken at low magnification (10×). Scale bar for **(A)**: 200 μm, for **(B)**: 500 μm and **(C–E)**: 50 μm.

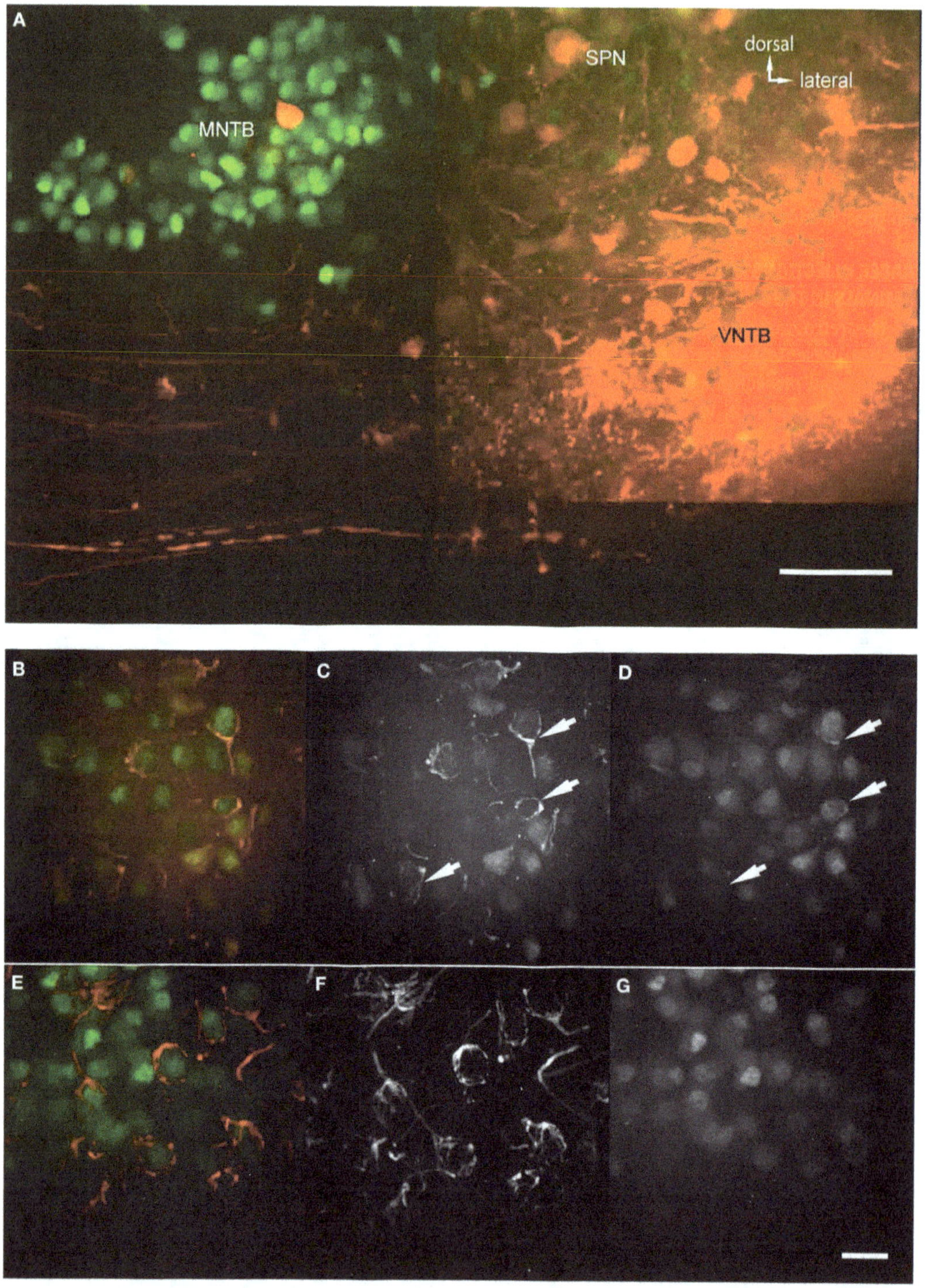

FIGURE 6 | Anterograde injections into VNTB reveal connections to MNTB neurons. (A) Brain stem section of a case where TMR was injected into the VNTB of a p14 GlyT2-GFP mouse. The image shows the injection site within the VNTB, as well as the ipsilateral MNTB. A number of axons projects from the injection area to the ipsilateral MNTB and appears to terminate there. The image consists of a total of 4 tiled confocal stacks; the image depth of the original stack was 300 μm. Before imaging, the section was cleared using the Clear^{T2}-protocol. **(B–D)** magnifications from the ipsilateral MNTB of a p14 brain that was cleared with the technique, showing a variety of labeled presynaptic elements. **(B)** Represents the overlay of both channels (red: TMR, green: GlyT2-GFP), **(C)** shows the red and **(D)** the green channel only. Double-labeled structures are highlighted with white arrows. **(E–G)** Since the majority of axons from AVCN to MNTB (innervating the calyces of Held) are passing through the injection area in the VNTB, typically some labeling of calyces of Held in the contralateral MNTB was observed as well. These were used as a control to compare to the labeled inhibitory endings in the ipsilateral MNTB. Note the structural differences between synapses labeled on the ipsilateral **(B–D)** and the contralateral side **(E–G)**, and the fact that at least some of the tracer-labeled ipsilateral structures are co-labeled with GFP, while the contralateral ones are not. Scale bar for **(A)**: 100 μm, for **(B–G)**: 50 μm.

acoustic stria where a number of fiber bundles run through the VNTB. Importantly, the injection resulted in labeling projections from VNTB to MNTB, as well as associated glycinergic presynaptic terminals surrounding *ipsilateral* MNTB principal neurons (**Figures 6B–D**). Since the area of the VNTB also contains fibers of the acoustic stria which run e.g., from the cochlear nucleus to the contralateral MNTB, some of these passing fibers were also labeled by the injection (**Figures 6E–G**). In the *contralateral* MNTB, calyces of Held are innervated by labeled fibers passing through the contralateral VNTB. Even though some inhibitory inputs appear to look somewhat like calyces (e.g., **Figure 6B**), calyces of Held branch much more extensively and surround MNTB postsynaptic neurons more completely (**Figures 6E,F**). More importantly, at least some of the *ipsilaterally* tracer-labeled presynaptic elements are GFP+ (**Figures 6B–D**), suggesting that these ipsilaterally labeled structures are of glycinergic nature. By contrast, the *contralaterally* labeled calyces of Held are *not GFP+* (**Figures 6F,G**), suggesting that these contralaterally labeled structures are *not* of glycinergic nature.

Figure 7 shows magnified examples of inputs to MNTB cells that arise from contralateral vs. ipsilateral nuclei which have significant structural differences. Firstly, the ipsilaterally labeled inputs branch much less than the contralaterally labeled inputs (**Figure 7A** vs. **Figure 7C**). Secondly, the ipsilaterally labeled structures are glycinergic while the contralaterally labeled structures are not (**Figure 7B** vs. **Figure 7D**). In total, we performed anterograde injections into 18 brainstem explants, and found labeled presynaptic terminals in ipsilateral MNTB in each case.

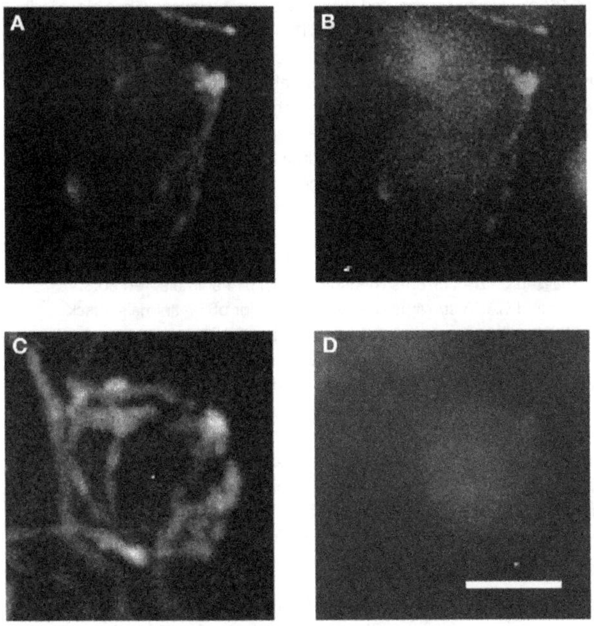

FIGURE 7 | Two magnified MNTB principal cells and their TMR-traced inputs. (A,B) are showing a cell located ipsilaterally to the injected VNTB, **(C,D)** a contralateral one. Note the structural differences between the two input types and the fact that the ipsilateral terminal can be seen in the green channel (coding for GlyT2-GFP). Scale bar: 25 μm.

IMMUNOHISTOCHEMICAL LABELING AGAINST GlyT2 REVEALED SIMILARLY SHAPED PRESYNAPTIC TERMINALS IN MNTB

Interestingly, the presynaptic terminals shown in **Figures 6B–D** suggest that several presynptic boutons may be innervated by the same fiber, which runs along the target neuron and makes several connections. While this finding is consistent with physiological results (Florian Mayer, unpublished data), we wanted to further interrogate this innervation pattern with immunohistochemistry against neuronal glycine transporter 2 (GlyT2). Thus, if the putative presynaptic terminals shown in **Figures 6B,C** are indeed presynaptic terminals and not simply axons or dendrites of glycinergic neurons, they should express GlyT2 protein.

We performed immunohistochemistry against GlyT2 protein in 5 brains obtained from both GlyT2-GFP negative (= wild type) and GlyT2-GFP mice (2 wild type and 3 GlyT2-GFP mice; data for wild type mice not shown). The distribution of GlyT2 protein in the boutons near MNTB principal neurons suggests that these boutons are indeed presynaptic terminals (**Figure 8**). The dense and complex structure of many of these terminals (**Figures 8A,D**) is reminiscent of the presynaptic elements labeled in our anterograde injections (**Figures 6B,C**), further supporting the notion that these structures might be glycinergic presynaptic terminals, several of which are innervated by the same fiber.

PARALLEL DEVELOPMENTAL CHANGES FROM GABA TO GLYCINE IN MNTB AND VNTB

Inhibitory inputs to MNTB undergo developmental changes. During early postnatal ages, inhibitory inputs to MNTB have both a GABAergic component and a glycinergic component. During postnatal development, the GABAergic contribution gets progressively smaller such that during later developmental stages, the inhibition to MNTB neurons is almost exclusively glycinergic. We assessed the sizes of the GABAergic and glycinergic components by using pharmacological blockers (**Figure 9**). From the amplitudes of the mixed and purely GABAergic/glycinergic currents, ratios were calculated. **Figure 9C** shows ratios of GABAergic and glycinergic currents at p14 (left group of data points, $n = 5$), and p55+ (right group of data points, $n = 4$), suggesting that at the younger age, 24% of the total inhibitory current is GABAergic. By age p55+, the contribution of GABA has dropped to 6%.

The data from the tracer injections shown above suggest that inhibitory projections from VNTB to MNTB may represent a major source of inhibition to MNTB. If that is the case, but inhibitory inputs to MNTB undergo a developmental change during which the contribution of GABA to the total inhibition decreases (**Figure 9**), one might postulate that VNTB neurons undergo a developmental switch from GABA to glycine that mirrors the switch observed at their target neurons in the MNTB. We addressed this question with immunohistochemical labeling against glutamic acid decarboxylase isoform 67 (GAD67) in both p14 mice and in p50+ mice (**Figure 10**). GAD67 protein catalyzes the decarboxylation of glutamate to GABA and CO_2 and thus is a marker of GABAergic neurons. In the younger age group, substantial amounts of GAD67 labeling can be observed within VNTB principal neurons (**Figures 10A–C**), while in the older age

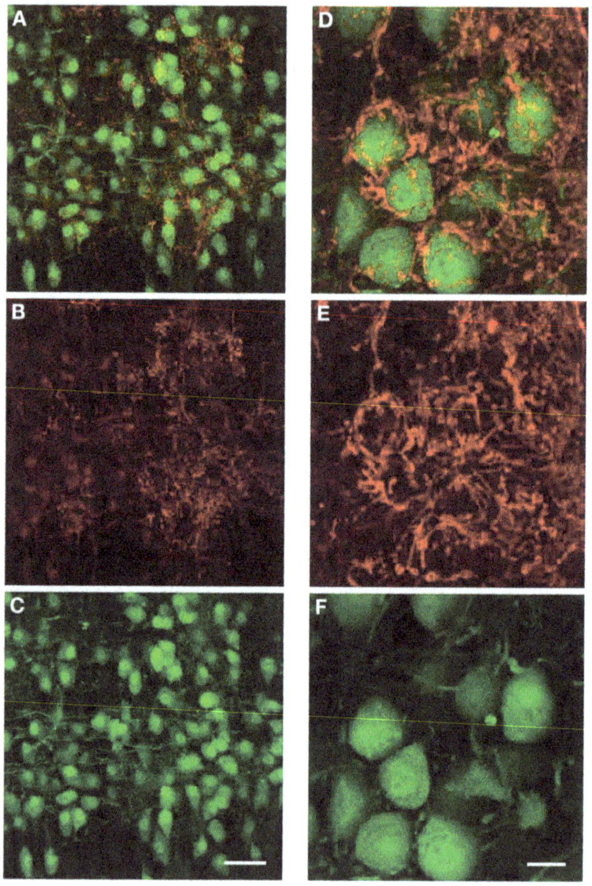

FIGURE 8 | Immunohistochemical labeling against GlyT2 protein reveals complex inhibitory synaptic structures surrounding MNTB principal neurons. All images are maximum projections of a confocal stack [image depth for **(A–C)**: 40 μm, for **(D–F)**: 20 μm]. The overlay of both channels is displayed in **(A)**. The antibody labeling against GlyT2 is shown in red **(B)** and the GFP-expression under the GlyT2-promoter in green **(C)**. Note that many of the presynaptic terminals labeled by the GlyT2 antibody are highly complex in their structure, and similar to the inhibitory synaptic inputs labeled with the anterograde TMR-injections into the ipsilateral VNTB shown in **Figures 6B–D**. **(D–F)**: Higher magnification image (3× digital zoom) taken in the MNTB of a different GlyT2-GFP mouse. Scale bar for **(A–C)**: 50 μm, for **(D–F)**: 10 μm. The age of the animal was p59.

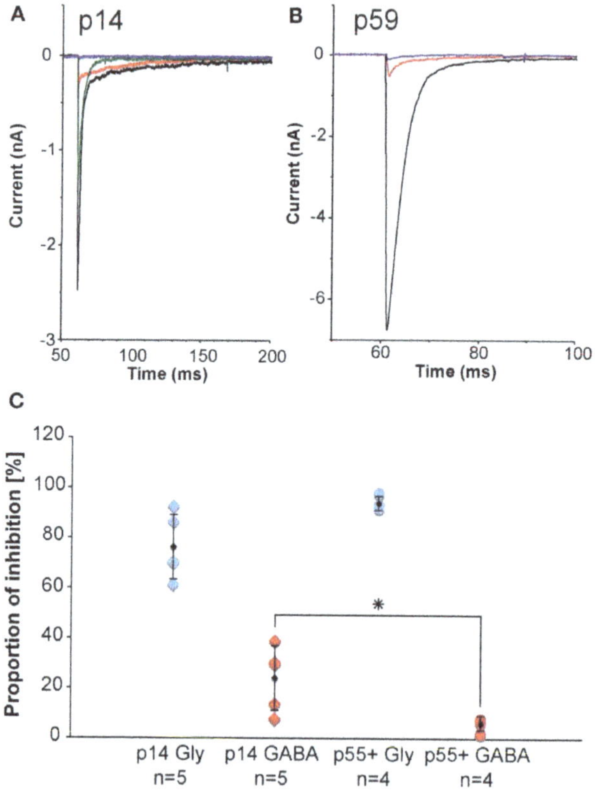

FIGURE 9 | *In-vitro* electrophysiology in the mouse reveals that the GABAergic contribution to the total inhibition at MNTB principal neurons declines with age. (A,B) are representative examples of pharmacologically isolated inhibitory currents observed in a p14 **(A)** and a p59 **(B)** mouse and measured while inhibitory synapses were electrically stimulated in the vicinity of the MNTB principal neuron. The black trace is the total inhibitory current following electrical stimulation, the red trace shows the residual GABAergic current after blocking the glycine component with strychnine, the blue trace is the complete block after an additional wash-in of SR-95531 (gabazine). The green trace shows a partial recovery after a successful washout of both drugs. **(C)** Normalized current amplitudes for glycine currents suggest a developmental decline of the GABAergic contribution to the total inhibition. Blue diamonds: normalized glycinergic currents measured from p14 animals; blue dots: normalized glycinergic currents measured from p55+ animals; red diamonds: normalized GABA currents measured from p14 animals; red dots: normalized GABA currents measured from for p55+ animals; black symbols: averages with error bars (SD). The GABA component declines significantly with age from almost 25% of total inhibitory current at postnatal day 14 down to about 6% in adult animals, whereas the glycine component does not experience statistically significant changes. All excitatory currents were blocked during these experiments with the glutamate receptor blockers DNQX and AP-V. All recordings were done near physiological temperature (35–37°C), which significantly speeds up channel kinetics (Leao et al., 2005). *The *p*-value is 0.032 (t-test).

group, much less label can be observed within the postsynaptic neurons (**Figures 10D–F**). Note that in both age groups there appears to be some small punctate GAD67 label outside of principal neurons. It is unclear whether these structures represent GABAergic synapses or other structures. However and importantly, GAD67 label inside the VNTB principal cells is highly reduced in the older age group.

To quantify this reduction, we performed Li's intensity correlation analysis to assess the extent of colocalization (Li et al., 2004) between the GFP signal and GAD immunoreactivity ($n =$ 11 of GlyT2-GFP brains). This intensity correlation analysis revealed a significant degree of colocalization at p14. However, at p50+, we calculated overall lower ICQ values between the GFP and GAD signals (see representative examples in **Figures 11A–D** and ICQ averages in **Figure 11E**). These results, together with the physiological recordings from MNTB principal neurons (**Figure 9**) suggest a parallel developmental switch from GABA to glycine in VNTB principal neurons (from which inhibitory inputs to MNTB originate) and inhibitory inputs to MNTB (where projections from VNTB terminate), providing further evidence for the idea that VNTB is a major source of inhibitory inputs to MNTB.

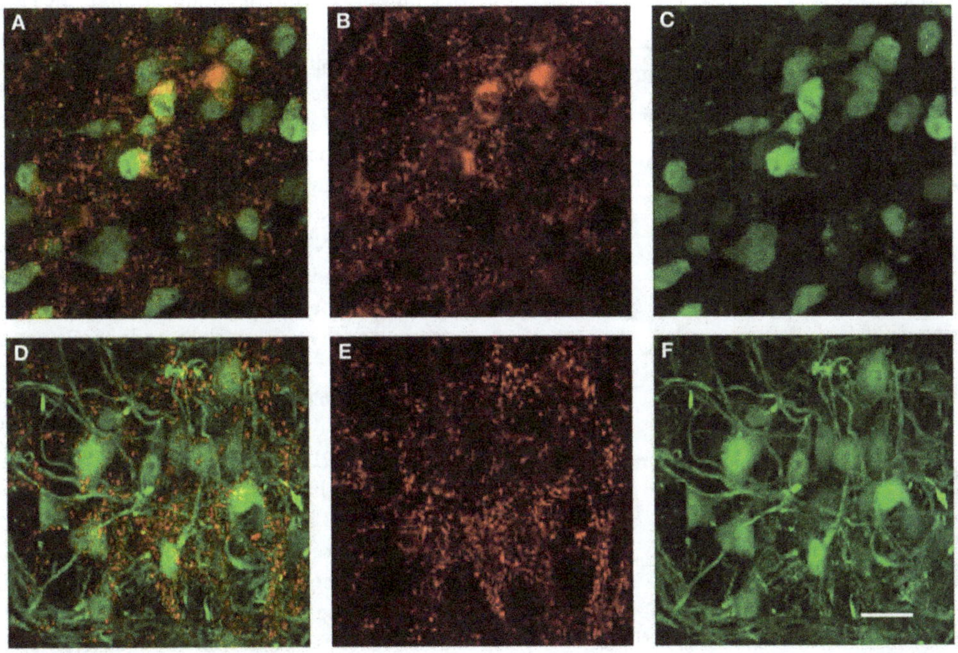

FIGURE 10 | Examples of immunohistochemical label against GAD67 in the VNTB of GlyT2-GFP mice. (A–C) show a representative anti-GAD67 labeling pattern in the VNTB of a p14 mouse, with **(A)** being the overlay of both channels, **(B)** the antibody labeling in red and **(C)** the GlyT2-GFP expression in green. Images shown in **(D–F)** show the same labeling in an adult animal aged p70 (color coding is the same as in **(A–C)**]. Note that at p14, many glycinergic neurons are co-labeled with GAD67, while almost none of the glycinergic neurons seen at the older age are co-labeled against GAD67. All images are maximum projections of confocal stacks. Scale bar: 20 μm.

DISCUSSION

The main conclusion from our study is that MNTB neurons in the mouse receive prominent glycinergic inputs from neurons in the VNTB. These neurons send projections to MNTB, which end in several synaptic boutons located on the somata of MNTB principal neurons. This conclusion is supported by several lines of evidence: retrograde tracer injections into MNTB label the somata of VNTB neurons intracellularly, anterograde tracer injections into VNTB label presynaptic glycinergic boutons on MNTB principal neurons, and the developmental switch of VNTB neurons from mixed GABAergic/glycinergic to almost exclusively glycinergic is matched by a parallel developmental switch of incoming inhibition to MNTB neurons from mixed GABAergic/glycinergic to almost exclusively glycinergic.

The method of injecting brain stem explants with tracer in a dish and subsequently incubating the tissue for a few hours *in-vitro* (Burger et al., 2005; Ford et al., 2009) greatly facilitated this study. Since both MNTB and VNTB are very close to the ventral surface of the brain stem, and are almost "surface structures" from a ventral view, tracer injections could be performed with great accuracy under visual guidance. Cell death during the relatively brief incubation time was very limited. The method of clearing brain tissue with the Clear^{T2} method (Kuwajima et al., 2013) worked relatively well in auditory brain stem sections, especially in those from younger animals. Fibers in the auditory brain stem myelinate extensively (Ryugo et al., 2006), which greatly impairs imaging quality both for physiological and anatomical studies. The brain clearing allowed us to prepare relatively thick sections of 200–500 micrometers, in which intact connections between VNTB and MNTB could be visualized. Nevertheless, in highly myelinated adult brain stem, this technique resulted in only incomplete clearing.

The results from the retrograde tracing studies alone, though conducted with two different tracers (CTB and TMR) would not be sufficient to demonstrate inhibitory connections between VNTB and MNTB because the VNTB also projects to *contralateral* SOC nuclei, such as the LSO (Spangler et al., 1985; Warr and Beck, 1996), the LNTB and DLPO (Warr and Beck, 1996; Thompson and Schofield, 2000), with associated fibers running close to or even through the ipsilateral MNTB. We therefore also performed anterograde injections into the VNTB, combined with subsequent brain clearing. In these experiments we were able to observe direct axonal connections running from VNTB to MNTB, as well as labeled presynaptic terminals within the MNTB. Though we cannot completely exclude the possibility of labeling potential *ipsilaterally* projecting calyces and/or collaterals of calyceal inputs that project to VNTB (Kuwabara et al., 1991), we think this possibility is unlikely for two reasons: First, a comparison to contralaterally labeled calyces of Held in the same brain slices revealed that the morphology of true calyces of Held is significantly different from the morphology of the putative inhibitory inputs. Second, contralaterally labeled calyces did not co-label for the GlyT2-GFP marker, but ipsilaterally labeled putative inhibitory inputs did. Although our data present evidence for a glycinergic projection from VNTB to MNTB, we cannot rule out other potential sources of inhibition to MNTB. Especially, intrinsic

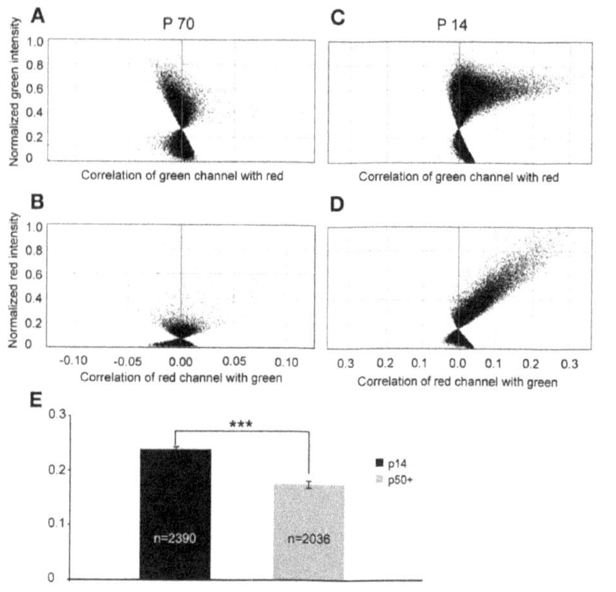

FIGURE 11 | Intrasomatic labeling against GAD67 in glycinergic VNTB neurons declines with age. (A–D) show pixel data from two single glycinergic VNTB neurons. Single glycinergic VNTB neurons were selected in a region of interest and analyzed for co-localization of signals in both channels. **(A,B)** display the normalized intensity correlation values of pixels in a p70 animal for the green and the red channel, respectively. Most of the values do not exceed the intensity correlation quotient (ICQ) range of −0.05 to 0.05 and are mostly distributed around the midline, indicating a largely uncorrelated or random distribution of overlapping green and red pixels (the resulting total ICQ was −0.001 in this case). By contrast, **(C,D)** show a strongly positive correlation of signals in the green and the red channels, respectively (with a resulting total ICQ value of 0.38 for this specific neuron). **(E)** Averaged total ICQ values for 2390 glycinergic VNTB neurons in p14 animals (black) and 2036 glycinergic VNTB neurons in p50+ (p59–70; gray) animals, respectively. $^{***}p < 0.001$ (Mann-Whitney rank-sum test).

connections within MNTB have been previously suggested as a second source of inhibition to MNTB neurons (Guinan and Li, 1990; Kuwabara and Zook, 1991). Our data does not address this possibility.

There are several pitfalls when using tracer injections to study connections between different brain nuclei. One of them is the difference between the *apparent* and the *effective* size of an injection site. One proven method to determine the effective size of an injection area consists of counting labeled neurons at the site of injection (e.g., Wang et al., 2014). There are several reasons, why we did not use this method in our study, and restricted ourselves to delineating only the *apparent* site of injection in the MNTB. Firstly, in our experiments the differences between the apparent and the effective sites of injection were presumably relatively small due to the fact that the brain stem explants were kept alive for relatively short amounts of time (1–4 h). In contrast, fluorescent dextran-based tracer labeling fades over days and weeks (Novikova et al., 1997; also see Köbbert et al., 2000 for a detailed review and comparison of neuroanatomical tracing techniques). More importantly, since TMR served as a *retrograde* tracer, the most accurate method to determine the effective size of injection would be counting the inhibitory synaptic inputs around MNTB cells. Determining labeled presynaptic terminals in the immensely bright area of the injection site proved to be impossible. Alternatively, assessing the effective injection site by labeled *post*synaptic cells would be less accurate because presynaptic terminals take up dye with different mechanisms as postsynaptic neurons do, resulting in inaccurate quantifications of the effective injection site. Moreover, a number of studies suggested intrinsic inhibitory connections within the MNTB (Guinan and Li, 1990; Kuwabara and Zook, 1991), making it impossible to distinguish between a postsynaptic neuron labeled by a "direct hit" and one that was labeled intrasomatically due to retrograde transport through recurrent collaterals.

Another potential pitfall to consider would include retrograde labeling of MNTB neurons projecting to VNTB (Kuwabara and Zook, 1991). If this was the case, observed label within the MNTB would have resulted from inhibitory terminals formed by (other) MNTB neurons that took up tracer material retrogradely through an axonal branch extending to VNTB, and subsequently transported the material from there to a collateral projecting to neighboring MNTB neurons. We think this possibility is unlikely because of the intensity differences of the fluorescent label between the labeled terminals surrounding MNTB cells and retrogradely labeled MNTB cell somata. While we could observe a subset of MNTB cells that were labeled retrogradely, their staining intensities were in most cases much lower than the staining intensities of the labeled inhibitory terminals surrounding principal cells.

GlyT2 has been shown to be a reliable marker of glycinergic neurons (Poyatos et al., 1997; Zeilhofer et al., 2005). Moreover, the GFP-expression pattern seen in the SOC of the GlyT2-GFP mouse line used here is consistent with observations made by Zeilhofer et al. (2005), as well as immunohistochemical and tracing studies from other investigators in different rodent species (MNTB, LNTB, MVPO/VNTB: Peyret et al., 1987; Helfert et al., 1989; SPN: Helfert et al., 1989; Saint Marie and Baker, 1990). Thus, the GFP expression in this mouse line is specific and reliably shows the (sub)populations of glycinergic cells in the auditory brainstem nuclei despite some variability in the *level* of GFP-expression between different nuclei and individual animals.

The nomenclature and the outlines of some auditory brainstem nuclei in rodents, especially the periolivary nuclei have been somewhat inconsistent. In the VNTB literature, at least six different names in three closely related rodent species (mouse, rat, and deermouse) have been used to describe the heterogeneous group of cells located ventrolaterally to the location of MNTB: VNTB appears to be the most commonly used term (see Thompson and Schofield, 2000 for a review). Other terms include IPN (internal parolivary nucleus in the deermouse; Ross, 1962) MPVO (medial preolivary nucleus in the deermouse, Ross, 1969), MVPO (e.g., Paxinos and Franklin Mouse Brain Atlas), VTN (ventral trapezoid nucleus in the rat; e.g., Brown and Howlett, 1972; see Ollo and Schwartz, 1979 for a review). Other investigators have subdivided the nucleus into VNTB and RPO (rostral periolivary region), based on morphology and basic electrophysiology in the rat (Robertson, 1996).

Whereas our study did not attempt to resolve these questions or define the outlines of the VNTB *in its entirety*, we did define the glycinergic subpopulation of VNTB principal cells that are GFP+ in the transgenic mouse line. We found that it closely matches the outlines defined by other authors who previously studied the anatomy of the mouse SOC more intensely (see Ollo and Schwartz, 1979; Franklin and Paxinos, 2008). Based on the patterns of GFP-expression and the morphology of GFP-positive, i.e., glycinergic cells, we were able to distinguish between the VNTB and other neighboring periolivary regions like the SPN and the LNTB with relative ease.

While connections between MNTB and VNTB have been suggested before (Kuwabara et al., 1991; Thompson and Schofield, 2000), the extent and the glycinergic nature of these projections have not been shown. VNTB contains several neuronal types, some of which are glycinergic (Helfert et al., 1989), while others are cholinergic or GABAergic (Helfert et al., 1989; Yao and Godfrey, 1998; Gómez-Nieto et al., 2008). We focused on the glycinergic subpopulation, because previous studies suggested that inhibitory inputs to MNTB principal cells are largely glycinergic (at least in the adult rodent; Awatramani et al., 2005). Moreover, glycinergic inhibition from VNTB and LNTB might play important roles in sound localization processing. For example, Roberts et al. (2013) showed that inhibition to the MSO (which originates from MNTB and LNTB; Thompson and Schofield, 2000) can arrive even *before* the excitation. This study and others are contributing to the idea that inhibition is playing a crucial, yet still not completely understood role in the auditory brain stem.

Lastly, Warr and Beck (1996) looked specifically at efferents of the VNTB and suggested that a projection from VNTB to MNTB "...does not appear to exist, at least in the rat, for VNTB neurons situated some distance away from the MNTB..." Our results are inconsistent with those findings from the rat, but support the findings of Kuwabara et al. (1991) in two other rodent species, the gerbil and the mouse, hinting at possible species-related differences in the intrinsic projection patterns within the SOC. Unfortunately, our anterograde injections into the VNTB could not discriminate between potential differences in the projection pattern between the medial and the lateral subpopulations of glycinergic VNTB neurons, which should be addressed in future studies (e.g., by using two different tracer colors for injections into the medial and the lateral portions of the VNTB).

Our data also confirm the idea that inhibitory inputs to MNTB are of auditory brainstem nature. This has been hypothesized by previous *in-vitro* studies due to the large synaptic amplitudes and fast decays produced by inhibitory synapses (Awatramani et al., 2004), as well as their ability to follow prolonged trains of ongoing stimulation. Although the amplitudes of the inhibitory currents do decrease with prolonged stimulation, the same has been shown by Hermann et al. (2007) for the excitation. Pharmacological manipulations performed *in-vivo*, however, have already seen evidence of the auditory nature of inhibitory inputs to MNTB neurons (Green and Sanes, 2005; Kopp-Scheinpflug et al., 2008; Tolnai et al., 2008). Since VNTB neurons receive excitatory input directly from the ventral cochlear nucleus on the contralateral side (Warr, 1972) their firing pattern most likely codes for relatively unprocessed auditory information, such as simple activity patterns and standard tuning curves.

We observed a developmental decrease in the contribution of GABA to the total inhibition innervating MNTB, as well as a parallel developmental decrease in GAD67 signal in glycinergic VNTB principal neurons. While the latter observation is novel, the first one is not. A similar decrease in the GABAergic contribution to total inhibition at MNTB neurons has been observed previously in the rat (Awatramani et al., 2005), suggesting that this decrease is a general mammalian phenomenon.

Both the anterograde tracer injections into VNTB and the GlyT2 immunolabels in MNTB revealed afferent fibers branching and terminating in several large synaptic boutons along MNTB principal cell somata. This innervation pattern suggests first of all that relatively few inhibitory synapses terminate on MNTB neurons and second of all that these boutons are connected to even fewer fibers. This result is consistent with our recent physiological data in which glycinergic input fibers were electrically stimulated in the vicinity of MNTB neurons in brain slices (Mayer et al., under review).

In summary, our data combining retrograde and anterograde tracing techniques, as well as demonstrating a simultaneous switch from GABA/glycine to mostly glycine in both the synaptic inputs to MNTB and the somata of glycinergic cells located in the VNTB, present a cumulative body of evidence suggesting that the glycinergic subset of VNTB neurons sends axonal connections to the MNTB, making the VNTB at least one major source of inhibition projecting to MNTB.

ACKNOWLEDGMENTS

Supported by NIH/NIDCD R01 DC 011582, the Rocky Mountain Neurological Disorders Core Center Grant NIH P30 NS048154, and the Rocky Mountain Taste and Smell Center Imaging Core Grant P30 DC004657. Imaging experiments were also performed in the University of Colorado Anschutz Medical Campus Advanced Light Microscopy Core supported in part by NIH/NCRR Colorado CTSI Grant Number UL1 RR025780. We would like to thank Dr. Tom Finger for many helpful discussions, and sharing his expertise in neuroanatomical tracing and immunohistochemical techniques. We would also like to thank Dr. Angie Ribera for critically reading a draft version of this manuscript and for providing helpful suggestions for improvements. Dr. Sascha du Lac from the Salk Institute provided us with the GlyT2-GFP mice.

REFERENCES

Awatramani, G., Turecek, R., and Trussell, L. (2004). Inhibitory control at a synaptic relay. *J. Neurosci.* 24, 2643–2647. doi: 10.1523/JNEUROSCI.5144-03.2004

Awatramani, G., Turecek, R., and Trussell, L. (2005). Staggered development of GABAergic and glycinergic transmission in the MNTB. *J. Neurophysiol.* 93, 819–828. doi: 10.1152/jn.00798.2004

Banks, M., and Smith, P. (1992). Intracellular recordings from neurobiotinlabeled cells in brain slices of the rat medial nucleus of the trapezoid body. *J. Neurosci.* 12, 2819–2837.

Borst, J. G. G., and van Hoeve, J. S. (2012). The calyx of Held synapse: From model synapse to auditory relay. *Annu. Rev. Physiol.* 74, 199–224. doi: 10.1146/annurev-physiol-020911-153236

Brown, J. C., and Howlett, B. (1972). The olivo-cochlear tract in the rat and its bearing on the homologies of some constituent cell groups of the mammalian superior olivary complex: a thiocholine study. *Acta Anat. (Basel)* 83, 505–526. doi: 10.1159/000143889

Burger, R. M., Cramer, K. S., Pfeiffer, J. D., and Rubel, E. W. (2005). Avian superior olivary nucleus provides divergent inhibitory input to parallel auditory pathways. *J. Comp. Neurol.* 481, 6–18. doi: 10.1002/cne.20334

Conte, W. L., Kamishina, H., Corvin, J. V., and Reep, R. L. (2008). Topography in the projections of lateral posterior thalamus with cingulate and medial agranular cortex in relation to circuitry for directed attention and neglect. *Brain Res.* 1240, 87–95. doi: 10.1016/j.brainres.2008.09.013

Conte, W. L., Kamishina, H., and Reep, R. L. (2009). Multiple neuroanatomical tract-tracing using fluorescent Alexa Fluor conjugates of cholera toxin subunit B in rats. *Nat. Protoc.* 4, 1157–1166. doi: 10.1038/nprot.2009.93

Dufour, A., Tell, F., Kessler, J. P., and Baude, A. (2010). Mixed GABA-glycine synapses delineate a specific topography in the nucleus tractus solitarii of adult rat. *J. Physiol.* 588, 1097–1115. doi: 10.1113/jphysiol.2009.184838

Ford, M. C., Grothe, B., and Klug, A. (2009). Fenestration of the calyx of Held occurs sequentially along the tonotopic axis, is influenced by afferent activity, and facilitates glutamate clearance. *J. Comp. Neurol.* 514, 92–106. doi: 10.1002/cne.21998

Forsythe, I. (1994). Direct patch recording from identified presynaptic terminals mediating glutamatergic EPSCs in the rat CNS, *in vitro*. *J. Physiol.* 479, 381–387.

Franklin, K. B. J., and Paxinos, G. (2008). *The Mouse Brain in Stereotaxic Coordinates. 3rd Edn.* New York, NY: Elsevier/Academic Press.

Gómez-Nieto, R., Rubio, M. E., and Lopez, D. E. (2008). Cholinergic input from the ventral nucleus of the trapezoid body to cochlear root neurons in rats. *J. Comp. Neurol.* 506, 452–468. doi: 10.1002/cne.21554

Green, J. S., and Sanes, D. H. (2005). Early appearance of inhibitory input to the MNTB supports binaural processing during development. *J. Neurophysiol.* 94, 3826–3835. doi: 10.1152/jn.00601.2005

Guinan, J. J. Jr., and Li, R. Y. (1990). Signal processing in brainstem auditory neurons which receive giant endings (calyces of Held) in the medial nucleus of the trapezoid body of the cat. *Hear. Res.* 49, 321–334. doi: 10.1016/0378-5955(90)90111-2

Hamann, M., Billups, B., and Forsythe, I. D. (2003). Non-calyceal excitatory inputs mediate low fidelity synaptic transmission in rat auditory brainstem slices. *Eur. J. Neurosci.* 18, 2899–2902. doi: 10.1111/j.1460-9568.2003.03017.x

Held, H. (1893). Die centrale Gehörleitung. *Arch. Anat. Physiol. Anat. Abt.* 17, 201–248.

Helfert, R. H., Bonneau, J. M., Wenthold, R. J., and Altschuler, R. A. (1989). GABA and glycine immunoreactivity in the guinea pig superior olivary complex. *Brain Res.* 501, 269–286. doi: 10.1016/0006-8993(89)90644-6

Hermann, J., Pecka, M., Von Gersdorff, H., Grothe, B., and Klug, A. (2007). Synaptic transmission at the calyx of Held under *in vivo* like activity levels. *J. Neurophysiol.* 98, 807–820. doi: 10.1152/jn.00355.2007

Ito, T., Hioki, H., Nakamura, K., Tanaka, Y., Nakade, H., Kaneko, T., et al. (2007). Gamma-aminobutyric acid-containing sympathetic preganglionic neurons in rat thoracic spinal cord send their axons to the superior cervical ganglion. *J. Comp. Neurol.* 502, 113–125. doi: 10.1002/cne.21309

Jaskolski, F., Mulle, C., and Manzoni, O. J. (2005). An automated method to quantify and visualize colocalized fluorescent signals. *J. Neurosci. Methods* 146, 42–49. doi: 10.1016/j.jneumeth.2005.01.012

Köbbert, C., Apps, R., Bechmann, I., Lanciego, J. L., Mey, J., and Thanos, S. (2000). Current concepts in neuroanatomical tracing. *Prog. Neurobiol.* 62, 327–351. doi: 10.1016/S0301-0082(00)00019-8

Kopp-Scheinpflug, C., Dehmel, S., Tolnai, S., Dietz, B., Milenkovic, I., and Rübsamen, R. (2008). Glycine-mediated changes of onset reliability at a mammalian central synapse. *Neuroscience* 157, 432–445. doi: 10.1016/j.neuroscience.2008.08.068

Kulesza, R. J. (2008). Cytoarchitecture of the human superior olivary complex: nuclei of the trapezoid body and posterior tier. *Hear. Res.* 241, 52–63. doi: 10.1016/j.heares.2008.04.010

Kuwabara, N., DiCaprio, R., and Zook, J. (1991). Afferents to the medial nucleus of the trapezoid body and their collateral projections. *J. Comp. Neurol.* 314, 684–706. doi: 10.1002/cne.903140405

Kuwabara, N., and Zook, J. (1991). Classification of the principal cells of the medial nucleus of the trapezoid body. *J. Comp. Neurol.* 314, 707–720. doi: 10.1002/cne.903140406

Kuwajima, T., Sitko, A. A., Bhansali, P., Jurgens, C., Guido, W., and Mason, C. (2013). ClearT: a detergent- and solvent-free clearing method for neuronal and non-neuronal tissue. *Development* 140, 1364–1368. doi: 10.1242/dev.091844

Leao, R. M., Kushmerick, C., Pinaud, R., Renden, R., Li, G. L., Taschenberger, H., et al. (2005). Presynaptic Na^+ channels: locus, development, and recovery from inactivation at a high-fidelity synapse. *J. Neurosci.* 25, 3724–3738. doi: 10.1523/JNEUROSCI.3983-04.2005

Li, Q., Lau, A., Morris, T. J., Guo, L., Fordyce, C. B., and Stanley, E. F. (2004). A syntaxin 1, Galpha(o), and N-type calcium channel complex at a presynaptic nerve terminal: analysis by quantitative immunocolocalization. *J. Neurosci.* 24, 4070–4081. doi: 10.1523/JNEUROSCI.0346-04.2004

Morest, D. (1968). The growth of synaptic endings in the mammalian brain: a study of the calyces of the trapezoid body. *Z. Anat. Entwicklungsgesch.* 127, 201–220. doi: 10.1007/BF00526129

Novikova, L., Novikov, L., and Kellerth, J. O. (1997). Persistent neuronal labeling by retrograde fluorescent tracers: a comparison between Fast Blue, Fluoro-Gold and various dextran conjugates. *J. Neurosci. Methods* 74, 9–15. doi: 10.1016/S0165-0270(97)02227-9

Ollo, C., and Schwartz, I. R. (1979). The superior olivary complex in C57BL/6 mice. *Am. J. Anat.* 155, 349–373. doi: 10.1002/aja.1001550306

Peyret, D., Campistron, G., Geffard, M., and Aran, J. M. (1987). Glycine immunoreactivity in the brainstem auditory and vestibular nuclei of the guinea pig. *Acta Otolaryngol.* 104, 71–76. doi: 10.3109/00016488709109049

Poyatos, I., Ponce, J., Aragón, C., Giménez, C., and Zafra, F. (1997). The glycine transporter GLYT2 is a reliable marker for glycine-immunoreactive neurons. *Brain Res. Mol. Brain Res.* 49, 63–70. doi: 10.1016/S0169-328X(97)00124-1

Roberts, M. T., Seeman, S. C., and Golding, N. L. (2013). A mechanistic understanding of the role of feedforward inhibition in the mammalian sound localization circuitry. *Neuron* 78, 923–935. doi: 10.1016/j.neuron.2013.04.022

Robertson, D. (1996). Physiology and morphology of cells in the ventral nucleus of trapezoid body and rostral periolivary regions of the rat superior olivary complex studied in slices. *Audit Neurosci.* 2, 15–31.

Rodríguez-Contreras, A., de Lange, R. P. J., Lucassen, P. J., and Borst, J. G. G. (2006). Branching of calyceal afferents during postnatal development in the rat auditory brainstem. *J. Comp. Neurol.* 496, 214–228. doi: 10.1002/cne.20918

Ross, M. D. (1962). Auditory pathway of the epileptic waltzing mouse. I. A comparison of the acoustic pathways of the normal mouse with those of the totally deaf epileptic waltzer. *J. Comp. Neurol.* 119, 317–339. doi: 10.1002/cne.901190305

Ross, M. D. (1969). The general visceral efferent component of the eighth cranial nerve. *J. Comp. Neurol.* 135, 453–477. doi: 10.1002/cne.901350405

Ryugo, D. K., Montey, K. L., Wright, A. L., Bennett, M. L., and Pongstaporn, T. (2006). Postnatal development of a large auditory nerve terminal: the endbulb of Held in cats. *Hear. Res.* 216–217, 100–115. doi: 10.1016/j.heares.2006.01.007

Saint Marie, R. L., and Baker, R. A. (1990). Neurotransmitter-specific uptake and retrograde transport of [3H]glycine from the inferior colliculus by ipsilateral projections of the superior olivary complex and nuclei of the lateral lemniscus. *Brain Res.* 524, 244–253. doi: 10.1016/0006-8993(90)90698-B

Schneggenburger, R., and Forsythe, I. D. (2006). The calyx of Held. *Cell Tissue Res.* 326, 311–337. doi: 10.1007/s00441-006-0272-7

Smith, P. H., Joris, P. X., Carney, L. H., and Yin, T. C. (1991). Projections of physiologically characterized globular bushy cell axons from the cochlear nucleus of the cat. *J. Comp. Neurol.* 304, 387–407. doi: 10.1002/cne.903040305

Spangler, K. M., Warr, W. B., and Henkel, C. K. (1985). The projections of principal cells of the medial nucleus of the trapezoid body in the cat. *J. Comp. Neurol.* 238, 249–262. doi: 10.1002/cne.902380302

Taschenberger, H., and von Gersdorff, H. (2000). Fine-tuning an auditory synapse for speed and fidelity: developmental changes in presynaptic waveform, EPSC kinetics, and synaptic plasticity. *J. Neurosci.* 20, 9162–9173.

Thompson, A., and Schofield, B. (2000). Afferent projections of the superior olivary complex. *Microsc. Res. Tech.* 51, 330–354. doi: 10.1002/1097-0029(20001115)51:4<330::AID-JEMT4>3.0.CO;2-X

Tolnai, S., Englitz, B., Kopp-Scheinpflug, C., Dehmel, S., Jost, J., and Rübsamen, R. (2008). Dynamic coupling of excitatory and inhibitory responses in the medial nucleus of the trapezoid body. *Eur. J. Neurosci.* 27, 3191–3204. doi: 10.1111/j.1460-9568.2008.06292.x von Gersdorff, H., and Borst, J. G. G. (2002). Short-term plasticity at the calyx of Held. *Nat. Rev. Neurosci.* 3, 53–64. doi: 10.1038/nrn705

Wang, Q., Henry, A. M., Harris, J. A., Oh, S. W., Joines, K. M., Nyhus, J., et al. (2014). Systematic comparison of adeno-associated virus and biotinylated dextran amine reveals equivalent sensitivity between tracers and novel projection targets in the mouse brain. *J. Comp. Neurol.* 522, 1989–2012. doi: 10.1002/cne.23567

Warr, W. (1972). Fiber degeneration following lesions in the multipolar and globular cell areas in the ventral cochlear nucleus of the cat. *Brain Res.* 40, 247–270. doi: 10.1016/0006-8993(72)90132-1

Warr, W. B., and Beck, J. E. (1996). Multiple projections from the ventral nucleus of the trapezoid body in the rat. *Hear. Res.* 93, 83–101. doi: 10.1016/0378-5955(95)00198-0

Webster, D. B., and Trune, D. R. (1982). Cochlear nuclear complex of mice. *Am. J. Anat.* 163, 103–130. doi: 10.1002/aja.1001630202

Yao, W., and Godfrey, D. A. (1998). Immunohistochemical evaluation of cholinergic neurons in the rat superior olivary complex. *Microsc. Res. Tech.* 41, 270–283.

Zeilhofer, H. U., Studler, B., Arabadzisz, D., Schweizer, C., Ahmadi, S., Layh, B., et al. (2005). Glycinergic neurons expressing enhanced green fluorescent protein in bacterial artificial chromosome transgenic mice. *J. Comp. Neurol.* 482, 123–141. doi: 10.1002/cne.20349

11

Inhibitory glycinergic neurotransmission in the mammalian auditory brainstem upon prolonged stimulation: Short-term plasticity and synaptic reliability

Florian Kramer[1], Désirée Griesemer[1], Dennis Bakker[1], Sina Brill[1], Jürgen Franke[2,3], Erik Frotscher[1] and Eckhard Friauf[1,3]*

[1] *Animal Physiology Group, Department of Biology, University of Kaiserslautern, Kaiserslautern, Germany*
[2] *Chair for Applied Mathematical Statistics, Department of Mathematics, University of Kaiserslautern, Kaiserslautern, Germany*
[3] *Center for Mathematical and Computational Modeling, University of Kaiserslautern, Kaiserslautern, Germany*

Correspondence:
Eckhard Friauf, Animal Physiology Group, Department of Biology, University of Kaiserslautern, POB 3049, D-67653 Kaiserslautern, Germany
e-mail: eckhard.friauf@biologie.uni-kl.de

Short-term plasticity plays a key role in synaptic transmission and has been extensively investigated for excitatory synapses. Much less is known about inhibitory synapses. Here we analyze the performance of glycinergic connections between the medial nucleus of the trapezoid body (MNTB) and the lateral superior olive (LSO) in the auditory brainstem, where high spike rates as well as fast and precise neurotransmission are hallmarks. Analysis was performed in acute mouse slices shortly after hearing onset (postnatal day (P)11) and 8 days later (P19). Stimulation was done at 37°C with 1–400 Hz for 40 s. Moreover, in a novel approach named marathon experiments, a very prolonged stimulation protocol was employed, comprising 10 trials of 1-min challenge and 1-min recovery periods at 50 and 1 Hz, respectively, thus lasting up to 20 min and amounting to >30,000 stimulus pulses. IPSC peak amplitudes displayed short-term depression (STD) and synaptic attenuation in a frequency-dependent manner. No facilitation was observed. STD in the MNTB-LSO connections was less pronounced than reported in the upstream calyx of Held-MNTB connections. At P11, the STD level and the failure rate were slightly lower within the ms-to-s range than at P19. During prolonged stimulation periods lasting 40 s, P19 connections sustained virtually failure-free transmission up to frequencies of 100 Hz, whereas P11 connections did so only up to 50 Hz. In marathon experiments, P11 synapses recuperated reproducibly from synaptic attenuation during all recovery periods, demonstrating a robust synaptic machinery at hearing onset. At 26°C, transmission was severely impaired and comprised abnormally high amplitudes after minutes of silence, indicative of imprecisely regulated vesicle pools. Our study takes a fresh look at synaptic plasticity and stability by extending conventional stimulus periods in the ms-to-s range to minutes. It also provides a framework for future analyses of synaptic plasticity.

Keywords: synaptic fidelity, fast-spiking cells, short-term depression, inhibitory postsynaptic currents, synaptic attenuation, lateral superior olive, medial nucleus of the trapezoid body, high-frequency neurotransmission

INTRODUCTION

Fast and reliable synaptic transmission at high frequencies is one of the hallmarks of the auditory system. In particular, it is a key feature for processing interaural time and intensity differences, the two major features for computation of sound localization (reviews: Yin, 2002; Borst and Soria van Hoeve, 2012). Central auditory relay synapses can follow high-frequency inputs (>100 Hz) with great fidelity, conveying signals with a high degree of precision and reliability (review: Klug, 2011). A great deal of knowledge concerning synaptic transmission has been obtained from principal neurons in the medial nucleus of the trapezoid body (MNTB) and their giant presynaptic partner structure, the calyx of Held, between which phase-locked transmission occurs in a failure-free, one-to-one fashion up to a frequency of 800 Hz, at least over a short period of 20 ms (Taschenberger and von Gersdorff, 2000). MNTB neurons provide the major inhibitory input to neurons in the lateral superior olive (LSO), and the MNTB-LSO pathway is a model system for investigating inhibitory neurotransmission (Sanes and Friauf, 2000; Kandler, 2004; Noh et al., 2010). In contrast to the well-characterized calyx of Held-MNTB synapses, however, much less is known about the reliability of downstream MNTB-LSO synapses.

Despite the demands concerning stable signal transmission, synapses display substantial, mostly temporary, alterations in strength during repetitive use. Distinctive types of synaptic plasticity are exhibited, such as depression and facilitation, or combinations of both. In the auditory system, calyceal input to MNTB neurons has been extensively analyzed (von Gersdorff et al., 1997; Taschenberger and von Gersdorff, 2000; Taschenberger et al., 2002; Trussell, 2002; von Gersdorff and Borst, 2002; Wong et al., 2003; Oleskevich et al., 2004). By contrast, in other auditory relay stations, short-term alterations are relatively unexplored (reviews: Bender and Trussell, 2011; MacLeod, 2011).

Short-term depression (STD) in a brief time window of <1 s has been described at specialized terminals of auditory nerve fibers, the endbulbs of Held, which contact bushy cells in the cochlear nuclear complex. Here, STD occurs upon stimulation with 100–300 Hz over a period of 150 ms (Oleskevich and Walmsley, 2002; Wang and Manis, 2006, 2008; Wang et al., 2010, 2011). STD was also reported in GABAergic synapses between the inferior colliculus and the medial geniculate body (Venkataraman and Bartlett, 2013). In the auditory cortex, GABAergic IPSCs display STD in a layer-specific manner (Humberto et al., 2011). In the only LSO studies so far, STD in the inhibitory MNTB-LSO path was described in P11–15 mice at 23–25°C with stimulus trains of 20 Hz lasting 1.05 s (Giugovaz-Tropper et al., 2011) and in P10–18 gerbils and P10–15 mice at 32°C with stimulus trains of 100 Hz lasting 200 ms (Walcher et al., 2011).

Here, we have functionally analyzed glycinergic MNTB-LSO synapses with the aims to characterize their performance and to determine their limits. To do so, IPSCs were recorded from mouse LSO neurons in brainstem slices at two ages (P11 and P19), two temperatures (37 and 26°C), and various frequencies (1–400 Hz). Moreover, "marathon experiments" involved very prolonged stimulation (20 min) comprising up to 30,600 stimuli, many-fold more than routinely used (cf. Galarreta and Hestrin, 1998). The rationale for this strategy is based on several arguments. First, continuous auditory stimulation is virtually ubiquitous in natural environments (Lalor et al., 2009). Second, brief tone bursts, commonly used stimuli for *in vivo* recordings, recruit bursts of action potentials (APs) at frequencies between 50 and 500 Hz (Klug, 2011). Finally, highly active conditions of prolonged stimulation are a better approximation of the *in vivo* situation than standard slice experiments. Our novel stimulus protocols address synaptic depression in both the milliseconds-to-seconds (STD) and the tens of seconds-to-minute range, for which we use the term "synaptic attenuation" as the counterpart to the term synaptic augmentation (Thompson, 2000; Regehr, 2012). Concerning the mechanisms underlying STD and synaptic attenuation, we provide some evidence in favor of presynaptic processes.

MATERIALS AND METHODS

ANIMALS

Experiments were performed on C57BL/6N mice of either sex at postnatal day (P)11 ± 1 or P19 ± 1. They were in accordance with the German law for conducting animal experiments and followed the NIH guide for the care and use of laboratory animals.

ELECTROPHYSIOLOGY

Patch-clamp recordings from LSO neurons were performed in the whole-cell configuration in acute brainstem slices generated as described previously (Balakrishnan et al., 2003). Slices were stored at room temperature in artificial cerebrospinal fluid (ACSF, in [mM]: NaCl 125; KCl 2.5; $NaHCO_3$ 25; NaH_2PO_4 1.25; Na-pyruvate 2; D-glucose 10; $CaCl_2$ 2; $MgCl_2$ 1; myo-inositol 3; ascorbic acid 0.44; pH = 7.3 when bubbled with 95% O_2-5% CO_2) before being transferred into a recording chamber in which they were continually superfused with ACSF (1–2 ml/min). Recordings were performed at near physiological temperature (37 ± 1°C, temperature controller III, Luigs&Neumann) or at room temperature (26 ± 2°C). The recording chamber was mounted on an upright microscope (Eclipse E600FN, Nikon) equipped with differential interference contrast optics (4× CFI Achromate, 0.1 NA; 60× CFI Fluor W, 1.0 NA, Nikon) and an infrared video camera system (CCD camera C5405-01, Hamamatsu). LSO principal neurons were identified by their location in the center of the nucleus, orientation, size, spindle-shaped somata, the presence of hyperpolarization-activated inward currents (Sterenborg et al., 2010) and of short-latency IPSCs upon stimulation of MNTB fibers. Membrane currents were digitized and stored using ClampEX 8.2 (Molecular Devices).

Patch pipettes were pulled from borosilicate glass capillaries (GB150(F)-8P, Science Products) with a horizontal puller (P-87, Sutter Instruments). They were connected to an Axopatch-1D patch-clamp amplifier (Molecular Devices) and had resistances of 3–7 MΩ when filled with intracellular solution (in [mM]: HEPES 10; EGTA 5; $MgCl_2$ 1; K-gluconate 140; Na_2ATP 2; Na_2GTP 0.3). The Cl^- concentration of 2 mM was slightly lower than the native 5 mM previously determined for P9–11 via perforated-patch clamp recordings (Ehrlich et al., 1999) and was chosen to increase the driving force for inward-directed Cl^- flow. With 2 mM $[Cl^-]_i$, E_{Cl} was −112 mV at 37°C and −108 mV at 26°C. Liquid junction potential was calculated using the program JPCalc (Barry, 1994); it amounted to 15.4 mV and was corrected offline. Data were sampled at 10 kHz, low-pass filtered at 5 kHz, and analyzed using ClampEX and ClampFit 8.2.0.235 (Molecular Devices) and Origin software (Origin Lab). Capacitive current transients were electronically compensated online, and the whole cell capacitance was estimated from this compensation. Throughout the experiments, the series resistance was monitored and ranged from 6 to 20 MΩ. It was routinely compensated by 60–80%. If it exceeded 20 MΩ, recordings were excluded from further analysis.

Recordings were performed in voltage clamp mode at a holding potential of −70 mV. To evoke inhibitory postsynaptic currents (IPSCs), a theta glass electrode (TST150-6, WPI) with a tip diameter of 10–20 μm was filled with ACSF and placed lateral to the MNTB (**Figure 1A**). Monopolar pulses (100 μs duration) were applied through a programmable pulse generator (Master 8, A.M.P.I.) connected to a stimulus isolator unit (A360, WPI). The amplitude of the stimulus pulses ranged from 0.1 to 4 mA and was set to achieve stable synaptic responses with a jitter in amplitude of <50 pA.

For normalization, 40 control stimuli were presented at 1 Hz during a baseline period and the peak amplitudes of the 40 IPSCs were averaged (= control value, set to 100%; cf. Galarreta and Hestrin, 1998). Two protocols were employed for determining the synaptic performance of the MNTB-LSO connection. For protocol 1, pulse trains were applied for 40 s each, with stimulation frequencies from 1 to 400 Hz in random order, and a 3-min pause was introduced between each pulse train (**Figure 1B$_1$**). For protocol 2, which assessed the performance over 20 min, 10 trials of stimulation were applied, alternating between 50 Hz stimulation for 60 s and 1 Hz stimulation for another 60 s (**Figure 1B$_2$**). 1 Hz stimulation for 60 s was chosen to describe the time course of recovery, rather than eliciting single test IPSCs at varying

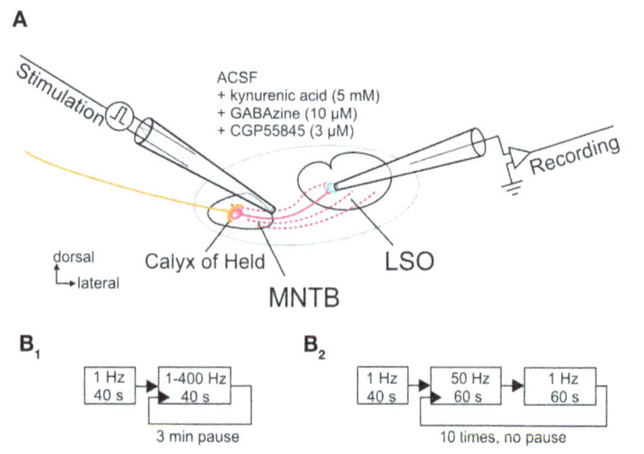

FIGURE 1 | Whole-cell patch clamp recordings from LSO neurons located in the central region of the nucleus upon electrical stimulation of their input fibers from the MNTB. (A) Schematic view of the circuit as seen in a coronal brainstem slice. A theta glass electrode was used for focal electrical stimulation and placed at the lateral border of the MNTB to reach the maximum number of connecting fibers (depicted in magenta). Glycinergic transmission was pharmacologically isolated with the depicted drugs. **(B_1,B_2)** Scheme of the two protocols used for prolonged and very prolonged stimulation, comprising up to 30,600 pulses.

time intervals (Giugovaz-Tropper et al., 2011). No pause was introduced between trials. In some control experiments, recordings were obtained from MNTB neurons in the current-clamp mode, and antidromic APs were evoked in the LSO by electrical stimulation of MNTB axons.

CHEMICALS AND PHARMACOLOGICAL COMPOUNDS

All chemicals were purchased from Sigma-Aldrich unless stated otherwise. Glycine-mediated receptor currents were isolated pharmacologically. To do so, N-methyl-D-aspartic acid (NMDA) and α-amino-3-hydroxy-5-methyl-4-isoxazole propionate (AMPA) receptor-mediated currents were blocked by kynurenic acid (5 mM). Furthermore, GABAzine (10 μM) and CGP55845 (3 μM) were used for blocking $GABA_A$ and $GABA_B$ receptor-mediated currents, respectively (purchased from Ascent Scientific and Tocris Bioscience). All drugs were added to the ACSF. In control experiments, the residual current could be completely abolished with strychnine (0.3 – 1 μM), thus verifying their glycinergic nature.

DATA ANALYSIS

Data analysis was performed with Mini Analysis 6.0.3 (Synaptosoft). At the beginning of each experiment, the control value of glycinergic IPSC peak amplitudes was obtained for each neuron (see above). The following peak amplitudes underwent statistical analysis: amplitudes of the 1st, 2nd, and 10th IPSC ($IPSC_1$, $IPSC_2$, $IPSC_{10}$), amplitudes after the 1st and the 40th s ($IPSC_{1\,s}$, $IPSC_{40\,s}$), and averaged amplitudes over several 10-s periods, namely 30–40 s, 50–60 s, and 110–120 s ($IPSC_{30-40\,s}$, $IPSC_{50-60\,s}$, $IPSC_{110-120\,s}$). When individual IPSC peak amplitudes were ≤5% of the control value, the event was considered a failure. A failure was also attributed if the peak amplitude was <15 pA, which equaled the noise level. For such failures, the peak amplitude was set to 0 pA. For kinetic measurements, the decay time constant τ (decay to 37% of peak amplitude) was determined by fitting a single exponential to the decay phase of the IPSC.

STATISTICS

Statistical analysis was performed on data sets if $n \geq 7$ (Winstat, R. Fitch Software). Outliers (more than four times standard deviation above/below mean) were excluded. Such outliers occurred in the range of 5.3–11.8% (median: 6.2%, mean: 8.0%). In absolute numbers, $n_{gross} = 19$ became $n_{net} = 18$ in the best case, and $n_{gross} = 17$ became $n_{net} = 15$ in the worst case. Samples with a Gaussian distribution (Kolmogorov–Smirnov) were compared using a paired or an unpaired two-tailed Student's *t*-test. A Wilcoxon-signed rank test was used for unequal variances. Equality of variances in unpaired samples Student's *t*-tests was assessed with an *F*-test. Values in bar charts are presented as mean ± s.e.m. Significance values were as follows: $^{*}p < 0.05$, $^{**}p < 0.01$, $^{***}p < 0.001$.

RESULTS

FREQUENCY-DEPENDENT SYNAPTIC DEPRESSION OF GLYCINERGIC IPSCs IN THE MILLISECONDS-TO-SECONDS RANGE

In a first series of experiments, synaptic current responses from LSO principal neurons were obtained by stimulating axons in the MNTB at P11, and glycinergic IPSCs were pharmacologically isolated at a holding potential of −70 mV (**Figure 1A**). Under these conditions, IPSCs comprised outward currents with a fast rising phase (<1 ms) and short decay times (<5 ms), corroborating that they were mediated through glycine receptors (GlyRs). The performance of the glycinergic MNTB-LSO synapses was assessed by prolonged stimulation for 40 s with frequencies of 1–400 Hz (in random order), inserting a 3-min pause in between (**Figure 1B$_1$**). As spontaneous discharges in this frequency and time range have been described for mouse MNTB neurons *in vivo* at P11–12 and thereafter (Sonntag et al., 2009), our stimuli resembled physiological conditions. We were further motivated to stimulate the MNTB-LSO synapses for prolonged periods with 1–400 Hz because mean spontaneous firing rates in this domain (25–100 Hz) have been recorded *in vivo* from auditory nerve fibers in several species, such as cats (Liberman, 1978), gerbils (Hermann et al., 2007), and chinchillas (Temchin et al., 2008).

Representative current traces from a P11 LSO neuron at 37 ± 1°C are illustrated in **Figure 2A**. At 1 Hz, every stimulus pulse elicited an IPSC (**Figures 2A$_1$,B$_1$**). As the stimulus frequency was increased, IPSC peak amplitudes declined, resulting in STD (**Figures 2A$_2$–B$_1$**). There was no indication of a short-term facilitation. Despite the frequency-dependent STD, the neuron displayed a detectable IPSC to each of the first 40 stimulus pulses, even at 333 Hz. STD was most prominent during the first 10 pulses (**Figure 2B$_1$**), whereas the peak amplitudes appeared to be quite stable after 5 s (**Figure 2B$_2$**). With time, however, some pulses remained unresponded, i.e., failures occurred (**Figure 2B$_2$**, five values at 100 Hz touching x axis after >10 s).

The STD behavior shown exemplarily in **Figure 2** was observed in the whole ensemble of P11/37°C LSO neurons

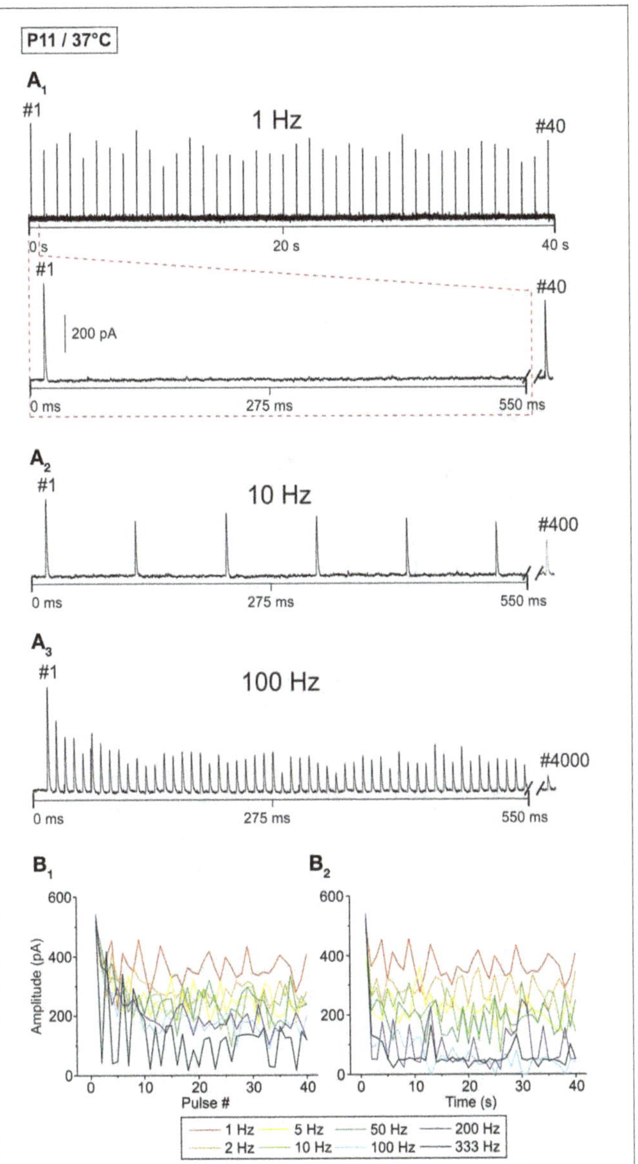

FIGURE 2 | Frequency-dependent changes in evoked glycinergic IPSCs obtained at P11 and physiological temperature (37 ± 1°C). (A1) Original 40 s recording of a representative LSO neuron during 1 Hz stimulation (top). The first 550 ms are time-expanded in the bottom trace (see red-stippled line). The last IPSC during the 40-s-period is shown on the right and depicted by its pulse number (#40). The 200 pA calibration bar is also valid for panels **(A2,A3)**. **(A2,A3)** IPSCs during 10 and 100 Hz stimulation, respectively, from the same neuron as in panel **(A1)**. Similar to **(A1)**, the very last IPSC during the 40-s-period is shown on the right (#400 and #4000, respectively). **(B1)** Time course of IPSC peak amplitudes from three LSO neurons at eight stimulation frequencies, ranging from 1 to 333 Hz (for color code, see inset). Peak values to the first 40 pulses (#1–40) are plotted. **(B2)** Like **(B1)**, but depicting the time course of IPSC peak amplitudes during the complete 40-s-periods. For each stimulation frequency, peak amplitudes were sampled at 1-s-intervals. Notice the frequency-dependent short-term depression (STD).

($n = 4$–22, depending on stimulus frequency; **Figure 3**). At each stimulus frequency and for virtually every neuron, the first IPSC ($IPSC_1$) had the highest peak amplitude (**Figure 3A**, see Methods for normalization to 100%). This was quantified by calculating the ratio between the mean peak amplitude of $IPSC_2$ and $IPSC_1$ ($IPSC_2/IPSC_1$). For example, at 1, 10, and 100 Hz, $IPSC_2/IPSC_1$ ratios amounted to 0.84, 0.85, and 0.80, respectively (**Table 1** and **Figure 3B1**). After the initial decline between $IPSC_1$ and $IPSC_2$, STD continued during the first 10 pulses, such that $IPSC_{10}$ was of significantly lower peak amplitude than $IPSC_2$ at stimulus frequencies ≥2 Hz (e.g., $IPSC_{10}/IPSC_2$ ratio at 50 Hz: 0.59; **Table 1**, **Figure 3B1**). Because of the prolonged stimulation period of 40 s, we extended the quantification from a pulse-based to a time-based analysis. During the first second of stimulation, peak amplitudes declined significantly and in a frequency-dependent manner >2 Hz (e.g., $IPSC_{1\,s}/IPSC_2$ at 50 Hz: 0.54; **Table 1**, **Figure 3B2**). No further decline occurred between $IPSC_{1\,s}$ and $IPSC_{40\,s}$, except for stimulus frequencies of 50 and 100 Hz, implying that stable inhibitory response amplitudes are maintained in the seconds-to-minutes range up to 10 Hz at P11/37°C (**Table 1**).

The frequency-dependent depression behavior was also evident in the mean peak amplitudes obtained during the last 10 s of recording, when a steady-state scenario appeared to be present (30–40 s; **Figures 3B2,C**). Peak amplitudes declined significantly with stimulus frequency up to 100 Hz, with no further decline at higher frequencies. The low mean amplitudes (<10% of the control) at ≥100 Hz are indicative of a massive depression in the P11/37°C MNTB-LSO connections in the seconds-to-minute range when the stimulus frequency is >50 Hz (**Figures 3B2,C**).

Concomitant with the frequency-dependent decline of peak amplitudes, LSO neurons were not able to respond reliably (i.e., failure-free) to high frequency stimulation, even during the first 40 pulses (**Table 2**, **Figures 3A1–A8**). Virtually 100% fidelity (no failures) was observed up to 50 Hz, because only a single failure occurred in a total of 2840 events, namely at 10 Hz (**Figure 3A4**). At 100 Hz, however, 27% of the neurons (4 of 15) displayed failures, and the average failure rate amounted to 0.8% (5 failures in 600 events), still a low value (**Figure 3A6**). The effect became more pronounced at even higher frequencies (333 Hz: 16.3% failure rate, 26 failures in 160 events, 3 of 4 neurons, **Figure 3A8**, **Table 2**). When analyzing the failure rate during the last 40 pulses, 100% fidelity was present only up to a stimulus frequency of 10 Hz (**Table 2**). At 50 Hz, 46% of the neurons (10 of 22) displayed failures with an average failure rate of 21% (188 failures in 880 events). Both the number of neurons with failures and the failure rate increased with stimulus frequency. Every neuron displayed failures at ≥100 Hz, and at 333 Hz, the failure rate amounted to 89.4% (**Table 2**). In summary, 50 Hz appears to be the maximal stimulus frequency to which P11/37°C MNTB-LSO synapses can continually respond within a time frame of milliseconds to tens of seconds.

TEMPERATURE-DEPENDENCY OF STD IN THE MILLISECONDS-TO-SECONDS RANGE

Next, we analyzed temperature effects on synaptic transmission. To do so, P11 LSO principal neurons were analyzed as described above, yet recordings were obtained at 26 ± 2°C. Representative recordings are illustrated in **Figure 4A**. Similar to the scenario at 37°C, IPSCs were reliably evoked at 1 Hz (**Figure 4A1**). IPSC amplitudes declined when the interpulse interval was shortened,

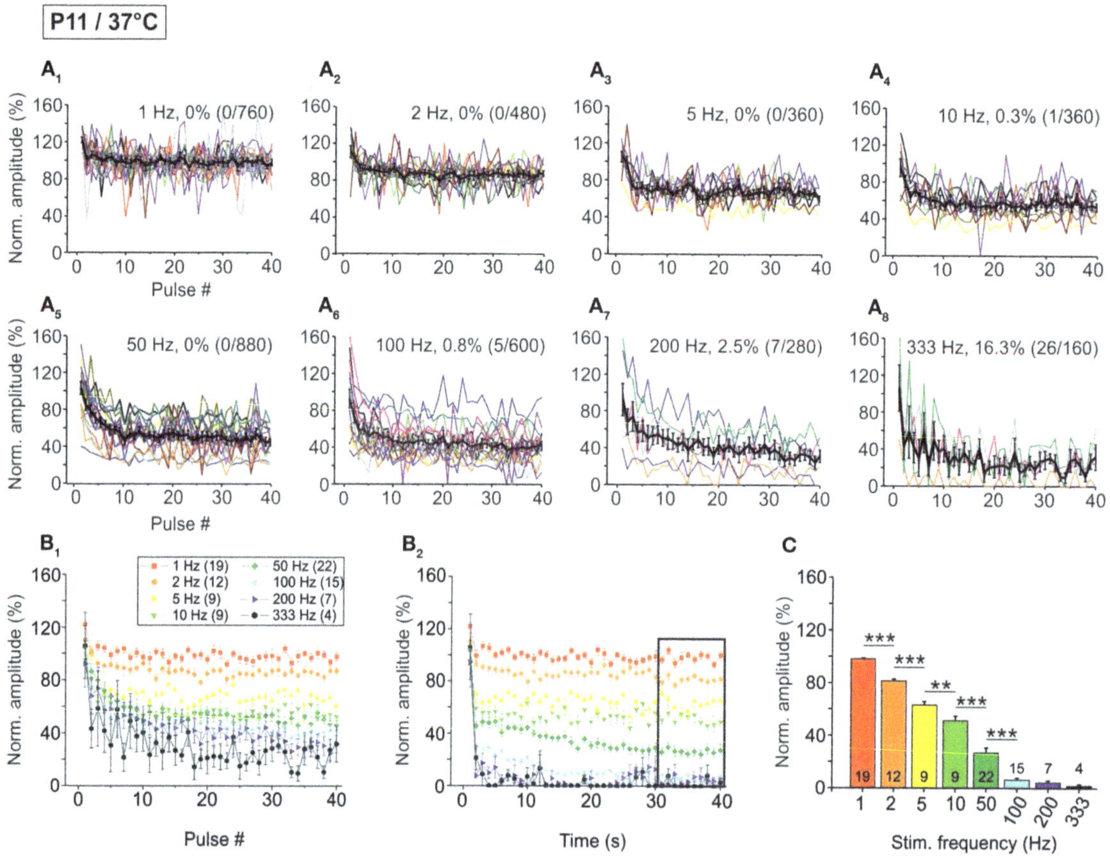

FIGURE 3 | Population data illustrating the frequency-dependent time course of glycinergic IPSC peak amplitudes at P11/37°C. (A_1–A_8) Color-coded plots for all recorded LSO neurons at eight stimulation frequencies ($n = 4$–22, cf. inset in panel **B_1**), depicting the time course of IPSC amplitudes in response to the first 40 stimuli. In each panel, the mean values ± s.e.m. are shown in black. The failure rate (%) and the ratio failures/events across neurons are also provided in each panel. **(B_1)** Mean values ± s.e.m. of the first 40 IPSCs obtained in response to the eight different stimulation frequencies. Notice the decline to <40% at frequencies ≥100 Hz. **(B_2)** Mean values ± s.e.m. obtained during the complete 40-s-periods of stimulation (sampled at 1-s-intervals). Color code as in panel **(B_1)**. Notice the decline to <20% at frequencies ≥100 Hz. Black frame depicts the last 10 data points in each trace that underwent statistical analysis shown in panel **(C)**. **(C)** IPSC peak amplitudes decreased with increasing stimulation frequency. *N* numbers in the inset of **(B_1)** correspond to all panels. $^{**}p < 0.01$; $^{***}p < 0.001$.

yet $IPSC_1$ to $IPSC_{40}$ were evoked reliably, even at a stimulus frequency of 200 Hz (**Figures 4A_2–B_1**). However, prolonged stimulation (40 s) resulted in drastically reduced peak amplitudes after 5 s at stimulus frequencies ≥50 Hz, and many failures occurred at 100 and 200 Hz (**Figure 4B_2**). Since the IPSCs decay time was >3 ms at 26°C (cf. **Figure 8**), we refrained from performing experiments with stimulus frequencies ≥333 Hz.

The analysis across the ensemble of P11/26°C LSO neurons ($n = 4$–18) revealed similarities as well as differences in STD behavior compared to 37°C (**Figure 5**). Similarly to 37°C, the mean $IPSC_2$ amplitude was significantly lower than the $IPSC_1$ amplitude at each frequency, with $IPSC_2/IPSC_1$ ratios amounting to 0.88, 0.69, and 0.61 at 1, 10, and 100 Hz, respectively (**Table 1**). Also similarly, further depression occurred from $IPSC_2$ to $IPSC_{10}$ (e.g., $IPSC_{10}/IPSC_2$ ratio at 50 Hz: 0.61; **Table 1**, **Figure 5B_1**), and the amount of depression was generally higher than at 37°C. The most prominent difference between 26 and 37°C became obvious only upon prolonged stimulation. For example at 100 Hz, the decline of peak amplitudes between $IPSC_2$ and $IPSC_{1\,s}$ (obtained after 1 s) was more pronounced at 26°C than at 37°C ($IPSC_{1\,s}/IPSC_2$ ratio: 0.24 vs. 0.39). The greater reduction with time at lower temperature was corroborated by the $IPSC_{40\,s}/IPSC_{1\,s}$ ratios. For example at 50 Hz, the ratio was 0.07 at 26°C, yet 0.61 at 37°C (**Table 1**). In line with this, the mean peak amplitudes obtained within 30–40 s at 50 Hz/26°C were drastically lower than those at 10 Hz/26°C, and there was no further decline beyond 50 Hz (**Figures 5B_2,C**). Together, a major temperature effect is that MNTB-LSO synapses can continually respond to 50 Hz stimulation at 37°C, yet only up to 10 Hz at 26°C.

Concerning the failure rate, P11/26°C MNTB-LSO synapses were able to respond with 100% fidelity to the first 40 pulses only up to a frequency of 5 Hz, because at 10 Hz, 1.1% failures occurred in 2 of 11 neurons (5 of 440 events; **Figures 5A_1–A_4**, **Table 2**). This was again in contrast to 37°C (0.3% failures) and further emphasized by a more than 10-fold higher failure rate at 100 Hz (26°C: 8.3%; 37°C: 0.8%, **Figure 5A_6**, **Table 2**). During the last 40 pulses, 100% fidelity was present only up to 5 Hz. Above 10 Hz, each neuron displayed failures, with a striking

Table 1 | Frequency-dependent changes in glycinergic IPSCs evoked in the MNTB-LSO connections.

Stimulus frequency (Hz)	*n*	$IPSC_1$ (%)	$IPSC_2$ (%)	$IPSC_{10}$ (%)	$IPSC_{1s}$ (%)	$IPSC_{40s}$ (%)	$IPSC_{30-40s}$ (%)	$IPSC_2/IPSC_1$ [*P*]	$IPSC_{10}/IPSC_2$ [*P*]	$IPSC_{1s}/IPSC_2$ [*P*]	$IPSC_{40s}/IPSC_{1s}$ [*P*]
P11/37°C											
1	19	122.1 ± 2.6	103.0 ± 2.6	99.3 ± 3.0	103.0 ± 2.6	100.4 ± 3.3	98.2 ± 0.6	0.84 [8E-06]	0.96 [0.449]	n.d.	1.0 [0.477]
2	12	110.5 ± 6.1	99.5 ± 1.9	92.7 ± 4.7	92.7 ± 3.7	83.6 ± 2.1	81.6 ± 1.3	0.90 [0.011]	0.93 [0.029]	0.93 [0.211]	0.90 [0.064]
5	9	104.7 ± 5.7	93.4 ± 4.6	71.1 ± 6.4	69.9 ± 4.5	65.4 ± 4.7	62.9 ± 2.6	0.89 [0.012]	0.76 [0.008]	0.75 [0.002]	0.94 [0.287]
10	9	94.9 ± 9.6	80.3 ± 6.5	53.2 ± 4.5	59.2 ± 5.7	49.4 ± 3.6	51.1 ± 3.0	0.85 [0.035]	0.66 [8E-04]	0.74 [0.005]	0.83 [0.089]
50	22	100.2 ± 5.1	83.9 ± 4.6	49.4 ± 3.2	45.6 ± 3.4	27.7 ± 4.8	26.8 ± 3.8	0.84 [5E-05]	0.59 [3E-08]	0.54 [2E-06]	0.61 [0.001]
100	15	92.1 ± 10.1	73.6 ± 7.5	46.5 ± 5.3	28.5 ± 4.6	7.5 ± 2.6	6.5 ± 1.3	0.80 [0.004]	0.63 [8E-04]	0.39 [1E-04]	0.26 [0.004]
200	7	94.6 ± 19.3	68.0 ± 14.0	49.2 ± 11.0	7.8 ± 1.5	3.6 ± 2.8	4.3 ± 1.3	0.72	0.72	0.11	0.46
333	4	106.1 ± 25.1	43.3 ± 14.6	40.4 ± 14.1	21.2 ± 9.2	2.8 ± 2.8	1.9 ± 1.0	0.41	0.93	0.49	0.13
P11/26°C											
1	11	140.2 ± 7.5	124.0 ± 3.3	100.0 ± 2.4	124.0 ± 3.3	99.2 ± 2.3	96.2 ± 1.5	0.88 [0.005]	0.81 [1E-05]	n.d.	0.80 [1E-06]
2	11	149.8 ± 5.6	119.1 ± 6.4	79.7 ± 6.6	94.6 ± 3.6	78.3 ± 4.7	78.3 ± 2.3	0.80 [0.012]	0.67 [3E-06]	0.79 [0.006]	0.83 [0.022]
5	11	147.1 ± 4.2	106.3 ± 5.9	62.4 ± 5.2	74.6 ± 4.6	69.1 ± 5.0	63.6 ± 3.8	0.72 [7E-05]	0.59 [2E-04]	0.70 [0.003]	0.93 [0.018]
10	11	163.0 ± 16.6	112.2 ± 11.6	71.1 ± 7.4	69.7 ± 6.9	47.3 ± 6.9	49.9 ± 4.5	0.69 [1E-05]	0.63 [3E-04]	0.62 [2E-04]	0.68 [0.014]
50	17	133.5 ± 6.7	113.7 ± 6.6	69.2 ± 8.2	40.7 ± 5.5	2.9 ± 1.4	2.2 ± 0.6	0.85 [0.027]	0.61 [1E-04]	0.36 [2E-08]	0.07 [2E-06]
100	18	133.8 ± 17.5	81.7 ± 10.7	40.4 ± 5.2	19.6 ± 3.3	0.0 ± 0.0	1.4 ± 0.5	0.61 [0.005]	0.49 [7E-04]	0.24 [1E-06]	0.00 [2E-04]
200	4	110.5 ± 30.0	48.6 ± 10.1	24.6 ± 6.6	5.5 ± 3.2	3.9 ± 2.7	1.3 ± 0.9	0.44	0.51	0.11	0.71
P19/37°C											
1	13	125.9 ± 6.7	101.6 ± 6.5	99.0 ± 7.7	101.6 ± 6.5	94.7 ± 5.7	99.7 ± 1.9	0.81 [0.063]	0.97 [0.790]	n.d.	0.93 [0.486]
2	12	111.8 ± 5.8	92.0 ± 7.5	72.0 ± 4.6	78.9 ± 7.7	72.9 ± 4.7	71.5 ± 3.7	0.82 [0.033]	0.76 [0.057]	0.86 [0.295]	0.92 [0.550]
5	12	93.9 ± 8.7	74.3 ± 7.6	60.6 ± 9.4	68.1 ± 6.8	56.5 ± 4.8	57.3 ± 3.8	0.79 [0.005]	0.82 [0.267]	0.92 [0.541]	0.83 [0.186]
10	11	101.0 ± 6.8	78.3 ± 7.1	42.8 ± 6.5	41.5 ± 4.3	64.6 ± 8.7	54.4 ± 3.0	0.78 [0.006]	0.55 [0.002]	0.53 [1E-04]	1.56 [0.055]
50	11	84.2 ± 8.7	72.9 ± 9.4	37.1 ± 5.5	33.2 ± 4.6	40.4 ± 7.5	36.1 ± 3.7	0.87 [0.156]	0.51 [0.001]	0.46 [2E-04]	1.21 [0.318]
100	15	88.2 ± 7.3	75.5 ± 9.6	44.8 ± 5.3	39.8 ± 7.5	21.0 ± 5.9	28.7 ± 5.2	0.86 [0.096]	0.59 [0.003]	0.53 [0.010]	0.53 [0.001]
200	8	96.2 ± 18.1	79.0 ± 9.5	49.0 ± 10.9	32.4 ± 8.7	10.2 ± 6.0	6.3 ± 2.7	0.82 [0.233]	0.77 [0.116]	0.86 [0.392]	0.15 [0.010]
333	7	84.9 ± 20.2	44.3 ± 14.3	34.2 ± 11.3	13.5 ± 7.8	0.0 ± 0.0	2.3 ± 1.1	0.52	0.77	0.31	0.00
400	7	83.7 ± 13.0	46.4 ± 18.5	3.7 ± 3.7	6.3 ± 4.3	0.0 ± 0.0	0.9 ± 0.7	0.55	0.08	0.14	0.00

Depicted are the mean values of IPSC peak amplitudes ± s.e.m. in relation to the control amplitude. The control amplitude is the average amplitude obtained for each neuron at the beginning of the experiment upon 40 stimuli at 1 Hz and was set to 100%. Statistical analysis (Student's t-test) was performed only on data sets with $n \geq 8$. P = significance value. Because $IPSC_{1s} = IPSC_2$ at 1 Hz stimulation, the ratio $IPSC_{1s}/IPSC_2$ is meaningless and, therefore, it was not determined at this frequency (n.d.).

Table 2 | Failure analysis of glycinergic IPSCs evoked in the MNTB-LSO connections.

Stimulus frequency (Hz)	First 40 pulses: Neurons with failures (%) [ratio]	First 40 pulses: Failure rate (%) [failures/events]	Last 40 pulses: Neurons with failures (%) [ratio]	Last 40 pulses: Failure rate (%) [failures/events]
P11/37°C				
1	0 [0/19]	0 [0/760]	0 [0/19]	0 [0/760]
2	0 [0/12]	0 [0/480]	0 [0/12]	0 [0/480]
5	0 [0/9]	0 [0/360]	0 [0/9]	0 [0/360]
10	11 [1/9]	0.3 [1/360]	0 [0/9]	0 [0/360]
50	0 [0/22]	0 [0/880]	46 [10/22]	21.4 [188/880]
100	27 [4/15]	0.8 [5/600]	93 [14/15]	55.5 [333/600]
200	29 [2/7]	2.5 [7/280]	100 [7/7]	71.1 [199/280]
333	75 [3/4]	16.3 [26/160]	100 [4/4]	89.4 [143/160]
P11/26°C				
1	0 [0/11]	0 [0/440]	0 [0/11]	0 [0/440]
2	0 [0/11]	0 [0/440]	0 [0/11]	0 [0/440]
5	0 [0/11]	0 [0/440]	0 [0/11]	0 [0/440]
10	18 [2/11]	1.1 [5/440]	9 [1/11]	3.2 [14/440]
50	12 [2/17]	2.8 [19/680]	100 [17/17]	76.2 [518/680]
100	44 [8/18]	8.3 [60/720]	100 [18/18]	89.4 [644/720]
200	25 [1/4]	12.5 [20/160]	100 [4/4]	100 [160/160]
P19/37°C				
1	0 [0/13]	0 [0/520]	0 [0/13]	0 [0/520]
2	0 [0/12]	0 [0/480]	0 [0/12]	0 [0/480]
5	8 [1/12]	0.2 [1/480]	0 [0/12]	0 [0/480]
10	9 [1/11]	0.2 [1/440]	9 [1/11]	0.2 [1/440]
50	18 [2/11]	0.5 [2/440]	46 [5/11]	4.1 [18/440]
100	40 [6/15]	3.7 [22/600]	60 [9/15]	26.2 [157/600]
200	38 [3/8]	4.1 [13/320]	100 [8/8]	78.4 [251/320]
333	86 [6/7]	28.9 [81/280]	100 [7/7]	93.2 [261/280]
400	100 [7/7]	45.4 [127/280]	100 [7/7]	96.1 [269/280]

Because of the long duration of IPSCs at P11/26°C, stimulus frequencies of 333 and 400 Hz were not applied.

difference to the corresponding failure rates at 37°C (**Table 2**). Together, these data show that 5–10 Hz is the highest stimulus frequency to which P11/26°C MNTB-LSO synapses can continually respond within a time frame of milliseconds to tens of seconds.

AGE-DEPENDENCY OF STD IN THE MILLISECONDS-TO-SECONDS RANGE

Although synaptic transmission in the rodent MNTB-LSO pathway appears to be quite mature by hearing onset (Kim and Kandler, 2003; Sonntag et al., 2011), some maturation steps still take place thereafter (Sanes and Friauf, 2000; Awatramani et al., 2005). To take this into consideration, we addressed synaptic transmission more than 1 week after hearing onset which, in mice, occurs at about P10 (Mikaelian and Ruben, 1965; Ehret, 1976; Ehret and Romand, 1992). We recorded from P19 LSO principal neurons at 37°C, essentially following the stimulus paradigms described above (highest stimulus frequency: 400 Hz). **Figure 6** shows representative data from two neurons. Similar to P11/37°C, amplitudes declined in a time- and frequency-dependent manner.

When analyzing the sample of all LSO neurons (n = 7–15), STD was consistently observed, progressing up to 200 Hz (**Figure 7**, **Table 1**). In slight contrast to P11/37°C, the mean $IPSC_2$ peak amplitude was significantly lower than that of $IPSC_1$ at only three of nine frequencies. For example, at 10 Hz, the $IPSC_2/IPSC_1$ ratio amounted to 0.78 ($p = 0.006$). At P11/37°C, the corresponding ratio was 0.85. A significant decline between $IPSC_2$ and $IPSC_{10}$ did not occur systematically. If there was one, it was moderate (e.g., $IPSC_{10}/IPSC_2$ at 100 Hz: 0.59; **Figure 7B$_1$**, **Table 1**) and similar to P11/37°C. STD between $IPSC_2$ and $IPSC_{1\,s}$ was significant only at $\geq$10 Hz (**Figure 7B$_2$**, **Table 1**). After the first second, peak amplitudes were quite stable and in a steady state, as evidenced by the finding that a statistically significant decline between $IPSC_{1\,s}$ and $IPSC_{40\,s}$ was evident only at 100 and 200 Hz (e.g., $IPSC_{40\,s}/IPSC_{1\,s}$ at 100 Hz: 0.53; **Table 1**). Thus, 1–40 s depression at P19 was slightly less pronounced than at

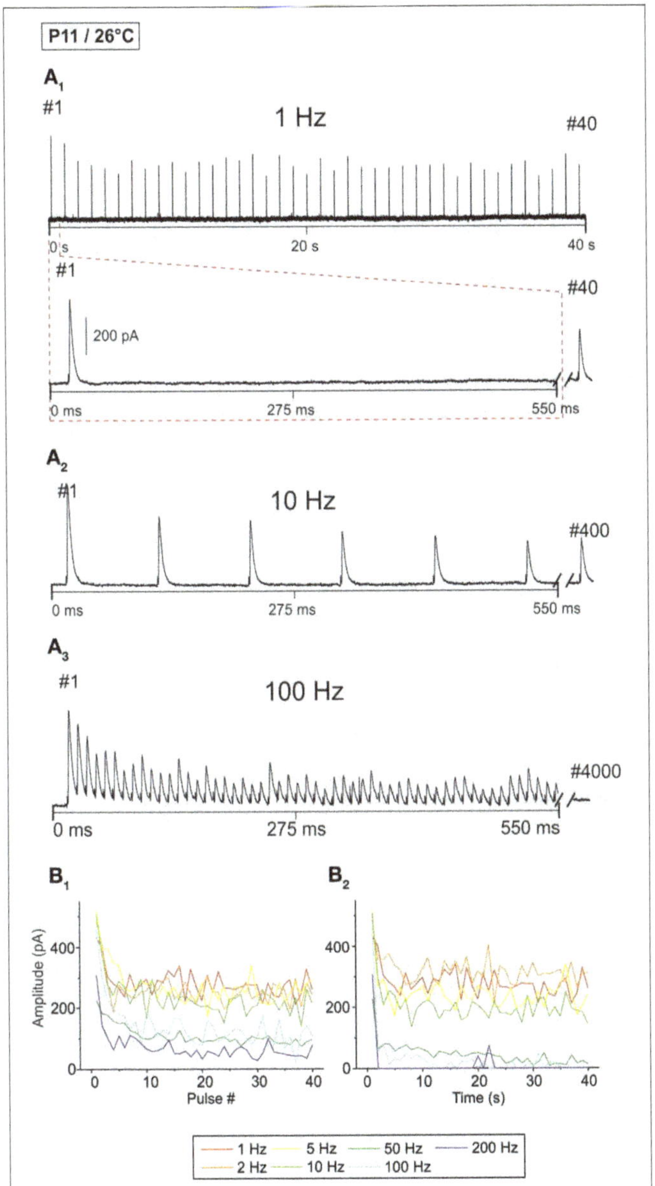

FIGURE 4 | Frequency-dependent changes in evoked glycinergic IPSCs obtained at P11 and room temperature (26 ± 2°C). (A_1) Original 40 s recording of a representative LSO neuron during 1 Hz stimulation (top). The first 550 ms are time-expanded in the bottom trace (see red-stippled line). The last IPSC during the 40-s-period is shown on the right and depicted by its pulse number (#40). The 200 pA calibration bar is also valid for panels **(A_2,A_3)**. **(A_2,A_3)** IPSCs during 10 and 100 Hz stimulation, respectively, from the same neuron as in panel **(A_1)**. Similar to **(A_1)**, the last IPSC during the 40-s-period is shown on the right (#400 and #4000, respectively). **(B_1)** Time course of IPSC peak amplitudes from two LSO neurons at stimulation frequencies ranging from 1–200 Hz (for color code, see inset). Peak values to the first 40 pulses (pulse #1–40) are plotted. **(B_2)**, Like **(B_1)**, but depicting the time course of IPSC peak amplitudes during the complete 40-s-periods. For each stimulation frequency, peak amplitudes were sampled at 1-s-intervals. Notice the stronger amount of STD than at 37°C, particularly at higher frequencies.

P11, because the latter displayed a statistically significant decline already at 50 Hz. Like at P11, mean peak $IPSC_{30-40\,s}$ amplitudes declined in a frequency-dependent manner in P19/37°C LSO neurons, but they remained above 25% of the control up to 100 Hz (**Figures 7B$_2$,C, Table 1**). Noticeably, this level was about 4-fold higher than at P11/37°C.

The moderate difference between P19/37°C and P11/37°C in STD behavior was also reflected by the failures. Interestingly, at virtually every stimulus frequency, both the percentage of neurons with failures and the failure rate were lower at P11 (**Table 2**). For example, at 100 Hz, 27% of the P11/37°C neurons displayed failures during the first 40 pulses (0.8% mean failure rate), whereas 40% of the P19/37°C neurons did so (3.5% mean failure rate). Thus, the performance of the MNTB-LSO connections shortly after hearing onset was surprisingly better in the millisecond range than that observed 1 week later. However, the opposite finding was achieved in the 40 s range, because P11 synapses displayed failure rates >20% at 50 Hz, whereas P19 synapses remained virtually failure-free up to 100 Hz (**Table 2**).

TEMPERATURE- AND AGE-DEPENDENCY OF IPSC KINETICS

IPSC kinetics at different temperatures and ages were determined from events obtained upon 1 Hz stimulation (**Figure 8A**; value for each neuron is the mean over 40 events). Concerning temperature dependency, the mean IPSC peak amplitude was 2-fold higher at 37°C than at 26°C (**Figure 8B**; P11/37°C: 303.8 ± 29.0 pA, $n = 31$; P11/26°C: 150.3 ± 16.9 pA, $n = 10$, $p = 4.8 \times 10^{-5}$). Noticeably, the absolute amplitudes should be treated carefully. First, they may have been reduced by the usage of kynurenic acid (Mok et al., 2009). Second, the driving force for inward-directed Cl-flow may have been slightly artificial because of the chloride concentration of 2 mM in the whole-cell patch pipettes.

The time course of the IPSCs was significantly shorter at 37°C, as evidenced by a 2-fold shorter rise time (37°C: 0.4 ± 0.02 ms, $n = 29$; 26°C: 0.8 ± 0.1 ms, $n = 10$; $p = 6.9 \times 10^{-5}$) and a 1.5-fold shorter decay time (37°C: 2.2 ± 0.1 ms, $n = 30$; 26°C: 3.4 ± 0.3 ms, $n = 10$; $p = 0.002$). Analysis of age-dependency (P19/37°C vs. P11/37°C) revealed significant differences for all three parameters tested (**Figure 8**), such that P19 MNTB-LSO synapses displayed a 30% lower peak amplitude (194.4 ± 27.0 pA, $n = 13$; $p = 0.030$), a 25% shorter rise time (10–90%: 0.3 ± 0.02 ms, $n = 13$; $p = 6 \times 10^{-7}$) and a 2-fold shorter decay time ($\tau = 1.2 \pm 0.1$ ms, $n = 13$; $p = 5.2 \times 10^{-10}$).

TEMPERATURE-DEPENDENCY OF SYNAPTIC ATTENUATION AND RECOVERY

In a next series of experiments, we assessed the capacity of P11 LSO neurons to recover from synaptic attenuation. To do so, we again obtained an initial baseline for normalization (1 Hz, 40 s) and then stimulated uniformly with 50 Hz, now extending the stimulus train to 60 s (**Figure 1B$_2$**). Immediately thereafter, the stimulus frequency was reduced to 1 Hz, and IPSCs were recorded for another 60 s. In the following, we refer to these two 60-s epochs as challenge period and recovery period, respectively. Recordings were performed at 37°C ($n = 22$) and 26°C ($n = 17$). Exemplary results from a neuron at 26°C and another at 37°C are illustrated in **Figures 9A$_1$,B$_1$**, respectively, and the ensemble data are shown in **Figures 9A$_2$,B$_2$**. As expected, synapses displayed synaptic attenuation during the first 40 s as shown before (cf. **Figures 3B$_2$, 5B$_2$**). By the very end of the challenge period, peak IPSC amplitudes ($IPSC_{60\,s}$) had completely collapsed to

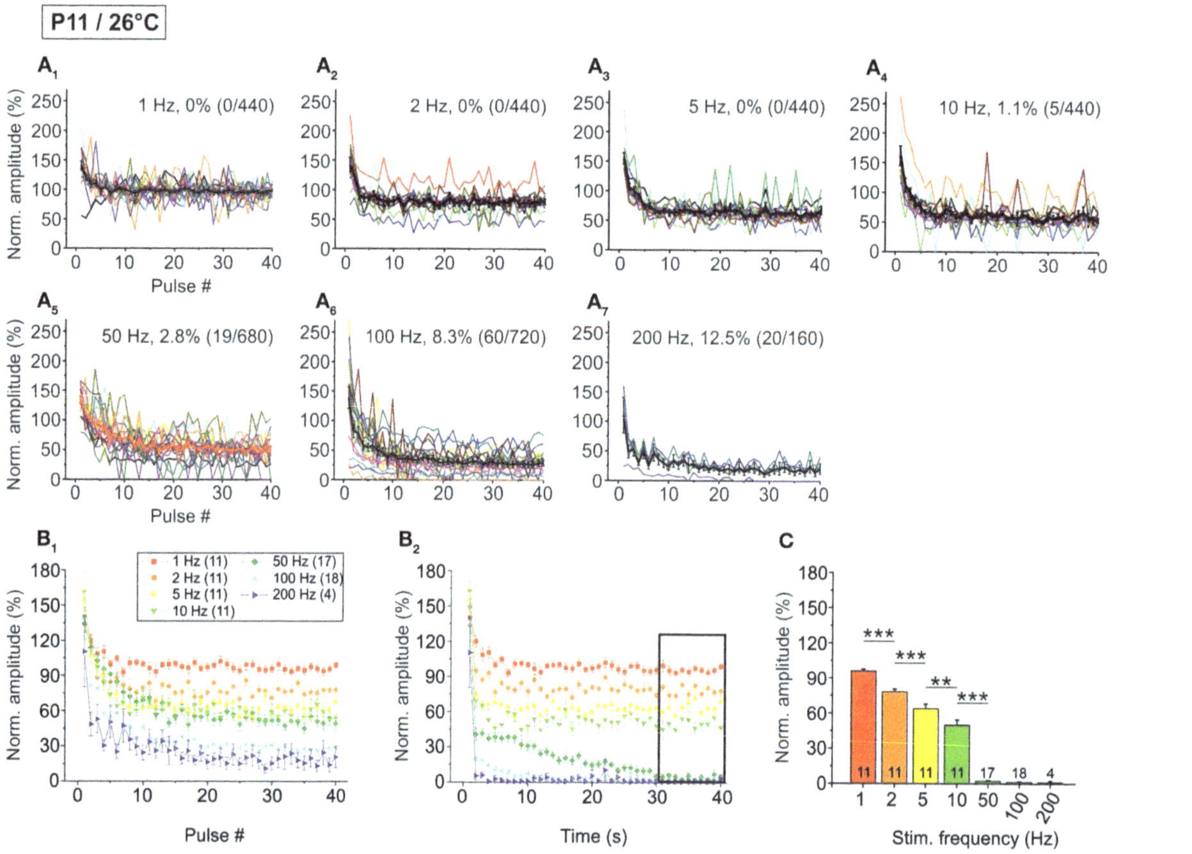

FIGURE 5 | Population data illustrating the frequency-dependent time course of glycinergic IPSC peak amplitudes at P11/26°C. (A_1–A_7) Color-coded plots for all recorded LSO neurons at seven stimulation frequencies ($n = 4$–18, cf. inset in panel B_1), depicting the time course of IPSC amplitudes during the first 40 stimulus pulses. In each panel, the mean values ± s.e.m. are shown in black. The failure rate (%) and the ratio failures/events across neurons are also provided in each panel. **(B_1)** Mean values ± s.e.m. of the first 40 IPSCs obtained in response to different stimulation frequencies. Notice the decline to <40% at frequencies ≥100 Hz. **(B_2)** Mean values ± s.e.m. obtained during the complete 40-s-periods of stimulation (sampled at 1-s-intervals). Color code as in panel **B_1**. Notice the virtual collapse to <10% at frequencies ≥50 Hz. Black frame depicts the last 10 data points in each trace that underwent statistical analysis shown in panel **(C)**. **(C)** IPSC peak amplitudes decreased with increasing stimulation frequency more profoundly than at P11/37°C. *N* numbers in the inset of **(B_1)** correspond to all panels. $^{**}p < 0.01$; $^{***}p < 0.001$.

0.0 ± 0.0% at 26°C, yet they remained at 20.6 ± 3.3% at 37°C (**Figures 9A$_2$,B$_2$**). The latter value did not differ significantly from that obtained after 40 s (27.7 ± 4.8%; $p = 0.226$), corroborating that 37°C responses are quite stable in the second-to-minute range. In contrast, IPSCs declined further between 40 and 60 s at 26°C ($IPSC_{40\,s}$: 2.9 ± 1.4%; $p = 0.049$). Together, this demonstrates that glycinergic MNTB-LSO neurotransmission is sustained at a steady-state level in the minute range only at physiological temperature. The better performance in the minute range at 37°C was also evident in drastically higher peak amplitudes during the last 10 s of the challenge period: at 37°C, the mean $IPSC_{50-60\,s}$ value was 23.3 ± 3.5%, but it was almost 40-fold lower at 26°C (0.6 ± 0.2%; $p = 1 \times 10^{-6}$; **Figures 9C,D**).

During the recovery period, several failures occurred within the first 10 s (60–70 s), albeit considerably fewer at 37°C (26°C: 16.5%; 37°C: 1.4%, **Figures 9A$_2$,B$_2$, Table 4**). Thereafter (70–120 s), only two failures occurred in the 26°C group (0.2%, 2/850) and three failures in the 37°C group (0.3%, 3/1100), indicating that neurotransmission recovered within a few seconds, regardless of temperature (**Figures 9A$_2$,B$_2$**). The course of recovery could be fitted with a mono-exponential function, resulting in τ-values of 9.1 ± 0.7 s at 26°C and 6.3 ± 0.9 s at 37°C (**Figures 9C,E**). Thus, the recovery at 26°C was almost 1.5-fold slower than at 37°C ($p = 0.016$). In comparison to recovery data obtained from IPSCs in other neuron types, the recovery of MNTB-LSO synapses was similarly fast (P14–14/32–33°C rat neocortex neurons: 4.3 s; (Galarreta and Hestrin, 1998); P10/room temp. rat spinal cord neurons: ca. 8 s; (Ingram et al., 2008); P13–15/31°C mouse cerebellar nucleus neurons: 10 s; (Telgkamp and Raman, 2002), ruling out that they are unusual or even unique in this respect.

At both temperatures, $IPSC_{110-120\,s}$ peak amplitudes of the P11 MNTB-LSO connections were significantly higher than $IPSC_{50-60\,s}$ amplitudes (**Table 3**; estimated recovery: 37°C: 3.6-fold; 26°C: 36.0-fold). $IPSC_{110-120\,s}$ values amounted to 107.7 ± 5.0% of the control value at 26°C and thus were overshooting (cf. Dinkelacker et al., 2000). At 37°C, the corresponding value was significantly lower (83.8 ± 6.4%, $p = 0.007$; **Table 3; Figure 9D**).

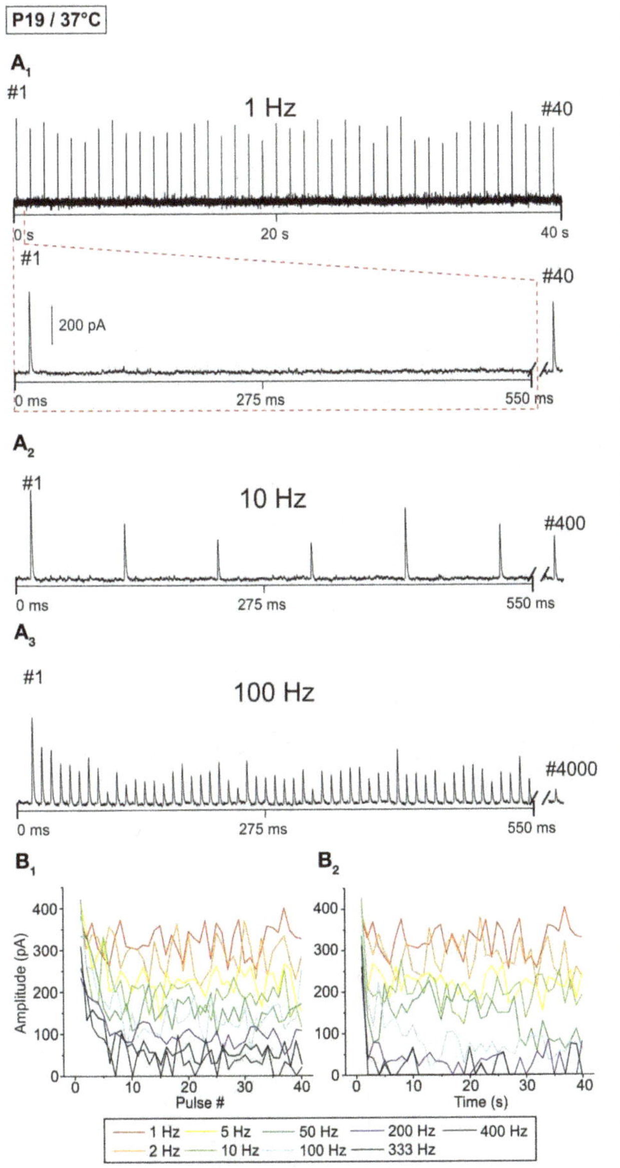

FIGURE 6 | Frequency-dependent changes in evoked glycinergic IPSCs obtained at P19/37°C. (A_1) Original 40 s recording of a representative LSO neuron during 1 Hz stimulation (top). The first 550 ms are time-expanded in the bottom trace (see red-stippled line). The last IPSC during the 40-s-period is shown on the right and depicted by its pulse number (#40). The 200 pA calibration bar is also valid for panels **(A_2,A_3)**. **(A_2,A_3)**, IPSCs during 10 and 100 Hz stimulation, respectively, from the same neuron as in panel **(A_1)**. Similar to **(A_1)**, the last IPSC during the 40-s-period is shown on the right (#400 and #4000, respectively). **(B_1)** Time course of IPSC peak amplitudes from two LSO neurons at eight stimulation frequencies, ranging from 1–400 Hz (for color code, see inset). Peak values to the first 40 pulses (pulse #1–40) are plotted. **(B_2)** Like **(B_1)**, but depicting the time course of IPSC peak amplitudes during the complete 40-s-periods. For each stimulation frequency, peak amplitudes were sampled at 1-s-intervals.

SYNAPTIC ATTENUATION DURING VERY PROLONGED STIMULATION AT P11/37°C (10 TRIALS, 20 MIN, 50 Hz)

As the glycinergic neurotransmission recovered robustly after a 60-s-stimulus train (cf. **Figure 9**), we decided to challenge the synapses even more with the aim to determine their limits. We extended the stimulation time and applied the 60 s/50 Hz challenge and 60 s/1 Hz recovery protocol for a total of ten times (Trial 1–10, **Figure 1B$_2$**), resulting in 30,600 pulses over a period of 20 min. The results from such "marathon experiments" are depicted in **Figure 10**. On average, the glycinergic MNTB-LSO neurotransmission was resistant to very prolonged stimulation, as evidenced by the fact that mean peak amplitudes did not decline below 15% (**Figures 10A,B**). Nevertheless, synaptic augmentation progressed, albeit only slightly, from trial to trial (**Figure 10B**, **Table 3**). For example, the mean $IPSC_{50-60\,s}$ in trial 10 was significantly lower than that in trial 1 (18.3 ± 3.6% vs. 23.3 ± 3.5%, $p = 0.020$). Likewise, the $IPSC_1$ amplitudes declined significantly, albeit only moderately, from trial 1 to trial 10 (**Table 3**). Similar effects were seen for $IPSC_2$, whereas $IPSC_{10}$ and $IPSC_{1\,s}$ did not decline during 20-min stimulation.

We also investigated the development of failures across trials during the challenge period. In a first step, we analyzed all IPSCs during the first 40 pulses. No failure was seen during trial 1, hardly any in trial 5 (0.4%), yet almost 10% in trial 10 (**Table 4**), indicative of some worsening with time. In a second step, we analyzed the failures during the last second of the challenge period (59–60 s). Whereas the percentage of neurons with failures increased only moderately (45.5% in trial 1, 57.1% in trial 5 and 10), the failure rate increased more than 2-fold (from 14.3% in trial 1 to 29.3% in trial 10; **Table 4**), again demonstrating some worsening performance with time.

SYNAPTIC ATTENUATION DURING VERY PROLONGED STIMULATION AT P11/26°C (10 TRIALS, 20 MIN, 50 Hz)

We next performed the "marathon experiments" at 26°C to assess temperature dependency (**Figure 11**). In contrast to 37°C, the mean $IPSC_1$ amplitude decreased drastically and highly significantly from trial 1–10, becoming more than 3-fold reduced (**Table 3**). Likewise, $IPSC_2$, $IPSC_{10}$, and $IPSC_{1\,s}$ decreased significantly with increasing trial number, and the effects were much more pronounced than at 37°C (**Table 3**). The time course of depression was similar across trials, resulting in almost completely collapsed amplitudes after about 35 s in each case. Mean $IPSC_{50-60\,s}$ peak amplitudes were <5% of the control, with a significant difference between trial 1 and 5 only (**Table 3**, **Figure 11B**), probably because amplitudes jittered considerably. This result was due to the almost complete collapse obvious already in trial 1.

Trial-to-trial development of the failures also displayed major differences between 26 and 37°C. During the first 40 pulses, the failure rate increased steadily from trial to trial, and much more rapidly than at 37°C. This was evidenced by a considerable increase from 14.3 to 22.3% between trial 1 and 5 at 26°C, yet a negligible increase from 0 to 0.4% at 37°C (**Table 4**). During the last second of the challenge period, however, there was no major difference in the failure rate between trials. Again, this can be explained by the fact that depression was already very robust in the first trial. Together, the failure rate was considerably higher than at 37°C.

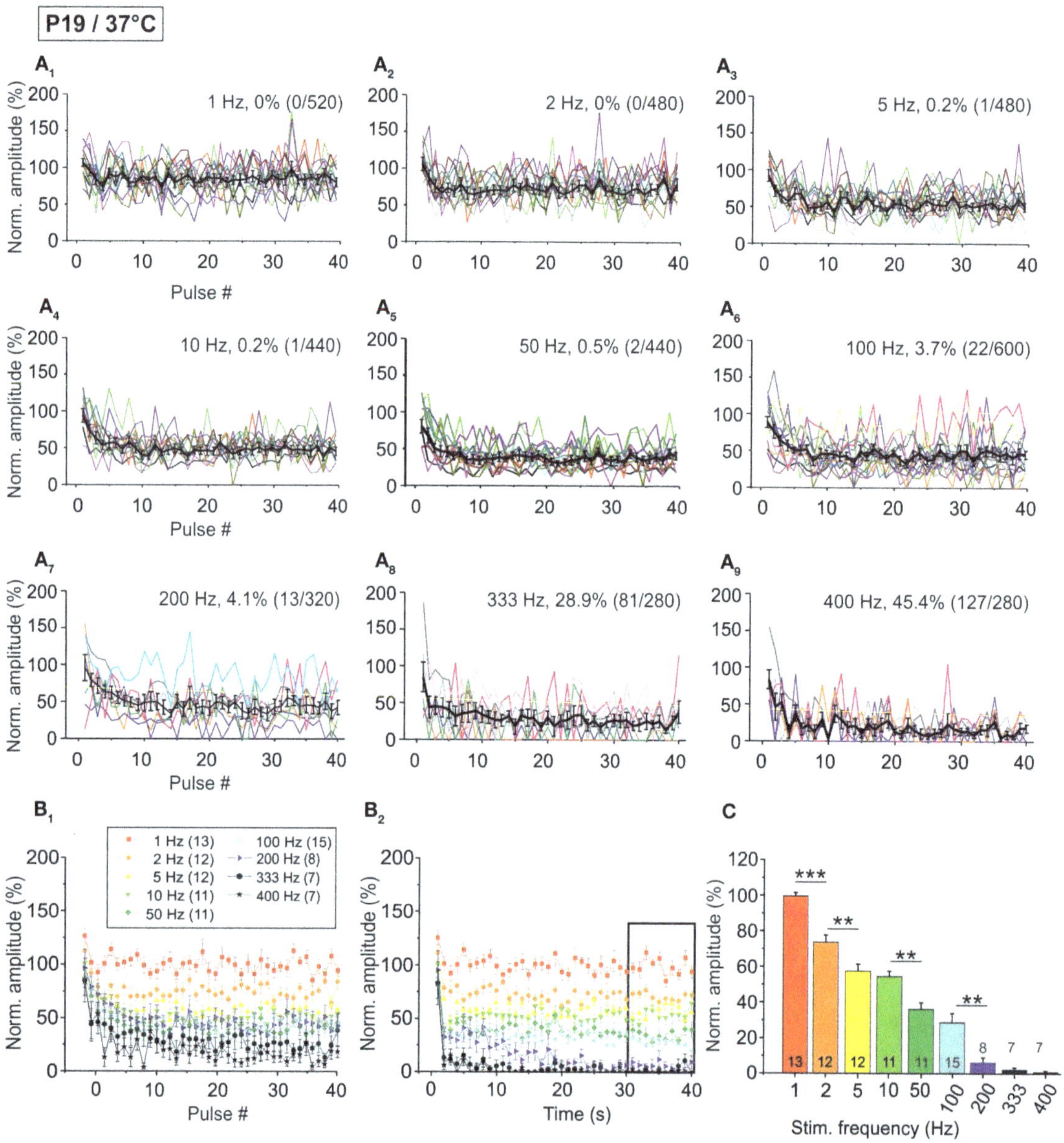

FIGURE 7 | Population data illustrating the frequency-dependent time course of glycinergic IPSC peak amplitudes at P19/37°C. (A_1–A_9), Color-coded plots for all recorded LSO neurons at nine stimulation frequencies ($n = 7$–15, cf. inset in panel B_1), depicting the time course of IPSC amplitudes during the first 40 stimulus pulses. In each panel, the mean values ± s.e.m. are shown in black. The failure rate (%) and the ratio failures/events across neurons are also provided in each panel. **(B_1)** Mean values ± s.e.m. of the first 40 IPSCs obtained in response to different stimulation frequencies. Notice the decline to <50% at frequencies ≥50 Hz. **(B_2)** Mean values ± s.e.m. obtained during the complete 40-s-periods of stimulation (sampled at 1-s-intervals). Color code as in panel **(B_1)**. Notice the gradual decline with frequency up to 200 Hz. Black frame depicts the last 10 data points in each trace that underwent statistical analysis shown in panel **(C)**. **(C)** IPSC peak amplitudes decreased with increasing stimulation frequency, yet stayed at >30% of the control amplitude up to 100 Hz. N numbers in the inset of **(B_1)** correspond to all panels. $^{**}p < 0.01$; $^{***}p < 0.001$.

TEMPERATURE DEPENDENCY OF RECOVERY DURING VERY PROLONGED STIMULATION (10 TRIALS, 20 MIN, 50 Hz)

At both 37 and 26°C, the course of recovery from synaptic attenuation was quite variable across neurons, particularly in later trials (**Figures 10A, 11A**). As assessed by the $IPSC_{50-60\,s}/IPSC_{110-120\,s}$ ratios, peak amplitudes recuperated significantly in all trials and at both temperatures (**Table 3**), but at 37°C, the recovery courses were much more reproducible (**Figures 10B, 11B**). At 37°C, mean $IPSC_{110-120\,s}$ amplitudes amounted to about 76.9–83.8% of the control value, with no significant differences between trial 1–5 and trial 1–10 (**Figure 10B, Table 3**). In contrast, mean $IPSC_{110-120\,s}$ amplitudes at 26°C became significantly reduced more than 2.5-fold (**Figure 11B, Table 3**, 107.7 ± 5.0% in trial 1, 43.9% ± 5.5 in trial 10). For a direct illustration of the temperature-dependent differences and for further quantification, we superimposed the curves obtained

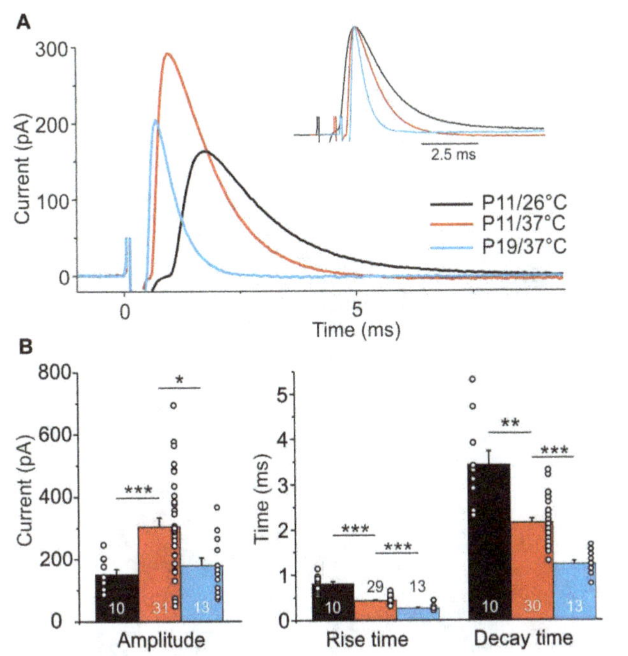

FIGURE 8 | Temperature dependency and age dependency of IPSC kinetics. (A) Average of 40 IPSCs obtained by 1 Hz stimulation at P11/26°C (black), P11/37°C (red), and P19/37°C (blue). Each trace is obtained from a single, representative MNTB-LSO connection. 0 ms corresponds to stimulus onset. Inset depicts traces with aligned peak amplitudes to better visualize differences in rise and decay time. **(B)** Statistical analysis of rise time, decay time, and peak amplitude. Numbers in bars depict the number of analyzed neurons, circles in bars depict single values. $^*p < 0.05$; $^{**}p < 0.01$; $^{***}p < 0.001$.

at both temperatures during trial 1, 5, and 10 (**Figure 12A**). At the end of each challenge period, $\text{IPSC}_{50-60\,\text{s}}$ values at 26°C were consistently lower than at 37°C (**Figures 12A,B**; $p = 1 \times 10^{-6}$, $p = 2 \times 10^{-4}$, $p = 1 \times 10^{-4}$ for trials 1, 5, 10). At the end of the recovery period, however, the situation was more diverse: at 37°C, $\text{IPSC}_{110-120\,\text{s}}$ values were significantly lower than those obtained at 26°C in trial 1, yet they were higher in trial 10. No difference occurred in trial 5 (**Figures 12A,C**; $p = 0.007$, $p = 0.188$, $p = 0.005$ for trials 1, 5, 10).

The temperature dependency of STD and amplitude recovery across trials was reflected by the time course of the failure rates. During the first 40 pulses at 37°C, failure rates of about 10% occurred in trial 10 only, whereas this level was reached already in trial 5 at 26°C (**Table 4**, **Figure 12D**). At the end of the challenge period (59–60 s), the temperature effect on the failure rate was even more pronounced, because values at 26°C exceeded 60% in all trials (**Table 4**, **Figure 12D**). In contrast, the failure rate during 59–60 s was drastically lower at 37°C (<30%), increasing moderately with trial number (**Table 4**, **Figure 12D**). Concerning the recovery at 37°C during the first 10 s (60–70 s), 9.1% of the neurons displayed failures in trial 1, whereas 14.3% did so both in trial 5 and trial 10, demonstrating a mild increase (**Table 4**). At 26°C, however, the percentage of neurons with failures was high already in trial 1 (52.9%) and remained high until the end (**Table 4**). Regarding the 60–70 s failure rate, the recovery of P11/37°C MNTB-LSO synapses was very good initially, yet it deteriorated from trial to trial and became 8.5-fold worse (trial 1: 1.4%; trial 10: 11.9%, **Table 4**, **Figure 12E**). In contrast, at 26°C the failure rate was much higher already from the beginning (trial 1: 16.5%) and remained at this high level during the "marathon experiment" (**Table 4**, **Figure 12E**). Thus, the performance at 37°C in the 20-min range was manifold superior to that at 26°C, but it also became less reliable with time. At the end of the recovery period (110–120 s) in trial 1, the failure rate was negligible at both temperatures (**Table 4**, **Figure 12E**). By the time trial 10 was finished, however, it had increased considerably at both temperatures, with a similar rate of about 10% in both cohorts. Still, the percentage of neurons displaying failures at 26°C was almost twice as high as at 37°C (17.6 vs. 9.5%). Together, these data demonstrate a relatively minor trial-to-trial deterioration of the glycinergic MNTB-LSO transmission at physiological temperature, whereas at lower temperature, the performance becomes impaired quickly.

POSSIBLE CONTRIBUTION OF MNTB AXON CONDUCTION PROBLEMS TO IPSC FAILURES

In a final series of experiments, we addressed the question whether possible AP conduction problems (Bucher and Goaillard, 2011) in axons of MNTB neurons may lead to the absence of neurotransmission and, therefore, to the absence of IPSCs. To do so, we compared our results obtained upon MNTB stimulation (orthodromic, synaptic) while recording from P11/37°C LSO neurons with those obtained via antidromic, non-synaptic stimulation of MNTB axons in the LSO while recording from MNTB neurons in the current-clamp mode. Orthodromic stimulation resulted in high-fidelity synaptic transmission during the first 40 pulses at stimulus frequencies from 1 to 200 Hz (**Figures 13A$_1$,B$_1$**). The great majority of neurons (6 of 8) displayed virtually no failures up to 100 Hz, but the fidelity declined to 98 ± 2% at 200 Hz and 84 ± 0.13% at 333 Hz (**Figure 13C$_1$**). During the last 40 pulses of the 40-s train, however, many more failures were apparent, and 100% fidelity was maintained only up to 10 Hz (**Figures 13A$_2$–C$_2$**). Above 10 Hz, the fidelity rate gradually declined to 83 ± 12% at 50 Hz and to 17 ± 10% at 333 Hz (**Figure 13C$_2$**). 90% fidelity (4 failures in 40 events) was computed at 280 Hz for the first 40 pulses and at 28 Hz for the last 40 pulses.

In the antidromic stimulation experiments, the pattern of successful responses (APs) and failures was quite similar to that obtained via orthodromic stimulation (**Figures 13D–F**). The performance declined with increasing stimulus frequency, such that APs occurred in response to the first 40 pulses in 93 ± 5% of cases at 100 Hz and 83 ± 11% at 200 Hz (**Figure 13F$_1$**). No failure occurred at frequencies ≤50 Hz. During the last 40 pulses, the performance was worse, the respective values being 45 ± 13% at 100 Hz and 6 ± 4% at 200 Hz (**Figure 13F$_2$**). Ninety percent fidelity occurred at 160 Hz during the first 40 pulses and at 55 Hz during the last 40 pulses. Thus, axons of P11/37°C MNTB neurons can conduct APs absolutely reliably up to 50 Hz, even upon very prolonged stimulation. Collectively, the results from orthodromic and antidromic stimulation show

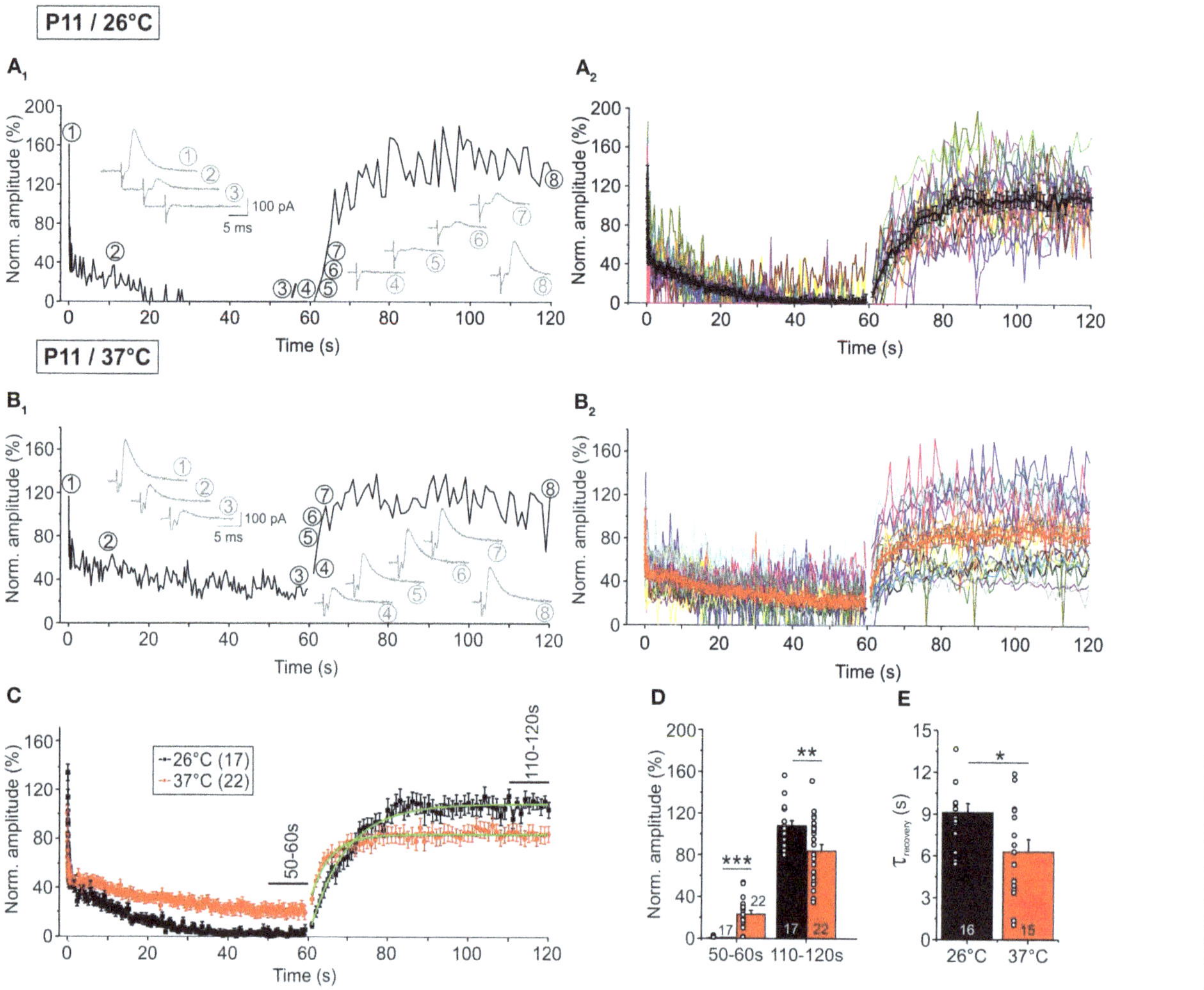

FIGURE 9 | Temperature dependency of STD and recovery of IPSC peak amplitudes at P11. Neurons were stimulated with 50 Hz for 60 s (depression phase) and subsequently stimulated with 1 Hz for another 60 s (recovery phase). **(A_1,B_1)** Time course of the IPSC peak amplitudes of two representative LSO neurons at 26°C **(A_1)** and 37°C **(B_1)**. Insets show eight original IPSCs at the positions marked by encircled numbers. **(A_2,B_2)**. Time course of the IPSC peak amplitudes of all recorded neurons. Mean values ± s.e.m. are shown in black (**A_2**: 26°C, $n = 17$) and red (**B_2**: 37°C, $n = 22$). The mean values represent the simple moving average of five data points, thus smoothing out short-term fluctuations and highlighting longer-term trends. **(C)** Superposition of average time courses to highlight the temperature effects. Mono-exponential fits during the recovery phase were obtained for each condition (green). Data obtained during seconds 50–60 and 110–120 (cf. bars) were used for the statistical analysis shown in panel **(D)**. **(D)** At 26°C, peak amplitudes declined significantly stronger during the depression phase. The opposite finding was obtained for the recovery phase. **(E)** The recovery was significantly faster at 37°C. τ-values were obtained by fitting the time course for each individual neuron. Numbers in bars depict numbers of neurons analyzed. $^*p < 0.05$; $^{**}p < 0.01$; $^{***}p < 0.001$.

that some fidelity decrease in synaptic transmission of the MNTB-LSO connection can be attributed to impaired AP conduction properties of MNTB neurons, rather than to deficits of the synaptic transmission machinery. However, the observed STD behavior is unlikely due to AP conduction problems and is rather a presynaptic effect (as further addressed in the Discussion).

DISCUSSION

Mature LSO neurons receive powerful inhibitory, glycinergic input from MNTB neurons, which are able to respond reliably to high frequency stimulation supplied via the excitatory calyx of Held, up to 800 Hz for brief trains lasting ca. 20 ms (Taschenberger and von Gersdorff, 2000; Mc Laughlin et al., 2008). Our results provide evidence that the subsequent glycinergic MNTB-LSO connections are less astounding in this time range, as they sustain faithful synaptic transmission merely to considerably lower frequencies (ca. 100 Hz at P11/37°C, cf. **Figure 3**). Although featuring robust STD and synaptic attenuation, the P11/37°C connections are nevertheless continuously functional in the 10 s-to-1 min range and, if recovery periods are introduced, neurotransmission is reliably sustained for at least 20 min upon 50 Hz stimulation. The performance crucially depends on temperature, as at 26°C, faithful neurotransmission falls close at >10 Hz, and collapses almost completely during prolonged stimulation with 50 Hz. Our data also demonstrate some moderate maturational changes from P11 to P19. The unusually short glycinergic IPSC decay time likely reflects specifically fast

Table 3 | IPSC peak amplitudes during challenge and recovery periods upon prolonged stimulation (20 min, 50 Hz).

	Challenge						Recovery				
	n	$IPSC_1$	$IPSC_2$	$IPSC_{10}$	$IPSC_{1s}$	$IPSC_{50-60s}$		n	$IPSC_{110-120s}$	$IPSC_{50-60s}/IPSC_{110-120s}$ [P]	Estimated recovery
P11/37°C											
Trial 1	22	100.2 ± 5.1	83.9 ± 4.6	49.4 ± 3.2	45.6 ± 3.4	23.3 ± 3.5	Trial 1	22	83.8 ± 6.4	0.277 ± 0.033 [0.00004]	3.6-fold
Trial 5	21	82.7 ± 7.4	70.0 ± 5.7	41.8 ± 3.4	42.5 ± 4.4	20.7 ± 3.8	Trial 5	21	81.4 ± 6.4	0.235 ± 0.031 [0.00006]	4.3-fold
Trial 10	21	78.1 ± 10.5	69.8 ± 8.5	41.1 ± 5.2	36.7 ± 4.7	18.3 ± 3.6	Trial 10	21	76.9 ± 9.4	0.227 ± 0.035 [0.0002]	4.4-fold
P: Trial 1 vs. Trial 5		0.014	0.013	0.158	0.581	0.048	*P*: Trial 1 vs. Trial 5		0.261		
P: Trial 1 vs. Trial 10		0.029	0.096	0.204	0.196	0.020	*P*: Trial 1 vs. Trial 10		0.385		
P11/26°C											
Trial 1	17	133.5 ± 6.7	113.7 ± 6.6	68.7 ± 8.1	43.8 ± 4.8	0.6 ± 0.2	Trial 1	17	107.7 ± 5.0	0.028 ± 0.017 [0.0003]	36.0-fold
Trial 5	17	59.5 ± 8.1	59.2 ± 6.4	45.9 ± 6.3	33.8 ± 5.2	4.1 ± 1.0	Trial 5	17	68.4 ± 7.2	0.050 ± 0.021 [0.0004]	20.0-fold
Trial 10	17	38.4 ± 5.6	37.6 ± 5.1	28.2 ± 3.6	25.3 ± 5.2	1.6 ± 0.5	Trial 10	17	43.9 ± 5.5	0.037 ± 0.011 [0.0004]	27.0-fold
P: Trial 1 vs. Trial 5		7E-06	3E-06	0.005	0.132	0.003	*P*: Trial 1 vs. Trial 5		3E-06		
P: Trial 1 vs. Trial 10		2E-08	4E-10	4E-05	0.003	0.069	*P*: Trial 1 vs. Trial 10		3E-09		

n, number of neurons. A Wilcoxon-signed rank test was used to account for obvious non-normality of the data, as, e.g., the mean $IPSC_{50-60s}$ equaled 0 in some neurons (complete collapse of responses). Due to the same reason, the ratio $IPSC_{50-60s}/IPSC_{110-120s}$ was determined, instead of the inverse ratio. The estimated recovery is the inverse ratio (e.g., 20-fold, if $IPSC_{50-60s}/IPSC_{110-120s} = 0.05$). Moreover, as some neurons featured mean IPSC values of 0 in the challenge and the recovery phase, they were excluded from the $IPSC_{50-60s}/IPSC_{110-120s}$ analysis. Consequently, n = 22, 21, 18 at 37°C and 17, 16, 16 at 26°C in the Wilcoxon-signed rank test.

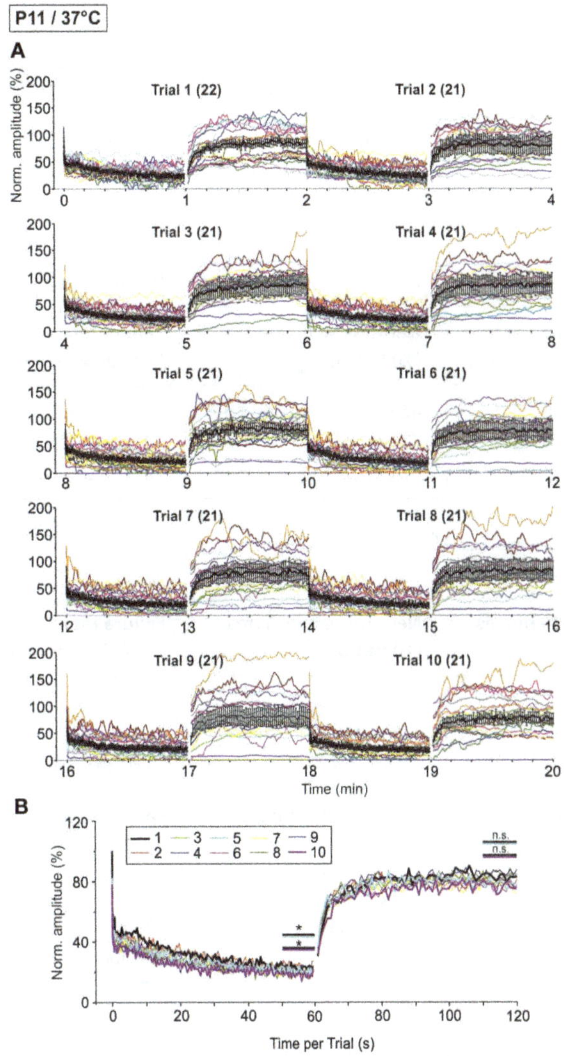

FIGURE 10 | Time course of depression and recovery of IPSC peak amplitudes at P11/37°C upon very prolonged stimulation, lasting 20 min (cf. Figure 1B$_2$). Ten trials of 50 and 1 Hz/60 s episodes were applied (Trial 1–10), amounting to a total of 30,600 stimuli. **(A)** Time course of the IPSC peak amplitudes (one color per neuron, n = 21–22). Mean values ± s.e.m. are shown in black (simple moving average of five data points). Due to the smoothing, failures are no longer discernable. **(B)** Superposition of the ten averaged time courses, illustrating the similarities across trials (traces for trials 1, 5, and 10 are highlighted by a thick black, turquoise, and magenta line, respectively). Statistical comparison was done between trials 1 and 5 and trails 1 and 10. *$p < 0.05$.

deactivation kinetics of GlyRs in LSO neurons, and thus rapid channel closure, which optimizes the integration of interaural intensity differences. On the other hand, the relatively normal recovery course from STD rules out a specific, ultrafast replenishment machinery in glycinergic MNTB-LSO synapses (Cho et al., 2011).

STD in glycinergic synapses is much less studied than in GABAergic synapses, and analyses are surprisingly limited to the auditory system, where they are only recent and rudimentary (Couchman et al., 2010; Kuo and Trussell, 2011). The present

Table 4 | Failure rate analysis during challenge and recovery periods upon prolonged stimulation (20 min, 50 Hz).

P11/37°C					
Challenge			**Recovery**		
First 40 pulses	**Neurons with failures (%) [ratio]**	**Failure rate (%) [failures/events]**	**60–70 s**	**Neurons with failures (%) [ratio]**	**Failure rate (%) [failures/events]**
Trial 1	0 [0/22]	0 [0/880]	Trial 1	9.1 [2/22]	1.4 [3/220]
Trial 5	9.5 [2/21]	0.4 [3/840]	Trial 5	14.3 [3/21]	3.3 [7/210]
Trial 10	23.8 [5/21]	9.9 [83/840]	Trial 10	14.3 [3/21]	11.9 [25/210]
59–60 s	**Neurons with failures (%) [ratio]**	**Failure rate (%) [failures/events]**	**110–120 s**	**Neurons with failures (%) [ratio]**	**Failure rate (%) [failures/events]**
Trial 1	45.5 [10/22]	14.3 [157/1100]	Trial 1	4.5 [1/22]	0.5 [1/220]
Trial 5	57.1 [12/21]	22.3 [234/1050]	Trial 5	0 [0/21]	0 [0/210]
Trial 10	57.1 [12/21]	29.3 [308/1050]	Trial 10	9.5 [2/21]	9.5 [20/210]
P11/26°C					
Challenge			**Recovery**		
First 40 pulses	**Neurons with failures (%) [ratio]**	**Failure rate (%) [failures/events]**	**60–70 s**	**Neurons with failures (%) [ratio]**	**Failure rate (%) [failures/events]**
Trial 1	11.8 [2/17]	2.8 [19/680]	Trial 1	52.9 [9/17]	16.5 [28/170]
Trial 5	17.6 [3/17]	10.4 [71/680]	Trial 5	29.4 [5/17]	14.1 [24/170]
Trial 10	35.3 [6/16]	14.0 [95/680]	Trial 10	47.1 [8/17]	20.0 [34/170]
59–60 s	**Neurons with failures (%)**	**Failure rate (%) [failures/events]**	**110–120 s**	**Neurons with failures (%) [ratio]**	**Failure rate (%) [failures/events]**
Trial 1	100 [17/17]	70.7 [601/850]	Trial 1	0 [0/17]	0 [0/170]
Trial 5	100 [17/17]	67.5 [574/850]	Trial 5	11.8 [2/17]	9.4 [16/170]
Trial 10	100 [17/17]	81.1 [689/850]	Trial 10	17.6 [3/17]	11.8 [20/170]

study provides the most extensive analysis of glycinergic short-term plasticity so far, and it also provides a fresh look into neurotransmission within a prolonged time window. In contrast to most studies, yet similar to two previous reports (Galarreta and Hestrin, 1998; Klyachko and Stevens, 2006), our analysis comprised normalization of the peak amplitude of $IPSC_1$ and all subsequent IPSCs to a control value (average from 40 IPSCs obtained at 1 Hz stimulus frequency prior to high frequency stimulation; **Figures 1B$_1$,B$_2$**). Under these conditions, mean peak amplitudes of $IPSC_1$, which was always evoked after a 3-min pause, exceeded 110% at every stimulus frequency when recordings were performed at 26°C (**Table 1**, **Figures 5B$_1$,B$_2$**). We propose that this initial overshoot may be due to disturbed and imprecise regulation of docking and/or priming processes, resulting in an increased number of fusion-competent vesicles after long periods of synaptic silence (cf. Hermann et al., 2007; Klug, 2011; Klug et al., 2012), for very similar treatises on the lack of chronic background activity on short-term plasticity). As such overshooting IPSCs were rare at 37°C, the disturbed regulation appears to be mainly a temperature artifact. It may also explain the overshooting recovery course in trial 1 at 26°C (**Table 3**, **Figures 9C,D**). Furthermore, our results add a general caveat to room temperature studies, because they overestimate the amplitude of the first event and, consequently, the amount of STD.

IPSC KINETICS

The decay times (P11/37°C: 2.2 ms; P19/37°C: 1.2 ms) were similar to estimated time constants described previously for rodent LSO principal neurons (mouse: 1.3 ms at P21–45/34°C, (Wu and Kelly, 1995); 4.6 ms at P9–19/25°C; (Sterenborg et al., 2010); gerbil: 2.6 ms at P17–23/31–32°C, (Sanes, 1990), yet it was considerably slower than the IPSC decay time constants reported for several other CNS neurons, e.g., P60/33–34°C mouse somatosensory cortex neurons (5.7 ms; Bragina et al., 2008), P7/30–32°C rat spinal cord motoneurons (7.2–17.0 ms; Sadlaoud et al., 2010), P28–35/29°C mouse amygdala neurons (24.1–41.4 ms; Song et al., 2013), P3/35°C chick nucleus laminaris neurons (10.4–54.8 ms; Tang and Lu, 2012), and P4/30°C chick vestibular nuclei neurons (10.5 ms; Shao et al., 2012).

CHARACTERISTICS OF STD

In virtually all of our recordings, IPSC peak amplitudes declined rapidly within the first 10 events, such that the $IPSC_{10}$ amplitudes

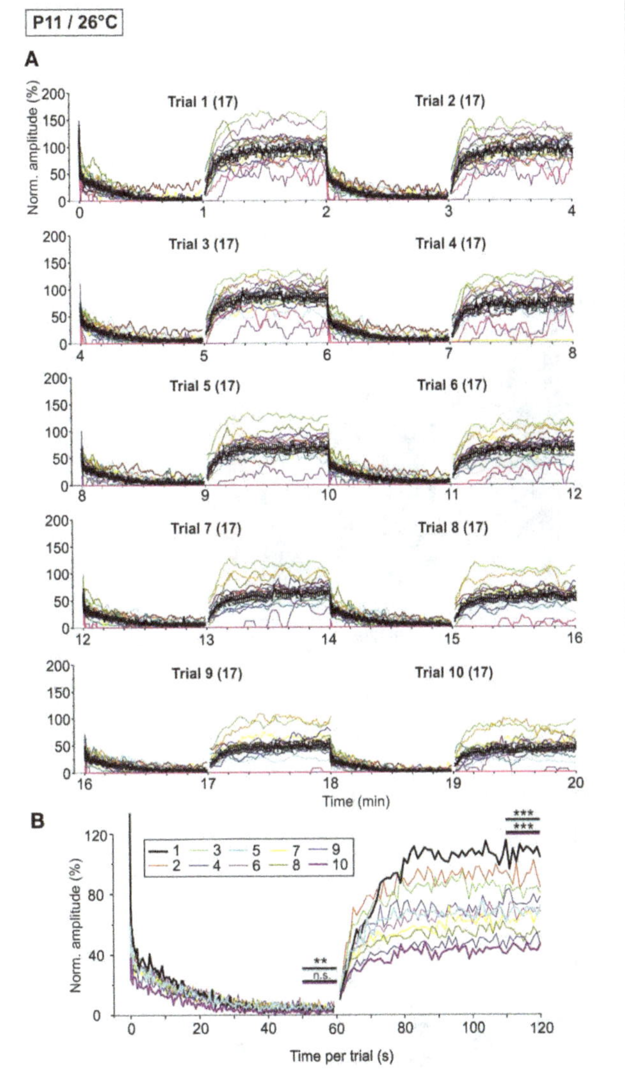

FIGURE 11 | Time course of depression and recovery of IPSC peak amplitudes at P11/26°C upon very prolonged stimulation. Same procedure as in **Figure 10**, except that recordings were obtained at 26°C. **(A)** Time course of the IPSC peak amplitudes (one color per neuron, $n = 17$). Mean values ± s.e.m. are shown in black (simple moving average of five data points). **(B)** Superposition of the ten averaged time courses, illustrating the differences between trials, particularly during the recovery phases (traces for trials 1, 5, and 10 are highlighted by a thick black, turquoise, and magenta line, respectively). Statistical comparison was done between trials 1 and 5 and trails 1 and 10. $^{**}p < 0.01$; $^{***}p < 0.001$.

reached a fraction of the control value at stimulus frequencies ≥5 Hz, regardless of age and temperature (cf. **Figures 3B$_1$, 5B$_1$, 7B$_1$**). Our results further show a prominent frequency dependency. When comparing the amount of STD observed in the present study with data obtained from various synapse types within and outside the auditory system, STD in the glycinergic MNTB-LSO connections is neither particularly high nor low, but tends to be on the low side (**Table 5**, cf. values for 100 Hz stimulus frequency). We found no indication for short-term facilitation, consistent with the idea that STD is key to maintaining temporal precision (Kuba et al., 2002; Cook et al., 2003). The absence of short-term facilitation at P11 and P19 in the MNTB-LSO synapses makes a developmental regulation of short-term plasticity unlikely within this time period, namely depression in younger and facilitation in mature synapses, as described for glutamatergic EPSPs in the rat neocortex between P14 and P18 (Reyes and Sakmann, 1999) and for GABAergic IPSCs in the gerbil auditory cortex after hearing onset (Takesian et al., 2010). Interestingly, preliminary results obtained from P30 MNTB-LSO connections also revealed no short-term facilitation, but STD, consistent with findings from mature endbulb of Held synapses (Wang and Manis, 2008).

PLATEAU PHASE DURING PROLONGED STIMULATION

An interesting observation in the course of STD was a plateau phase, which was centered at 3–4 s and lasted several seconds. This plateau phase was particularly evident at P11/37°C during 50 Hz stimulation (**Figure 9C**). A similar phenomenon, named delayed response enhancement, has been described in glutamatergic hippocampal synapses, where it depends on presynaptic synapsins I and II, is temperature-dependent, and most prominent in adults "marathon experiments." The underlying mechanism of this plateau phase in the glycinergic MNTB-LSO connections needs to be characterized in future studies.

RELIABILITY DURING VERY PROLONGED STIMULATION

The present study is quite novel in that the vast majority of studies so far have assessed synaptic depression with very few tetanic pulses (ca. 20), whereas we have stimulated over a period of 60 s and in 10 trials, resulting in 30,600 stimuli total (marathon experiments). We did so because the IPSC peak amplitudes had not reached a steady state after 20 pulses. Rather, they further declined considerably, e.g., reaching values of <30% after 40 s at 50Hz/P11/37°C (cf. **Table 1**, **Figure 3B$_2$**). These results are consistent with the rare results described elsewhere for such IPSCs, namely in the hippocampus (Klyachko and Stevens, 2006). EPSCs in this intermediate range have been analyzed more extensively, for example in the calyx-MNTB synapse (deLange et al., 2003), primary hippocampal neurons (Sara et al., 2002), autaptic hippocampal neurons (Lambert et al., 2010), and the neuromuscular junction (Richards et al., 2003). Together the results, like ours, show that STD does not reach a plateau level during the first 1–2 s of tetanic stimulation. In our case, steady state was not reached until about 30 s into the experiment.

Glycinergic IPSC peak amplitudes of the MNTB-LSO connection were not depressed below 20%, and the failure rate was remarkably low, even when stimulation lasted ≥1 min (P11/37°C/50 Hz; cf. **Figure 10B**, **Table 4**). As our stimulus paradigm included a 1-min-long recovery period between subsequent 1-min challenge epochs, we cannot rule out that IPSC peak amplitudes will diminish further when the stimulus train is extended beyond 1 min. Preliminary results (Bakker and Friauf, unpublished) indeed demonstrate a further decline when stimulation lasts 10 min, yet the transmission stays functional, with mean peak amplitudes amounting to about 15% during the last minute.

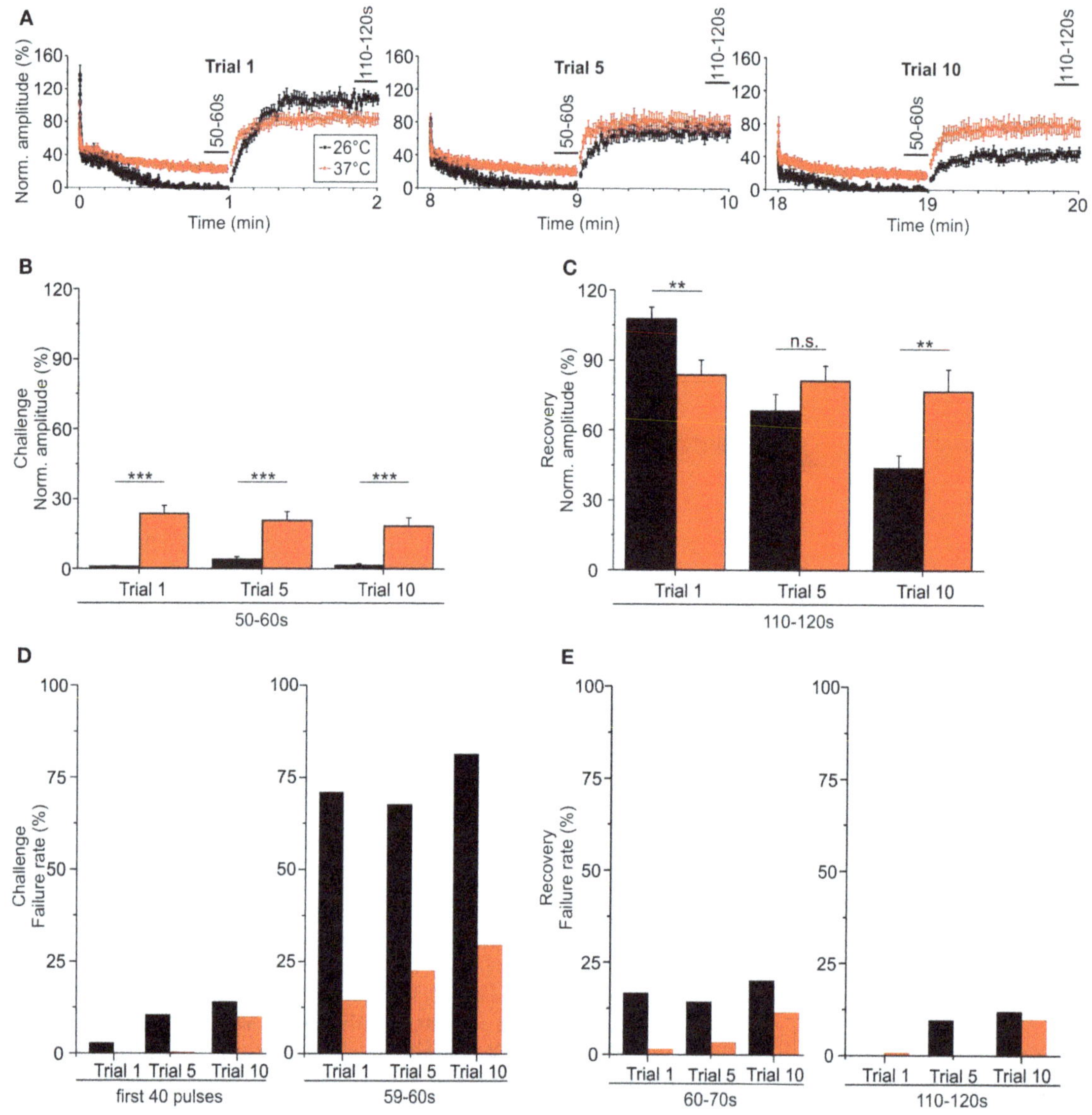

FIGURE 12 | Temperature effect on synaptic attenuation and recovery as assessed during very prolonged stimulation (20 min). (A) Superposition of averaged time courses depicted in **Figures 10, 12** (26°C in black, 37°C in red), highlighting the temperature-dependent differences. **(B)** Statistical analysis of IPSC peak amplitudes at the end of the challenge periods (50–60 s). **(C)** As in **(B)**, but for the end of the recovery periods (110–120 s). **(D)** Failure rate analysis at the beginning (0–800 ms) and end (59–60 s) of the challenge periods. **(E)** As in **(D)**, but at the beginning (60–70 s) and end (110–120 s) of the recovery periods. $^{**}p < 0.01$; $^{***}p < 0.001$.

PARTICIPATION OF GABA$_B$ RECEPTORS?

As shown in gerbils, LSO neurons release GABA during spiking activity which acts as a retrograde transmitter at presynaptic GABA$_B$ receptors, leading to an adjustment of the synaptic strength (Magnusson et al., 2008) and rendering the system more dynamic (Grothe and Koch, 2011). Such a scenario can be ruled out in our experiments which were done under voltage-clamp conditions, thus preventing spike generation. Moreover, in current-clamp conditions, the glycinergic MNTB-LSO neurotransmission would have been hyperpolarizing because of the chloride concentrations used in the bath and pipette solutions. Therefore, we conclude that retrograde signaling via presynaptic GABA$_B$ receptors was not confounded by our pharmacological blockade of these receptors with CGP55845. Still, GABA may have been co-released together with glycine from the axon terminals of MNTB neurons (Kotak et al., 1998; Nabekura et al., 2004; Wojcik et al., 2006) and, thereby, GABA$_B$ receptors may have been affected. However, control experiments in the absence of CGP55845 (not shown) did not reveal any effect on the time course of synaptic depression and recovery. Thus, we exclude a considerable role of GABA$_B$ receptor signaling from our experiments.

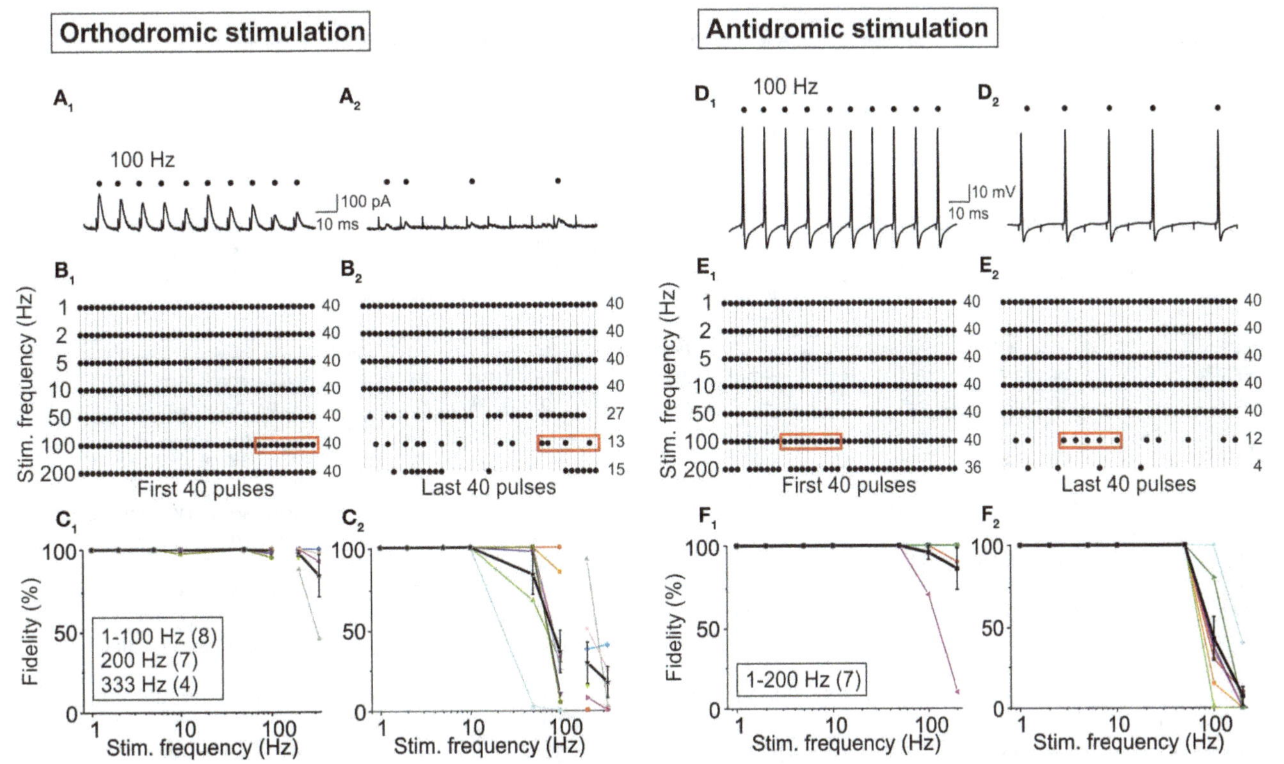

FIGURE 13 | Fidelity analysis of action potentials evoked through orthodromic (A–C) and antidromic (D–F) stimulation of P11/37°C MNTB axons. Orthodromic stimulation was performed as in **Figure 1B$_1$**, and recordings were obtained from LSO neurons. **(A$_1$,A$_2$)** Original current traces from a neuron stimulated with 100 Hz, depicting IPSCs to stimulus number 31–40 **(A$_1$)** and to stimulus number 3991–4000 **(A$_2$)**. Dots mark reliable synaptic transmission; note six failures in **(A$_2$)**. **(B$_1$)** Dot plots from the LSO neuron in **(A)** stimulated with seven frequencies (1–200 Hz), illustrating fidelity behavior to stimulus number 1–40. Frame at 100 Hz depicts the scenario shown in **(A$_1$)**. Numbers to the right are the numbers of successful responses. **(B$_2$)** Dot plots from the same LSO neuron, again stimulated at seven frequencies (1–200 Hz), but now illustrating fidelity behavior to stimulus number 3961–4000. Frame at 100 Hz depicts the scenario shown in **(A$_2$)**. Notice the occurrence of failures at frequencies ≥50 Hz. **(C$_1$,C$_2$),** Fidelity data of the population of LSO neurons as a function of stimulus frequency. 100% fidelity means 40 successful responses to 40 stimuli (40/40). Individual neurons are depicted in different colors, and mean values ± s.e.m. are shown in black. For antidromic stimulation, MNTB axons were stimulated in the LSO and somatic recordings were obtained from MNTB neurons. **(D$_1$,D$_2$)** Original voltage traces from a neuron stimulated with 100 Hz, depicting action potentials to stimulus number 11–20 **(D$_1$)** and to stimulus number 3971–3980 **(D$_2$)**. Dots mark successful antidromic propagation; note five failures in **(D$_2$)**. **(E$_1$)** Dot plots from the MNTB neuron in **(D)** stimulated with seven frequencies (1–200 Hz), illustrating fidelity behavior to stimulus number 1–40. Frame at 100 Hz depicts the scenario shown in **(D$_1$)**. Numbers to the right are the numbers of successful spike propagation. **(E$_2$)** Dot plots from the same MNTB neuron, again stimulated at seven frequencies (1–200 Hz), but now illustrating fidelity behavior to stimulus number 3961–4000. Frame at 100 Hz depicts the scenario shown in **(D$_2$)**. Notice the occurrence of an increasing number of failures at frequencies ≥100 Hz. **(F$_1$,F$_2$)** Fidelity data of the population of LSO neurons ($n = 7$) as a function of stimulus frequency. 100% fidelity means 40 successful responses to 40 stimuli (40/40). Mean values ± s.e.m. are shown by black squares. Notice that the course is similar to that seen upon orthodromic stimulation.

PRE- OR POSTSYNAPTIC MECHANISM OF DEPRESSION?

STD can be caused by depletion of transmitter release (von Gersdorff and Matthews, 1997). Likewise, postsynaptic receptors can be desensitized (Jones and Westbrook, 1996; Overstreet et al., 2000) or saturated (Kirischuk et al., 2002) by repetitive exposure to neurotransmitter. However, in contrast to $GABA_A$ receptors (Jones and Westbrook, 1995), GlyRs do not desensitize heavily, i.e., they do not enter long-lived closed states in the prolonged presence of glycine (Akaike and Kaneda, 1989; Lewis et al., 1991; Melnick and Baev, 1993; Harty and Manis, 1996; Breitinger et al., 2004; Mørkve and Hartveit, 2009). Therefore, we conclude that the observed STD is a presynaptic phenomenon. STD is often ascribed to depletion of the readily releasable vesicle pool (Rizzoli and Betz, 2005). Inactivation of presynaptic Ca^{2+} channels (Forsythe et al., 1998; Xu and Wu, 2005; Hennig et al., 2008; Mochida et al., 2008) or the refractoriness of release sites during repetitive activation (Dittman et al., 2000) are also feasible (see González-Inchauspe et al., 2007, for counterarguments). In contrast, feedback activation of presynaptic autoreceptors, as shown for GABA, glutamate, and adenosine (Takahashi et al., 1998; Zucker and Regehr, 2002), appears to be unlikely, because high-affinity metabotropic GlyRs are unknown. Quite to the contrary, activation of presynaptic ionotropic GlyRs opens presynaptic Cl^- channels, which in turn depolarizes the terminal, resulting in opening of voltage-operated Ca^{2+} channels, elevated presynaptic $[Ca^{2+}]_i$, and, ultimately, enhanced neurotransmitter release (Turecek and Trussell, 2001; Zucker and Regehr, 2002). Our

Table 5 | Comparison of STD in several neuronal systems.

	Synapse type	System	Species	Age	Temperature (°C)	Stimulus frequency (Hz)	Amount of STD (%)	References
1	Glycinergic IPSCs	MNTB-LSO	Mouse	P11 P19 P11	37 37 26	50, 100	51, 50 48, 70 68, 49	Present study
2	Glycinergic IPSCs	MNTB-LSO	Mouse	P11–15	23–25	20	42	Giugovaz-Tropper et al., 2011
3	IPSCs	MNTB-LSO	Gerbil, Mouse	P10–18	32	100	73	Walcher et al., 2011
4	GABAergic IPSPs	IC-MGB	Rat	P8 P16 P27	35	5, 10, 50	77, 77, 93 37, 49, 91 51, 62, 89	Venkataraman and Bartlett, 2013
5	EPSCs	Calyx-MNTB	Mouse	P12–15	20–22	100, 200, 300	50, 65, 85	Wang and Kaczmarek, 1998
6	EPSCs	Calyx-MNTB	Rat	P8–11	21–25	0.5, 10, 100	33, 75, 92	von Gersdorff et al., 1997
7	EPSCs	Calyx-MNTB	Rat	P5–7 P12–14	35	10, 100, 300	85, 95, 95 55, 70, 80	Taschenberger and von Gersdorff, 2000
8	EPSCs	Calyx-MNTB	Rat	P6–10	22–25	20	75	deLange et al., 2003
9	EPSCs	Calyx-MNTB	Mouse	P11–16	22–25	100	70	Oleskevich et al., 2004
10	EPSCs	Endbulb-VCN	Mouse	P11–16	22–25	100	>80	Oleskevich and Walmsley, 2002; Oleskevich et al., 2004
11	EPSCs	Endbulb-VCN	Mouse	P15–21	34	100	>67	Yang and Xu-Friedman, 2008
12	EPSCs	Endbulb-VCN	Mouse	P15–21	34	100	35	Wang and Manis, 2008
13	EPSCs and IPSCs	MSO	Gerbil	P60–100	35	100	70	Couchman et al., 2010
14	EPSCs	Ncl. magnocellularis	Chick	E16–17	31–35	200	85	Zhang and Trussell, 1994
15	EPSCs	Ncl. laminaris	Chick	E18–21	37	100	75	Cook et al., 2003
16	GABAergic IPSCs	Ncl. laminaris	Chick	E17–P3	35	50, 100, 200	40, 75, 85	Tang and Lu, 2012
17	GABAergic IPSCs	Auditory cortex	Gerbil	P8–11 P17–22 P25–30	32	25	87 27 5	Takesian et al., 2010
18	GABAergic IPSCs	Neocortex	Rat	P14–17	32–33	20	60	Galarreta and Hestrin, 1998
19	GABAergic IPSCs	Visual cortex	Rat	P13–19	32–35	20, 50	45, 55	Varela et al., 1999
20	GABAergic IPSCs	Hypothalamus	Rat	P21–27	32.5	10, 20, 50	51, 59, 72	Baimoukhametova et al., 2004
21	GABAergic IPSCs	Hippocampus	Rat	P20–24	34	50	64	Hefft et al., 2002
22	GABAergic IPSCs	Hippocampus	Rat	P14–25	33.5	40	40	Klyachko and Stevens, 2006
22	GABAergic IPSCs	Purkinje cells-Cerebellar nuclei	Mouse	P13–15	31	50	50	Telgkamp and Raman, 2002
24	GABAergic IPSCs	Amygdala	Mouse	P28–35	29	20	66–84	Song et al., 2013
25	GABAergic IPSCs	Spinal cord	Rat	P3–21	Room temp.	10	40	Ingram et al., 2008
26	GABAergic IPSCs	Visual cortex	Rat	P35	Room temp.	30	60	Jiang et al., 2010
27	GABAergic IPSCs	Somatosensory cortex	Mouse	P15–23	32	20	63–87	Ma et al., 2012

Publications 1–17 have analyzed STD in inhibitory and excitatory synapses in the auditory system, publications 18–27 in inhibitory, GABAergic synapses outside the auditory system. For the sake of clarity, the Table does not list any data on short-term facilitation. In each case, the amount of STD is given by: $100x(1 - PSC_{10}/PSC_1)$. In order to allow for a direct comparison between our data and those published, we have recalculated our data listed in ***Table 1*** *accordingly. Abbreviations: IC, inferior colliculus; LSO, lateral superior olive; MGB, medial geniculate body; MNTB, medial nucleus of the trapezoid body; MSO, medial superior olive; VCN, ventral cochlear nucleus.*

results of increased STD at lower temperature are also in line with a presynaptic effect, because physiological temperatures accelerate vesicle recruitment and reduce STD (Kushmerick et al., 2006). Finally, we can rule out a collapse of the chloride driving force in the LSO neurons during repetitive stimulation (Ehrlich et al., 1999), and thus a postsynaptic effect, because we performed our experiments in the whole-cell mode, thereby clamping E_{Cl} to −112 mV and generating a constant driving force.

Our results from antidromic stimulation experiments imply that AP conduction failures, which occurred only at stimulus frequencies ≥100 Hz, do not at all contribute to impaired transmission at frequencies ≤50 Hz. Rather, the presynaptic release machinery cannot faithfully follow such frequencies, resulting in failures. Furthermore, as the fidelity of AP conduction at 100 Hz was 45% (**Figure 13F$_2$**), and as about eight MNTB neurons converge onto a single LSO neuron (Noh et al., 2010; Hirtz et al., 2012), the probability that all of these eight neurons simultaneously display a conduction failure calculates to 1% ($55\%^8$). This low value does not explain the 64% failures in IPSCs (cf. **Figure 13C$_2$**). Only at 200 Hz, AP conduction failures appear to contribute to IPSC failures, because the probability of an AP conduction failure in all eight converging MNTB neurons ($94\%^8 = 61\%$) comes close to the observed IPSC failure rate of

71%. Finally, also the course of recovery cannot be explained by spike failures.

In sum, although glycinergic MNTB-LSO connections undergo STD and synaptic attenuation, they can sustain high frequency transmission at hearing onset over long periods (minutes) and thousands of stimuli if stimulus frequency does not exceed 50 Hz. They also recover robustly ($\tau = 6.3$ s). At P11, connections appear to function quite reliably, yet sustained transmission at 100 Hz is reached only by P19. If the physiological temperature is reduced by 11°C, the performance worsens drastically, in that 10 Hz is now the upper frequency for reliable transmission. Depletion of transmitter release is the most likely cause of the depression behavior. It is important to assess the impact of glycine recycling in replenishing the transmitter pool. One aspect is neuronal and glial re-uptake from the synaptic cleft, which is mediated by glycine transporters 1 and 2, respectively. The role of these transporters may be addressed in pharmacological (Jeong et al., 2010; Jiménez et al., 2011) and genetic knock-out experiments (Gomeza et al., 2003a,b), employing the same battery of stimuli as used in the present study.

AUTHOR CONTRIBUTIONS

Eckhard Friauf, Florian Kramer, and Désirée Griesemer designed the study; Florian Kramer, Dennis Bakker, Sina Brill, and Erik Frotscher performed the experiments; Eckhard Friauf, Désirée Griesemer, Jürgen Franke, and Florian Kramer analyzed data and wrote the paper.

ACKNOWLEDGMENTS

This work was supported by the Deutsche Forschungsgemeinschaft (DFG Grant FR 1784/17-1 to Eckhard Friauf) and the DFG Research Training Group "Molecular, physiological and pharmacological analysis of cellular membrane transport" (GRK 845, Florian Kramer and Eckhard Friauf). Further support was provided by the Center for Mathematical and Computational Modeling, Kaiserslautern. We thank Jennifer Winkelhoff for excellent technical support and Dr. Marco Rust, Dr. Jonathan Stephan, and Alex Fischer for valuable comments on an earlier version of the manuscript.

REFERENCES

Akaike, N., and Kaneda, M. (1989). Glycine-gated chloride current in acutely isolated rat hypothalamic neurons. *J. Neurophysiol.* 62, 1400–1409.

Awatramani, G. B., Turecek, R., and Trussell, L. O. (2005). Staggered development of GABAergic and glycinergic transmission in the MNTB. *J. Neurophysiol.* 93, 819–828. doi: 10.1152/jn.00798.2004

Baimoukhametova, D. V., Hewitt, S. A., Sank, C. A., and Bains, J. S. (2004). Dopamine modulates use-dependent plasticity of inhibitory synapses. *J. Neurosci.* 24, 5162–5171. doi: 10.1523/JNEUROSCI.4979-03.2004

Balakrishnan, V., Becker, M., Löhrke, S., Nothwang, H. G., Güresir, E., and Friauf, E. (2003). Expression and function of chloride transporters during development of inhibitory neurotransmission in the auditory brainstem. *J. Neurosci.* 23, 4134–4145.

Barry, P. H. (1994). JPCalc, a software package for calculating liquid junction potential corrections in patch-clamp, intracellular, epithelial and bilayer measurements and for correcting junction potential measurements. *J. Neurosci. Methods* 51, 107–116. doi: 10.1016/0165-0270(94)90031-0

Bender, K. J., and Trussell, L. O. (2011). Synaptic plasticity in inhibitory neurons of the auditory brainstem. *Neuropharmacology* 60, 774–779. doi: 10.1016/j.neuropharm.2010.12.021

Borst, J. G. G., and Soria van Hoeve, J. (2012). The calyx of Held synapse: from model synapse to auditory relay. *Annu. Rev. Physiol.* 74, 199–224. doi: 10.1146/annurev-physiol-020911-153236

Bragina, L., Marchionni, I., Omrani, A., Cozzi, A., Pellegrini-Giampietro, D. E., Cherubini, E., et al. (2008). GAT-1 regulates both tonic and phasic GABA(A) receptor-mediated inhibition in the cerebral cortex. *J. Neurochem.* 105, 1781–1793. doi: 10.1111/j.1471-4159.2008.05273.x

Breitinger, H. G., Lanig, H., Vohwinkel, C., Grewer, C., Breitinger, U., Clark, T., et al. (2004). Molecular dynamics simulation links conformation of a pore-flanking region to hyperekplexia-related dysfunction of the inhibitory glycine receptor. *Chem. Biol.* 11, 1339–1350. doi: 10.1016/j.chembiol.2004.07.008

Bucher, D., and Goaillard, J. M. (2011). Beyond faithful conduction: short-term dynamics, neuromodulation, and long-term regulation of spike propagation in the axon. *Prog. Neurobiol.* 94, 307–346. doi: 10.1016/j.pneurobio.2011.06.001

Cho, S., Li, G. L., and von Gersdorff, H. (2011). Recovery from short-term depression and facilitation is ultrafast and Ca^{2+} dependent at auditory hair cell synapses. *J. Neurosci.* 31, 5682–5692. doi: 10.1523/JNEUROSCI.5453-10.2011

Cook, D. L., Schwindt, P. C., Grande, L. A., and Spain, W. J. (2003). Synaptic depression in the localization of sound. *Nature* 421, 66–70. doi: 10.1038/nature01248

Couchman, K., Grothe, B., and Felmy, F. (2010). Medial superior olivary neurons receive surprisingly few excitatory and inhibitory inputs with balanced strength and short-term dynamics. *J. Neurosci.* 30, 17111–17121. doi: 10.1523/JNEUROSCI.1760-10.2010

deLange, R. P. J., deRoos, A. D. G., and Borst, J. G. G. (2003). Two modes of vesicle recycling in the rat calyx of Held. *J. Neurosci.* 23, 10164–10173.

Dinkelacker, V., Voets, T., Neher, E., and Moser, T. (2000). The readily releasable pool of vesicles in chromaffin cells is replenished in a temperature-dependent manner and transiently overfills at 37°C. *J. Neurosci.* 20, 8377–8383.

Dittman, J. S., Kreitzer, A. C., and Regehr, W. G. (2000). Interplay between facilitation, depression, and residual calcium at three presynaptic terminals. *J. Neurosci.* 20, 1374–1385.

Ehret, G. (1976). Development of absolute auditory thresholds in the house mouse. *J. Am. Audiol. Soc.* 1, 179–184.

Ehret, G., and Romand, R. (1992). Development of tone response thresholds, latencies and tuning in the mouse inferior colliculus. *Dev. Brain Res.* 67, 317–326. doi: 10.1016/0165-3806(92)90233-M

Ehrlich, I., Löhrke, S., and Friauf, E. (1999). Shift from depolarizing to hyperpolarizing glycine action in rat auditory neurons is due to age-dependent Cl^- regulation. *J. Physiol. (Lond.)* 520, 121–137. doi: 10.1111/j.1469-7793.1999.00121.x

Forsythe, I. D., Tsujimoto, T., BarnesDavies, M., Cuttle, M. F., and Takahashi, T. (1998). Inactivation of presynaptic calcium current contributes to synaptic depression at a fast central synapse. *Neuron* 20, 797–807. doi: 10.1016/S0896-6273(00)81017-X

Galarreta, M., and Hestrin, S. (1998). Frequency-dependent synaptic depression and the balance of excitation and inhibition in the neocortex. *Nat Neurosci.* 1, 587–594. doi: 10.1038/2882

Giugovaz-Tropper, B., González-Inchauspe, C., Di Guimi, M. N., Urbano, F. J., Forsythe, I. D., and Uchitel, O. D. (2011). P/Q-type calcium channel ablation in a mice glycinergic synapse mediated by multiple types of Ca(2+) channels alters transmitter release and short term plasticity. *Neuroscience* 192, 219–230. doi: 10.1016/j.neuroscience.2011.06.021

Gomeza, J., Hülsmann, S., Ohno, K., Eulenburg, V., Szöke, K., Richter, D., et al. (2003a). Inactivation of the glycine transporter 1 gene discloses vital role of glial glycine uptake in glycinergic inhibition. *Neuron* 40, 785–796. doi: 10.1016/S0896-6273(03)00672-X

Gomeza, J., Ohno, K., Hülsmann, S., Armsen, W., Eulenburg, V., Richter, D. W., et al. (2003b). Deletion of the mouse glycine transporter 2 results in a hyperekplexia phenotype and postnatal lethality. *Neuron* 40, 797–806. doi: 10.1016/S0896-6273(03)00673-1

González-Inchauspe, C., Forsythe, I. D., and Uchitel, O. D. (2007). Changes in synaptic transmission properties due to the expression of N-type calcium channels at the calyx of Held synapse of mice lacking P/Q-type calcium channels. *J. Physiol.* 584, 835–851. doi: 10.1113/jphysiol.2007.139683

Grothe, B., and Koch, U. (2011). Dynamics of binaural processing in the mammalian sound localization pathway - The role of GABA(B) receptors. *Hear. Res.* 279, 43–50. doi: 10.1016/j.heares.2011.03.013

Harty, T. P., and Manis, P. B. (1996). Glycine-evoked currents in acutely dissociated neurons of the guinea pig ventral cochlear nucleus. *J. Neurophysiol.* 75, 2300–2311.

Hefft, S., Kraushaar, U., Geiger, J. R., and Jonas, P. (2002). Presynaptic short-term depression is maintained during regulation of transmitter release at a GABAergic synapse in rat hippocampus. *J. Physiol.* 539, 201–208. doi: 10.1113/jphysiol.2001.013455

Hennig, M. H., Postlethwaite, M., Forsythe, I. D., and Graham, B. P. (2008). Interactions between multiple sources of short-term plasticity during evoked and spontaneous activity at the rat calyx of Held. *J. Physiol.* 586, 3129–3146. doi: 10.1113/jphysiol.2008.152124

Hermann, J., Pecka, M., von Gersdorff, H., Grothe, B., and Klug, A. (2007). Synaptic transmission at the calyx of Held under *in vivo*-like activity levels. *J. Neurophysiol.* 98, 807–820. doi: 10.1152/jn.00355.2007

Hirtz, J. J., Braun, N., Griesemer, D., Hannes, C., Janz, K., Löhrke, S., et al. (2012). Synaptic refinement of an inhibitory topographic map in the auditory brainstem requires functional Cav1.3 calcium channels. *J. Neurosci.* 32, 14602–14616. doi: 10.1523/JNEUROSCI.0765-12.2012

Humberto, S., Garcia-Oscos, F., Lu, D., and Atzori, M. (2011). Dynamic modulation of short term synaptic plasticity in the auditory cortex: the role of norepinephrine. *Hear. Res.* 271, 26–36. doi: 10.1016/j.heares.2010.08.014

Ingram, R. A., Fitzgerald, M., and Baccei, M. L. (2008). Developmental changes in the fidelity and short-term plasticity of GABAergic synapses in the neonatal rat dorsal horn. *J. Neurophysiol.* 99, 3144–3150. doi: 10.1152/jn.01342.2007

Jeong, H. J., Vandenberg, R. J., and Vaughan, C. W. (2010). N-arachidonyl-glycine modulates synaptic transmission in superficial dorsal horn. *Br. J. Pharmacol.* 161, 925–934. doi: 10.1111/j.1476-5381.2010.00935.x

Jiang, B., Huang, S., Pasquale, R., Millman, D., Song, L., Lee, H. K., et al. (2010). The maturation of GABAergic transmission in visual cortex requires endocannabinoid-mediated LTD of inhibitory inputs during a critical period. *Neuron* 66, 248–259. doi: 10.1016/j.neuron.2010.03.021

Jiménez, E., Zafra, F., Pérez-Sen, R., Delicado, E. G., Miras-Portugal, M. T., Aragón, C., et al. (2011). P2Y purinergic regulation of the glycine neurotransmitter transporters. *J. Biol. Chem.* 286, 10712–10724. doi: 10.1074/jbc.M110.167056

Jones, M. V., and Westbrook, G. L. (1995). Desensitized states prolong $GABA_A$ channel responses to brief agonist pulses. *Neuron* 15, 181–191. doi: 10.1016/0896-6273(95)90075-6

Jones, M. V., and Westbrook, G. L. (1996). The impact of receptor desensitization on fast synaptic transmission. *Trends Neurosci.* 19, 96–101. doi: 10.1016/S0166-2236(96)80037-3

Kandler, K. (2004). Activity-dependent organization of inhibitory circuits: lessons from the auditory system. *Curr. Opin. Neurobiol.* 14, 96–104. doi: 10.1016/j.conb.2004.01.017

Kim, G., and Kandler, K. (2003). Elimination and strengthening of glycinergic/GABAergic connections during tonotopic map formation. *Nat. Neurosci.* 6, 282–290. doi: 10.1038/nn1015

Kirischuk, S., Clements, J. D., and Grantyn, R. (2002). Presynaptic and postsynaptic mechanisms underlie paired pulse depression at single GABAergic boutons in rat collicular cultures. *J. Physiol.* 543, 99–116. doi: 10.1113/jphysiol.2002.021576

Klug, A. (2011). Short-term synaptic plasticity in the auditory brain stem by using *in-vivo*-like stimulation parameters. *Hear. Res.* 279, 51–59. doi: 10.1016/j.heares.2011.05.011

Klug, A., Borst, J. G., Carlson, B. A., Kopp-Scheinpflug, C., Klyachko, V. A., and Xu-Friedman, M. A. (2012). How do short-term changes at synapses fine-tune information processing? *J. Neurosci.* 32, 14058–14063. doi: 10.1523/JNEUROSCI.3348-12.2012

Klyachko, V. A., and Stevens, C. F. (2006). Excitatory and feed-forward inhibitory hippocampal synapses work synergistically as an adaptive filter of natural spike trains. *PLoS Biol.* 4:e207. doi: 10.1371/journal.pbio.0040207

Kotak, V. C., Korada, S., Schwartz, I. R., and Sanes, D. H. (1998). A developmental shift from GABAergic to glycinergic transmission in the central auditory system. *J. Neurosci.* 18, 4646–4655.

Kuba, H., Koyano, K., and Ohmori, H. (2002). Synaptic depression improves coincidence detection in the nucleus laminaris in brainstem slices of the chick embryo. *Eur. J. Neurosci.* 15, 984–990. doi: 10.1046/j.1460-9568.2002.01933.x

Kuo, S. P., and Trussell, L. O. (2011). Spontaneous spiking and synaptic depression underlie noradrenergic control of feed-forward inhibition. *Neuron* 71, 306–318. doi: 10.1016/j.neuron.2011.05.039

Kushmerick, C., Renden, R., and von Gersdorff, H. (2006). Physiological temperatures reduce the rate of vesicle pool depletion and short-term depression via an acceleration of vesicle recruitment. *J. Neurosci.* 26, 1366–1377. doi: 10.1523/JNEUROSCI.3889-05.2006

Lalor, E. C., Power, A. J., Reilly, R. B., and Foxe, J. J. (2009). Resolving precise temporal processing properties of the auditory system using continuous stimuli. *J. Neurophysiol.* 102, 349–359. doi: 10.1152/jn.90896.2008

Lambert, T. J., Storm, D. R., and Sullivan, J. M. (2010). MicroRNA132 modulates short-term synaptic plasticity but not basal release probability in hippocampal neurons. *PLoS ONE* 29:e15182. doi: 10.1371/journal.pone.0015182

Lewis, C. A., Ahmed, Z., and Faber, D. S. (1991). A characterization of glycinergic receptors present in cultured rat medullary neurons. *J. Neurophysiol.* 66, 1291–1303.

Liberman, M. C. (1978). Auditory nerve response from cats raised in a low-noise chamber. *J. Acoust. Soc. Am.* 63, 442–455. doi: 10.1121/1.381736

Ma, Y. Y., Hu, H., and Agmon, A. (2012). Short-term plasticity of unitary inhibitory-to-inhibitory synapses depends on the presynaptic interneuron subtype. *J. Neurosci.* 32, 983–988. doi: 10.1523/JNEUROSCI.5007-11.2012

MacLeod, K. M. (2011). Short-term synaptic plasticity and intensity coding. *Hear. Res.* 279, 13–21. doi: 10.1016/j.heares.2011.03.001

Magnusson, A. K., Park, T. J., Pecka, M., Grothe, B., and Koch, U. (2008). Retrograde GABA signaling adjusts sound localization by balancing excitation and inhibition in the brainstem. *Neuron* 59, 125–137. doi: 10.1016/j.neuron.2008.05.011

Mc Laughlin, M., van der Heijden, M., and Joris, P. X. (2008). How secure is *in vivo* synaptic transmission at the calyx of Held? *J. Neurosci.* 28, 10206–10219. doi: 10.1523/JNEUROSCI.2735-08.2008

Melnick, I. V., and Baev, K. V. (1993). Glycine conductance changes in chick spinal cord neurons developing in culture. *Neuroscience* 52, 347–360. doi: 10.1016/0306-4522(93)90162-9

Mikaelian, D., and Ruben, R. J. (1965). Development of hearing in the normal CBA-J mouse. *Acta Oto-Laryngol.* 59, 451–461. doi: 10.3109/00016486509124579

Mochida, S., Few, A. P., Scheuer, T., and Catterall, W. A. (2008). Regulation of presynaptic $Ca_V2.1$ channels by Ca^{2+} sensor proteins mediates short-term synaptic plasticity. *Neuron* 57, 210–216. doi: 10.1016/j.neuron.2007.11.036

Mok, S. M. H., Fricker, A. C., Weil, A., and Kew, J. N. C. (2009). Electrophysiological characterisation of the actions of kynurenic acid at ligand-gated ion channels. *Neuropharmacology* 57, 242–249. doi: 10.1016/j.neuropharm.2009.06.003

Mørkve, S. H., and Hartveit, E. (2009). Properties of glycine receptors underlying synaptic currents in presynaptic axon terminals of rod bipolar cells in the rat retina. *J. Physiol. (Lond.)* 587, 3813–3830. doi: 10.1113/jphysiol.2009.173583

Nabekura, J., Katsurabayashi, S., Kakazu, Y., Shibata, S., Matsubara, A., Jinno, S., et al. (2004). Developmental switch from GABA to glycine release in single-central synaptic terminals. *Nat. Neurosci.* 7, 17–23. doi: 10.1038/nn1170

Noh, J., Seal, R. P., Garver, J. A., Edwards, R. H., and Kandler, K. (2010). Glutamate co-release at GABA/glycinergic synapses is crucial for the refinement of an inhibitory map. *Nat. Neurosci.* 13, 232–238. doi: 10.1038/nn.2478

Oleskevich, S., and Walmsley, B. (2002). Synaptic transmission in the auditory brainstem of normal and congenitally deaf mice. *J. Physiol.* 540, 447–455. doi: 10.1113/jphysiol.2001.013821

Oleskevich, S., Youssoufian, M., and Walmsley, B. (2004). Presynaptic plasticity at two giant auditory synapses in normal and deaf mice. *J. Physiol.* 560, 709–719. doi: 10.1113/jphysiol.2004.066662

Overstreet, L. S., Jones, M. V., and Westbrook, G. L. (2000). Slow desensitization regulates the availability of synaptic GABA(A) receptors. *J. Neurosci.* 20, 7914–7921.

Regehr, W. G. (2012). Short-term presynaptic plasticity. *Cold Spring Harb. Perspect. Biol.* 4:a005702. doi: 10.1101/cshperspect.a005702

Reyes, A., and Sakmann, B. (1999). Developmental switch in the short-term modification of unitary EPSPs evoked in layer 2/3 and layer 5 pyramidal neurons of rat neocortex. *J. Neurosci.* 19, 3827–3835.

Richards, D. A., Guatimosim, C., Rizzoli, S. O., and Betz, W. J. (2003). Synaptic vesicle pools at the frog neuromuscular junction. *Neuron* 39, 529–541. doi: 10.1016/S0896-6273(03)00405-7

Rizzoli, S. O., and Betz, W. J. (2005). Synaptic vesicle pools. *Nat. Rev. Neurosci.* 6, 57–69. doi: 10.1038/nrn1583

Sadlaoud, K., Tazerart, S., Brocard, C., Jean-Xavier, C., Partalier, P., Brocard, F., et al. (2010). Differential plasticity of the GABAergic and glycinergic synaptic transmission to rat lumbar motoneurons after spinal cord injury. *J. Neurosci.* 30, 3358–3369. doi: 10.1523/JNEUROSCI.6310-09.2010

Sanes, D. H. (1990). An *in vitro* analysis of sound localization mechanisms in the gerbil lateral superior olive. *J. Neurosci.* 10, 3494–3506.

Sanes, D. H., and Friauf, E. (2000). Development and influence of inhibition in the lateral superior olivary nucleus. *Hear. Res.* 147, 46–58. doi: 10.1016/S0378-5955(00)00119-2

Sara, Y., Mozhayeva, M. G., Liu, X., and Kavalali, E. T. (2002). Fast vesicle recycling supports neurotransmission during sustained stimulation at hippocampal synapses. *J. Neurosci.* 22, 1608–1617.

Shao, M., Hirsch, J. C., and Peusner, K. D. (2012). Plasticity of spontaneous excitatory and inhibitory synaptic activity in morphologically defined vestibular nuclei neurons during early vestibular compensation. *J Neurophysiol.* 107, 29–41. doi: 10.1152/jn.00406.2011

Song, C., Xu, X. B., He, Y., Liu, Z. P., Wang, M., Zhang, X., et al. (2013). Stuttering interneurons generate fast and robust inhibition onto projection neurons with low capacity of short term modulation in mouse lateral amygdala. *PLoS ONE* 8:e60154. doi: 10.1371/journal.pone.0060154

Sonntag, M., Englitz, B., Kopp-Scheinpflug, C., and Rübsamen, R. (2009). Early postnatal development of spontaneous and acoustically evoked discharge activity of principal cells of the medial nucleus of the trapezoid body: an *in vivo* study in mice. *J. Neurosci.* 29, 9510–9520. doi: 10.1523/JNEUROSCI.1377-09.2009

Sonntag, M., Englitz, B., Typlt, M., and Rübsamen, R. (2011). The calyx of Held develops adult-like dynamics and reliability by hearing onset in the mouse *in vivo*. *J. Neurosci.* 31, 6699–6709. doi: 10.1523/JNEUROSCI.0575-11.2011

Sterenborg, J. C., Pilati, N., Sheridan, C. J., Uchitel, O. D., Forsythe, I. D., and Barnes-Davies, M. (2010). Lateral olivocochlear (LOC) neurons of the mouse LSO receive excitatory and inhibitory synaptic inputs with slower kinetics than LSO principal neurons. *Hear. Res.* 270, 119–126. doi: 10.1016/j.heares.2010.08.013

Takahashi, T., Kajikawa, Y., and Tsujimoto, T. (1998). G-protein-coupled modulation of presynaptic calcium currents and transmitter release by a $GABA_B$ receptor. *J. Neurosci.* 18, 3138–3146.

Takesian, A. E., Kotak, V. C., and Sanes, D. H. (2010). Presynaptic $GABA_B$ receptors regulate experience-dependent development of inhibitory short-term plasticity. *J. Neurosci.* 30, 2716–2727. doi: 10.1523/JNEUROSCI.3903-09.2010

Tang, Z. Q., and Lu, Y. (2012). Two GABAA responses with distinct kinetics in a sound localization circuit. *J. Physiol.* 590, 3787–3805. doi: 10.1113/jphysiol.2012.230136

Taschenberger, H., Leao, R. M., Rowland, K. C., Spirou, G. A., and von Gersdorff, H. (2002). Optimizing synaptic architecture and efficiency for high-frequency transmission. *Neuron* 36, 1127–1143. doi: 10.1016/S0896-6273(02)01137-6

Taschenberger, H., and von Gersdorff, H. (2000). Fine-tuning an auditory synapse for speed and fidelity: developmental changes in presynaptic waveform, EPSC kinetics, and synaptic plasticity. *J. Neurosci.* 20, 9162–9173.

Telgkamp, P., and Raman, I. M. (2002). Depression of inhibitory synaptic transmission between Purkinje cells and neurons of the cerebellar nuclei. *J. Neurosci.* 22, 8447–8457.

Temchin, A. N., Rich, N. C., and Ruggero, M. A. (2008). Threshold tuning curves of chinchilla auditory nerve fibers. II. Dependence on spontaneous activity and relation to cochlear nonlinearity. *J. Neurophysiol.* 100, 2899–2906. doi: 10.1152/jn.90639.2008

Thompson, A. M. (2000). Facilitation, augmentation and potentiation at central synapses. *Trends Neurosci.* 23, 305–312. doi: 10.1016/S0166-2236(00)01580-0

Trussell, L. O. (2002). Modulation of transmitter release at giant synapses of the auditory system. *Curr. Opin. Neurobiol.* 12, 400–404. doi: 10.1016/S0959-4388(02)00335-5

Turecek, R., and Trussell, L. O. (2001). Presynaptic glycine receptors enhance transmitter release at a mammalian central synapse. *Nature* 411, 587–590. doi: 10.1038/35079084

Varela, J. A., Song, S., Turrigiano, G. G., and Nelson, S. B. (1999). Differential depression at excitatory and inhibitory synapses in visual cortex. *J Neurosci.* 19, 4293–4304.

Venkataraman, Y., and Bartlett, E. L. (2013). Postnatal development of synaptic properties of the GABAergic projection from inferior colliculus to auditory thalamus. *J. Neurophysiol.* 109, 2866–2882. doi: 10.1152/jn.00021.2013

von Gersdorff, H., and Borst, J. G. G. (2002). Short-term plasticity at the calyx of Held. *Nat. Rev. Neurosci.* 3, 53–64. doi: 10.1038/nrn705

von Gersdorff, H., and Matthews, G. (1997). Depletion and replenishment of vesicle pools at a ribbon-type synaptic terminal. *J Neurosci.* 17, 1919–1927.

von Gersdorff, H., Schneggenburger, R., Weis, S., and Neher, E. (1997). Presynaptic depression at a calyx synapse: the small contribution of metabotropic glutamate receptors. *J. Neurosci.* 17, 8137–8146.

Walcher, J., Hassfurth, B., Grothe, B., and Koch, U. (2011). Comparative post-hearing development of inhibitory inputs to the lateral superior olive in gerbils and mice. *J. Neurophysiol.* 106, 1443–1453. doi: 10.1152/jn.01087.2010

Wang, L. Y., and Kaczmarek, L. K. (1998). High-frequency firing helps replenish the readily releasable pool of synaptic vesicles. *Nature* 394, 384–388. doi: 10.1038/28645

Wang, Y., and Manis, P. B. (2006). Temporal coding by cochlear nucleus bushy cells in DBA/2J mice with early onset hearing loss. *J. Assoc. Res. Otolaryngol.* 7, 412–424. doi: 10.1007/s10162-006-0052-9

Wang, Y., and Manis, P. B. (2008). Short-term synaptic depression and recovery at the mature mammalian endbulb of Held synapse in mice. *J. Neurophysiol.* 100, 1255–1264. doi: 10.1152/jn.90715.2008

Wang, Y., O'Donohue, H., and Manis, P. (2011). Short-term plasticity and auditory processing in the ventral cochlear nucleus of normal and hearing-impaired animals. *Hear. Res.* 279, 131–139. doi: 10.1016/j.heares.2011.04.018

Wang, Y., Ren, C., and Manis, P. B. (2010). Endbulb synaptic depression within the range of presynaptic spontaneous firing and its impact on the firing reliability of cochlear nucleus bushy neurons. *Hear. Res.* 270, 101–109. doi: 10.1016/j.heares.2010.09.003

Wojcik, S. M., Katsurabayashi, S., Guillemin, I., Friauf, E., Rosenmund, C., Brose, N., et al. (2006). A shared vesicular carrier allows synaptic corelease of GABA and glycine. *Neuron* 50, 575–587. doi: 10.1016/j.neuron.2006.04.016

Wong, A. Y., Graham, B. P., Billups, B., and Forsythe, I. D. (2003). Distinguishing between presynaptic and postsynaptic mechanisms of short-term depression during action potential trains. *J. Neurosci.* 23, 4868–4877.

Wu, S. H., and Kelly, J. B. (1995). Inhibition in the superior olivary complex: pharmacological evidence from mouse brain slice. *J. Neurophysiol.* 73, 256–269.

Xu, J., and Wu, L. G. (2005). The decrease in the presynaptic calcium current is a major cause of short-term depression at a calyx-type synapse. *Neuron* 46, 633–645. doi: 10.1016/j.neuron.2005.03.024

Yang, H., and Xu-Friedman, M. A. (2008). Relative role of different mechanims of depression at the mouse endbulb of Held. *J. Neurophysiol.* 99, 2510–2521. doi: 10.1152/jn.01293.2007

Yin, T. C. T. (2002). "Neural mechanisms of encoding binaural localization cues in the auditory brainstem," in *Integrative Functions in the Mammalian Auditory Pathway,* eds Oertel, Fay, and Popper (New York, NY: Springer-Verlag), 99–159.

Zhang, S., and Trussell, L. O. (1994). Voltage clamp analysis of excitatory synaptic transmission in the avian nucleus magnocellularis. *J. Physiol.* 480, 123–136.

Zucker, R. S., and Regehr, W. G. (2002). Short-term synaptic plasticity. *Annu. Rev. Physiol.* 64, 355–405. doi: 10.1146/annurev.physiol.64.092501.114547

12

Distribution of glycine receptors on the surface of the mature calyx of Held nerve terminal

Johana Trojanova[1], Akos Kulik[2,3], Jiri Janacek[4], Michaela Kralikova[1], Josef Syka[1] and Rostislav Turecek[1]*

[1] *Department of Auditory Neuroscience, Laboratory of Synaptic Transmission, Institute of Experimental Medicine, Academy of Sciences of the Czech Republic, Prague, Czech Republic*
[2] *Department of Physiology II, University of Freiburg, Freiburg, Germany*
[3] *BIOSS Centre for Biological Signalling Studies, University of Freiburg, Freiburg, Germany*
[4] *Department of Biomathematics, Institute of Physiology, Academy of Sciences of the Czech Republic, Prague, Czech Republic*

***Correspondence:**
Rostislav Turecek, Department of Auditory Neuroscience, Laboratory of Synaptic Transmission, Institute of Experimental Medicine, Academy of Sciences of the Czech Republic, Videnska 1083, Prague 4 - Krc, Czech Republic
e-mail: turecek@biomed.cas.cz

The physiological functions of glycine receptors (GlyRs) depend on their subcellular locations. In axonal terminals of the central neurons, GlyRs trigger a slow facilitation of presynaptic transmitter release; however, their spatial relationship to the release sites is not known. In this study, we examined the distribution of GlyRs in the rat glutamatergic calyx of Held nerve terminal using high-resolution pre-embedding immunoelectron microscopy. We performed a quantitative analysis of GlyR-associated immunogold (IG) labeling in 3D reconstructed calyceal segments. A variable density of IG particles and their putative accumulations, inferred from the frequency distribution of inter-IG distances, indicated a non-uniform distribution of the receptors in the calyx. Subsequently, increased densities of IG particles were found in calyceal swellings, structures characterized by extensive exocytosis of glutamate. In swellings as well as in larger calyceal stalks, IG particles did not tend to accumulate near the glutamate releasing zones. On the other hand, GlyRs in swellings (but not in stalks) preferentially occupied membrane regions, unconnected to postsynaptic cells and presumably accessible by ambient glycine. Furthermore, the sites with increased GlyR concentrations were found in swellings tightly juxtaposed with GABA/glycinergic nerve endings. Thus, the results support the concept of an indirect mechanism underlying the modulatory effects of calyceal GlyRs, activated by glycine spillover. We also suggest the existence of an activity-dependent mechanism regulating the surface distribution of α homomeric GlyRs in axonal terminals of central neurons.

Keywords: presynaptic, glycine receptor, MNTB, calyx of Held, pre-embedding immunoelectron microscopy, spillover

INTRODUCTION

The subcellular distribution of ligand-gated ion channels (LGICs) in neuronal cells is tightly correlated with the physiological functions of the receptors. Somatodendritic receptors reside at subsynaptic sites, generating fast and phasic responses to synaptic transmitters, as well as in extrasynaptic compartments, where they mediate slow or tonic modulation of neuronal activity (Farrant and Nusser, 2005; Muller et al., 2008; Hardingham and Bading, 2010; Vizi et al., 2010; Brickley and Mody, 2012; Kopach and Voitenko, 2013). Numerous immunohistochemistry examinations have shown that synaptic receptors typically form intrasynaptic clusters while extrasynaptic receptors are mostly dispersed (Bernard et al., 1997; Caruncho et al., 1997; Kharazia and Weinberg, 1997; Nusser et al., 1998; Walmsley et al., 1998; Zarei et al., 1999; Kieval et al., 2001; Rubio and Soto, 2001; Geiman et al., 2002; Wei et al., 2003; Masugi-Tokita et al., 2007; Petralia, 2012). Little is known about the localization of LGIC in the plasma membrane of presynaptic nerve terminals. These receptors mediate relatively slow modulation of presynaptic exocytosis and plasticity, and their physiological activation often results from the spillover of neurotransmitters (Danbolt, 2001; Kullmann, 2001; Boehm and Kubista, 2002; Engelman and MacDermott, 2004; Pinheiro and Mulle, 2008; Trigo et al., 2008; Verhoog and Mansvelder, 2011). The surface distribution of LGIC in presynaptic nerve terminals would therefore be expected to be similar to that of extrasynaptic receptors in somatodendritic compartments (Kieval et al., 2001; Belenky et al., 2003; Darstein et al., 2003; Ruiz et al., 2003; Jourdain et al., 2007).

Receptors for inhibitory neurotransmitter glycine form chloride permeable ion channels and belong to the Cys-loop family of LGIC (Lester et al., 2004). Native GlyRs are expressed in both pre- and postsynaptic parts of mature neurons. GlyRs on nerve terminals form homomers of α1 subunits which disperse onto the presynaptic plasma membrane (Turecek and Trussell, 2002; Jeong et al., 2003; Deleuze et al., 2005; Morkve and Hartveit, 2009; Kubota et al., 2010; Hruskova et al., 2012; Xiong et al., 2014) and mediate a slow modulation of neurotransmitter release (Turecek and Trussell, 2001; Jeong et al., 2003; Chu et al., 2012;

Hruskova et al., 2012). GlyRs potentiate exocytosis of glutamate in the calyx of Held, a large axonal terminal of globular bushy cells located in the anteroventral cochlear nucleus and projecting to principal cells (PC) in the medial nucleus of trapezoid body (MNTB). Physiological activation of calyceal GlyRs involves heterosynaptic cross-talk and/or glycine spillover from surrounding glial cells (Turecek and Trussell, 2001; Kopp-Scheinpflug et al., 2008). A mature calyx of Held is comprised of morphologically and functionally distinct parts (Rowland et al., 2000; Wimmer et al., 2006) suggesting an appropriate compartmentalization of calyceal GlyRs. However, the subcellular distribution of GlyRs in the calyx has not yet been reported. By using high resolution immunoelectron microscopy, we show that GlyRs occur in calyceal swellings and stalks, compartments responsible for glutamate release. Moreover, the data show that GlyRs are not just randomly dispersed on the surface of calyx and that their localization pattern depends on the presence of endogenous sources of agonists.

MATERIALS AND METHODS

ANIMALS

Experiments were performed on three adult male Wistar rats (~250 g) obtained from Charles River, Freiburg, Germany or Institute of Physiology, ASCR, Prague, Czech Republic. The care and handling of animals before and during the experimental procedures followed European Union regulations and was approved by the Animal Care and Use Committees of the authors' institutions.

TISSUE PREPARATION

Animals were deeply anesthetized using ketamine-xylazin (100 mg/kg, 16 mg/kg body weight; Calypsol, Gedeon Richter, Hungary; Xylapan, Vétoquiol, UK) and perfused transcardially with 0.9% saline followed by a fixative containing 4% (w/v) paraformaldehyde (Sigma-Aldrich, USA), 15% (v/v) picric acid (saturated aqueous solution; 1.3% in H_2O; Sigma-Aldrich, USA) and 0.05% (v/v) glutaraldehyde (conc. 25%; TAAB, UK) in 0.1 M phosphate buffer (PB). Brains were excised, postfixed, washed in PB, and 50 μm thick coronal sections were cut using the VT100S slicer (Leica, Germany).

PRE-EMBEDDING IMMUNOELECTRON MICROSCOPY

Brainstem sections were cryoprotected in solution containing 25% (w/v) sucrose and 10% (v/v) glycerol in 50 mM PB. The sections were freeze-thawed and incubated in a blocking solution containing 20% (v/v) Chemiblocker (Chemicon, Millipore, USA) in 50 mM Tris-buffered saline (TBS, pH 7.4) for 4 h, followed by incubation with primary antibodies diluted in TBS containing 5% (v/v) Chemiblocker overnight at 4°C. We used polyclonal rabbit antibodies recognizing the second intracellular loop of the α1 subunit of GlyR (0.75 μg/ml) or vesicular GABA transporter (vGAT; 1.7 μg/ml), and polyclonal guinea pig antibodies, against vesicular glutamate transporter 1 (vGluT1; 1.25 μg/ml) (all from Synaptic Systems, Germany). The sections were then incubated in a mixture of biotinylated goat anti-guinea pig IgG antibody (Jackson ImmunoResearch Laboratories, USA) and goat anti-rabbit IgG antibodies coupled to 1.4 nm gold particles (Nanoprobes, USA) overnight at 4°C. After several washes in 25 mM phosphate-buffered saline (PBS), the sections were post-fixed in 1% (v/v) glutaraldehyde in PBS, followed by intensification with HQ Silver Enhancement kit (Nanoprobes) and then incubation in the Vectastain ABC Kit (Vector Laboratories, USA). Sections were further treated with 1% osmium tetroxide (TAAB, UK), stained with 1% (w/v) uranyl acetate (Polysciences, USA), dehydrated in a graded series of ethanol and propylene oxid (Polysciences), and flat-embedded in epoxy resin (Durcupan ACM, Sigma-Aldrich, Gillingham, UK). After polymerization, 70–80 nm thick sections were cut using an ultramicrotome Reichert Ultracut S (Leica, Germany). The slices were examined using the LEO 906E transmission electron microscope (Carl Zeiss, Germany). Images were acquired by BioVision/VarioVision 3.2 software (Soft Imaging System; Olympus).

ANALYSIS OF GlyR IMMUNOLABELING

Calyces of Held were identified as vGluT1 positive structures containing round synaptic vesicles and forming asymmetric synaptic contacts with MNTB PC (**Figures 1A,B,C**; Billups, 2005). Calyceal stalks and swellings were distinguished based on their different morphological properties. Stalks were identified as first order branches of the myelin-free pre-terminal axons (also called axonal heminodes; Leão et al., 2005), extending over the surface of postsynaptic neuron (Rowland et al., 2000; Sätzler et al., 2002; **Figures 1A,F**). Swellings were smaller processes with round cross sections containing numerous synaptic vesicles (Rowland et al., 2000; Wimmer et al., 2006; **Figures 1A,E**). Inhibitory nerve terminals were distinguished as vGluT1-immunonegative and vGAT-immunoreactive boutons that contained pleomorphic vesicles and formed symmetric synaptic contacts with a PC (**Figures 1B,D**; Hruskova et al., 2012). Plasma membrane GlyR-associated IG labeling was analyzed in electron micrographs using ImageJ software,[1] Reconstruct™ software (Fiala, 2005) and IRIS Explorer (NAG, UK). We analyzed images of 2304 cross-sections through calyceal processes. The presynaptic plasma membrane surrounding each section was depicted with a contour line (**Figure 2A**; Tamaru et al., 2001). 11–69 contoured serial sections were used to compile each of the 72 calyceal segments in total (an example of a segment is shown in **Figure 2B**). The surface area of a segment was estimated using the Cavalieri principle (Duerstock et al., 2003). All data are presented as mean ± SD. Statistical significance was assessed using the non-parametric two-tailed Mann-Whitney test, two-tailed Kolmogorov-Smirnov test, unpaired and paired two-tailed Students's *t*-tests or one-way ANOVA followed by Dunnett's or Bonferroni's multiple comparison test, using Prism 5.04 (GraphPad, USA) or XLStat 2014.4.07 (Addinsoft).

RESULTS

NON-UNIFORM DISTRIBUTION OF GlyRs AT THE CALYX OF HELD NERVE TERMINAL

To reveal the surface distribution of presynaptic GlyRs, we performed a quantitative analysis of their plasma membrane-associated labeling with anti-GlyRα1-coupled IG particles in

[1] http://rsbweb.nih.gov/ij/

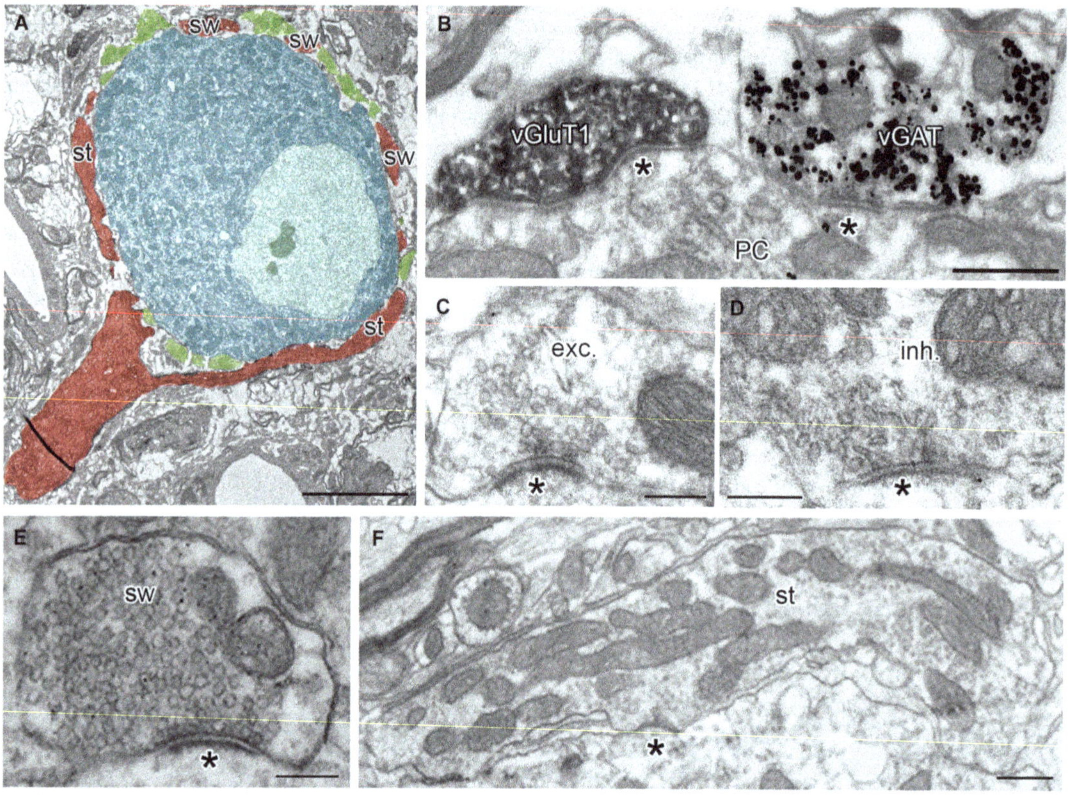

FIGURE 1 | Identification of presynaptic terminals and postsynaptic neurons in adult MNTB. **(A)** A single ultrathin section through the calyx of Held terminal (red) and inhibitory boutons (green) surrounding the soma of the MNTB PC (blue). Note that the pre-calyceal axon branches to large stalks (st) and smaller calyceal swellings (sw). **(B)** An electron micrograph showing a calyceal process, immunostained for vGluT1 (peroxidase reaction end product), and an inhibitory bouton, immunopositive for vGAT (gold particles). Asterisks indicate synaptic contacts between the calyx or the inhibitory ending and a PC. **(C,D)** Examples of putative excitatory (exc.) and putative inhibitory (inh.) active zones (AZ) at synaptic contacts (asterisk) formed by the calyceal or presumed inhibitory nerve terminals on somata of the PC. Note round vs. pleomorphic synaptic vesicles in excitatory vs. inhibitory terminals. **(E,F)** Electron micrographs of cross-sections through calyceal processes considered as swelling (sw) or stalk (st). Scale bars: 5 μm **(A)**, 0.5 μm **(B,F)**, 0.2 μm **(C,D,E)**.

calyceal segments (as illustrated in **Figures 2A,B**). Presynaptic IG particles appeared to have a dispersed distribution (see an example in **Figure 2B**) which contrasted with a clustered distribution of the particles at postsynaptic sites (**Figure 2C**). The latter staining pattern is typical for somatodendritic GlyRs that accumulate in synaptic contacts between inhibitory boutons and MNTB PC (Hruskova et al., 2012). The average surface density of the presynaptic IG particles varied from 0.4 to 39.1 per μm^2 (mean ± S.D. = 9.3 ± 7.2 IG/μm^2, N = 72 segments). The calyx of Held is a complex structure comprising of larger stalks that branch via tiny necks into swellings of various sizes (Rowland et al., 2000; Perkins et al., 2010). To assess the distribution of labeling among differently sized parts of the compartments, we plotted the number of IG particles on each calyceal cross-section against its perimeter length (**Figure 3A**). The number of the particles roughly correlated with the size of each section. A sorting of sections into the six size groups revealed that the number of IG particles increases until the perimeters reach the range of 16–20 μm and then it remains similar in sections with perimeters >20 μm (**Figure 3B**). This implies lower average densities of IG particles in larger sections and suggests that calyces do not have a simply random distribution of GlyRs. To further test this, we measured distances between IG particles (inter-IG distances) along the plasma membrane and compared them across the three sectional size groups (**Figure 3C**). Cumulative frequency histograms of the distances for each group indicate that shorter inter-IG distances (<2 μm) dominate in about 70% of the sections, irrespective of their size. Thus the results indicate sites with increased densities of IG particles implying a preferential localization of GlyRs at some compartments of the calyx.

INCREASED DENSITY OF GlyRs IN CALYCEAL SWELLINGS

Morphologically distinct calyceal compartments were found to differ in number and composition of presynaptic ion channels (Dodson et al., 2003; Elezgarai et al., 2003; Leão et al., 2005; Spirou et al., 2008). We next tested whether two main calyceal structures, stalks and swellings, responsible for the release of glutamate, contain different amounts of presynaptic GlyRs. Calyceal segments were reconstituted

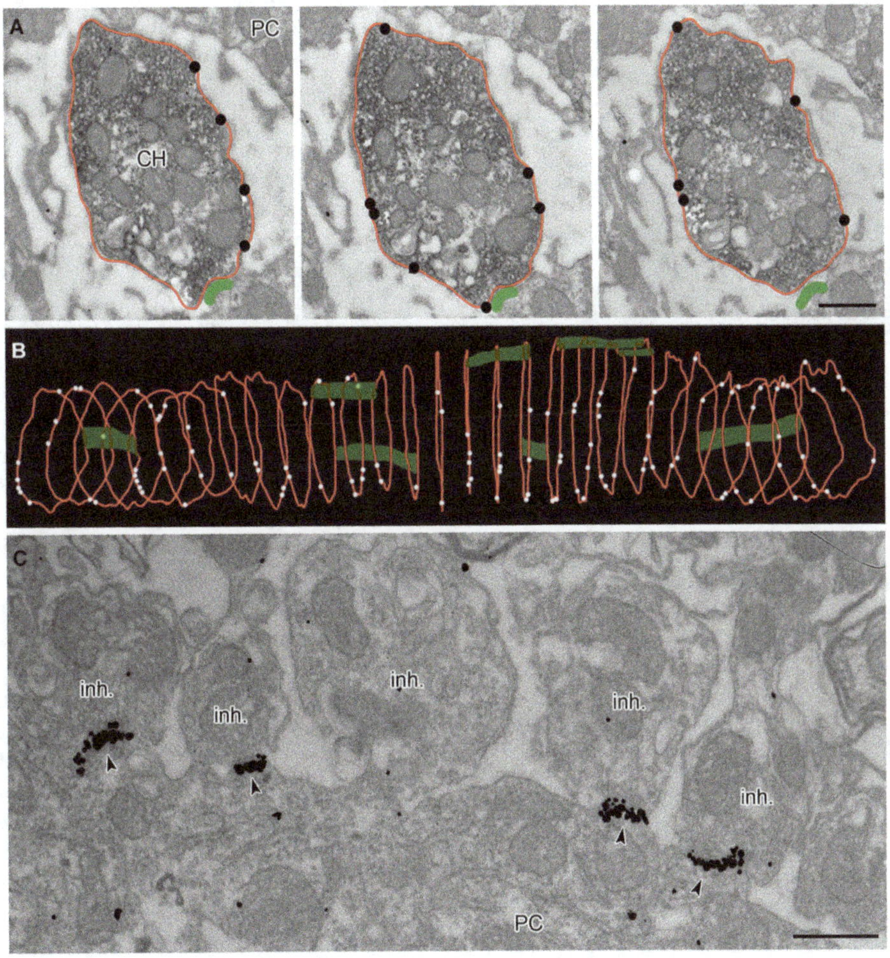

FIGURE 2 | Analysis of membrane-localized GlyR α1-immunoreactivity in 3D reconstructed calyceal processes. (A) Three consecutive ultrathin sections through a calyceal swelling (CH) and a PC. The calyx is immunostained for vGluT1 (peroxidase) and for GlyR α1 (IG particles; indicated by black circles) along the presynaptic plasma membrane (outlined red). The postsynaptic density (PSD) of synaptic contacts between the calyx and PC are labeled green. **(B)** 3D alignment of digital contours of 29 serial sections (each 70 nm thick) of the same calyceal segment as in **(A)**, showing the dispersed distribution of presynaptic GlyRs (white dots) and synaptic contacts (green). **(C)** Electron micrograph showing clusters of GlyR-associated IG particles (arrowheads) at postsynaptic sites juxtaposed with putative inhibitory terminals (inh.). Scale bars: 0.5 μm **(A,C)**.

using 11–69 (33 on average) serial sections through each identified stalk ($N = 11$) (**Figures 4C,D,D'**) or swelling ($N = 51$) (**Figures 4A,A',B,B'**). To estimate the surface density of GlyRs, the number of membrane localized IG particles was counted in each segment and normalized to its surface area value. We found a higher relative density of the particles in swellings (10.8 ± 7.5 IG/μm^2) compared to stalks (5.9 ± 2.7 IG/μm^2, $P < 0.001$; unpaired Student's t-test with Welch's correction for unequal variances) indicating that GlyRs are more frequent in swellings than in stalks.

Some of the presynaptic LGICs were localized near the neurotransmitter releasing active zones (AZ; Jaskolski et al., 2005; Pinheiro and Mulle, 2008; Trigo et al., 2010). Consistent with this, the 3D reconstructions of calyceal stalks and swellings show numerous IG particles near the synaptic junctions (**Figures 4B',D'**). As noted previously (Hermida et al., 2010), calyceal swellings form more synaptic contacts with the postsynaptic cell than stalks do. It is therefore possible that an accumulation of GlyRs over the glutamatergic AZ accounts for the more frequent occurrence of the receptors in the swellings. To test this, we compared densities of IG particles in calyceal segments containing various numbers of synaptic junctions. Consistent with the literature we found more junctions in swellings (0.4 ± 0.1 per μm^2) than in stalks (0.3 ± 0.2 per μm^2, $P < 0.05$; unpaired Student's t-test). Serial sections of each calyceal segment were then sorted into five groups based on the number of synaptic junctions (0–4) and IG particles were counted in these subsegments. As shown in **Figure 5A**, IG particle density was similar between the groups indicating that the number of GlyRs did not correlate with the amount of junctions in the subsegments. Furthermore, we tested whether GlyRs show preferential location around the

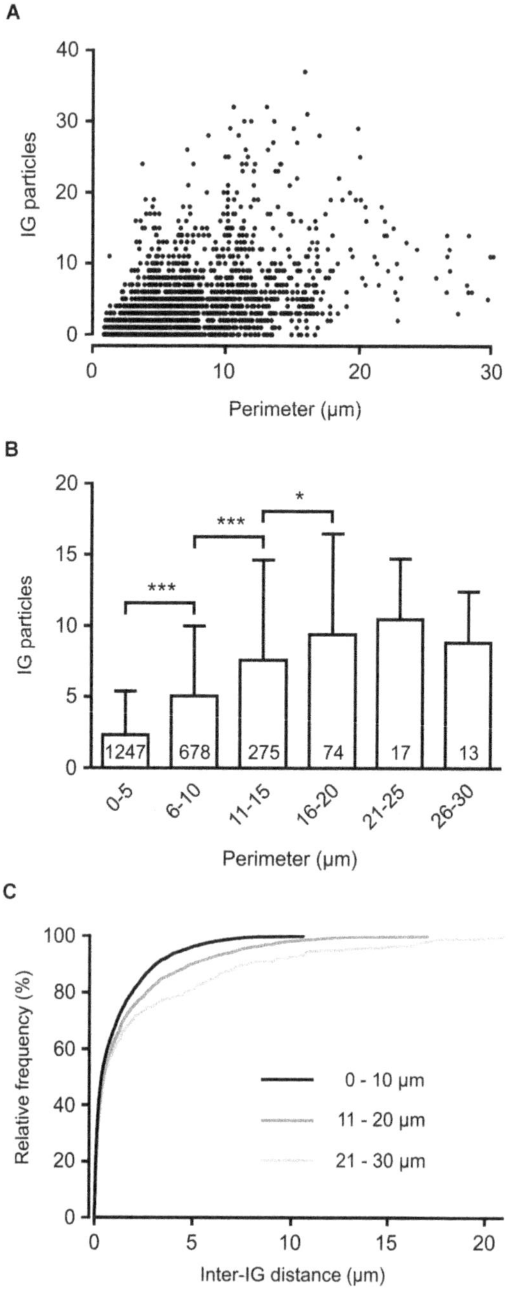

FIGURE 3 | Non-homogenous distribution of GlyRs in the calyx of Held terminal. **(A)** The plot shows IG particle numbers found in variously sized calyceal cross-sections ($N = 2304$). Each perimeter value is derived from the length of a contour line drawn along the presynaptic plasma membrane (as illustrated in **Figure 2A**). **(B)** Bar graph comparing IG particle numbers in sections sorted into six groups based on their perimeter length. *** $P < 0.001$; * $P < 0.05$; Bonferroni's multiple comparison test. The number inside each column indicates sample size of the group. **(C)** Cumulative histograms of inter-IG distances measured in the sections sorted into three size groups as indicated. Note that shorter inter-IG distances dominate in all distributions.

AZ. Perisynaptic heteroreceptors are observed to lie within tens to hundreds of nanometers from the edges of synaptic contacts (Jones and Wonnacott, 2004; Nyíri et al., 2005; Paspalas and Goldman-Rakic, 2005). The length of the postsynaptic density (PSD) in sections through the calyx of Held synapses appears to be quite variable and spans the range of several hundreds of nanometers (Rowland et al., 2000; Sätzler et al., 2002; Taschenberger et al., 2002; Hermida et al., 2010). To estimate proportions of GlyRs spatially related to the AZ, we therefore compared IG particle densities in 2 µm-long, PSD containing membrane regions (left and right borders of the region were placed 1 µm aside from the middle of PSD; see inset in **Figure 5B**), and in the rest of the membrane in sections containing a single synaptic contact. The data in **Figure 5B** show that the relative amounts of particles in membrane parts adjacent to an AZ (Perisynaptic) are not significantly different from the amounts found in more distant parts (Extrasynaptic) (9.0 ± 6.2 IG/µm^2 vs. 10.8 ± 9.2 IG/µm^2; paired Student's *t*-test). Thus the results do not indicate an elevated intrasynaptic or perisynaptic IG labeling, which argues against the possibility that a higher density of GlyRs in swellings is caused by their preferential location around the AZ.

The 3D reconstructions shown in **Figure 4** also suggest that IG particles could distribute on the surface of swellings and stalks differently. In swellings, IG particles appear to be more frequent on the side which is not contacting the postsynaptic soma (**Figures 4B,B'**). In stalks, the particles seem to prefer the side which is facing the PC (**Figures 4D,D'**). To test this, we compared distributions of IG particles along the perimeters of cross-sections obtained from stalks and swellings. In each section we measured perimeter distances between every IG particle and a point which was arbitrarily set at the horizontal edge of a section (see inset in **Figure 5C**). The cumulative frequency distributions of the distances normalized against the perimeter length are shown in **Figure 5C** (black lines). Differences between the histograms are consistent with the assumption that in swellings, IG particles occupy more frequently locations that roughly correspond to the plasma membrane that is not in contact with the postsynaptic cell ($P < 0.001$; Kolmogorov-Smirnov test). This is supported by more pronounced difference between the distributions after exclusion of sections without clear contacts between calyces and PC (**Figure 5C**, gray lines).

The assumption was further tested by counting IG particles in two parts of the surface of calyceal segments (see inset in **Figure 5D**). The first part comprised the plasma membranes that contacted the postsynaptic cell body (including those enclosing the extended extracellular spaces; Rowland et al., 2000) while the second part included membranes that were not in contact with the postsynaptic cell. The borders separating these membrane parts are indicated by white arrowheads in **Figure 4A**. As shown in **Figure 5D**, IG particle density was significantly higher in the latter part of the surface of swellings but not of stalks. Thus the data support a differential distribution of GlyRs in stalks and swellings and suggest that increased densities of GlyRs in calyceal swellings could at least partially be explained by an accumulation of the receptors at the side that faces away from the body of the MNTB principal neuron.

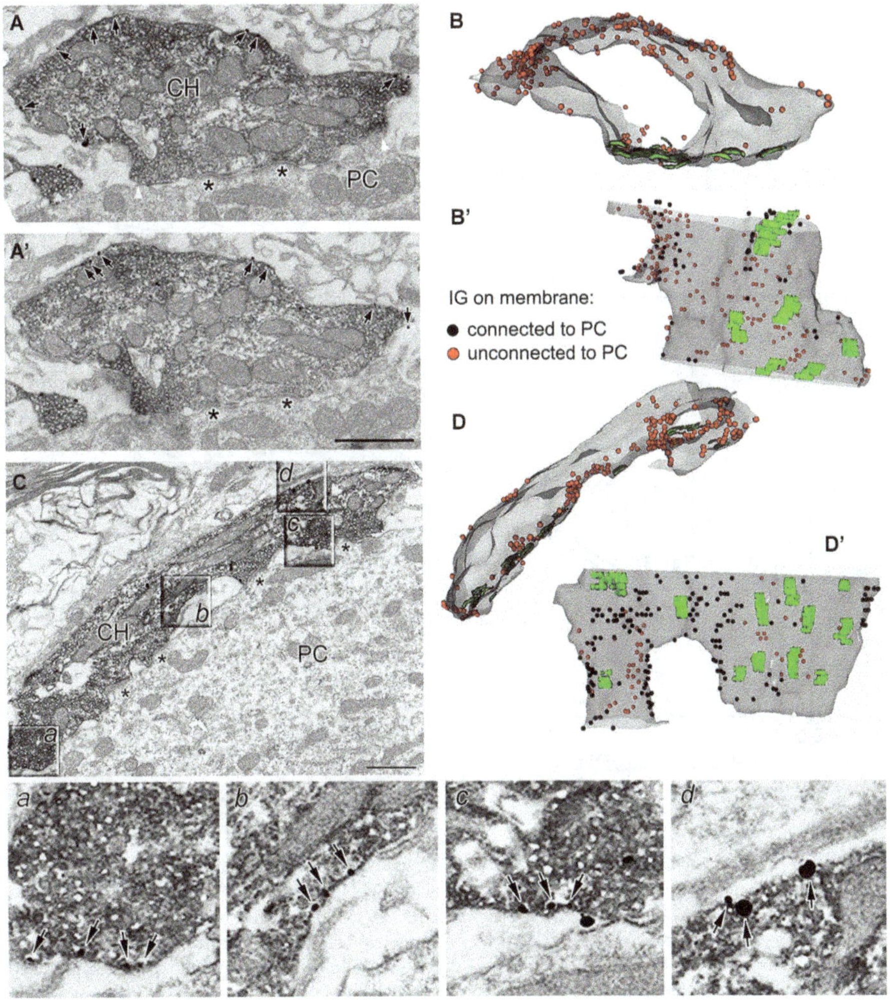

FIGURE 4 | Localization of GlyRs in identified calyceal processes. **(A,A')** Two consecutive sections through a calyceal swelling (CH) double labeled with antibodies against vGluT1 (peroxidase) and GlyR α1 (IG particles; arrows). Asterisks denote synaptic contacts between the calyx and a PC. White arrowheads in panel A indicate borders between membrane regions that are either connected or unconnected to the soma of a PC. **(B)** A semitransparent superposition of 29 contoured sections as in **(A)** to reconstruct a segment of swelling with several synaptic junctions (green areas) and numerous GlyRs (red dots). **(B')** The same stack of contoured sections as in **(B)** viewed from a different angle (the PC facing side). Black and red dots illustrate GlyRs localized in the calyceal membrane that is either connected or unconnected to the soma of a PC. **(C)** EM image of anti-vGluT1 labeled calyceal stalk immunoreactive for GlyR α1. Sectors in boxes **(a–d)**, displayed on an expanded scale below, show examples of GlyRs (arrows) on plasma membrane that is unconnected **(a,d)** to the postsynaptic cell or that encloses extended extracellular spaces **(b,c)**. **(D)** The 3D reconstruction of 28 serial sections as in **(C)** illustrating a semitransparent segment of calyceal stalk forming synaptic contacts (green areas) with a PC and containing numerous GlyRs (red dots). **(D')** The same stack of contours as in **(D)** viewed from a different angle (the PC facing side). Scale bar: 1 μm **(A',C)**.

ACCUMULATION OF GlyRs IN SWELLINGS IN CLOSE PROXIMITY TO GLYCINERGIC BOUTONS

High-frequency stimulation of glycinergic fibers evokes strychnine-sensitive facilitation of glutamate release from the calyx (Turecek and Trussell, 2001). The heterosynaptic nature of the facilitation led to the proposition that it results from presynaptic GlyR activation by glycine spillover. This mechanism of activation requires the receptors to be located at sites accessible by ambient agonist (Rusakov et al., 1999). Consistent with this assumption, findings in our study (**Figure 5**) indicated GlyRs on the side of the calyx that is exposed to the extracellular space. To provide further insight into the mechanism of presynaptic GlyR activation by endogenous glycine, we analyzed the distribution of the receptors in swellings adjacent to glycinergic boutons. **Figures 6A,B** show numerous IG particles in calyceal parts proximal to putative inhibitory terminal (vGluT1-negative structure that contains pleomorphic synaptic vesicles and forms synaptic contacts with a PC). Using 3D reconstructed segments we measured the spatial distances between each IG particle and the middle of the PSD under the inhibitory AZ (see scheme in **Figure 6D**). The cumulative probability histogram of these distances indicates that most of IG particles lie within ~1.5 μm from the AZ, the distance that roughly matches a small molecule transmitter spillover range (Faber and Korn, 1988;

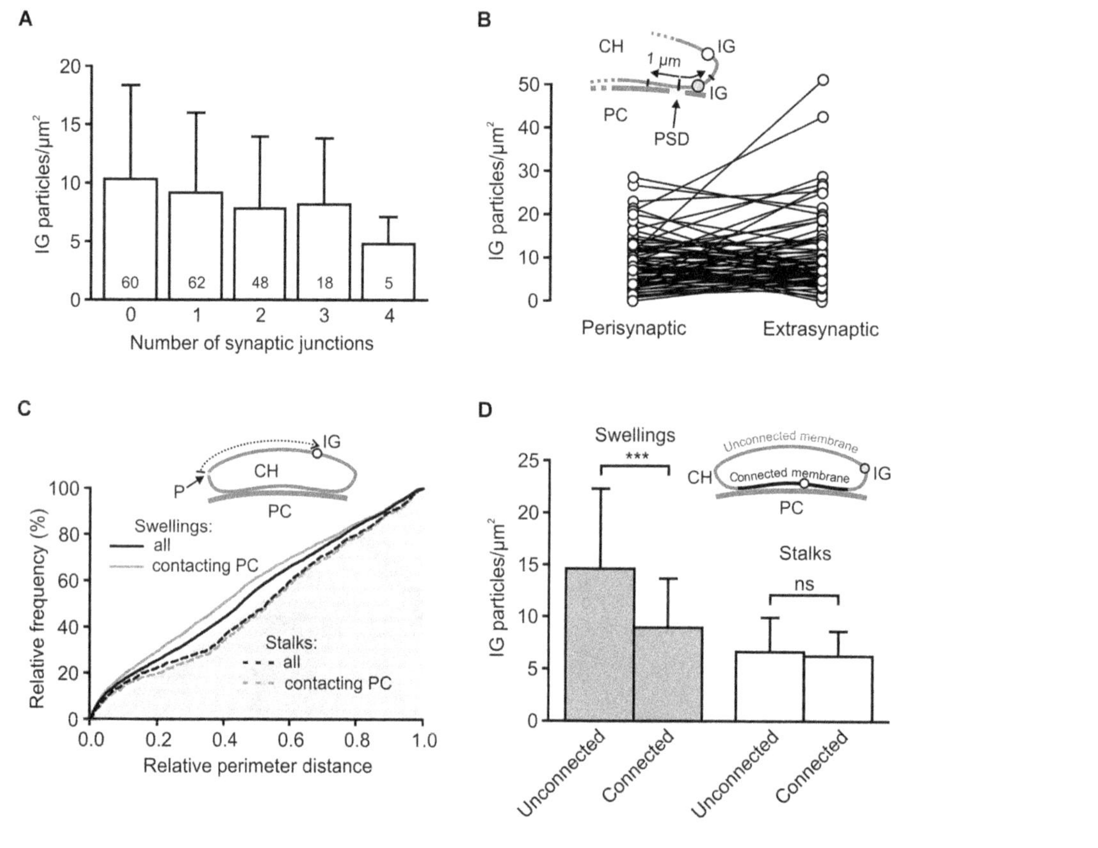

FIGURE 5 | Differential distribution of GlyRs in calyceal swellings and stalks. (A) Bar graph showing the average densities of IG particles in calyceal subsegments containing various numbers (0–4) of synaptic contacts with a PC (see Results). The differences between the groups are not significant (data from all 72 calyceal segments; Bonferroni's Multiple Comparison Test). Numbers inside the columns indicate sample size for each group. **(B)** The plot compares densities of IG particles that lie in two 1 μm-long membrane parts, left and right from the middle of PSD (Perisynaptic), and those that are distributed in remaining parts of sections (Extrasynaptic) constituting subsegments ($N = 71$) containing a single synaptic junction. Sections without any IG particles were excluded from the analysis. Inset illustrates a part of the calyx of Held (CH) process that is apposed to the PSD of the PC and is bearing extrasynaptic (empty circle) and perisynaptic (gray circle) IG particles (IG). **(C)** Cumulative histograms of distances between IG particles and a reference point (P) to compare IG particle distribution along perimeters of sections through stalks (dashed lines) or swellings (solid lines). The reference point was arbitrarily set at the left horizontal edge of a section and the distances were measured in a clockwise direction (see scheme in inset). The histograms were constructed using unbinned data either from all sections (black lines) constituting 51 swellings (6746 distances from 1101 sections) and 11 stalks (1425 distances from 236 sections) or from a selection of sections in which calyceal processes clearly contacted somata of PC (gray lines; swellings: 4572 distances from 628 sections; stalks: 1063 distances from 202 sections) while sections without the contacts were excluded. In all histograms, distributions of IG particles are not random as they significantly differ from the distribution of perimeter distances of surface points, which lie on the hypotenuse of the gray triangle ($P < 0.001$ for all distributions; Kolmogorov-Smirnov test). The exclusion of sections without the contacts led to significant changes in the distribution for swellings (solid gray line; $P < 0.001$; Kolmogorov-Smirnov test) but not for stalks (dashed gray line; Kolmogorov-Smirnov test). **(D)** Bar graph comparing the average densities of IG particles in two regions of the segments from swellings (gray; $N = 36$) and stalks (empty; $N = 11$). The plasma membrane of each section was divided into two parts: membrane connected or unconnected to the soma of a PC (as illustrated by scheme in inset; IG particle in the connected or unconnected membrane is indicated by empty or gray circle). *** $P < 0.001$; paired *t*-test.

Barbour and Hausser, 1997; **Figure 6C**). Interestingly, a comparison between the distribution of IG particles and the distribution of contoured surface points of the segments showed a significant difference (Kolmogorov-Smirnov test, $P < 0.001$) (**Figure 6D**) and suggested a more frequent incidence of GlyRs in parts closer to the inhibitory AZ. Similar differences were not observed in swellings without glycinergic terminals in their vicinity (**Figure 6E**) implying that the surface distribution of GlyRs is affected by the presence of an endogenous agonist.

This hypothesis was further tested by comparing the IG particle distributions along perimeters of calyceal cross-sections in the presence or absence of the inhibitory terminals. Perimeters of sections constituting swellings with or without the inhibitory terminals were similar (7.2 ± 3.1 μm vs. 7.5 ± 3.9 μm; 25%/75% percentiles: 4.6/9.8 μm vs. 4.8/9.3 μm). We therefore analyzed the distribution of IG particles among membrane regions that were proportional to the perimeter length. The perimeter of every section was subdivided to five even intervals and the number of IG particles was counted in each of them (see schemes in **Figures 6F,G**). The data showed a significantly increased amount of particles in a partition adjacent to the inhibitory terminal (**Figure 6F**). In sections without an identified inhibitory bouton

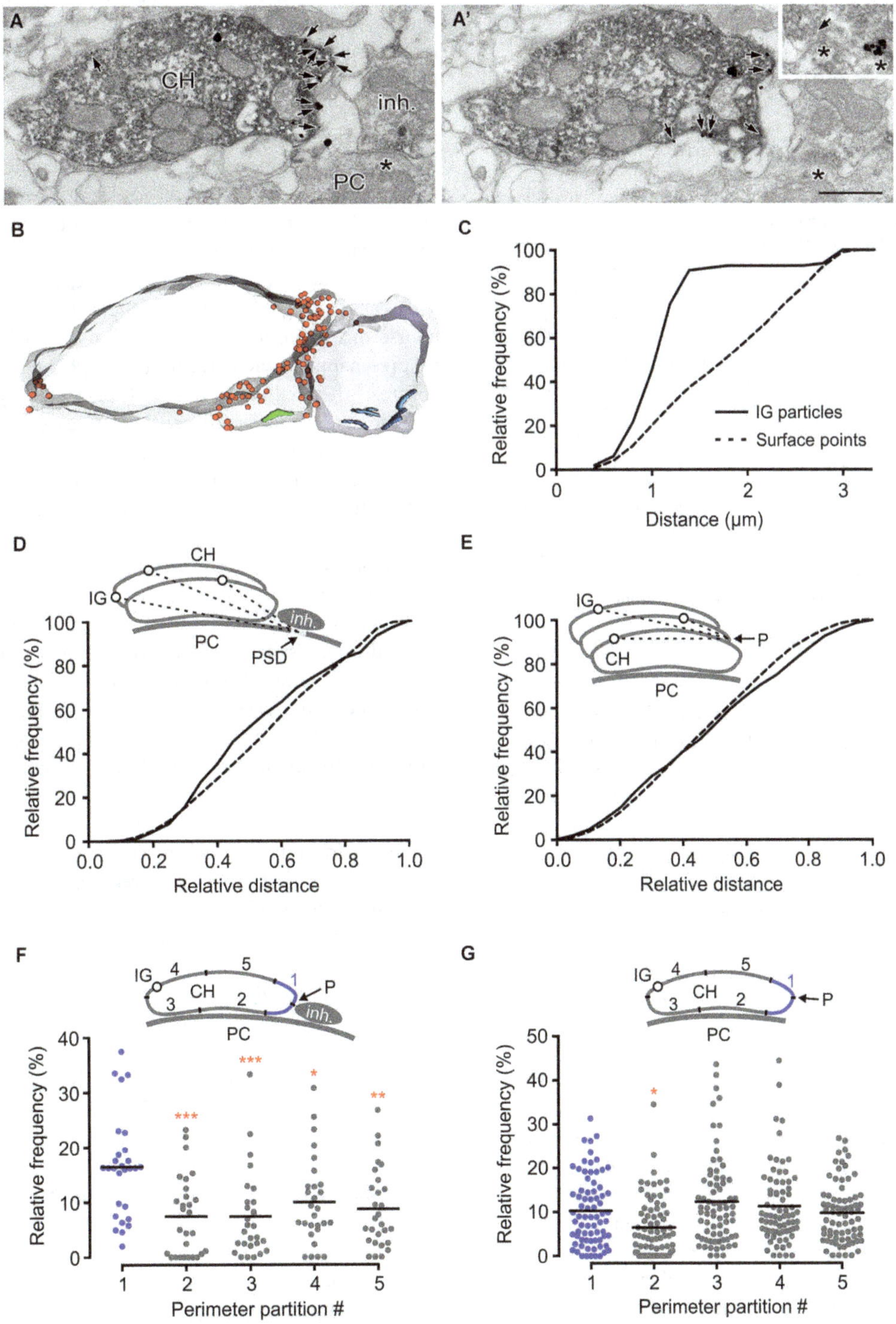

FIGURE 6 | GlyRs tend to accumulate in calyceal swellings proximal to inhibitory boutons. (A,A′) Two consecutive sections through a calyceal swelling (CH), immunoreactive for vGluT1 (peroxidase) and GlyR α1 (IG particles; arrows), and vGluT1-immunonegative, putatively inhibitory bouton (inh.). Asterisks denote synaptic contacts between the bouton and a PC. Inset shows an example of a flat vesicle (arrow) at the inhibitory AZ and a cluster of IG particles at the inhibitory synaptic contact. Scale bar: 0.5 μm. **(B)** Stack of contours from 17 serial EM images of sections shown in **(A)**. Note an accumulation of GlyRs (red dots) in calyceal compartments adjacent to the bouton. Synaptic contacts made by the calyx or by the bouton with a PC are shown in green or blue. **(C)** Cumulative histogram showing the distribution of spatial distances between each IG particle (solid line) on the calyceal segment shown in **(B)** and the middle of the PSD of the nearest synaptic contact between the inhibitory bouton and a PC (see inset in panel **D**). For comparison, the distribution of the distances between digitized points delineating the surface of the swelling and the middle of the PSD is shown (dotted line). The distributions significantly differ ($P < 0.001$; Kolmogorov-Smirnov test; bin width = 0.2 μm). **(D)** The distribution of distances provided by similar measurements as in **(C)**.

(Continued)

FIGURE 6 | Continued
The data was collected from 12 segments of swellings adjacent to an inhibitory bouton. The lengths are plotted relative to the longest distance in a segment. The distributions of IG particles and surface points are significantly different ($P < 0.001$; Kolmogorov-Smirnov test; bin width = 0.05). **(E)** The histogram shows spatial distances between each IG particle (solid line) or each digitized surface point (dotted line) of a calyceal segment and a reference point (P) which was arbitrarily set at the horizontal edge of a section that is placed in the middle of the segment (see inset).The data was collected from 21 swellings without any detectable inhibitory bouton in their proximity. Note that the distribution of IG particles in these segments is not random ($P < 0.001$; Kolmogorov-Smirnov test; bin width = 0.05). **(F,G)** The plots show relative frequencies of IG particles in five partitions of perimeters of sections constituting segments of swellings with (**F**; $N = 14$) or without (**G**; $N = 37$) an inhibitory bouton in their proximity. Each data point represents the sum of IG particles found in one of the partitions of sections constituting a segment (see schemes in insets). Mean values are indicated by horizontal bars. The quantity of IG particles in each partition was normalized to the total number of the particles in a segment. The partitions are labeled 1–5 while that containing a reference point (blue in each inset) is the partition #1. The reference point was set either as an intersection of the calyceal membrane and a link between midpoints of cross-sections through a swelling and a bouton **(F)** or at the horizontal edge of a swelling **(G)**. Note significantly increased amounts of IG particles in the partition adjacent to the inhibitory bouton. *** $P < 0.001$; ** $P < 0.01$; * $P < 0.05$; Dunnett's multiple comparison test (data from the partition #1 were used as a control).

this localization pattern was not observed (**Figure 6G**). Thus the data shows that the surface distribution of presynaptic GlyRs is consistent with the activation of the receptors by glycine spillover from inhibitory terminals. Moreover, the data suggests that the distribution of the receptors in calyceal processes depends on the presence of glycinergic nerve terminals. The average density of IG particles in swellings with or without an inhibitory bouton in their proximity was not significantly different (11.9 ± 8.3 IG/μm^2 vs. 10.0 ± 7.4 IG/μm^2; unpaired Student's t-test). This indicated that the presence of inhibitory AZ affects the location of GlyRs rather than their overall expression level in calyceal swellings.

DISCUSSION

In this study we analyzed the distribution of GlyR-associated IG particles in the mature calyx of Held nerve terminal. To discriminate between the presynaptic and postsynaptic labeling, we used antibodies that recognize an intracellular part of the receptor (Hruskova et al., 2012). Our data suggests that the locations of presynaptic GlyRs correlate with both the function of the receptors and their accessibility for endogenous agonists. We found the strongest labeling in calyceal swellings, compartments releasing glutamate and characterized by high density of voltage-gated Ca^{2+} channels (VGCC; Spirou et al., 2008). This observation would be thus consistent with the role of the receptors in Ca^{2+}-dependent enhancement of the presynaptic release probability by glycine (Turecek and Trussell, 2001; Awatramani et al., 2005). Calyceal GlyRs, however, do not preferentially locate near the glutamate release sites in domains typical for analogous presynaptic autoreceptors. These include ionotropic glutamate receptors that form Ca^{2+}-permeable channels able to facilitate exocytosis of glutamate by delivering Ca^{2+} directly into the presynaptic AZ (see Engelman and MacDermott, 2004; Pinheiro and Mulle, 2008; Ruiz and Kullmann, 2013 for review). GlyRs elevate presynaptic Ca^{2+} concentration indirectly, via chloride efflux leading to nerve terminal depolarization and subsequent activation of presynaptic VGCC (Turecek and Trussell, 2001; Price and Trussell, 2006; Huang and Trussell, 2008). Moreover, the mechanism downstream of the presynaptic calcium signals was observed to include protein kinase C-dependent enhancement of the number of the readily releasable vesicles (Chu et al., 2012). Hence, the synaptic location of GlyRs does not seem to be strictly required for an effective modulation of glutamate release. In fact, the extrasynaptic incidence of GlyRs acting via a cascade of signaling events might be expected as the time course of glycine-induced facilitation is much slower than that of presynaptic GlyR currents (Turecek and Trussell, 2001). In contrast, the facilitatory effect of GlyRs on glycinergic boutons at dissociated spinal cord neurons appears to have a faster time course (Jeong et al., 2003), suggesting a more direct mechanism operating closer to the glycine release sites. Thus the subcellular distributions of GlyRs on glutamatergic and glycinergic terminals likely differ and match the common distribution patterns proposed for presynaptic heteroreceptors vs. autoreceptors (Pinheiro and Mulle, 2008).

Heterosynaptic modes of activation have been well documented for presynaptic GABA-A receptors inducing facilitation of glutamate release from hippocampal mossy fibers (Ruiz et al., 2003; Alle and Geiger, 2007). GlyRs, analogously operating at the calyx of Held synapse, could therefore also be activated by agonists diffusing from the inhibitory release sites. In agreement with this hypothesis, a repetitive stimulation of glycinergic fibers innervating MNTB PC was observed to enhance the release of glutamate from the calyx (Turecek and Trussell, 2001). Moreover, here we show that GlyRs preferentially occupy those parts of calyceal swellings that are not in contact with the postsynaptic cell body and that the receptors tend to align close to glycinergic boutons. Thus the spatial distribution of the receptors seems to be well adjusted to sense the extracellular agonist concentration dropping as a cubic function of the distance from the inhibitory AZ (Vizi et al., 2010). At this point it is not clear whether such activation of calyceal GlyRs is under the control of glycine transporters, similarly to how presynaptic GABA-A spillover currents recorded from the mossy fibers are shaped by the GABA uptake system (Alle and Geiger, 2007). The sequestration of glycine might indeed be expected as MNTB cells are strongly immunopositive for type 1 and 2 glycine transporters (GlyT1 and GlyT2; Zafra et al., 1995; Friauf et al., 1999; Zeilhofer et al., 2005). Glia-specific GlyT1 might be of particular interest as calyces are surrounded by astrocytic processes and GlyT1 inhibitors have been found to affect a sound-evoked activity in gerbil MNTB (Sätzler et al., 2002; Kopp-Scheinpflug et al., 2008; Reyes-Haro et al., 2010; Uwechue et al., 2012). The reversal of the glial uptake of glycine might in turn activate those calyceal GlyRs that could not be reached by the spillover from glycinergic terminals.

The non-homogenous distribution of presynaptic GlyRs spatially related to inhibitory release sites suggests the presence of the use-dependent mechanism of receptor relocation. It is well established that excitatory synaptic activity can exert changes in the subcellular distribution of ionotropic glutamate receptors via numerous molecular mechanisms (reviewed by Triller and Choquet, 2005; Newpher and Ehlers, 2008; Gladding and Raymond, 2011). Likewise, an elevation in cytoplasmic Ca^{2+} concentration has been shown to stimulate GlyR accumulation at postsynaptic sites via a mechanism involving protein-protein interactions with synaptic scaffolds (Lévi et al., 2008). The interactions largely build upon the GlyR β subunit-binding protein gephyrin which reduces the lateral diffusibility of heteromeric GlyRs and connects them to cytoskeletal components (Kneussel and Betz, 2000; Meier et al., 2001). Gephyrin was not found in the calyx of Held terminal (Hruskova et al., 2012), indicating relatively mobile presynaptic α1 homomeric GlyRs (Turecek and Trussell, 2002; Hruskova et al., 2012; Xiong et al., 2014) with a potential of use-dependent redistribution by gephyrin-independent mechanisms. More experiments would be needed to find out whether these processes involve receptor-stimulated sorting of presynaptic membrane to specialized zones with subsets of GlyRs confined in their lateral movement (Sheets et al., 1995; Kusumi et al., 2012). Such activity-regulated changes in presynaptic GlyR distribution could underlie plasticity of glycine-mediated signaling in MNTB.

ACKNOWLEDGMENTS

We thank Elisa Brann for comments on our manuscript. This study was supported by grants from the Grant Agency of the Czech Republic (P303/11/0131 and P304/12/G069) to Michaela Kralikova or Josef Syka, the Wellcome Trust (WT073966) to Rostislav Turecek, and by BIOSS-2 Project A6 to Akos Kulik.

REFERENCES

Alle, H., and Geiger, J. R. (2007). GABAergic spill-over transmission onto hippocampal mossy fiber boutons. *J. Neurosci.* 27, 942–950. doi: 10.1523/jneurosci.4996-06.2007

Awatramani, G. B., Price, G. D., and Trussell, L. O. (2005). Modulation of transmitter release by presynaptic resting potential and background calcium levels. *Neuron* 48, 109–121. doi: 10.1016/j.neuron.2005.08.038

Barbour, B., and Hausser, M. (1997). Intersynaptic diffusion of neurotransmitter. *Trends Neurosci.* 20, 377–384.

Belenky, M. A., Sagiv, N., Fritschy, J. M., and Yarom, Y. (2003). Presynaptic and postsynaptic GABAA receptors in rat suprachiasmatic nucleus. *Neuroscience* 118, 909–923. doi: 10.1016/s0306-4522(03)00062-9

Bernard, V., Somogyi, P., and Bolam, J. P. (1997). Cellular, subcellular and subsynaptic distribution of AMPA-type glutamate receptor subunits in the neostriatum of the rat. *J. Neurosci.* 17, 819–833.

Billups, B. (2005). Colocalization of vesicular glutamate transporters in the rat superior olivary complex. *Neurosci. Lett.* 382, 66–70. doi: 10.1016/j.neulet.2005.02.071

Boehm, S., and Kubista, H. (2002). Fine tuning of sympathetic transmitter release via ionotropic and metabotropic presynaptic receptors. *Pharmacol. Rev.* 54, 43–99. doi: 10.1124/pr.54.1.43

Brickley, S. G., and Mody, I. (2012). Extrasynaptic GABA(A) receptors: their function in the CNS and implications for disease. *Neuron* 73, 23–34. doi: 10.1016/j.neuron.2011.12.012

Caruncho, H. J., Guidotti, A., Lindstrom, J., Costa, E., and Pesold, C. (1997). Subcellular localization of the alpha 7 nicotinic receptor in rat cerebellar granule cell layer. *Neuroreport* 8, 1431–1433. doi: 10.1097/00001756-199704140-00021

Chu, Y., Fioravante, D., Thanawala, M., Leitges, M., and Regehr, W. G. (2012). Calcium-dependent isoforms of protein kinase C mediate glycine-induced synaptic enhancement at the calyx of held. *J. Neurosci.* 32, 13796–13804. doi: 10.1523/JNEUROSCI.2158-12.2012

Danbolt, N. C. (2001). Glutamate uptake. *Prog. Neurobiol.* 65, 1–105. doi: 10.1016/S0301-0082(00)00067-8

Darstein, M., Petralia, R. S., Swanson, G. T., Wenthold, R. J., and Heinemann, S. F. (2003). Distribution of kainate receptor subunits at hippocampal mossy fiber synapses. *J. Neurosci.* 23, 8013–8019.

Deleuze, C., Runquist, M., Orcel, H., Rabié, A., Dayanithi, G., Alonso, G., et al. (2005). Structural difference between heteromeric somatic and homomeric axonal glycine receptors in the hypothalamo-neurohypophysial system. *Neuroscience* 135, 475–483. doi: 10.1016/j.neuroscience.2005.05.024

Dodson, P. D., Billups, B., Rusznák, Z., Szûcs, G., Barker, M. C., and Forsythe, I. D. (2003). Presynaptic rat Kv1.2 channels suppress synaptic terminal hyperexcitability following action potential invasion. *J. Physiol.* 550, 27–33. doi: 10.1113/jphysiol.2003.046250

Duerstock, B. S., Bajaj, C. L., and Borgens, R. B. (2003). A comparative study of the quantitative accuracy of three-dimensional reconstructions of spinal cord from serial histological sections. *J. Microsc.* 210, 138–148. doi: 10.1046/j.1365-2818.2003.01130.x

Elezgarai, I., Díez, J., Puente, N., Azkue, J. J., Benítez, R., Bilbao, A., et al. (2003). Subcellular localization of the voltage-dependent potassium channel Kv3.1b in postnatal and adult rat medial nucleus of the trapezoid body. *Neuroscience* 118, 889–898. doi: 10.1016/s0306-4522(03)00068-x

Engelman, H. S., and MacDermott, A. B. (2004). Presynaptic ionotropic receptors and control of transmitter release. *Nat. Rev. Neurosci.* 5, 135–145. doi: 10.1038/nrn1297

Faber, D. S., and Korn, H. (1988). Synergism at central synapses due to lateral diffusion of transmitter. *Proc. Natl. Acad. Sci. U S A* 85, 8708–8712. doi: 10.1073/pnas.85.22.8708

Farrant, M., and Nusser, Z. (2005). Variations on an inhibitory theme: phasic and tonic activation of GABA(A) receptors. *Nat. Rev. Neurosci.* 6, 215–229. doi: 10.1038/nrn1625

Fiala, J. C. (2005). Reconstruct: a free editor for serial section microscopy. *J. Microsc.* 218, 52–61. doi: 10.1111/j.1365-2818.2005.01466.x

Friauf, E., Aragón, C., Löhrke, S., Westenfelder, B., and Zafra, F. (1999). Developmental expression of the glycine transporter GLYT2 in the auditory system of rats suggests involvement in synapse maturation. *J. Comp. Neurol.* 412, 17–37. doi: 10.1002/(sici)1096-9861(19990913)412:1<17::aid-cne2>3.3.co;2-5

Geiman, E. J., Zheng, W., Fritschy, J. M., and Alvarez, F. J. (2002). Glycine and GABA(A) receptor subunits on Renshaw cells: relationship with presynaptic neurotransmitters and postsynaptic gephyrin clusters. *J. Comp. Neurol.* 444, 275–289. doi: 10.1002/cne.10148

Gladding, C. M., and Raymond, L. A. (2011). Mechanisms underlying NMDA receptor synaptic/extrasynaptic distribution and function. *Mol. Cell. Neurosci.* 48, 308–320. doi: 10.1016/j.mcn.2011.05.001

Hardingham, G. E., and Bading, H. (2010). Synaptic versus extrasynaptic NMDA receptor signalling: implications for neurodegenerative disorders. *Nat. Rev. Neurosci.* 11, 682–696. doi: 10.1038/nrn2911

Hermida, D., Mateos, J. M., Elezgarai, I., Puente, N., Bilbao, A., Bueno-López, J. L., et al. (2010). Spatial compartmentalization of AMPA glutamate receptor subunits at the calyx of held synapse. *J. Comp. Neurol.* 518, 163–174. doi: 10.1002/cne.22189

Hruskova, B., Trojanova, J., Kulik, A., Kralikova, M., Pysanenko, K., Bures, Z., et al. (2012). Differential distribution of glycine receptor subtypes at the rat calyx of held synapse. *J. Neurosci.* 32, 17012–17024. doi: 10.1523/JNEUROSCI.1547-12.2012

Huang, H., and Trussell, L. O. (2008). Control of presynaptic function by a persistent Na(+) current. *Neuron* 60, 975–979. doi: 10.1016/j.neuron.2008.10.052

Jaskolski, F., Coussen, F., and Mulle, C. (2005). Subcellular localization and trafficking of kainate receptors. *Trends Pharmacol. Sci.* 26, 20–26. doi: 10.1016/j.tips.2004.11.008

Jeong, H. J., Jang, I. S., Moorhouse, A. J., and Akaike, N. (2003). Activation of presynaptic glycine receptors facilitates glycine release from presynaptic terminals synapsing onto rat spinal sacral dorsal commissural nucleus neurons. *J. Physiol.* 550, 373–383. doi: 10.1113/jphysiol.2003.041053

Jones, I. W., and Wonnacott, S. (2004). Precise localization of alpha7 nicotinic acetylcholine receptors on glutamatergic axon terminals in the rat ventral tegmental area. *J. Neurosci.* 24, 11244–11252. doi: 10.1523/jneurosci.3009-04.2004

Jourdain, P., Bergersen, L. H., Bhaukaurally, K., Bezzi, P., Santello, M., Domercq, M., et al. (2007). Glutamate exocytosis from astrocytes controls synaptic strength. *Nat. Neurosci.* 10, 331–339. doi: 10.1038/nn1849

Kharazia, V. N., and Weinberg, R. J. (1997). Tangential synaptic distribution of NMDA and AMPA receptors in rat neocortex. *Neurosci. Lett.* 238, 41–44. doi: 10.1016/s0304-3940(97)00846-x

Kieval, J. Z., Hubert, G. W., Charara, A., Paré, J. F., and Smith, Y. (2001). Subcellular and subsynaptic localization of presynaptic and postsynaptic kainate receptor subunits in the monkey striatum. *J. Neurosci.* 21, 8746–8757.

Kneussel, M., and Betz, H. (2000). Clustering of inhibitory neurotransmitter receptors at developing postsynaptic sites: the membrane activation model. *Trends Neurosci.* 23, 429–435. doi: 10.1016/s0166-2236(00)01627-1

Kopach, O., and Voitenko, N. (2013). Extrasynaptic AMPA receptors in the dorsal horn: evidence and functional significance. *Brain Res. Bull.* 93, 47–56. doi: 10.1016/j.brainresbull.2012.11.004

Kopp-Scheinpflug, C., Dehmel, S., Tolnai, S., Dietz, B., Milenkovic, I., and Rübsamen, R. (2008). Glycine-mediated changes of onset reliability at a mammalian central synapse. *Neuroscience* 157, 432–445. doi: 10.1016/j.neuroscience.2008.08.068

Kubota, H., Alle, H., Betz, H., and Geiger, J. R. (2010). Presynaptic glycine receptors on hippocampal mossy fibers. *Biochem. Biophys. Res. Commun.* 393, 587–591. doi: 10.1016/j.bbrc.2010.02.019

Kullmann, D. M. (2001). Presynaptic kainate receptors in the hippocampus: slowly emerging from obscurity. *Neuron* 32, 561–564. doi: 10.1016/s0896-6273(01)00507-4

Kusumi, A., Fujiwara, T. K., Morone, N., Yoshida, K. J., Chadda, R., Xie, M., et al. (2012). Membrane mechanisms for signal transduction: the coupling of the meso-scale raft domains to membrane-skeleton-induced compartments and dynamic protein complexes. *Semin. Cell Dev. Biol.* 23, 126–144. doi: 10.1016/j.semcdb.2012.01.018

Leão, R. M., Kushmerick, C., Pinaud, R., Renden, R., Li, G. L., Taschenberger, H., et al. (2005). Presynaptic Na+ channels: locus, development and recovery from inactivation at a high-fidelity synapse. *J. Neurosci.* 25, 3724–3738. doi: 10.1523/jneurosci.3983-04.2005

Lester, H. A., Dibas, M. I., Dahan, D. S., Leite, J. F., and Dougherty, D. A. (2004). Cys-loop receptors: new twists and turns. *Trends Neurosci.* 27, 329–336. doi: 10.1016/s0166-2236(04)00109-2

Lévi, S., Schweizer, C., Bannai, H., Pascual, O., Charrier, C., and Triller, A. (2008). Homeostatic regulation of synaptic GlyR numbers driven by lateral diffusion. *Neuron* 59, 261–273. doi: 10.1016/j.neuron.2008.05.030

Masugi-Tokita, M., Tarusawa, E., Watanabe, M., Molnár, E., Fujimoto, K., and Shigemoto, R. (2007). Number and density of AMPA receptors in individual synapses in the rat cerebellum as revealed by SDS-digested freeze-fracture replica labeling. *J. Neurosci.* 27, 2135–2144. doi: 10.1523/jneurosci.2861-06.2007

Meier, J., Vannier, C., Sergé, A., Triller, A., and Choquet, D. (2001). Fast and reversible trapping of surface glycine receptors by gephyrin. *Nat. Neurosci.* 4, 253–260. doi: 10.1038/85099

Morkve, S. H., and Hartveit, E. (2009). Properties of glycine receptors underlying synaptic currents in presynaptic axon terminals of rod bipolar cells in the rat retina. *J. Physiol.* 587, 3813–3830. doi: 10.1113/jphysiol.2009.173583

Muller, E., Le-Corronc, H., and Legendre, P. (2008). Extrasynaptic and postsynaptic receptors in glycinergic and GABAergic neurotransmission: a division of labor? *Front. Mol. Neurosci.* 1:3. doi: 10.3389/neuro.02.003.2008

Newpher, T. M., and Ehlers, M. D. (2008). Glutamate receptor dynamics in dendritic microdomains. *Neuron* 58, 472–497. doi: 10.1016/j.neuron.2008.04.030

Nusser, Z., Sieghart, W., and Somogyi, P. (1998). Segregation of different GABAA receptors to synaptic and extrasynaptic membranes of cerebellar granule cells. *J. Neurosci.* 18, 1693–1703.

Nyíri, G., Cserép, C., Szabadits, E., Mackie, K., and Freund, T. F. (2005). CB1 cannabinoid receptors are enriched in the perisynaptic annulus and on preterminal segments of hippocampal GABAergic axons. *Neuroscience* 136, 811–822. doi: 10.1016/j.neuroscience.2005.01.026

Paspalas, C. D., and Goldman-Rakic, P. S. (2005). Presynaptic D1 dopamine receptors in primate prefrontal cortex: target-specific expression in the glutamatergic synapse. *J. Neurosci.* 25, 1260–1267. doi: 10.1523/jneurosci.3436-04.2005

Perkins, G. A., Tjong, J., Brown, J. M., Poquiz, P. H., Scott, R. T., Kolson, D. R., et al. (2010). The micro-architecture of mitochondria at active zones: electron tomography reveals novel anchoring scaffolds and cristae structured for high-rate metabolism. *J. Neurosci.* 30, 1015–1026. doi: 10.1523/JNEUROSCI.1517-09.2010

Petralia, R. S. (2012). Distribution of extrasynaptic NMDA receptors on neurons. *ScientificWorldJournal* 2012:267120. doi: 10.1100/2012/267120

Pinheiro, P. S., and Mulle, C. (2008). Presynaptic glutamate receptors: physiological functions and mechanisms of action. *Nat. Rev. Neurosci.* 9, 423–436. doi: 10.1038/nrn2379

Price, G. D., and Trussell, L. O. (2006). Estimate of the chloride concentration in a central glutamatergic terminal: a gramicidin perforated-patch study on the calyx of held. *J. Neurosci.* 26, 11432–11436. doi: 10.1523/jneurosci.1660-06.2006

Reyes-Haro, D., Müller, J., Boresch, M., Pivneva, T., Benedetti, B., Scheller, A., et al. (2010). Neuron-astrocyte interactions in the medial nucleus of the trapezoid body. *J. Gen. Physiol.* 135, 583–594. doi: 10.1085/jgp.200910354

Rowland, K. C., Irby, N. K., and Spirou, G. A. (2000). Specialized synapse-associated structures within the calyx of held. *J. Neurosci.* 20, 9135–9144.

Rubio, M. E., and Soto, F. (2001). Distinct localization of P2X receptors at excitatory postsynaptic specializations. *J. Neurosci.* 21, 641–653.

Ruiz, A., Fabian-Fine, R., Scott, R., Walker, M. C., Rusakov, D. A., and Kullmann, D. M. (2003). GABAA receptors at hippocampal mossy fibers. *Neuron* 39, 961–973. doi: 10.1016/s0896-6273(03)00559-2

Ruiz, A. J., and Kullmann, D. M. (2013). Ionotropic receptors at hippocampal mossy fibers: roles in axonal excitability, synaptic transmission and plasticity. *Front. Neural Circuits* 6:112. doi: 10.3389/fncir.2012.00112

Rusakov, D. A., Kullmann, D. M., and Stewart, M. G. (1999). Hippocampal synapses: do they talk to their neighbours? *Trends Neurosci.* 22, 382–388. doi: 10.1016/s0166-2236(99)01425-3

Sätzler, K., Söhl, L. F., Bollmann, J. H., Borst, J. G., Frotscher, M., Sakmann, B., et al. (2002). Three-dimensional reconstruction of a calyx of held and its postsynaptic principal neuron in the medial nucleus of the trapezoid body. *J. Neurosci.* 22, 10567–10579.

Sheets, E. D., Simson, R., and Jacobson, K. (1995). New insights into membrane dynamics from the analysis of cell surface interactions by physical methods. *Curr. Opin. Cell Biol.* 7, 707–714. doi: 10.1016/0955-0674(95)80113-8

Spirou, G. A., Chirila, F. V., von Gersdorff, H., and Manis, P. B. (2008). Heterogeneous Ca2+ influx along the adult calyx of held: a structural and computational study. *Neuroscience* 154, 171–185. doi: 10.1016/j.neuroscience.2008.04.002

Tamaru, Y., Nomura, S., Mizuno, N., and Shigemoto, R. (2001). Distribution of metabotropic glutamate receptor mGluR3 in the mouse CNS: differential location relative to pre- and postsynaptic sites. *Neuroscience* 106, 481–503. doi: 10.1016/s0306-4522(01)00305-0

Taschenberger, H., Leão, R. M., Rowland, K. C., Spirou, G. A., and von Gersdorff, H. (2002). Optimizing synaptic architecture and efficiency for high-frequency transmission. *Neuron* 36, 1127–1143. doi: 10.1016/s0896-6273(02)01137-6

Trigo, F. F., Bouhours, B., Rostaing, P., Papageorgiou, G., Corrie, J. E., Triller, A., et al. (2010). Presynaptic miniature GABAergic currents in developing interneurons. *Neuron* 66, 235–247. doi: 10.1016/j.neuron.2010.03.030

Trigo, F. F., Marty, A., and Stell, B. M. (2008). Axonal GABAA receptors. *Eur. J. Neurosci.* 28, 841–848. doi: 10.1111/j.1460-9568.2008.06404.x

Triller, A., and Choquet, D. (2005). Surface trafficking of receptors between synaptic and extrasynaptic membranes: and yet they do move! *Trends Neurosci.* 28, 133–139. doi: 10.1016/j.tins.2005.01.001

Turecek, R., and Trussell, L. O. (2001). Presynaptic glycine receptors enhance transmitter release at a mammalian central synapse. *Nature* 411, 587–590. doi: 10.1038/35079084

Turecek, R., and Trussell, L. O. (2002). Reciprocal developmental regulation of presynaptic ionotropic receptors. *Proc. Natl. Acad. Sci. U S A* 99, 13884–13889. doi: 10.1073/pnas.212419699

Uwechue, N. M., Marx, M. C., Chevy, Q., and Billups, B. (2012). Activation of glutamate transport evokes rapid glutamine release from perisynaptic astrocytes. *J. Physiol.* 590, 2317–2331. doi: 10.1113/jphysiol.2011.226605

Verhoog, M. B., and Mansvelder, H. D. (2011). Presynaptic ionotropic receptors controlling and modulating the rules for spike timing-dependent plasticity. *Neural Plast.* 2011:870763. doi: 10.1155/2011/870763

Vizi, E. S., Fekete, A., Karoly, R., and Mike, A. (2010). Non-synaptic receptors and transporters involved in brain functions and targets of drug treatment. *Br. J. Pharmacol.* 160, 785–809. doi: 10.1111/j.1476-5381.2009.00624.x

Walmsley, B., Alvarez, F. J., and Fyffe, R. E. (1998). Diversity of structure and function at mammalian central synapses. *Trends Neurosci.* 21, 81–88. doi: 10.1016/s0166-2236(97)01170-3

Wei, W., Zhang, N., Peng, Z., Houser, C. R., and Mody, I. (2003). Perisynaptic localization of delta subunit-containing GABA(A) receptors and their activation by GABA spillover in the mouse dentate gyrus. *J. Neurosci.* 23, 10650–10661.

Wimmer, V. C., Horstmann, H., Groh, A., and Kuner, T. (2006). Donut-like topology of synaptic vesicles with a central cluster of mitochondria wrapped into membrane protrusions: a novel structure-function module of the adult calyx of held. *J. Neurosci.* 26, 109–116. doi: 10.1523/jneurosci.3268-05.2006

Xiong, W., Chen, S. R., He, L., Cheng, K., Zhao, Y. L., Chen, H., et al. (2014). Presynaptic glycine receptors as a potential therapeutic target for hyperekplexia disease. *Nat. Neurosci.* 17, 232–239. doi: 10.1038/nn.3615

Zafra, F., Aragón, C., Olivares, L., Danbolt, N. C., Giménez, C., and Storm-Mathisen, J. (1995). Glycine transporters are differentially expressed among CNS cells. *J. Neurosci.* 15, 3952–3969.

Zarei, M. M., Radcliffe, K. A., Chen, D., Patrick, J. W., and Dani, J. A. (1999). Distributions of nicotinic acetylcholine receptor alpha7 and beta2 subunits on cultured hippocampal neurons. *Neuroscience* 88, 755–764. doi: 10.1016/s0306-4522(98)00246-2

Zeilhofer, H. U., Studler, B., Arabadzisz, D., Schweizer, C., Ahmadi, S., Layh, B., et al. (2005). Glycinergic neurons expressing enhanced green fluorescent protein in bacterial artificial chromosome transgenic mice. *J. Comp. Neurol.* 482, 123–141. doi: 10.1002/cne.20349

13

Superficial stellate cells of the dorsal cochlear nucleus

Pierre F. Apostolides† and Laurence O. Trussell*

Oregon Hearing Research Center and Vollum Institute, Oregon Health and Science University, Portland, OR, USA

Correspondence:
Laurence O. Trussell, Oregon Hearing Research Center and Vollum Institute, Oregon Health and Science University, 3181 SW Sam Jackson Park Rd, L335A, Portland, OR 97221, USA
e-mail: trussell@ohsu.edu

†Present address:
Pierre F. Apostolides, Janelia Farm Research Campus, Howard Hughes Medical Institute, 19700 Helix Drive, Ashburn, VA 20147, USA

The dorsal cochlear nucleus (DCN) integrates auditory and multisensory signals at the earliest levels of auditory processing. Proposed roles for this region include sound localization in the vertical plane, head orientation to sounds of interest, and suppression of sensitivity to expected sounds. Auditory and non-auditory information streams to the DCN are refined by a remarkably complex array of inhibitory and excitatory interneurons, and the role of each cell type is gaining increasing attention. One inhibitory neuron that has been poorly appreciated to date is the superficial stellate cell. Here we review previous studies and describe new results that reveal the surprisingly rich interactions that this tiny interneuron has with its neighbors, interactions which enable it to respond to both multisensory and auditory afferents.

Keywords: interneurons, auditory pathways, glycine, gap junctions, electrical synapses

INTRODUCTION

The dorsal cochlear nucleus (DCN) is an auditory structure unique to mammals, with anatomical, physiological and molecular similarities to the cerebellar cortex and the electrosensory lobe of mormyrid electric fish (ELL; Oertel and Young, 2004; Bell et al., 2008). Fusiform principal cells receive auditory input onto their basal dendrites and multisensory input onto their apical dendrites (**Figure 1**). Each type of input signal is preprocessed by a system of interneurons. The function of some of these interneurons (tuberculoventral or vertical cell, and the cartwheel cell) have been established through a combination of *in vivo* and *in vitro* studies over many years. Others (granule, Golgi and unipolar brush cell) are currently under study but their basic function may be generally understood by analogy to their counterparts in the cerebellar cortex and ELL.

However, one cell type, the superficial stellate cell (SSC), has received little attention over the years. Several reasons may account for this neglect: SSCs are sparse, tiny cells positioned just under the ependymal cell layer, features that all present challenges for targeting during *in vivo* recordings. However *in vitro* brain slice preparations have recently made it easier to visualize and reach these cells with electrodes, particular in mouse lines in which genetically-encoded fluorophores are expressed in SSCs. Through our studies, several surprising features have come to light about the SSCs that inspire a renewed effort to understand the function of these neurons. Indeed, while in some ways homologous to cerebellar molecular layer stellate cells, SSCs exhibit properties that place them in a computationally unique position in the entire cochlear nucleus. Their size heightens their sensitivity to small inputs and their location optimizes their ability to communicate with specific dendrites of DCN principal cells. Most interestingly, gap junctions in SSCs are used to communicate both excitatory and inhibitory signals between the auditory and multisensory domains.

METHODS

Methods are for new data presented in **Figures 2**, **3**, and **6**.

SLICE PREPARATION

Experimental procedures were approved by OHSU's Institutional Animal Care and Use Committee. C57/Bl6 mice P15-P24 were anesthetized with isofluorane, decapitated, and slices (200–250 μm thick) containing the DCN were cut in an ice-cold sucrose solution which contained (in mM): 87 NaCl, 25 $NaHCO_3$, 25 glucose, 75 sucrose, 2.5 KCl, 1.25 NaH_2PO_4, 0.5 $CaCl_2$, 7 $MgCl_2$, bubbled with 5% CO_2/95% O_2. Slices subsequently recovered for 30–45 min at 34°C in artificial cerebrospinal fluid (ACSF) solution which contained (in mM): 130 NaCl, 2.1 KCl, 1.7 $CaCl_2$, 1 $MgSO_4$, 1.2 KH_2PO_4, 20 $NaHCO_3$, 3 Na-HEPES, 10–12 glucose, bubbled with 5% CO_2/95% O_2 (300–310 mOsm). This solution was also used as the standard perfusate for all experiments. In some experiments 5 μM 3-((R)-2-Carboxypiperazin-4-yl)-propyl-1-phosphonic acid (R-CPP) or 50 μM D-2-amino-5-phosphonovalerate (D-APV) were added to the cutting solution and/or recovery chamber. After recovery, slices were maintained at 22°C until recording, typically within 5 h of slice preparation.

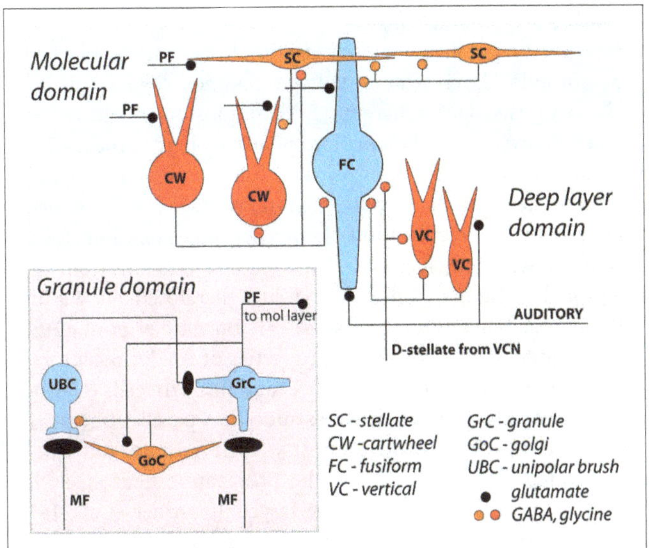

FIGURE 1 | General circuit diagram of the DCN, divided into three computational domains. The auditory domain comprises the auditory input to fusiform cell basal dendrites, and its modification by vertical and D-stellate interneurons. The non-auditory domain receives mossy fiber input to granule cells, and is modified by Golgi and unipolar brush cells. The molecular layer domain comprises the parallel fiber input from granule cells, terminating on fusiform cell apical dendrites and onto cartwheel and SSC cells, both of which in turn control fusiform activity. Omitted here are the giant cells, whose local synaptic circuitry is not well understood.

ELECTROPHYSIOLOGY

Slices mounted in the recording chamber were continuously perfused at 3–5 ml/min with ACSF (31–33°C) and visualized using Dodt contrast optics using either a 40x or 63x objective on a Zeiss Axioskcop 2 microscope. Patch pipette solution contained (in mM) 113 K-gluconate, 4.8 $MgCl_2$, 4 ATP, 0.5 GTP, 10 Tris-phosphocreatine, 0.1–0.2 EGTA, 10 HEPES, pH adjusted between 7.2–7.3 with KOH (~290 mOsm). Pipette resistances for fusiform and stellate cells were typically 2–3 and 3–5 MOhm, respectively, when filled with the K-gluconate solution. Pipette capacitance was cancelled and series resistance effects adjusted with bridge balance.

CELL IDENTIFICATION

Stellate cells were identified by their small size and location in the slice at the outer edge of the molecular layer just below the ependymal surface. In experiments with transgenic mice, GFP fluorescence was observed with a 100 W Hg bulb placed in the epi-fluorescence port of the microscope and passed through a GFP filter. Fusiform neurons were identified as large cells situated in the DCN cell body layer, and showed spike characteristics as previously described (Zhang and Oertel, 1993; Golding and Oertel, 1997).

DATA ACQUISITION AND ANALYSIS

Data were recorded with a Multiclamp 700B amplifier and a Digidata 1322A analog-digital converter board using pClamp 9 software. Signals were low-pass filtered at 10–20 kHz and digitized at 20–50 kHz. Data were analyzed offline after filtering the traces at 2–10 kHz. All values are reported as mean ± SEM.

GlyT2-GFP MICE

Recordings were initially made from mice expressing GFP under the control of the promoter for the neuronal glycine transporter GlyT2 (Zeilhofer et al., 2005), to aid in learning to identify SSCs in our slices. To examine the distribution of this GFP label among cells in the cochlear nucleus, mice were transcardially perfused with warm (38°C) 100 mM phosphate buffered saline (PBS) solution, pH 7.4, followed by ice-cold 4% paraformaldehyde in PBS. The brains were dissected from the skull and incubated overnight in 4% paraformaldehyde for complete tissue fixation. Brains were rinsed in PBS and coronal sections were cut at 30 μm using a vibratome. The sections were washed in PBS solution for 30 min and then slide mounted and coverslipped in Fluoromount G medium (Southern Biotechnology Associates).

REAGENTS

2, 3- Dioxo -6- nitro-1, 2, 3, 4- tetrahydrobenzo[f]quinoxaline -7-sulfonamide (NBQX), APV, CPP, SR95531 were purchased from Ascent Scientific/Abcam. Strychnine was purchased from Sigma-Aldrich.

RESULTS

PREVIOUS STUDIES

Cells resembling SSCs in the DCN have been described in anatomical studies stretching back over a century (Cajal, 1911; Brawer et al., 1974; Kane, 1974; Disterhoft et al., 1980; Nó, 1981; Webster and Trune, 1982). However, it was not until the landmark Golgi and electron microscopy (EM) study of Wouterlood et al. (1984) that we had a comprehensive approach specifically to the SSCs. Those authors described small cells whose soma, dendrites and axons were restricted to the outermost, molecular layer of the DCN, and in this sense resembled the stellate cells of the molecular layer of the cerebellar cortex. Ultrastructurally, Gray's Type II terminals made by SSCs suggested that these cells were inhibitory, a conclusion supported by a subsequent paper showing expression of glutamic acid decarboxylase (GAD) in SSCs (Mugnaini, 1985). Terminals of stellate cells were seen on dendrites restricted largely to the DCN molecular layer, dendrites belonging to the fusiform principal cells, cartwheel interneurons, and other SSCs. With this description, a picture emerges of domains of inhibition in the DCN, and most interestingly of subcellular domains of individual fusiform cells. Synapses made by SSCs terminate on apical dendrites, boutons of inhibitory cartwheel cells terminate on the soma and proximal dendrites (Wouterlood et al., 1984; Rubio and Juiz, 2004), and the terminals of inhibitory tuberculoventral (vertical) cells occupy the soma and basal dendrite (**Figure 5;** Rubio and Juiz, 2004) Thus, the fusiform cells are controlled by three classes of interneuron having partially overlapping domains of inhibition, with the SSC controlling primarily the apical dendrites.

Wouterlood et al. (1984) also described putative excitatory inputs to SSCs, and ascribed these to the *en passant* terminals of the parallel fiber axons of granule cells. Given the diverse, multimodal control of granule cells by mossy fibers, these observations suggest that SSCs are activated predominately by non-auditory rather than auditory fibers. This conclusion, however, is not entirely accurate, as shown in a brain slice study of Zhang and Oertel (1993), who observed EPSPs in a putative SSC following stimulation of the auditory nerve root in the ventral cochlear nucleus, even though auditory nerve fibers do not reach the DCN molecular layer. Moreover, those authors showed that puffs of glutamate in the ventral cochlear nucleus (VCN) also evoked EPSPs in the SSC, suggesting the possibility that excitatory neurons in the VCN, possibly the T-stellate cells, contact SSCs. As discussed in a later section, we suggest an alternative explanation by which auditory nerve activity may excite SSCs in the absence of direct contact from auditory nerve fibers.

RECENT WORKS

In this section we will summarize our recent publications and include some new observations regarding the synaptic and intrinsic properties of SSCs. Studies on mouse SSCs in our lab have focused on cells in the very outermost part of the molecular layer. Such cells are visible in mouse lines in which GFP is expressed under the control of promoters for GAD or for the neuronal plasma membrane glycine transporter GlyT2 (Apostolides and Trussell, 2014a; **Figure 2** shows an example). The GlyT2 mouse line in particular reveals the striking abundance of glycinergic neurons in the DCN, and highlights that the SSC appears as the primary interneuron in the outer region of the DCN molecular layer (**Figure 2**, inset, arrows). In our published works, as well as the new work described below, we have recorded from SSCs in these locations in coronal slices of mouse DCN.

SSCs had membrane input resistances of about 1 GOhm (Apostolides and Trussell, 2013b) and therefore were sensitive to relatively small current injections as compared to cartwheel or fusiform cells. In a set of 29 neurons studied in current clamp, we now find that when cell membrane potentials were held between -55 and -80 mV, hyperpolarizing current injection revealed a small "sag" in membrane potential typically attributed to an I_H conductance (**Figures 3A,B**). When the negative bias current was small (-71 ± 1 mV with -9 ± 2 pA bias), most cells (24/29) tested fired one or several rebound spikes (mean spike number 1.45 ± 0.12) followed by an after-depolarization (**Figure 3A**). By contrast, with larger negative bias to maintain a more negative voltage (-88 ± 1 mV with -73 ± 10 pA bias) this rebound spike behavior was absent (0 of 21 tested cells; **Figure 3B**). The drive for rebound firing has previously been attributed to I_H and/or T-type Ca^{2+} channels (e.g., Aizenman and Linden, 1999; Kopp-Scheinpflug et al., 2011), and suggests that post-inhibitory rebound firing of SSCs depends on membrane potential history. When held between -55 and -70 mV, SSCs fired repetitively upon positive current injection, and could sustain firing at >100 Hz during 150–200 pA current steps (**Figure 3A**). By contrast, depolarizations from more hyperpolarized levels (**Figure 3B**) resulted in either spike bursts or an adapting spike pattern. Notably, during evoked or spontaneous spike activity, small, ~ 1 mV spikelets, were often visible in the traces (**Figure 3A** insets), reflecting electrical coupling to neighboring spiking neurons, as described below. With no added bias current, 14/29 (48%) of SSCs tested fired spontaneous action potentials in current clamp with an average frequency of 6.7 ± 1.8 Hz (**Figures 3C,D**).

Excitatory glutamatergic inputs

Activation of parallel fibers by a stimulus electrode placed in the molecular layer near a voltage clamped SSC resulted in excitatory postsynaptic currents (EPSCs; Apostolides and Trussell, 2014a). Analysis of the kinetics and pharmacology of these AMPA receptor-mediated responses revealed features similar to those of cerebellar stellate cells, in particular submillisecond EPSC decay times and inward rectification of current voltage relations for the glutamate activated channels. These features are consistent with receptors lacking the GluR2 subunit and therefore having a high Ca^{2+} permeability (Hume et al., 1991; Burnashev et al., 1992) and are quite distinct from the properties of AMPA receptors at parallel fiber synapses onto cartwheel and fusiform cells (Gardner et al., 1999, 2001). Thus, if we assume that parallel fibers constitute a uniform population, postsynaptic receptor subtype is not dictated by the identity of the presynaptic neuron, as has been proposed for auditory nerve targets (Gardner et al., 1999, 2001). Interestingly, the similarities to cerebellar stellate cells suggests that excitatory synapses onto SSCs may exhibit long-term synaptic plasticity (Liu and Cull-Candy, 2000). The possibility of plasticity at these synapses is also hinted at by a distinct difference from cerebellar stellate cells in the expression of NMDA receptors. In the cerebellum, NMDA receptors onto stellate cells appear to be expressed extrasynaptically, and activated only when multiple parallel fibers are fired or when they are fired at high rates (Clark and Cull-Candy, 2002; Nahir and Jahr, 2013). However, single action potentials in single parallel fibers are sufficient to activate NMDA receptors on SSCs (Apostolides and Trussell, 2014a); thus there are two synaptic sources of intracellular Ca^{2+} to SSCs, AMPA and NMDA receptors. It will be of interest to test whether activation of parallel fiber synapses can trigger long-term plasticity, as has been shown at synapses onto cartwheel cells and fusiform cells (Tzounopoulos et al., 2004).

Inhibitory synapses

As predicted by the studies from Mugnaini and colleagues (Wouterlood et al., 1984; Mugnaini, 1985), we found that SSCs make GABAergic synapses onto cartwheel cells, fusiform cells, onto other SSCs, and even autaptic contacts onto themselves (Apostolides and Trussell, 2013b, 2014a). However, it was clear that these same synapses also released glycine, because an antagonist of $GABA_A$ receptors, SR95531, did not fully eliminate inhibitory transmission, but transmission was blocked by a mixture of SR95531 and strychnine. Such co-release and co-transmission is common in auditory brainstem interneurons, but varies according to cell type, possibly due to differential receptor distribution (Dugué et al., 2005; Lu et al., 2008; Apostolides and Trussell, 2013a). We examined co-transmission quantitatively by activating autaptic connections and found that 70% of the IPSC was blocked by SR95531 and the remainder by the glycine receptor antagonist strychnine (Apostolides and Trussell, 2014a). This was then confirmed in experiments in which nearby SSCs were selectively excited and the IPSCs those SSCs then made onto a recorded SSC were analyzed pharmacologically. This approach avoided the potential problem of dialysis of GABA during presynaptic recordings which might otherwise diminish the magnitude of GABAergic transmission (Apostolides and Trussell, 2013a).

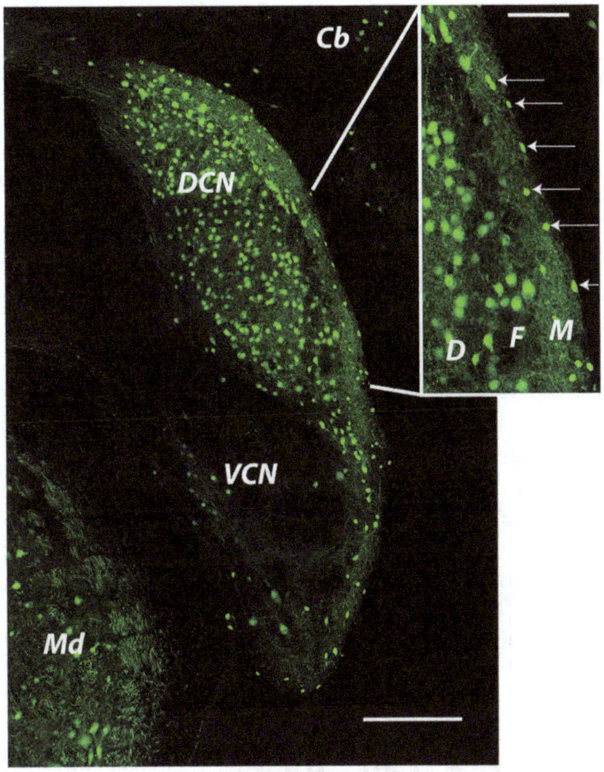

FIGURE 2 | Distribution of glycinergic neurons in the cochlear nucleus as revealed by GFP labeling in a GlyT2-GFP mouse. The image was produced from tiled images captured at a single focal plane with a 20x objective. Cells identified as SSCs (arrows in inset) were small bright cells located in the DCN molecular layer. Cells used for recordings were most often those closest to the edge of the brain stem at the ependymal layer. Cb: cerebellum; DCN: dorsal cochlear nucleus; Md: medulla; VCN: ventral cochlear nucleus. Inset: D: deep layer; F: fusiform cell layer; M: molecular layer.

As the IPSC components produced by the two transmitters had distinct kinetic signatures, the results imply that co-transmission might enable both fast and slow phases of inhibition.

Gap junction coupling

Wouterlood et al. (1984) predicted on the basis of ultrastructural evidence that gap junctions may form between SSCs, again in alignment with observations from cerebellar stellate cells (Sotelo and Llinas, 1972; Mann-Metzer and Yarom, 1999). In Apostolides and Trussell (2013b) we therefore searched for electrical coupling between cells by making paired recordings between adjacent SSCs in 2–4 week-old mice, and found that indeed voltage displacements in one SSC led to voltage changes in neighboring SSCs in 21% of pairs, with coupling coefficients (the ratio of postjunctional to prejunctional response) of a few percent (Apostolides and Trussell, 2013b). More frequent coupling with similar strength was observed between adjacent fusiform neurons (71% of pairs). However, most striking was the observation that SSCs were also electrically coupled to fusiform cells (45% of pairs), with an apparent preferred direction of communication from principal cell to interneuron (**Figures 4A,C**). Thus, coupling coefficients for connected pairs were ~4-fold higher for signals passing from fusiform cells to SSCs than for the reverse direction, and this range of values was maintained in mice at least up to 9 weeks of age (**Figure 4C**). This developmentally stable, heterotypic electrical connection was blocked by the gap junction blocker meclofenamic acid and was absent in connexin 36 knockout mice (**Figure 4B**). The basis of the rectification was most likely a simple outcome of "impedance mismatch", as SSCs had input resistances about tenfold higher than fusiform cells. Thus, gap junctions between SSCs and fusiform cells facilitate non-chemical, rapid synaptic communication, with a direction that in principle would lead to activation of SSCs when fusiform cells are activated by their parallel fiber or auditory nerve input. **Figure 5** summarizes the pattern of electrical contacts observed among fusiform and SSCs, and contrasts these contacts with the pattern of chemical synapses made by SSCs and the other interneurons. In the next sections we will overview what are the functional outcomes of this novel neural pathway.

Fusiform → SSC transmission

Transmission of biological signals from fusiform to SSCs is evident by the presence of spikelets in SSCs which were shown to originate in fusiform cells (Apostolides and Trussell, 2013b). When spikes in fusiform cells are triggered at high frequency, spikelets in SSCs summated to a low depolarizing plateau. Reasoning that fusiform cells might converge on SSCs, and thus drive them more effectively, two types of experiments were performed. In the first, auditory nerve fibers leading to fusiform cells were

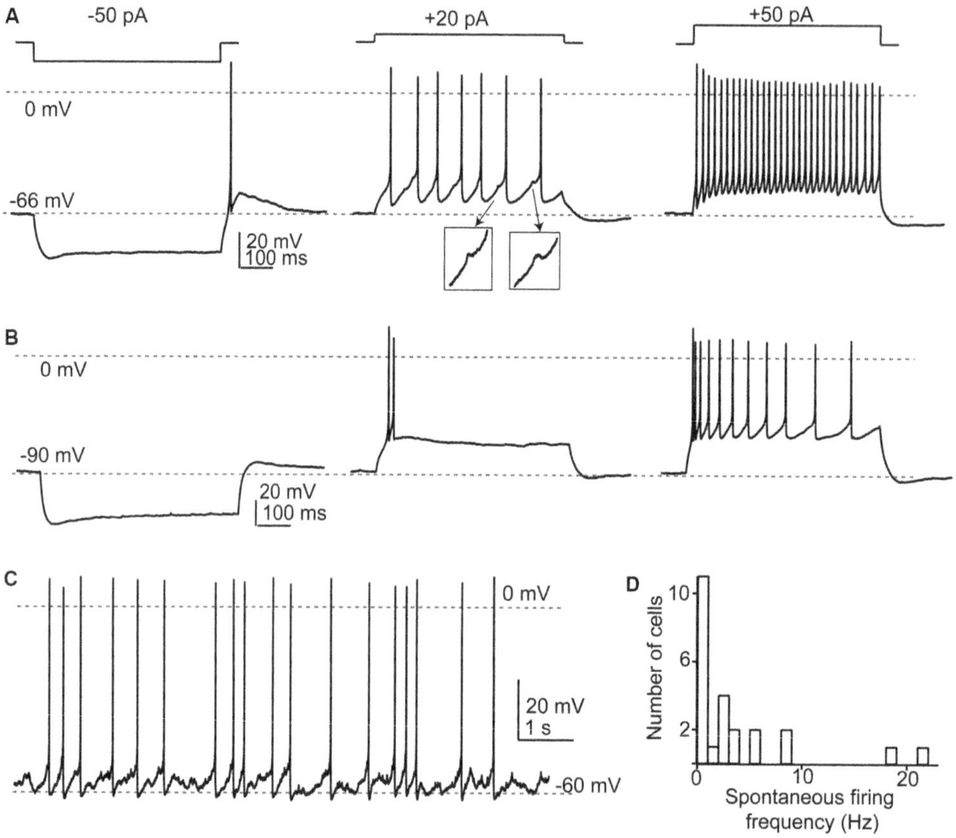

FIGURE 3 | Response properties of SSCs. (A) Responses to current injections to three different levels illustrating a regular firing pattern. Note that in the middle panel spikelets (shown in insets) were apparent between the full-amplitude spikes. **(B)** When depolarized from more negative membrane potentials, SSCs generated spike bursts or exhibited an adapting profile of spiking. **(C)** Example of spontaneous spike activity that was apparent in about half of recorded SSCs. **(D)** Broad frequency distribution of spontaneous spiking in a population of 29 SSCs.

activated, and this led to a substantial depolarization of SSCs. This result might at least partially account for the observation of Zhang and Oertel (1993), that stimulation of the nerve produced an apparent EPSP in an SSC. In the second, groups of fusiform cells were activated following light exposure in slices taken from mice expressing channelrhodopsin2 (ChR2) specifically in fusiform cells, which in turn drove action potentials in SSCs.

Three consequences of transmission in this direction were observed. Depolarization of fusiform cells could enhance the potency of depolarizing stimuli delivered directly to SSCs. Moreover, following a period of depolarization, fusiform cells showed a prominent afterhyperpolarization (AHP) which was potently transmitted to SSCs, and could block excitation of SSCs. Finally, spikes triggered in SSCs by fusiform excitation led to synaptic inhibition of all three targets of SSCs: cartwheel cells, neighboring fusiform cells, and other SSCs (Apostolides and Trussell, 2013b, 2014a). Overall, the results suggested the possibility that *in vivo*, SSCs may be driven by auditory nerve activity, not because of direct synaptic input, or even indirect input via mossy fibers and parallel fibers, but rather because auditory signaling in the fusiform cell would be conveyed to the molecular layer through gap junctions.

Besides the modification of SSC firing by fusiform spikes and their AHPs, it was also found that subthreshold EPSPs in fusiform cells are communicated to SSCs, but in a very remarkable manner. In Apostolides and Trussell (2014b), EPSPs generated either by parallel fiber stimulation or by injection of synaptic like current waveforms, were converted to long lasting depolarizations by activation of a subthreshold Na^+ conductance. This broad EPSP deactivated I_H, thus leading to an obligatory AHP. The resulting biphasic waveform lasted hundreds of ms and was effectively transmitted to the SSCs through gap junctions. Indeed, given the filtering properties of gap junctions, these results showed that EPSPs in fusiform cells may more effectively modulate the activity of the SSC network than spikes.

SSC → Fusiform transmission

While the electrical coupling coefficient in the SSC-to-fusiform cell direction was low, we now find that long-lasting hyperpolarizing signals in SSCs may inhibit activity in fusiform cells. **Figure 6A** shows a recording from an electrically coupled SSC and fusiform cell, as defined by the bi-directional transmission of electrotonic pulses across the two cells (described in Apostolides and Trussell, 2013b). The fusiform cell in this

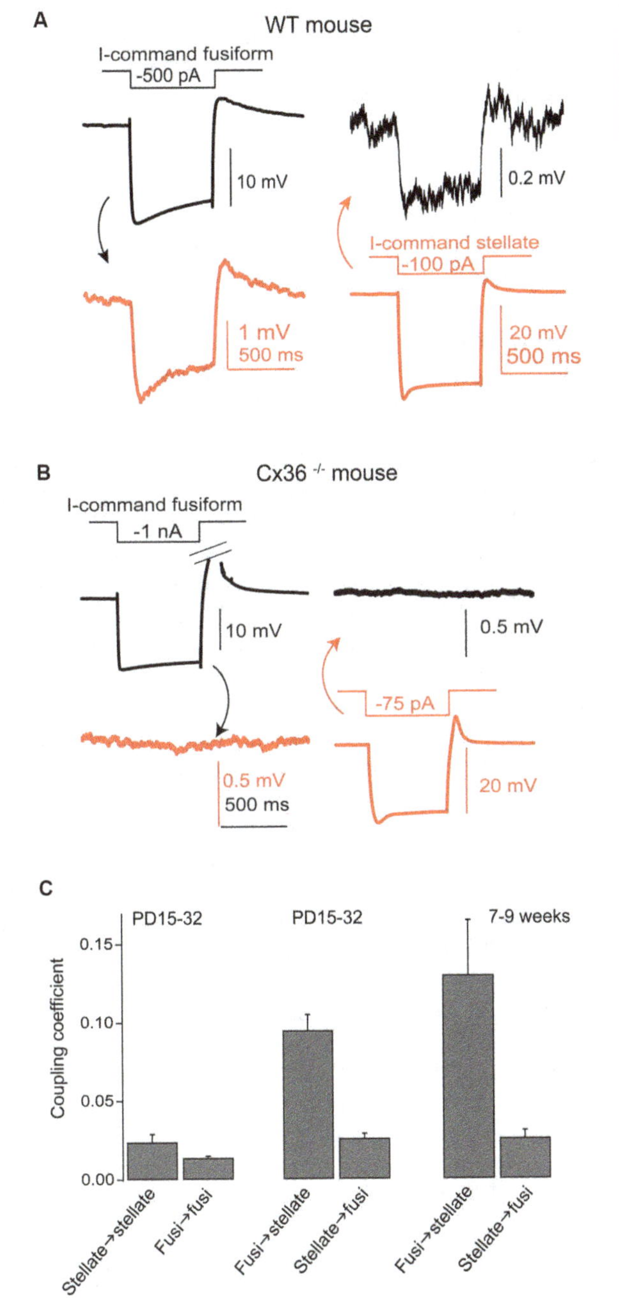

FIGURE 4 | Gap junctions couple SSCs and fusiform cells. **(A)** Coupling between a recorded SSC and fusiform pair was tested by injection of hyperpolarizing currents in one cell and then the other, as indicated. Hyperpolarizations of smaller amplitude in the postjunctional cell was taken as evidence of coupling. **(B)** A similar experiment was performed in a Cx36 knockout mouse, and showed no evidence of coupling. **(C)** Average coupling coefficients reveal bias for transmission from fusiform cell to SSC. This coupling was present in mice up to 9 weeks postnatal. Data adapted from Apostolides and Trussell (2013b).

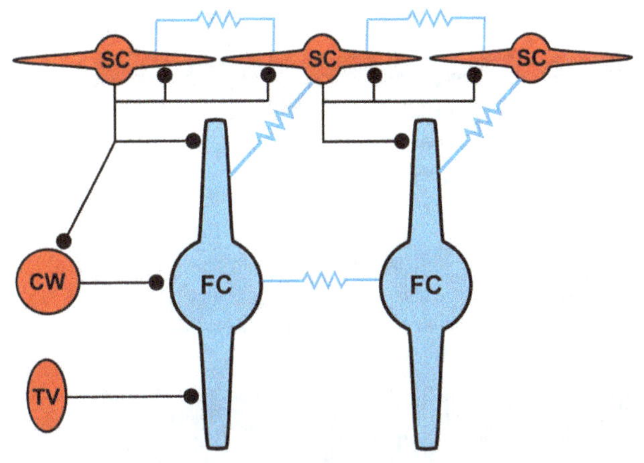

FIGURE 5 | Proposed circuit diagram for inhibitory inputs to fusiform cells and the gap junction connectivity (represented by resistors) between SSCs and fusiform cells. SSCs, cartwheel and tuberculoventral cells occupy distinct domains of the fusiform somatodendritic space. SSCs are unique among the three inhibitory cell types in their additional electrical connectivity with fusiform cells and with one another.

example was spontaneously active, as typical of these cells *in vitro* and *in vivo* (Rhode et al., 1983; Hancock and Voigt, 2002; Leao et al., 2012), and spikelet activity was readily apparent in the adjoining SSC. Negative displacements of the SSC membrane potential from the resting potential had a clear inhibitory effect on the spontaneous firing rate of fusiform cell. Among average data (**Figure 6B**), spike rate had a nearly linear dependence on SSC membrane voltage between 0 to −30 mV negative to the resting potential. While this effect required relatively large hyperpolarizations, it might be more potent if multiple SSCs were to converge on fusiform cells and were hyperpolarized as a group, perhaps occurring when SSCs receive inhibition from neighboring cells or through the actions of a neuromodulator. In any case, these data complement our previous studies, and show that SSCs inhibit fusiform cells through both chemical and electrical contacts, whereas fusiform cells both excite and inhibit SSCs through electrical contacts.

DISCUSSION

The network of SSCs in the DCN shares several features with that of stellate cells of the cerebellar cortex, including expression of Ca^{2+}-permeable AMPA receptors, formation of GABAergic contacts between stellate cells, autapses, and inhibitory contacts on principal cells (fusiform and Purkinje cells), as well as electrical coupling between stellate cells. But the parallels seem to end there, as SSCs show additional features that are quite distinct from their cerebellar counterparts. Excitatory chemical synapses onto SSCs utilize both AMPA and NMDA receptors, and inhibitory chemical synapses release glycine along with GABA and activate both GABA and glycine receptors. Electrical synapses between stellate cells and Purkinje cells of the cerebellum have not been reported, although one study described dye-coupling between these neurons following exposure to nicotine (Middleton et al., 2008). These and other physiological and molecular differences highlight the different natures of computation in DCN and cerebellum. It will be of interest to contrast the properties of SSCs in these structures with their

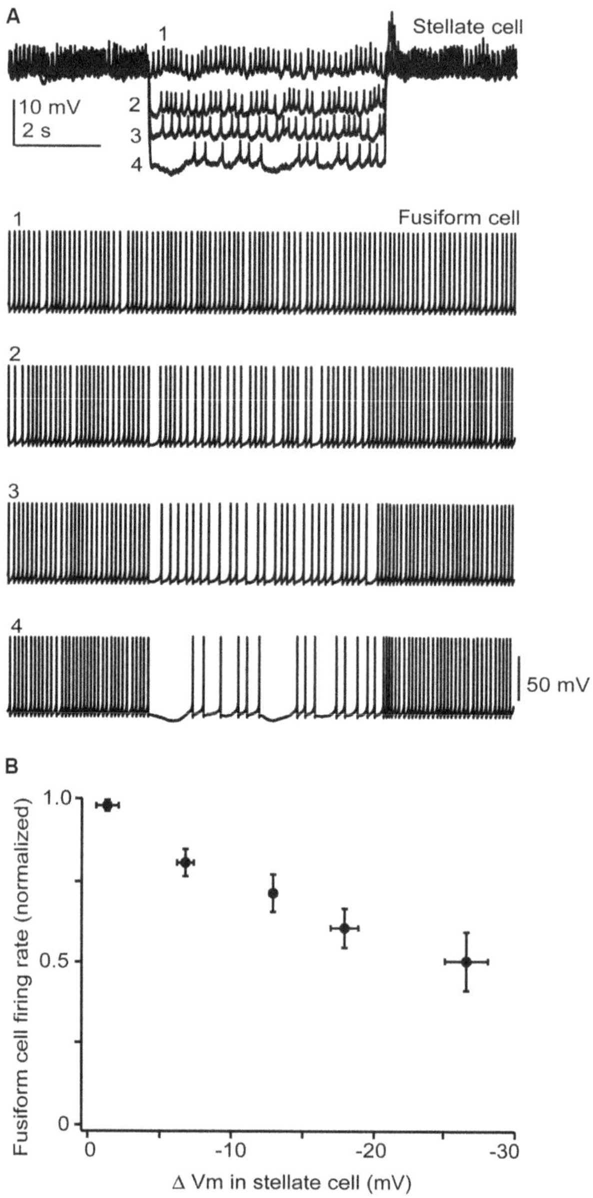

FIGURE 6 | Stellate membrane potential modulates fusiform spontaneous spike rate. (A) In an electrically coupled cell pair, injection of hyperpolarizing current steps into the SSC shifted the SSC potential up to 20 mV negative to the resting potential of −65 mV and had a clear inhibitory effect on fusiform spontaneous spiking. **(B)** Average data from 5 cell pairs shows a near linear dependence of fusiform cell spike rate on SSC membrane potential. Firing rates varied widely among fusiform cells and so were normalized in each cell to the rate during the baseline condition where no hyperpolarizing current step was injected into the stellate cell.

counterparts in the electrosensory lobe of mormyrid electric fish, which share many of key features with the DCN (Bell et al., 2008).

The positioning of SSCs in the DCN, combined with their unusual synaptic connectivity, suggest interesting potential roles in multisensory integration. Their restriction to the molecular layer, in many cases the very edge of the molecular layer, point to a domain of control limited to the outermost dendritic fields of fusiform and cartwheel cells (**Figure 5**). Presumably, SSCs have the capacity to suppress excitatory synaptic signals to those dendrites in a region specific manner. As noted above, SSCs thus stand in contrast to the domains of influence of cartwheel and tuberculoventral cells, and this anatomical relationship points to a picture of complex computational subregions in the fusiform cell (**Figure 5**). Moreover, the observation that cartwheel cells and SSCs contact one another, combined with the possibility of cartwheel-tuberculoventral interconnections (Kuo and Trussell, unpublished observations), suggests that temporal patterns of input to the three interneuronal subtypes could dictate how these subregions of the fusiform cell are recruited and utilized.

Future studies will need to examine several important aspects of SSC function and synaptic topology. Given the precedent of plasticity at cerebellar stellate cell synapses (Liu and Cull-Candy, 2000) and at parallel fiber to cartwheel and fusiform cell synapses (Fujino and Oertel, 2003; Tzounopoulos et al., 2004), it will be of interest to examine use-dependent changes in strength of parallel fiber to SSC contacts. Indeed, given the complex relationships between SSCs and their targets, such plasticity might potently shift the balance between multisensory (via parallel fibers) and auditory nerve (via the fusiform cell and electrical synapses) control of inhibition in the molecular layer.

Just as important is the question of how stellate cells are "hooked up". Are electrical and chemical contacts random or are there preferential synaptic targets? What is the layout of SSC axons vs. dendrites in relation to fusiform cells, SSCs, and the tonotopic axis along which fusiform cells are distributed? Recent studies have highlighted the concept of "structured connectivity", and a recent example showed evidence for preferential connectivity among cerebellar stellate cells (Rieubland et al., 2014). In the DCN this question may be particularly interesting given the orthogonal directions of parallel fibers and the tonotopic axis: do gap junctions connect cells receiving common auditory input or common multisensory input? If SSCs form a more broad electrically coupled network, could electrical connections generate synchronized firing among them? If so, then the AHP communicated by the fusiform cells might serve to upset such synchronous firing, as shown for AHPs in cerebellar Golgi cells (Vervaeke et al., 2010). Beyond the SSC itself is the question of whether electrical synapses play a broader role in auditory processing. A likely target for future physiological studies will be the bushy cells of the ventral cochlear nucleus, in which ultrastructural studies have revealed the presence of gap junctions linking adjacent cell bodies and their dendrites (Sotelo et al., 1976; Gómez-Nieto and Rubio, 2009).

Lastly, it will be of important to examine stellate cell function in animal models of tinnitus, a condition characterized by heightened excitability of fusiform cells and the perception of a subjective sound. This has suggested a causal relationship between the two, although it is likely that other cell types and other brain regions are involved. Middleton et al. (2011) used brain slices to show that excitation of cells in the molecular layer generated a flavoprotein autofluorescence image indicative of cell firing. This signal could be enhanced by a $GABA_A$ receptor antagonist, suggesting that cell firing was controlled by a local GABAergic input. In noise treated animals that tested positive in a behavioral assay for tinnitus, autofluoresence signals were less well controlled by the antagonist, suggesting that GABAergic inhibition was diminished in the animal model. It is possible that the source of this GABAergic inhibition is the SSC, since the only other inhibitory cell in that region is the cartwheel cell, whose transmission is dominated 80–90% by glycine and glycine receptors (Roberts et al., 2008). Thus, the remarkably rich physiological features of the SSC may warrant a shift in standing from a neglected tiny cell type to a prominent component in multisensory integration and disease.

ACKNOWLEDGMENTS

Funding was provided by NIH Grants R01DC004450 to Laurence O. Trussell and F31DC012222 to Pierre F. Apostolides and P30 DC005983.

REFERENCES

Aizenman, C. D., and Linden, D. J. (1999). Regulation of the rebound depolarization and spontaneous firing patterns of deep nuclear neurons in slices of rat cerebellum. *J. Neurophysiol.* 82, 1697–1709.

Apostolides, P. F., and Trussell, L. O. (2013a). Rapid, activity-independent turnover of vesicular transmitter content at a mixed glycine/GABA synapse. *J. Neurosci.* 33, 4768–4781. doi: 10.1523/JNEUROSCI.5555-12.2013

Apostolides, P. F., and Trussell, L. O. (2013b). Regulation of interneuron excitability by gap junction coupling with principal cells. *Nat. Neurosci.* 16, 1764–1772. doi: 10.1038/nn.3569

Apostolides, P. F., and Trussell, L. O. (2014a). Chemical synaptic transmission onto superficial stellate cells of the mouse dorsal cochlear nucleus. *J. Neurophysiol.* 111, 1812–1822. doi: 10.1152/jn.00821.2013

Apostolides, P. F., and Trussell, L. O. (2014b). Control of interneuron firing by subthreshold synaptic potentials in principal cells of the dorsal cochlear nucleus. *Neuron*, in press.

Bell, C. C., Han, V., and Sawtell, N. B. (2008). Cerebellum-like structures and their implications for cerebellar function. *Annu. Rev. Neurosci.* 31, 1–24. doi: 10.1146/annurev.neuro.30.051606.094225

Brawer, J. R., Morest, D. K., and Kane, E. C. (1974). The neuronal architecture of the cochlear nucleus of the cat. *J. Comp. Neurol.* 155, 251–300. doi: 10.1002/cne.901550302

Burnashev, N., Monyer, H., Seeburg, P. H., and Sakmann, B. (1992). Divalent ion permeability of AMPA receptor channels is dominated by the edited form of a single subunit. *Neuron* 8, 189–198. doi: 10.1016/0896-6273(92)90120-3

Cajal, S. R. Y. (1911). *Histologie du système Nerveux de l'Homme et des Vertébrés.* Paris: Maloine.

Clark, B. A., and Cull-Candy, S. G. (2002). Activity-dependent recruitment of extrasynaptic NMDA receptor activation at an AMPA receptor-only synapse. *J. Neurosci.* 22, 4428–4436.

Disterhoft, J. F., Perkins, R. E., and Evans, S. (1980). Neuronal morphology of the rabbit cochlear nucleus. *J. Comp. Neurol.* 192, 687–702. doi: 10.1002/cne.901920405

Dugué, G. P., Dumoulin, A., Triller, A., and Dieudonne, S. (2005). Target-dependent use of co-released inhibitory transmitters at central synapses. *J. Neurosci.* 25, 6490–6498. doi: 10.1523/jneurosci.1500-05.2005

Fujino, K., and Oertel, D. (2003). Bidirectional synaptic plasticity in the cerebellum-like mammalian dorsal cochlear nucleus. *Proc. Natl. Acad. Sci. U S A* 100, 265–270. doi: 10.1073/pnas.0135345100

Gardner, S. M., Trussell, L. O., and Oertel, D. (1999). Time course and permeation of synaptic AMPA receptors in cochlear nuclear neurons correlate with input. *J. Neurosci.* 19, 8721–8729.

Gardner, S. M., Trussell, L. O., and Oertel, D. (2001). Correlation of AMPA receptor subunit composition with synaptic input in the mammalian cochlear nuclei. *J. Neurosci.* 21, 7428–7437.

Golding, N. L., and Oertel, D. (1997). Physiological identification of the targets of cartwheel cells in the dorsal cochlear nucleus. *J. Neurophysiol.* 78, 248–260.

Gómez-Nieto, R., and Rubio, M. E. (2009). A bushy cell network in the rat ventral cochlear nucleus. *J. Comp. Neurol.* 516, 241–263. doi: 10.1002/cne.22139

Hancock, K. E., and Voigt, H. F. (2002). Intracellularly labeled fusiform cells in dorsal cochlear nucleus of the gerbil. I. Physiological response properties. *J. Neurophysiol.* 87, 2505–2519.

Hume, R. I., Dingledine, R., and Heinemann, S. F. (1991). Identification of a site in glutamate receptor subunits that controls calcium permeability. *Science* 253, 1028–1031. doi: 10.1126/science.1653450

Kane, E. C. (1974). Synaptic organization in the dorsal cochlear nucleus of the cat: a light and electron microscopic study. *J. Comp. Neurol.* 155, 301–329. doi: 10.1002/cne.901550303

Kopp-Scheinpflug, C., Tozer, A. J., Robinson, S. W., Tempel, B. L., Hennig, M. H., and Forsythe, I. D. (2011). The sound of silence: ionic mechanisms encoding sound termination. *Neuron* 71, 911–925. doi: 10.1016/j.neuron.2011.06.028

Leao, R. M., Li, S., Doiron, B., and Tzounopoulos, T. (2012). Diverse levels of an inwardly rectifying potassium conductance generate heterogeneous neuronal behavior in a population of dorsal cochlear nucleus pyramidal neurons. *J. Neurophysiol.* 107, 3008–3019. doi: 10.1152/jn.00660.2011

Liu, S. Q., and Cull-Candy, S. G. (2000). Synaptic activity at calcium-permeable AMPA receptors induces a switch in receptor subtype. *Nature* 405, 454–458. doi: 10.1038/35013064

Lu, T., Rubio, M. E., and Trussell, L. O. (2008). Glycinergic transmission shaped by the corelease of GABA in a mammalian auditory synapse. *Neuron* 57, 524–535. doi: 10.1016/j.neuron.2007.12.010

Mann-Metzer, P., and Yarom, Y. (1999). Electrotonic coupling interacts with intrinsic properties to generate synchronized activity in cerebellar networks of inhibitory interneurons. *J. Neurosci.* 19, 3298–3306.

Middleton, J. W., Kiritani, T., Pedersen, C., Turner, J. G., Shepherd, G. M., and Tzounopoulos, T. (2011). Mice with behavioral evidence of tinnitus exhibit dorsal cochlear nucleus hyperactivity because of decreased GABAergic inhibition. *Proc. Natl. Acad. Sci. U S A* 108, 7601–7606. doi: 10.1073/pnas.1100223108

Middleton, S. J., Racca, C., Cunningham, M. O., Traub, R. D., Monyer, H., Knopfel, T., et al. (2008). High-frequency network oscillations in cerebellar cortex. *Neuron* 58, 763–774. doi: 10.1016/j.neuron.2008.03.030

Mugnaini, E. (1985). GABA neurons in the superficial layers of the rat dorsal cochlear nucleus: light and electron microscopic immunocytochemistry. *J. Comp. Neurol.* 235, 61–81. doi: 10.1002/cne.902350106

Nahir, B., and Jahr, C. E. (2013). Activation of extrasynaptic NMDARs at individual parallel fiber-molecular layer interneuron synapses in cerebellum. *J. Neurosci.* 33, 16323–16333. doi: 10.1523/JNEUROSCI.1971-13.2013

Nó, L. D. (1981). *The Primary Acoustic Nuclei.* New York: Raven Press.

Oertel, D., and Young, E. D. (2004). What's a cerebellar circuit doing in the auditory system? *Trends Neurosci.* 27, 104–110. doi: 10.1016/j.tins.2003.12.001

Rhode, W. S., Smith, P. H., and Oertel, D. (1983). Physiological response properties of cells labeled intracellularly with horseradish peroxidase in cat dorsal cochlear nucleus. *J. Comp. Neurol.* 213, 426–447. doi: 10.1002/cne.902130407

Rieubland, S., Roth, A., and Hausser, M. (2014). Structured connectivity in cerebellar inhibitory networks. *Neuron* 81, 913–929. doi: 10.1016/j.neuron.2013.12.029

Roberts, M. T., Bender, K. J., and Trussell, L. O. (2008). Fidelity of complex spike-mediated synaptic transmission between inhibitory interneurons. *J. Neurosci.* 28, 9440–9450. doi: 10.1523/JNEUROSCI.2226-08.2008

Rubio, M. E., and Juiz, J. M. (2004). Differential distribution of synaptic endings containing glutamate, glycine and GABA in the rat dorsal cochlear nucleus. *J. Comp. Neurol.* 477, 253–272. doi: 10.1002/cne.20248

Sotelo, C., and Llinas, R. (1972). Specialized membrane junctions between neurons in the vertebrate cerebellar cortex. *J. Cell Biol.* 53, 271–289. doi: 10.1083/jcb.53.2.271

Sotelo, C., Gentschev, T., and Zamora, A. J. (1976). Gap junctions in ventral cochlear nucleus of the rat. A possible new example of electrotonic junctions in the mammalian C.N.S. *Neuroscience* 1, 5–7. doi: 10.1016/0306-4522(76)90041-5

Tzounopoulos, T., Kim, Y., Oertel, D., and Trussell, L. O. (2004). Cell-specific, spike timing-dependent plasticities in the dorsal cochlear nucleus. *Nat. Neurosci.* 7, 719–725. doi: 10.1038/nn1272

Vervaeke, K., Lorincz, A., Gleeson, P., Farinella, M., Nusser, Z., and Silver, R. A. (2010). Rapid desynchronization of an electrically coupled interneuron network with sparse excitatory synaptic input. *Neuron* 67, 435–451. doi: 10.1016/j.neuron.2010.06.028

Webster, D. B., and Trune, D. R. (1982). Cochlear nuclear complex of mice. *Am. J. Anat.* 163, 103–130. doi: 10.1002/aja.1001630202

Wouterlood, F. G., Mugnaini, E., Osen, K. K., and Dahl, A. L. (1984). Stellate neurons in rat dorsal cochlear nucleus studies with combined Golgi impregnation and electron microscopy: synaptic connections and mutual coupling by gap junctions. *J. Neurocytol.* 13, 639–664. doi: 10.1007/bf01148083

Zeilhofer, H. U., Studler, B., Arabadzisz, D., Schweizer, C., Ahmadi, S., Layh, B., et al. (2005). Glycinergic neurons expressing enhanced green fluorescent protein in bacterial artificial chromosome transgenic mice. *J. Comp. Neurol.* 482, 123–141. doi: 10.1002/cne.20349

Zhang, S., and Oertel, D. (1993). Cartwheel and superficial stellate cells of the dorsal cochlear nucleus of mice: intracellular recordings in slices. *J. Neurophysiol.* 69, 1384–1397.

14

Activity-dependent modulation of inhibitory synaptic kinetics in the cochlear nucleus

Jana Nerlich[1], Christian Keine[1], Rudolf Rübsamen[1], R. Michael Burger[2] and Ivan Milenkovic[3]*

[1] Department of Neurobiology, Faculty of Biosciences, Pharmacy and Psychology, University of Leipzig, Leipzig, Germany
[2] Department of Biological Sciences, Lehigh University, Bethlehem, PA, USA
[3] Department of Physiology, Faculty of Medicine, Carl Ludwig Institute for Physiology, University of Leipzig, Leipzig, Germany

***Correspondence:**
Ivan Milenkovic, Department of Physiology, Faculty of Medicine, Carl Ludwig Institute for Physiology, University of Leipzig, Liebigstrasse 27, Leipzig, 04103, Germany
e-mail: Ivan.Milenkovic@medizin.uni-leipzig.de

Spherical bushy cells (SBCs) in the anteroventral cochlear nucleus respond to acoustic stimulation with discharges that precisely encode the phase of low-frequency sound. The accuracy of spiking is crucial for sound localization and speech perception. Compared to the auditory nerve input, temporal precision of SBC spiking is improved through the engagement of acoustically evoked inhibition. Recently, the inhibition was shown to be less precise than previously understood. It shifts from predominantly glycinergic to synergistic GABA/glycine transmission in an activity-dependent manner. Concurrently, the inhibition attains a tonic character through temporal summation. The present study provides a comprehensive understanding of the mechanisms underlying this slow inhibitory input. We performed whole-cell voltage clamp recordings on SBCs from juvenile Mongolian gerbils and recorded evoked inhibitory postsynaptic currents (IPSCs) at physiological rates. The data reveal activity-dependent IPSC kinetics, i.e., the decay is slowed with increased input rates or recruitment. Lowering the release probability yielded faster decay kinetics of the single- and short train-IPSCs at 100 Hz, suggesting that transmitter quantity plays an important role in controlling the decay. Slow transmitter clearance from the synaptic cleft caused prolonged receptor binding and, in the case of glycine, spillover to nearby synapses. The GABAergic component prolonged the decay by contributing to the asynchronous vesicle release depending on the input rate. Hence, the different factors controlling the amount of transmitters in the synapse jointly slow the inhibition during physiologically relevant activity. Taken together, the slow time course is predominantly determined by the receptor kinetics and transmitter clearance during short stimuli, whereas long duration or high frequency stimulation additionally engage asynchronous release to prolong IPSCs.

Keywords: inhibition, activity-dependent decay, re-uptake, intersynaptic pooling, asynchronous release, spherical bushy cell, cochlear nucleus

INTRODUCTION

Synaptic inhibition is mainly mediated by glycine and $GABA_A$ receptors (GlyR and $GABA_AR$, respectively) which tightly regulate neuronal and network activities. While the GlyR-generated inhibitory postsynaptic current (IPSC) is generally endowed with fast decay kinetics (Takahashi et al., 1992; Awatramani et al., 2004), GABA provides slow and in some cases tonic inhibition (Farrant and Nusser, 2005; Capogna and Pearce, 2011; Tang et al., 2011). Notably, there are presynaptic terminals in the sensory systems (Wentzel et al., 1993; Protti et al., 1997; Apostolides and Trussell, 2014), cerebellum (Dumoulin et al., 2001; Rousseau et al., 2012; Husson et al., 2014) and in the spinal cord (Jonas et al., 1998; O'Brien and Berger, 1999; Keller et al., 2001; Seddik et al., 2007) that release both transmitters beyond the early postnatal development. This allows for an additional variability, through activity-dependent use of transmitters (Nerlich et al., 2014), differential distribution of respective receptors at the same cell (Chéry and de Koninck, 1999), at different cells (Dugué et al., 2005; Kuo et al., 2009), or shaping the IPSC decay through action of both glycine and GABA on GlyR (Lu et al., 2008).

The postsynaptic responses in neurons expressing both GlyR and $GABA_AR$ usually represent a mixture of respective fast and slow synaptic currents (Russier et al., 2002; Awatramani et al., 2005; González-Forero and Alvarez, 2005; Coleman et al., 2011; Apostolides and Trussell, 2013). The relative contribution of both physiologically important components can change according to the activity pattern (Fischl et al., 2014). Such activity-dependent inhibitory control, mediated by dual glycine-GABA signaling, has been recently shown for the spherical bushy cells (SBCs) in the central auditory system (Nerlich et al., 2014). SBCs receive acoustically evoked excitatory input from auditory nerve fibers through large calyceal terminals, the endbulds of Held (Ryugo and Sento, 1991; Isaacson and Walmsley, 1996; Nicol and Walmsley, 2002), and non-primary inhibition from neurons within the cochlear nucleus (Wickesberg and Oertel,

1990; Saint Marie et al., 1991; Campagnola and Manis, 2014). The amplitude of IPSCs is dominated by GlyRs, while the initially small GABAergic component successively enhances the inhibitory strength and shapes its duration at physiologically relevant rates (Nerlich et al., 2014). Unlike other central auditory synapses that utilize phasic inhibition even at high rates (Awatramani et al., 2004; Kramer et al., 2014), IPSCs in SBCs summate due to slow kinetics (Xie and Manis, 2013, 2014; Nerlich et al., 2014), thereby providing a functionally tonic inhibition, similar to inhibition acting on the granule cells in the dorsal cochlear nucleus (DCN) and nucleus magnocellularis neurons in the cochlear nucleus of the chick (Lu and Trussell, 2000; Monsivais et al., 2000; Balakrishnan et al., 2009). To date, the synaptic mechanisms that determine the slow kinetics of the mixed glycine-GABA transmission in SBCs remained elusive.

We examined the mechanisms underlying the slow activity-dependent IPSC kinetics in SBCs by performing whole-cell recordings in acute slice preparations of juvenile Mongolian gerbils in combination with synaptic stimulation of inhibitory inputs. Our results demonstrate that the low capacity of glycine and GABA uptake allows transmitter rebinding, particularly at input rates above 100 Hz. The activity-driven transmitter spillover possibly engaged distant GlyR but not $GABA_AR$. Synaptic activity largely desynchronized the release of glycine and GABA, which had a significant contribution to the slow IPSC profile.

MATERIALS AND METHODS

The experimental procedures were approved by the Saxonian district Government Leipzig (T 84/12, T 67/13) and conducted according to the European Communities Council Directive (86/609/EEC).

SLICE PREPARATION

Coronal slices (180 μm) containing the rostral anteroventral cochlear nucleus (AVCN) were cut from P22-P30 gerbils of either sex. The brainstem was sliced with a vibratome in low-calcium artificial cerebrospinal fluid (ACSF) solution containing (in mM): 125 NaCl, 2.5 KCl, 0.1 $CaCl_2$, 3 $MgCl_2$, 1.25 NaH_2PO_4, 25 $NaHCO_3$, 25 glucose, 2 sodium pyruvate, 3 myo-inositol, 0.5 ascorbic acid, continuously bubbled with 5% CO_2 and 95% O_2, pH 7.4. Slices were incubated in the standard recording solution (ACSF same as for slicing, except $CaCl_2$ and $MgCl_2$ were changed to 2 mM and 1 mM, respectively) for 30 min at 37°C and stored at room temperature until recording. Experiments were performed at nearly physiological temperature (33.5 ± 0.5°C).

ELECTROPHYSIOLOGICAL RECORDINGS

Whole-cell patch clamp recordings were performed on SBCs in the rostral pole of the AVCN. Due to their large soma size and localization in the low-frequency area of the gerbil AVCN, these neurons can be visually distinguished from globular bushy cells. Morphological verification of SBCs was done during the recording by intracellular labeling with ATTO 488 and visualization by a CCD camera (IMAGO Typ VGA; TILL Photonics). The pipettes had resistances of 3–4 MΩ when filled with (mM): 125 $CsMeSO_3$, 18 TEA-Cl, 3 $MgCl_2$, 10 HEPES, 0.1 EGTA, 4.5 QX-314-Cl, 5 phosphocreatine, 2 ATP disodium salt, 0.3 GTP disodium salt, and 50 μM ATTO 488 (pH 7.3 with CsOH). The resulting inward currents with larger amplitudes enabled more accurate analyses compared to the small events occurring with physiological $[Cl^-]_{pip}$. Consistent with slow inhibitory kinetics in the present study, the synaptically evoked hyperpolarizations acquired with gramicidin perforated patch recordings also exhibited slow activity-dependent synaptic decays (gramicidin perforated patch: t_{wd} single: 18.5 ± 4.0 ms, 100 Hz 10th IPSC: 42.6 ± 4.1 ms, n = 6, see Nerlich et al., 2014). IPSCs were evoked by electrical stimulation of afferent fibers through a bipolar theta glass electrode (Science Products, tip Ø 5 μm) filled with bath solution and placed at distances of 30–60 μm from the cell. Pulse stimuli (100 μs, 15–90 V) were generated by a stimulator (Master 8) and delivered via a stimulus isolation unit (AMPI Iso-flex) to evoke either single events or train-responses at different frequencies. Voltage clamp measurements were done from V_{hold} = −71 mV, (Nerlich et al., 2014), except in cases where the amplitudes of the small asynchronous events were increased for precise event detection by holding the cell at −81 mV (**Figure 5**). To isolate glycine- and $GABA_A$ receptor mediated signals, a pharmacological inhibition of glutamate (50 μM AP-5, 10 μM NBQX) and $GABA_B$receptors (3 μM CGP 55845) was performed in all experiments. Offline correction of voltages was done for junction potentials of 11 mV. For some experiments, the extracellular calcium concentration in the ACSF was reduced to 1.2 mM in order to decrease the release probability. In such cases, the magnesium concentration was simultaneously increased to 1.8 mM to maintain the concentration of divalent cations.

DATA AQUISITION AND ANALYSIS

The recordings were acquired using a Multiclamp 700B amplifier (Molecular Devices). The mean capacitance of the cells was 23.15 ± 4.34 pF (mean ± SD, n = 52). The average series resistance was 11.25 ± 1.56 MΩ (n = 52), which was compensated by 50% to a remaining Rs of 3–7 MΩ. During experiments the series resistance changed on average by 2.6% (n = 52). Cells with series resistance changes >10% were excluded from analysis. There was no correlation between the IPCS amplitudes and decay time constants (r_s = 0.17, p = 0.22, n = 53). Together with the previously reported lack of correlation between the IPSC amplitudes and rise times (r_s = 0.04, p = 0.78, n = 43, Nerlich et al., 2014), these data rule out the possible contribution of series resistance error to decay time constant measurements. Recorded signals were digitized at 50 kHz and filtered with a 6 kHz Bessel low-pass filter. Data were examined with pClamp 10 software (Molecular Devices) followed by analyses using custom-written Matlab routines (version 8.3, Mathworks, Natick). Mean amplitudes, 10–90% rise times and decay time constants of IPSCs were analyzed from averaged traces (>5 repetitions). For detection of asynchronous release events, the current traces were band-pass filtered between 50 and 1500 Hz using a zero-phase forward and reverse digital IIR filter to remove the decay component (see **Figure 5A**). Statistical analysis by means of z-test revealed events with current amplitudes exceeding 1.96 times (p < 0.05) the standard deviation of the baseline. To avoid multiple triggers of the same event, all triggers occurring within 5 ms after the preceding event were excluded from the analysis. The results were visually controlled to ensure the correct detection of spontaneous events. The events occurring prior to electrical stimulation (spontaneous IPSCs) were quantified and compared to events emerging after the end of synaptic stimulation of inhibitory inputs. Asynchronous events were clearly visible during the decay phase of the last evoked IPSC. Events detected by the software during the first 20 ms of the current decay were not included into the analysis to avoid false positive results. Data from 3 repetitions for each condition were pooled and presented for each cell.

IPSC decay phase was fitted with mono- or bi-exponential functions based on an increase in adjusted R^2 values. The weighted τ decay was calculated as $\tau_{wd} = (A_{fast} \times \tau_{fast} + A_{slow} \times \tau_{slow})/(A_{fast} + A_{slow})$, where A_{fast} and A_{slow} are amplitudes at $t = 0$ and τ_{fast} and τ_{slow} are the fast and slow time constants, respectively. In cases of mono-exponential fits, one exponential component was set to 0.

STATISTICS

Data sets were compared with the appropriate *t*-test or analysis of variance (ANOVA). The *p*-values of multiple comparisons were adjusted by the Dunn-Šidak procedure. Within-subject comparisons were performed by repeated-measures (RM) ANOVA after testing for sphericity using Mauchly test, and Greenhouse-Geissner correction applied as appropriate. ANOVA was used to test for effects of drugs and possible interactions of input frequency and drug superfusion. The changes in asynchronous release evoked by different input frequencies were tested for significance by a *z*-test, $z = (A - BL)/SD_{BL}$, with A being the average number of events/bin 20–60 ms after stimulation, BL the mean of the baseline (1 s prior to stimulation = spontaneous IPSC level) and SD_{BL} the standard deviation of the baseline. All data are reported as mean ± SEM, unless otherwise stated.

RESULTS

IPSC DECAY RATE IS ACTIVITY-DEPENDENT

SBCs exhibit slow inhibitory synaptic decays (**Figure 1A**) mediated by GlyR and $GABA_AR$ (gerbil: spontaneous IPSCs: τ_{wd} = 16.7 ± 1.2 ms, synaptically evoked IPSCs τ_{wd} = 23.7 ± 5.3 ms, Nerlich et al., 2014; mouse: spontaneous IPSCs: τ_{wd} = 8.75 ± 0.6 ms, synaptically evoked IPSCs τ_{wd} = 11.1 ± 0.8 ms, Xie and Manis, 2013). Both the glycinergic and the GABAergic components were observed in all pharmacology experiments acquiring IPSCs with suprathreshold stimulation to evoke reliable responses (see also Nerlich et al., 2014). Notably, the pharmacologically isolated glycinergic and GABAergic single events were previously shown to have similar kinetics (Nerlich et al., 2014), thus arguing against the hypothesis that in SBCs the fast decay component can be accounted to glycine and the slow component to GABA. In the present study we investigated the underlying mechanism determining such inhibitory current kinetics. The decay phase of synaptically evoked single IPSCs was best fit with a bi-exponential function with a fast decay time constant τ_{fast} = 8.7 ± 2.1 ms, a slow decay time constant τ_{slow} = 38.9 ± 7.2 ms and their respective

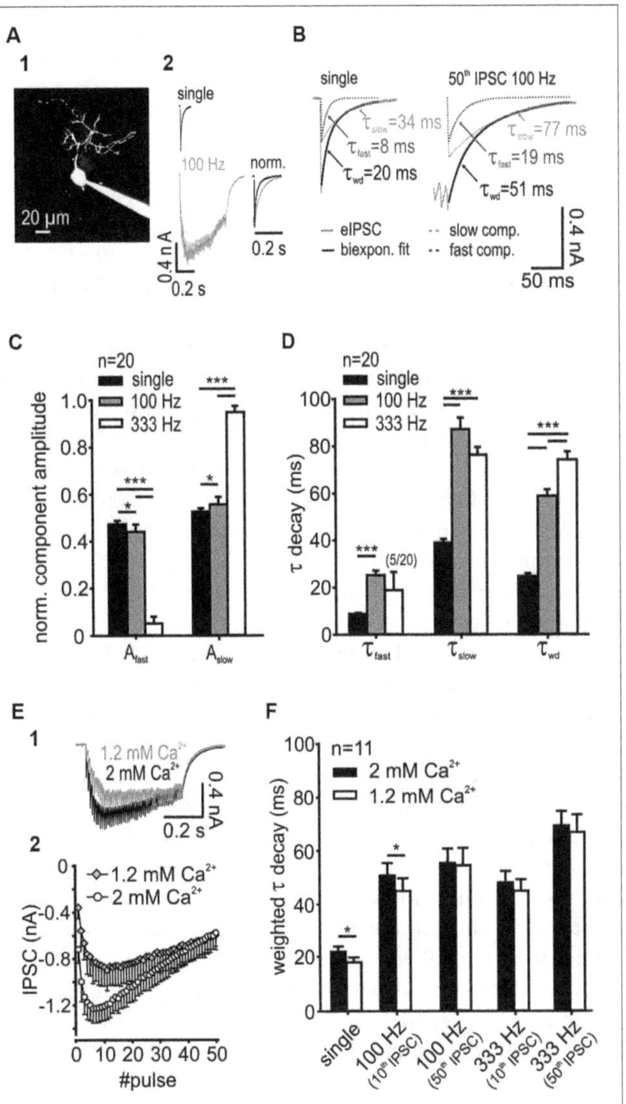

FIGURE 1 | IPSC decay kinetics are activity-dependent. (A1) SBC labeled with ATTO 488 reveals its characteristic morphology. **(A2)** Exemplary IPSCs elicited by single and 100 Hz stimulation of synaptic inputs. Right: Superimposed normalized IPSC from single-pulse, and 50-pulse responses, the latter showing decay times prolonged by train stimulation. **(B)** IPSCs decay was best fit with a bi-exponential function with the decay time constants τ_{fast} and τ_{slow}; also shown are the respective weighted decay time constants τ_{wd} **(C)** The respective component amplitudes A_{fast} and A_{slow} varied systematically with stimulation frequency. The fraction of the slow exponential component increased at higher input frequencies ($n = 20$, $^*p < 0.05$, $^{***}p < 0.001$, RM ANOVA) with a complementary decrease in the fast component amplitude. **(D)** Fast and slow decay time constants at different input frequencies ($n = 20$). Compared to single pulse stimulation, the increased input rate prolonged τ_{fast} at 100 Hz ($p < 0.001$, paired *t*-test) and τ_{slow} at both 100 Hz and 333 Hz ($p < 0.001$, RM ANOVA). Activity-dependent change of the τ_{fast} and τ_{slow} and the respective amplitudes at 100 Hz and 333 Hz (see panel **C**) resulted in a prolonged τ_{wd} of repetitive IPSCs ($p < 0.001$, RM ANOVA). **(E)** The release probability determines the temporal profile and the inhibitory strength at the onset of an IPSC train. **(E1)** Traces of IPSCs under standard (2 mM, used for slice recordings) and reduced (1.2 mM) extracellular calcium concentration. **(E2)** Mean baseline amplitudes of 50 IPSCs in a 100 Hz train under different

(Continued)

FIGURE 1 | Continued
extracellular calcium concentrations ($n = 6$). **(F)** For single IPSCs and the 10th IPSC at 100 Hz the weighted decay time constant was shorter under 1.2 mM extracellular calcium. $[Ca^{2+}]_o$ had no influence on τ_{wd} at longer trains of IPSCs (50 pulses) or at higher input frequency (333 Hz) ($n = 11$, single and 100 Hz 10th $p < 0.05$, 100 Hz 50th, 333 Hz 10th and 50th, $p > 0.27$, RM ANOVA).

relative amplitudes $A_{fast} = 0.47 \pm 0.06$ and $A_{slow} = 0.53 \pm 0.06$. The resulting average weighted decay time constant for 20 SBCs was $\tau_{wd} = 24.7 \pm 5.4$ ms (mean $\pm$ SD). The synaptic current decays were progressively slower after repetitive stimulation of inputs and with increasing input frequencies (**Figures 1B,D**). Also, the relative amplitude of the slow exponential component increased with input rates (**Figure 1C**; A_{slow} single $= 0.53 \pm 0.06$, 100 Hz $= 0.56 \pm 0.03$; 333 Hz $= 0.95 \pm 0.03$, single vs. 100 Hz $p < 0.05$; 100 Hz vs. 333 Hz $p < 0.001$, $n = 20$, RM ANOVA). Complementary decrease in amplitude of the fast component occurred over the same range of stimuli (A_{fast} single $= 0.47 \pm 0.06$, 100 Hz $= 0.44 \pm 0.03$, 333 Hz $= 0.05 \pm 0.03$). The slow decay time constant was prolonged substantially at 100 Hz and 333 Hz (**Figure 1D**; τ_{slow} single $= 38.9 \pm 1.6$ ms, 100 Hz $= 87.1 \pm 5.0$ ms, 333 Hz $= 76.3 \pm 3.3$ ms, $n = 20$, $p < 0.001$ for single vs. 100 Hz and 333 Hz, RM ANOVA). At 333 Hz, the decay phase was best fit with a mono-exponential function excluding the fast exponential component in 75% of recorded SBCs (in these cells A_{fast} was set to 0). Due to the rare occurrence of τ_{fast} at 333 Hz (only in 5 out of 20 cells), this parameter was statistically compared only for the single and 100 Hz stimulation. The τ_{fast} was prolonged at 100 Hz compared to single pulse stimulation (τ_{fast} single $= 7.1 \pm 0.6$, 100 Hz $= 21.4 \pm 3.0$, $n = 20$, single vs. 100 Hz $p < 0.001$, paired t-test). Activity-dependent change of τ_{fast}, τ_{slow} and the respective amplitudes resulted in a prolongation of τ_{wd} with increasing input frequency (**Figure 1D**; τ_{wd} single $= 24.7 \pm 1.2$ ms, 100 Hz $= 58.8 \pm 2.8$ ms, 333 Hz $= 74.2 \pm 3.5$ ms, $n = 20$, $p < 0.001$ for all comparisons, RM ANOVA). However, the longer decays were not associated with larger IPSC amplitudes (τ_{wd} single $= 22.8 \pm 0.8$ ms, 50th 100 Hz $= 61.8 \pm 2.5$ ms, $n = 25$, $p < 0.001$, paired t-test; IPSC amplitude single $= 0.56 \pm 0.5$ nA, 50th 100 Hz $= 0.55 \pm 0.04$ nA, $n = 25$, $p = 0.81$, paired t-test), thus suggesting that activity-dependent synaptic mechanisms, rather than series resistance errors cause the decay time prolongation. Together, these data indicate that the increase in input rates increases the transmitter quantity in the cleft which particularly prolongs the τ_{slow} through transmitter rebinding.

Studies at the calyx of Held-MNTB principal neuron synapse revealed that *in vivo* release probability may be approximated in slice recordings by using 1.2 mM Ca^{2+} in the extracellular solution (Borst, 2010). The dependance of the IPSC decay times on the release probability was shown at other auditory synapses (Balakrishnan et al., 2009; Tang and Lu, 2012). Although the *in vivo* release probability for the endbulb of Held-SBC synapse remains to be elucidated, we still addressed the question, whether the slow decay of inhibitory currents measured in SBCs is due to an increased release probability in the slice recordings. For this, the weighted decay time constant was measured from the last event within trains consisting of different numbers of pulses and the results were compared for 1.2 mM and 2 mM external calcium concentration (**Figure 1F**). Single IPSCs and short trains (10 pulses at 100 Hz) revealed faster decay time constants under the lower release probability condition. However, with increasing stimulus number and frequency, the weighted decay time constant of the last pulse in the train was similar between the two calcium conditions, (**Figure 1F**; main effect calcium $p = 0.04$, 1.2 vs. 2 mM: single, 100 Hz 10th IPSC $p < 0.05$, 100 Hz 50th IPSC $p = 0.72$, 333 Hz 10th $p = 0.27$ and 50th IPSC $p = 0.33$, $n = 11$, RM ANOVA). The slower IPSC at the higher release probability could either be due to transmitter pooling or to multivesicular release. The latter mechanism could explain the data for the single and short IPSC trains. The reduction of extracellular calcium to 1.2 mM decreased the IPSCs amplitudes, especially at the onset of a 100 Hz train (50 pulses) (**Figure 1E**). However, at the end of the train the baseline IPSC amplitudes were similar to those measured under 2 mM $[Ca^{2+}]_o$ (IPSC amplitudes 2 mM vs. 1.2 mM: onset = 1st IPSC, $p < 0.001$; maximum = mean 6–8th IPSC vs. mean 10–12th IPSC, $p < 0.01$; end = mean 48–50th IPSC, $p = 0.88$, $n = 6$, RM ANOVA). Thus, the release probability is unlikely to play a role for longer trains of stimuli or high frequency stimulation pointing to transmitter pooling as a mechanism contributing to slow decays.

RECRUITMENT OF FIBERS SLOWS THE IPSC DECAY

Recruitment of nearby inputs can lead to spillover of transmitter to remote synaptic or extrasynaptic sites, and thereby to intersynaptic pooling. Thus, it is conceivable that the slow IPSC decay in SBCs is caused by ongoing rebinding of transmitter and activation of extrasynaptic receptors, as shown earlier (Balakrishnan et al., 2009; Tang and Lu, 2012). To determine whether synaptic recruitment influences the kinetics of inhibition in SBCs, IPSCs were evoked with increasing stimulus intensities (**Figure 2A**). The low intensity was set slightly above the threshold with IPSC amplitudes reaching $38.5 \pm 16\%$ (mean $\pm$ SD, $n = 7$) of the maximal amplitude evoked by high stimulation intensity. With an increase in stimulus intensity, the amplitude of a single evoked IPSC and the last IPSC in a 100 Hz train increased threefold (**Figure 2B**; low vs. high intensity: single, $n = 7$, $p < 0.01$; 100 Hz 10th IPSC, $n = 5$, $p < 0.01$, paired t-test). Furthermore, the weighted decay time constants of single and repetitive IPSCs were prolonged at high stimulus intensities (**Figure 2C**; τ_{wd} single: low $= 21.6 \pm 0.6$ ms, high $= 26.3 \pm 0.6$ ms, $n = 7$, $p < 0.01$, 100 Hz 10th IPSC: low $= 35.4 \pm 0.8$ ms, high $= 46.0 \pm 0.8$ ms, $n = 5$, $p < 0.01$, paired t-tests). On the other hand, the rise time of single IPSCs was not dependent on stimulus intensity, suggesting the recruitment of nearby synaptic inputs (**Figure 2D**; low $= 0.44 \pm 0.03$ ms, high $= 0.46 \pm 0.03$ ms, $n = 7$, $p = 0.79$, paired t-test). As we neither observed a build-up, nor a run-down of IPSC amplitudes during repetitions at a given stimulus intensity, it is unlikely that the number of activated inputs changed. Therefore, these data suggest that the transmitter quantity substantially contributes to slow inhibitory kinetics.

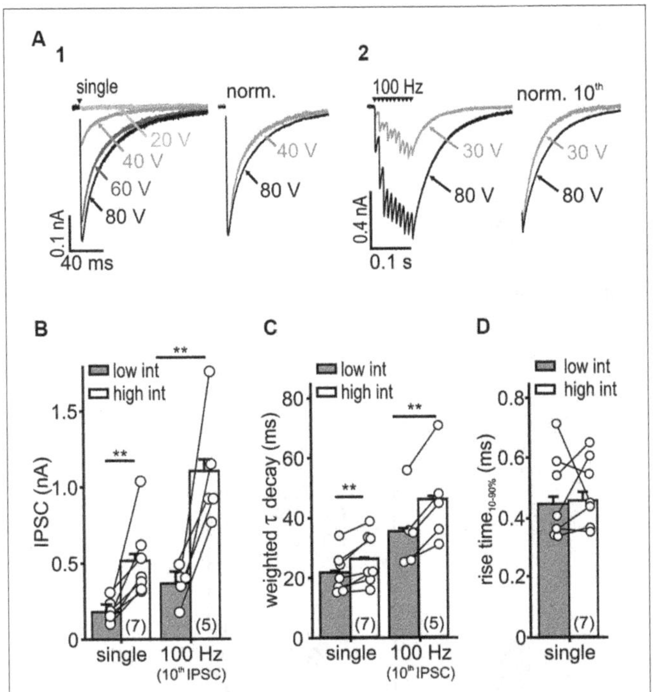

FIGURE 2 | IPSC kinetics depends on stimulus intensity.
(A) Representative IPSC traces evoked by a single **(A1)** or repetitive stimulation **(A2)** at varying stimulus intensities. Higher stimulus intensities evoked IPSCs of longer decays during single and repetitive stimulations (right: normalized last IPSCs). **(B,C)** Both IPSC amplitude **(B)** and τ_{wd} **(C)** increased with stimulation intensity (cell numbers are given in parentheses, $p < 0.01$, paired t-test). **(D)** The IPSC rise-time was unaffected by the stimulus intensity ($n = 7$, $p = 0.79$, paired t-test).

TRANSMITTER UPTAKE CONTRIBUTES TO THE IPSC KINETICS

If transmitter spillover and its clearance from the synaptic cleft shape the IPSC decay in an activity-dependent manner, the postsynaptic currents should be sensitive to a blockade of re-uptake transporters (Otis et al., 1996; Balakrishnan et al., 2009; Tang and Lu, 2012). Bath application of the glycine transporter 2 (GlyT2) inhibitor ORG 25543 (20 μM, Bradaïa et al., 2004; Balakrishnan et al., 2009) slowed down the decay of both single and train IPSCs (**Figures 3A,B**; $n = 6$, RM ANOVA). The fast decay time constant, the respective amplitudes of the exponential components and the IPSC rise time were not affected by the glycine re-uptake block ($n = 6$, control vs. +ORG, τ_{fast}: $p = 0.15$; A_{slow} and A_{fast}: $p = 0.37$, RM ANOVA, rise time: $p = 0.99$, paired t-test). Therefore, it can be concluded that the τ_{wd} prolongation (**Figure 3B**) is caused by the significantly longer τ_{slow} (**Figure 3B**). Given the similar IPSC decays of the isolated glycinergic and GABAergic single events (Nerlich et al., 2014), the τ_{fast} probably describes the intrinsic kinetics of receptor activation and de-activation, whereas the transmitter clearance, relief from saturation and delayed release determine τ_{slow}.

In addition to the sensitivity to glycine re-uptake, the IPSC decay phase was also shaped by GABA clearance. Simultaneous inhibition of the respective neuronal- and glial-GABA transporters with 20 μM NO 711 (Szabadics et al., 2007; Tang and Lu, 2012) and 100 μM SNAP 5114 (Keros and Hablitz, 2005; Song et al., 2013) extended the weighted decay time constant of the last IPSC in 100 Hz trains. Again, the prolongation of τ_{slow} during re-uptake blockade underlie the slowing of train IPSCs (**Figures 3C,D**; $n = 8$, control vs. +NO/SNAP, τ_{slow}: $p < 0.001$, τ_{wd}: $p < 0.01$, RM ANOVA). Notably, the GABA uptake is apparently only contributing to the decay during ongoing activity, as single evoked IPSC decays were not affected ($p > 0.45$) (**Figure 3D**). Similar to the effects seen after blockade of glycine re-uptake, GABA re-uptake inhibition did not change the fast decay time constants, the respective amplitudes of the exponential components and the IPSC rise times ($n = 8$, control vs. +NO/SNAP, τ_{fast}: $p = 0.11$, A_{slow} and A_{fast}: $p = 0.43$, RM ANOVA, rise time: $p = 0.40$, paired t-test). Together, these data suggest that glycine rebinding caused by transmitter pooling due to slow clearance is an important factor in shaping the inhibitory current profile. On the other hand, the GABA re-uptake only contributes at high stimulus input rates to the decay kinetics, when it presumably accumulates in the synaptic cleft.

To investigate transmitter rebinding and the possible contribution of spillover to inhibitory kinetics, we assessed the effects of low affinity GlyR and $GABA_AR$ antagonists. The rationale to use weak competitive antagonists to probe for putative remote synapses arises from studies showing that the receptors distant to the release site are likely to encounter a lower transmitter concentration during a synaptic event (Diamond, 2001; Chen and Diamond, 2002). Hence, the low-affinity competitive antagonists are progressively more effective at receptors facing low transmitter concentrations through spillover (Overstreet and Westbrook, 2003; Szabadics et al., 2007; Balakrishnan et al., 2009; Tang and Lu, 2012). Bath application of a high concentration of SR 95531 (200 μM), employed as a low affinity antagonist of GlyR (Wang and Slaughter, 2005; Beato, 2008; Balakrishnan et al., 2009), reduced the IPSC amplitudes considerably and accelerated the weighted decay time constant of single and repetitive IPSCs (**Figures 4A–C**; $n = 6$, RM ANOVA). Low concentrations of SR 95531 (10 and 20 μM) specifically blocked $GABA_A$ receptors on SBCs and reduced the IPSC amplitudes by 18 ± 2% and 16 ± 3%, respectively (Nerlich et al., 2014). At the concentration of 200 μM, a 76 ± 5% reduction of the IPSC amplitude was observed (**Figure 4D**; 200 μM vs. 10 μM ($n = 6$), $p < 0.001$; 200 μM ($n = 6$) vs. 20 μM ($n = 11$), $p < 0.001$, ANOVA). This result is consistent with an additional antagonistic action of a high SR 95531 concentration at GlyR, as opposed to specific $GABA_AR$ blockade at concentrations of 10 and 20 μM (Nerlich et al., 2014). To further confirm the competitive antagonistic action of SR 95531 at GlyR, the glycine concentration in the cleft was increased by co-applying the glycine re-uptake inhibitor ORG 25543. This partially reversed the long τ_{wd} confirming that the current decay is regulated by the amount of available glycine (**Figure 4D**; change of τ_{wd}: +20 μM SR = −8.1 ± 2.4%, $n = 13$; +200 μM SR = −35.3 ± 2.5%, $n = 6$; +200 μM SR+ORG = −21.2 ± 5.5%, $n = 6$; 20 μM vs. 200 μM SR $p < 0.001$, 200 μM SR vs. 200 μM SR+ORG $p = 0.01$, ANOVA). As the uptake blockers reveal transmitter spillover by increasing its quantity and enabling distant

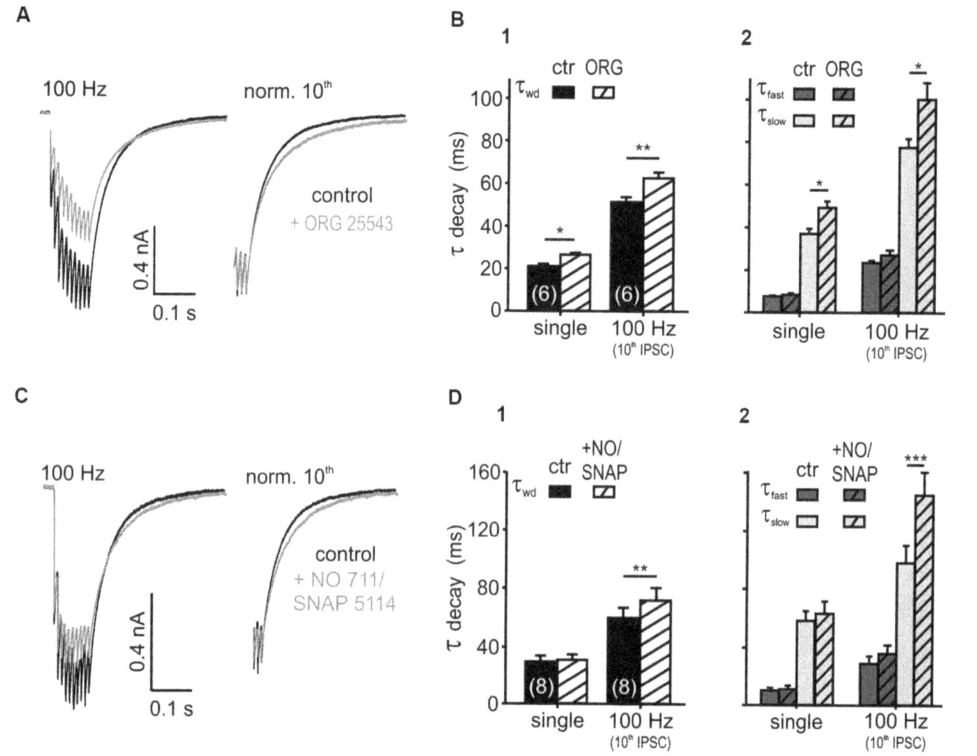

FIGURE 3 | Glycine and GABA re-uptake contributes to the IPSC kinetics. **(A)** Average traces of 100 Hz IPSC trains, before and after the bath application of the GlyT2 blocker ORG 25543 (20 μM). The weighted time constant increased under the glycine re-uptake block (right: traces normalized to the last IPSC). **(B)** Inhibition of GlyT2 prolonged the τ_{wd} **(B1)** upon single ($p < 0.05$) and repetitive ($p < 0.01$) synaptic stimulation due to an increase in τ_{slow} ($p < 0.05$). The fast exponential component was unaffected **(B2)** ($n = 6$, $p = 0.15$, RM ANOVA). **(C)** IPSCs evoked at 100 Hz, before and after the bath application of 20 μM NO 711 and 100 μM SNAP 5114. The weighted decay time constant increased under the GABA re-uptake block (right: traces normalized to the last IPSC). **(D)** Inhibition of GABA uptake prolonged the weighted decay of IPSCs at 100 Hz ($p < 0.01$) **(D1)** by increasing τ_{slow} ($p < 0.001$) **(D2)**. The IPSC kinetics of single events were not affected ($p > 0.45$, $n = 8$, RM ANOVA).

receptors to encounter a lower concentration of an agonist (Chen and Diamond, 2002; Thomas et al., 2011), our data showing a decay time prolongation under ORG 25543 are consistent with glycine spillover.

Inhibitory currents in SBCs show an activity-dependent depression of the IPSC peak amplitudes (I_{peak}, **Figure 4E**). Yet, under the low affinity GlyR antagonist (200 μM SR 95531), the peak amplitudes showed a weaker depression which in some cells even changed into facilitation (**Figures 4E,F**). This result is consistent with a relief from receptor saturation and/or desensitization (Chanda and Xu-Friedman, 2010). Thus, the peak IPSC depression at high input rates is presumably caused by postsynaptic receptor saturation and/or desensitization, rather than presynaptic short-term plasticity.

Contrary to glycine signaling, GABA is apparently not activating nearby synapses. Even at high stimulation rates, the low affinity $GABA_AR$ antagonist TPMPA (Szabadics et al., 2007; Tang and Lu, 2012) neither affected the IPSC decay nor the amplitudes, suggesting that the postsynaptic $GABA_AR$ could be tightly coupled to release sites of the transmitter and, thus, encounter consistently high GABA concentration (**Figures 4G–I**; control vs. TPMPA τ_{wd}: single $p = 0.97$; 100 Hz 10th IPSC $p = 0.62$; IPSC amplitude: single $p = 0.67$; 100 Hz 10th IPSC $p = 0.19$; $n = 8$, RM ANOVA). In summary, the apparently low uptake capacity of glycine and GABA transporters slows the decay of IPSCs, thereby enabling spillover of glycine. While we found no evidence for spillover of GABA, the transmitter quantity and intrinsic receptor properties probably account for the slow GABAergic transmission.

ACTIVITY-DEPENDENT ASYNCHRONOUS RELEASE

A further mechanism putatively contributing to IPSC decay time in SBCs could be an activity-induced desynchronization of vesicle release, as shown for several inhibitory synapses (Lu and Trussell, 2000; Hefft and Jonas, 2005; Tang and Lu, 2012). To test this hypothesis, high frequency stimulation (100 and 333 Hz) of inhibitory inputs to SBCs was employed to evoke small asynchronous events in the decay phase following the IPSC trains (**Figure 5A**). The quantity of asynchronous IPSCs increased with stimulus duration (**Figures 5B,E**) and frequency (**Figures 5C,F**). To compare the spontaneously occurring IPSCs (sIPSC, without input stimulation) and delayed IPSCs following repetitive input stimulation, the events were detected during 1 s before synaptic stimulation and 2 s after the last evoked IPSC

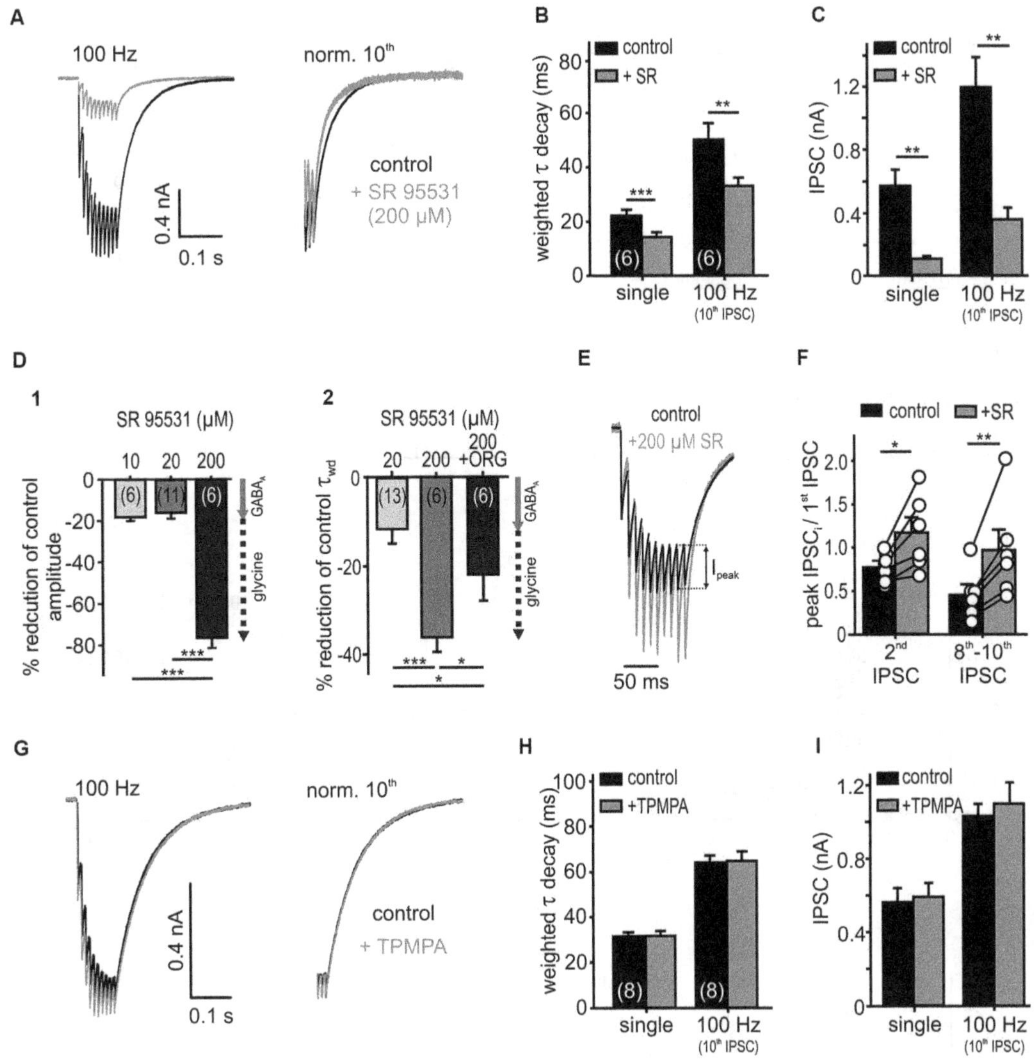

FIGURE 4 | Low affinity antagonist reveals spillover and rebinding of glycine. **(A)** Responses to 10 stimuli at 100 Hz, under the control condition and in the presence of a weak glycine receptor antagonist SR 95531 (200 μM). The weighted decay decreased under SR 95531 (right: traces normalized to the last IPSC). **(B,C)** Summary data showing faster IPSC decay time constants **(B)** and substantially reduced amplitudes **(C)** under the weak antagonism of SR95531 for single and 100 Hz stimulation ($n = 6$, RM ANOVA). **(D)** Percentage reduction of amplitudes **(D1)** and decay values **(D2)** of single IPSCs under different SR 95531 concentrations and SR 95531+ ORG 25543 compared to control condition (100%). At concentrations of 10 μM and 20 μM, SR 95531 had similar inhibitory effects on IPSC amplitude, due to a specific $GABA_AR$ antagonism (Nerlich et al., 2014) (gray arrow = $GABA_A$ receptor contribution). At a concentration of 200 μM, SR 95531 further reduced the amplitude and accelerated the IPSCs decay time. The faster IPSCs under 200 μM SR 95531, were again prolonged after the additional inhibition of GlyT2 by ORG 25543 (20 μM) **(D2)** suggesting a low-affinity inhibition of glycine receptors by 200 μM SR 95531 (dashed arrow = putative glycine receptor blockade). Cell numbers are given in parentheses; ANOVA. **(E)** Representative traces (10 IPSCs at 100 Hz) for control condition and superfusion of 200 μM SR 95531 normalized to the first event. I_{peak}: difference between steady state of the preceding event and peak of the successive event. **(F)** The peak amplitude of the second IPSC and the mean of the 8th–10th peak IPSCs relative to the first IPSC increased in the presence of SR 95531 (2nd/1st IPSC ratio increased by 0.46 ± 0.12, $p < 0.05$; 8th–10th/1st IPSC ratio increased by 0.96 ± 0.23, $p < 0.01$, paired t-test, symbols: single cell data, bars: mean ± SEM). The low affinity antagonism of GlyR counteracts depression. **(G)** Low affinity $GABA_AR$ antagonist (200 μM TPMPA) had no effect on IPSCs (normalized to the 10th IPSC: right). **(H,I)** Summary data showing a lack of TPMPA effect on the IPSC decays (single: $p = 0.96$, 100 Hz: $p = 0.62$) and the amplitudes (single: $p = 0.66$, 100 Hz: $p = 0.19$, $n = 8$, RM ANOVA). $^{*}p < 0.05$, $^{**}p < 0.01$, $^{***}p < 0.001$.

(see methods). The number of asynchronous events increased significantly after the 333 Hz stimulation (**Figure 5E** summary data for 4 cells and respective presentation of 10, 25 and 50 stimuli at 333 Hz z values > 10.1, $p < 0.001$, z-test), compared to the rate of sIPSC before stimulation (**Figure 5D**; mean # of sIPSCs/20 ms bin = 0.56 ± 0.08, $n = 4$). This result suggests

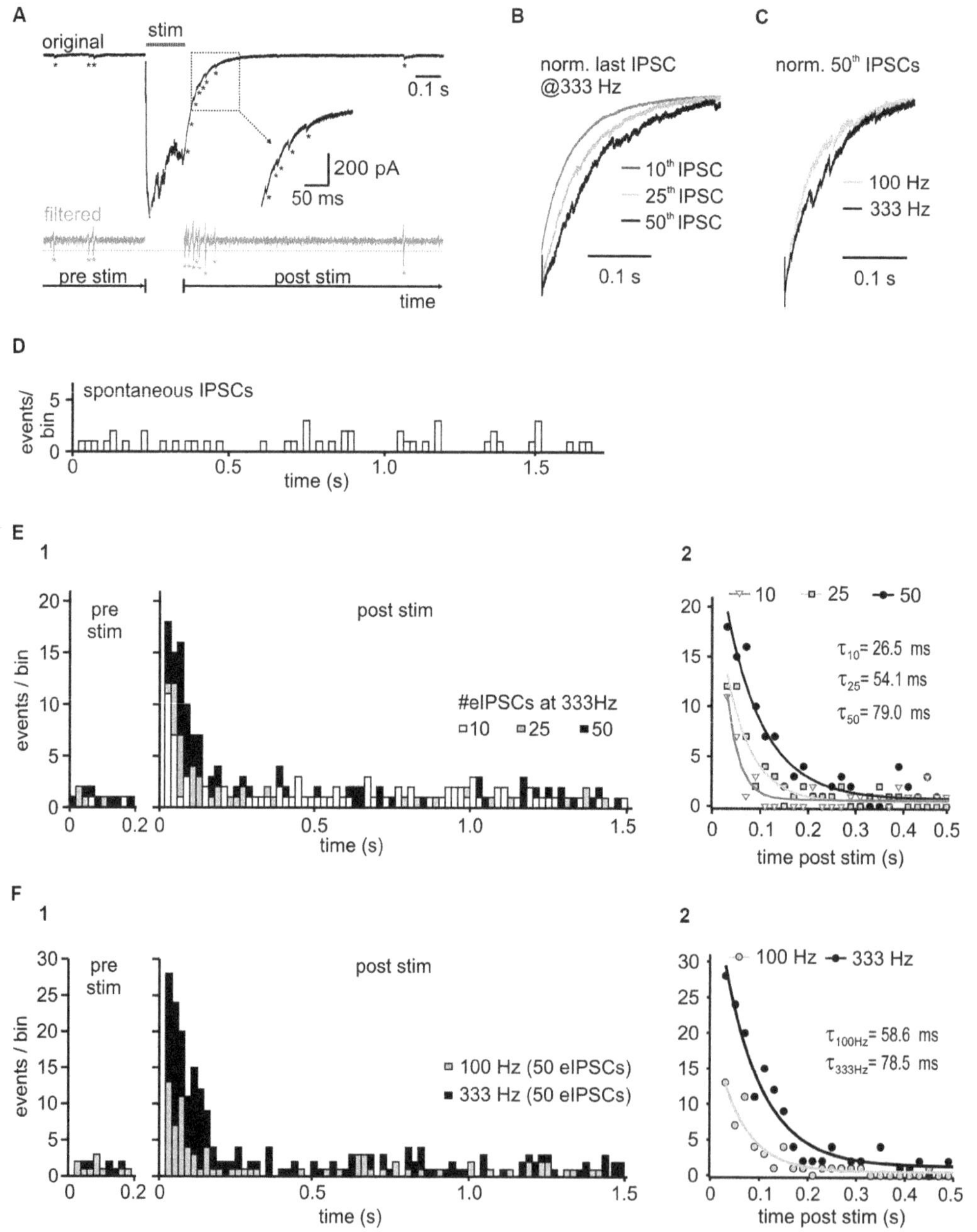

FIGURE 5 | Activity-dependence of asynchronous release. (A) Representative trace with detected asynchronous release events, before and after 50 stimuli at 333 Hz (upper panel). For event detection the signal was bandpass filtered between 50 and 1500 Hz (bottom panel). Potential events were detected when the filtered current amplitude exceeded 1.96 times ($p < 0.05$) the standard deviation of the noise (dashed gray line). Note the increased incidence of events in the decay phase of the last IPSC. **(B)** Normalized last IPSCs elicited by different numbers of stimuli in a 333 Hz train. **(C)** Superimposed normalized last IPSCs in a 50-pulse train at 100 Hz and 333 Hz. **(D)** Histogram of spontaneous IPSCs before synaptic stimulation of inhibitory inputs ($n = 4$ cells, bin width: 20 ms). **(E1)** Histograms of asynchronous release events before (= spontaneous events, pre stim) and after the 333 Hz input stimulation (= asynchronous and spontaneous events, post stim) with different number of stimuli ($n = 4$ cells, bin width: 20 ms, post stim $t = 0$ refers to the time of the last IPSC in the train). Following synaptic stimulation, the time course of asynchronous events relaxed back to the resting state with a mono-exponential function. The increase of asynchronous events during the decay phase depends on the presynaptic activity. **(E2)** Mono-exponential fits to the data from **(E1)**. The initial incidence of events, and the time constant (τ) depend on stimulus number (10 vs. 25 vs. 50 stimuli $p < 0.05$ for each comparison). **(F)** Input frequency determines the amount of asynchronous release. **(F1)** Summary histograms of asynchronous events from 6 cells, before and after 50-pulse stimulation at 100 Hz and 333 Hz. **(F2)** Mono-exponential fits to the data from F1. The initial incidence of events was increased and the exponential time constant prolonged with higher input frequency (100 Hz vs. 333 Hz $p < 0.05$).

the occurrence of activity induced asynchronous events in the decay phase of IPSC trains. Detailed analyses revealed the time course of incidence of asynchronous events which was best fit with a mono-exponential function relaxing back to the resting state. The following parameters were used to quantify the delayed release: initial amplitude (peak incidence of asynchronous events (A), an exponential time constant (τ) and a steady state value (c) (**Figure 5E**; fit comparison 10 vs. 25 vs. 50 stimuli $p < 0.001$, F-test). The peak incidence of asynchronous events after stimulation at 333 Hz increased almost 2-fold by extending the train from 10 to 50 pulses ($A_{\#eIPSC}$ 95% CI [lower, upper]: $A_{10} = 10.6$ [9.1, 12.2] events, $A_{25} = 12.9$ [11.7, 14.0] events, $A_{50} = 18.8$ [17.3, 20.3] events, 10 vs. 25 vs. 50 stimuli $p < 0.05$). The exponential time constant was also prolonged ($\tau_{\#eIPSC}$ 95% CI [lower, upper]: $\tau_{10} = 26.5$ [20.5, 37.4] ms, $\tau_{25} = 54.1$ [46.8, 64.4] ms, $\tau_{50} = 79.0$ [69.7, 91.1] ms, 10 vs. 25 vs. 50 stimuli $p < 0.05$), whereas the steady state values were similar to the mean sIPSC levels 1 s before stimulation ($c_{\#eIPSC}$ 95% CI [lower, upper]: $c_{10} = 0.63$ [0.52, 0.75] events/bin, $c_{25} = 0.43$ [0.33, 0.53] events/bin, $c_{50} = 0.73$ [0.59, 0.87] events/bin; sIPSCs ± SEM: prior to 10 eIPSCs = 0.54 ± 0.12 sIPSCs/bin, prior to 25 eIPSCs = 0.48 ± 0.10 sIPSCs/bin, prior to 50 eIPSCs = 0.74 ± 0.10 sIPSCs/bin, $p > 0.05$).

The rate of delayed release was not only dependent on the stimulus duration, but also on the stimulation frequency (**Figure 5C,F** summary data for 6 cells). **Figure 5F**, shows that presynaptic activity determines the quantity and duration of asynchronous release (A or τ, 95% CI [lower, upper]: $A_{100Hz} = 12.4$ [10.8, 13.9] events, $A_{333Hz} = 28.3$ [26.0, 30.5] events, $p < 0.05$; $\tau_{100Hz} = 58.6$ [48.3, 74.7] ms, $\tau_{333Hz} = 78.5$ [69.3, 90.7] ms, $p < 0.05$, $n = 6$, fit comparison 100 Hz vs. 333 Hz $p < 0.001$, *F*-test).

The putative cause for the delayed asynchronous transmitter release is the accumulation of presynaptic calcium during high frequency IPSC trains. This can be experimentally enhanced by replacing the extracellular calcium with strontium, or alternatively, the effect can be reduced by applying a cell permeable calcium chelator that accelerates the decay of presynaptic calcium transients (Goda and Stevens, 1994; Atluri and Regehr, 1996, 1998; Lu and Trussell, 2000; Xu-Friedman and Regehr, 2000; Hefft and Jonas, 2005; Best and Regehr, 2009; Tang and Lu, 2012). To test whether the delayed asynchronous events can prolong the IPSCs decay times, their incidence was increased by replacing 2 mM extracellular calcium by 8 mM strontium (**Figures 6A–C**). In addition to a higher frequency of asynchronous events (A) shortly after the 100 Hz stimulation (10 eIPSCs), strontium also caused a prolongation of the time course (τ) of the last IPSC (**Figures 6B,C**; $n = 6$, mono-exponential fit comparison: $p < 0.001$, *F*-Test; A or τ 95 % CI [lower, upper]: $A_{Ca^{2+}} = 6.8$ [5.7, 7.9] events, $A_{Sr^{2+}} = 21.2$ [19.4, 23.0] events; $\tau_{Ca^{2+}} = 13.5$ [9.4, 23.9] ms, $\tau_{Sr^{2+}} = 47.2$ [40.9, 55.8] ms, Ca^{2+} vs. Sr^{2+} $p < 0.05$). Consistent with the observation that asynchronous release strongly depends on synaptic activity (**Figure 5**), 8 mM strontium was more potent in prolonging the IPSC τ_{wd} following higher stimulation rate and longer stimulation (**Figure 6C**; Ca^{2+} vs. Sr^{2+} 100 Hz 10th $p < 0.05$; 333 Hz 50th $p < 0.01$, $n = 6$, RM ANOVA). Notably, single IPSC decays were not affected by the Ca^{2+} replacement ($p = 0.8$). These results suggest that the slow decay of IPSCs is indeed shaped by the asynchronous release which in turn is determined by the rate of presynaptic activity.

To further address this issue, the contribution of the delayed vesicle release to IPSC decay times was determined through reduction of presynaptic calcium with the calcium chelator EGTA-AM (100 μM) (**Figures 6D–G**). The IPSC amplitudes strongly decreased under EGTA-AM by 55 ± 8% for single IPSC, 71 ± 4% for the 10th IPSC at 100 Hz and 55 ± 10% for 50th IPSC at 333 Hz, presumably due to a reduction in the peak Ca^{2+} concentration in the presynaptic terminal (Atluri and Regehr, 1996). The significant increase of asynchronous events observed in control condition after 333 Hz stimulation (50 IPSCs) vanished completely under EGTA-AM (**Figure 6E**; change of asynchronous events after stimulation compared to baseline level before stimulation: control $z = 29.2$, $p < 0.001$; +EGTA-AM $z = -1.01$, $p = 0.16$, *z*-test). Moreover, the weighted decay time constant was shortened by 30 ± 3% regardless of stimulus condition (**Figure 6F**; EGTA-AM effect vs. frequency $p = 0.9$, $n = 5$, RM ANOVA) and transmitter type (glycine, GABA or both) (**Figure 6G**; EGTA-AM effect vs. transmission type $p = 0.59$, $n = 5$ for each condition, ANOVA). Together, these data suggest that both glycine and GABA contribute to the delayed release and thereby shape the inhibitory current profile in an activity-dependent manner.

DISCUSSION

The mixed glycine-GABA transmission observed in SBCs is for the most part dominated by glycine but it still exhibits slow synaptic decays resulting in a long lasting, tonic-like inhibition. While glycine primarily contributes to the IPSC amplitudes, GABA enhances and prolongs the total inhibitory conductance, especially at higher firing rates (Nerlich et al., 2014). Here we demonstrate that the resulting IPSC decay strongly depends on both the synaptic activity and the number of recruited inhibitory fibers, each increasing the amount of transmitters released. The slow glycine and GABA clearance permits a longer availability of the transmitters in the synaptic cleft, thereby enabling transmitter rebinding and glycine spillover. Moreover, the IPSC kinetics is dynamically shaped by the delayed release of glycine and GABA. In addition to the shift towards slower GABAergic transmission at higher input rates (Nerlich et al., 2014), these activity-dependent mechanisms jointly determine the remarkably slow inhibition in SBCs.

TRANSMITTER REBINDING AND SPILLOVER CONTRIBUTE TO THE IPSC DECAY

The SBCs of the cochlear nucleus are the first synaptic center where primary auditory input from the cochlea is integrated with a higher-order, acoustically-evoked inhibition to preserve or improve temporal precision on the sub-millisecond scale (Gai and Carney, 2008; Dehmel et al., 2010; Kuenzel et al., 2011). Such synaptic inhibition is likely to contribute to the temporal synchronization of AP discharges to a particular phase of a low frequency tone burst (Joris et al., 1994; Paolini et al., 2001; Dehmel et al., 2010). Saying this, it should not be disregarded that also other previously discussed mechanisms (Nerlich et al., 2014), such as coincidence of presynaptic inputs also add to the synchronicity of postsynaptic SBC discharges (Kuhlmann et al., 2002; Xu-Friedman and Regehr, 2005). With

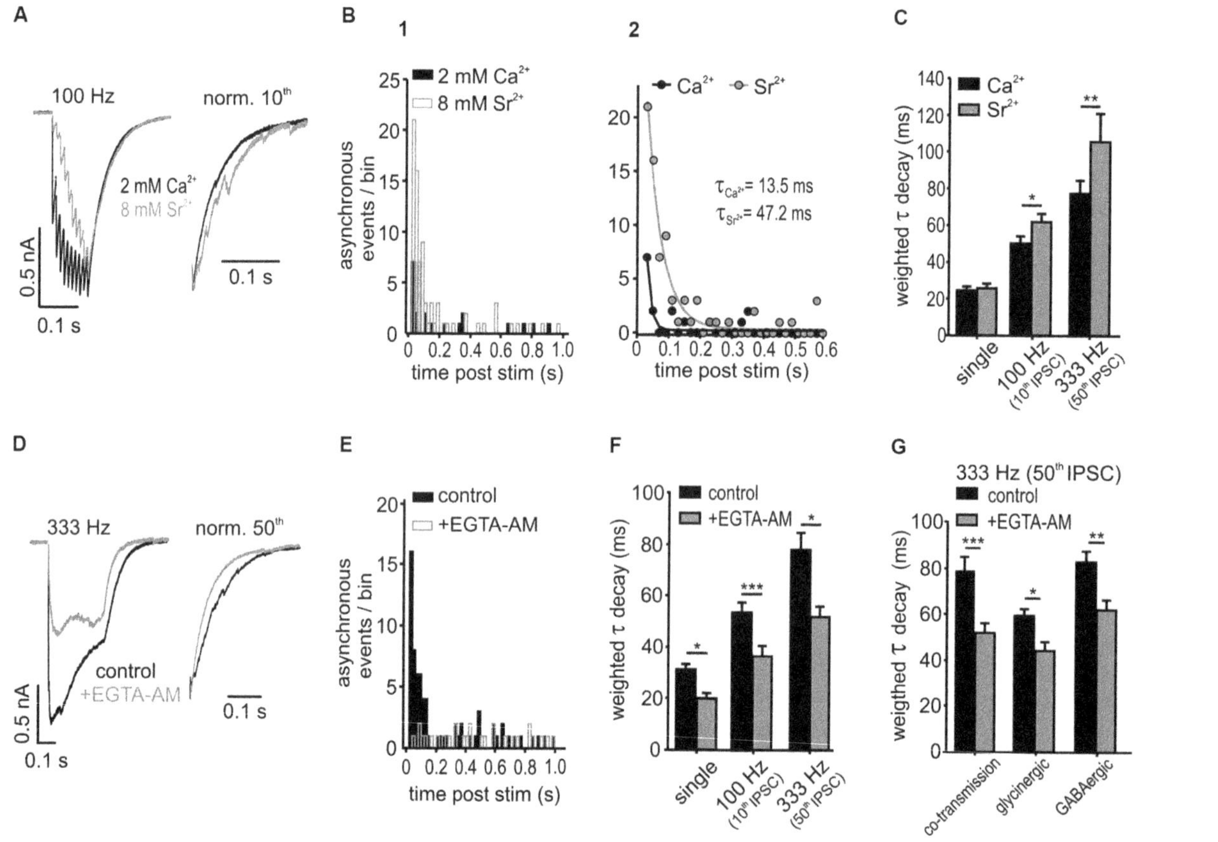

FIGURE 6 | Asynchronous release influences IPSC decay in SBCs. **(A)** Superimposed responses to a 100 Hz stimulation in 2 mM calcium- and 8 mM strontium-ACSF. Right: Normalized last IPSCs showing an increased incidence of asynchronous release events under strontium. **(B1)** Summary histograms of asynchronous release events, before and after a 10 pulse stimulation at 100 Hz for both conditions (n = 6). **(B2)** Mono-exponential fits to the data in B1. The amount of asynchronous events after stimulation was increased and the time of increased incidence prolonged under 8 mM Sr^{2+} (A and τ: Ca^{2+} vs. Sr^{2+} $p < 0.05$). **(C)** Substitution of Ca^{2+} by Sr^{2+} prolonged the weighted decay time of IPSCs after 100 Hz and 333 Hz stimulation, but not of single IPSCs (n = 6, single: p = 0.8, 100 Hz: $p < 0.05$, 333 Hz: $p < 0.01$, RM ANOVA). **(D)** Averaged trains of 50 IPSCs at 333 Hz before and after bath application of 100 μM EGTA-AM. Right: normalized last IPSCs. **(E)** Summary histograms of asynchronous release events before and after application of EGTA-AM. Note the lack of the increase in asynchronous release after stimulation in EGTA-AM (n = 5, bin width: 20 ms; control: z = 29.2 $p < 0.001$; +EGTA-AM: z = −1.01 p = 0.16, z-test). **(F)** EGTA-AM shortened τ_{wd} by about 30 % regardless of stimulation frequency (n = 5, *$p < 0.05$, ***$p < 0.001$, RM ANOVA). **(G)** EGTA-AM equally affects the control (mixed glycine/GABA) IPSCs, isolated glycinergic (+20 μM SR 95531), and GABAergic IPSCs (+0.5 μM strychnine) in terms of decreasing the weighted decay time constants (co-transmission: n = 5, $p < 0.001$; glycinergic: n = 5, $p < 0.05$; GABAergic: n = 5, $p < 0.01$; ANOVA).

respect to the inhibitory effects, it was shown that an activity-dependent regulation of inhibitory strength mediated trough a slow glycine-GABA transmission adjusts the fidelity at the endbulb of Held synapse towards fast rising and large EPSPs (Kuenzel et al., 2011; Xie and Manis, 2013; Nerlich et al., 2014). The present data further demonstrate that the inhibitory strength crucially depends on the presynaptic firing rate, which is of particular physiological importance given the weak inhibition at lower sound intensities, i.e., low firing rates (Kuenzel et al., 2011). Following strong inhibitory stimulation, slow glycine and GABA clearance from the synaptic cleft appears to enable ongoing rebinding of transmitters and intersynaptic pooling of glycine. A similar mechanism was previously shown to mediate prolonged inhibition of granule cells in the rat DCN (Balakrishnan et al., 2009) and of the nucleus laminaris neurons in the chick auditory brainstem (Tang and Lu, 2012). Several lines of evidence suggest that both the GlyT2 and the GABA transporters GAT1/3 contribute to the kinetics of activity-dependent inhibition at SBCs. Particularly, the slow decay phase (τ_{slow}) was affected by increasing stimulus frequencies, suggesting longer availability of transmitters. Similar τ_{slow} prolongation was also observed in the presence of glycine and GABA transporter antagonists. As the respective slowly decaying current is most likely due to slow transmitter clearance (Otis et al., 1996; Williams et al., 1998), our data are consistent with transporter saturation during higher neuronal activity. In line with this, the vesicular inhibitory amino acid transporter (VGAT), which depends on the supply of cytosolic transmitter to enable synaptic corelease of glycine and GABA (Wojcik et al., 2006), is apparently not the rate limiting factor for efficient refilling of inhibitory vesicles (Apostolides and Trussell, 2013).

At mixed glycine-GABA synapses, several factors determine the characteristics of the postsynaptic response: (i) the glycine/GABA ratio in synaptic vesicles which is not only determined by the higher VGAT affinity for glycine than for GABA (McIntire et al., 1997; Bedet et al., 2000); but also crucially depends on the availability of glycine through GlyT2 activity (Rousseau et al., 2008); and (ii) the postsynaptic receptor expression levels, clustering, and localizations (Todd et al., 1996; Dugué et al., 2005). In our recent study, we described a relative increase of the GABAergic component from 5 to 12% of the mixed IPSC amplitude during ongoing synaptic activity (Nerlich et al., 2014). When glycine and GABA were puff-applied (equimolar concentrations of 500 μM), the current amplitude ratio was ~3:2 (1.7:1.2 nA), indicating that $GABA_AR$ availability is probably not the rate limiting factor for restricted GABAergic contribution to the IPSC. Presently, we found no evidence for GABA spillover to distant receptors that could account for the activity-dependent increase in the GABAergic proportion. Thus, the slow glycine clearance by GlyT2 and its low intracellular availability may possibly explain the progressively higher GABAergic signaling at *in vivo*-like firing rates.

Compared to the events elicited in 1.2 mM $[Ca^{2+}]_o$, IPSCs measured under the standard 2 mM $[Ca^{2+}]_o$ condition were found to be slower after shorter stimulus trains or at lower input rates, possibly indicating a contribution of multivesicular release. However, longer or high frequency stimulation (50 pulses at 100 Hz, 10 or 50 pulses at 333 Hz) evoked IPSC of comparable amplitudes towards the end of the train and the similar decay kinetics of the last event. This suggests that prolonged neuronal activity at physiological-like rates leads to a steady state transmitter level in the cleft, independent of the initial release probability. The data also argue against the prominent receptor desensitization, because its effect would render IPSCs faster with increasing transmitter concentrations at higher rates (Jones and Westbrook, 1996), which was not observed in our experiments.

Glycine receptor saturation and spillover onto nearby or distant receptors probably shapes the IPSC kinetics at physiologically relevant firing rates. Due to the lack of effect of the low-affinity $GABA_A$ antagonist, we conclude that the respective receptors are probably tightly coupled to the release sites and unlikely to saturate. In line with this notion, is the lack of $GABA_A$ α6 and δ subunit expression on SBCs (Campos et al., 2001) which were shown to constitute the extrasynaptic receptors (Nusser et al., 1998; Kullmann et al., 2005). The slow IPSC kinetics measured at SBCs contrast with respective data for other inhibitory auditory synapses with decay time constants <5 ms, in which GABA is either not engaged or plays a minor role in determining the response decay time (Awatramani et al., 2004; Magnusson et al., 2005; Chirila et al., 2007; Couchman et al., 2010). As the SBC IPSCs progressively resembled the kinetics of pharmacologically isolated GABAergic events at increasing input frequencies, the mechanisms engaged with GABA release are likely to regulate the duration of inhibition at physiologically relevant rates (Nerlich et al., 2014). One possible contributing mechanism, though not a focus of the present study, is the kinetics of the $GABA_A$ receptor itself. The α3 subunit, linked to slow kinetics, deactivation- and desensitization rates (Verdoorn, 1994; Gingrich et al., 1995) is coexpressed with the subunits α1, α5, β3 and γ2L in the rat AVCN (Campos et al., 2001). In olfactory bulb neurons of juvenile rats, the deactivation kinetics of GABA-evoked mIPSCs can span a τ_{wd} range of 3–30 ms through the expression of different compositions of the fast α1 and the slow α3 subunits in the receptor heteromers (Eyre et al., 2012). Therefore, it is conceivable that the specific composition of $GABA_A$ subunits in SBCs partially contributes to an increase in τ_{wd} which ranged between 20–90 ms in an activity-dependent manner. Notably, even the isolated glycinergic spontaneous- and evoked-IPSCs exhibit slow synaptic decays (Xie and Manis, 2013, 2014; Nerlich et al., 2014). This may be surprising, given the general developmental down-regulation of the GlyR α2 subunit, associated with slower receptor kinetics (Veruki et al., 2007) in the cochlear nucleus and in the superior olivary compex (Sato et al., 1995; Friauf et al., 1997). However, the developmental replacement by the α1 subunit in the AVCN seems in the AVCN, as low levels of α2 mRNA were found up to the third postnatal week (Piechotta et al., 2001). Our data substantiate the hypothesis of a persistent α2 subunit expression throughout adulthood by showing that single pulse stimulation evokes IPSCs of similar τ_{wd} for pharmacologically isolated glycinergic, GABAergic, and mixed glycine-GABA events (Nerlich et al., 2014). Here, further corroboration is provided by showing comparable slow kinetics of the spontaneous IPSCs and IPSCs synaptically elicited in low release probability conditions. In both cases, the amount of released transmitters is presumed low, thus reducing the contribution of activity-dependent mechanisms. Although our results argue for a role of slow GlyR and $GABA_AR$, this still seems to be only an additional mechanism shaping the overall kinetic profile.

INHIBITORY KINETICS IS SHAPED BY THE ACTIVITY-INDUCED DELAYED RELEASE

Asynchronous (or delayed) transmitter release is another mechanism to generate a long-long lasting inhibition in the brain (Lu and Trussell, 2000; Hefft and Jonas, 2005; Tang and Lu, 2012). The ongoing synaptic activity can lead to Ca^{2+} accumulation in the presynaptic terminal, thereby causing the loss of coupling between the presynaptic AP and the release machinery (Chen and Regehr, 1999). Our data from the present and previous study (Nerlich et al., 2014) consistently show the activity-dependent change of release mode. The individual IPSCs were clearly segregated at 100 Hz, indicating synchronized quantal release, whereas the 333 Hz stimulation evoked a large plateau current caused by asynchronous release. Notably, the delayed asynchronous release events, mediated by both glycine and GABA, were observed at both frequencies during the decay phase of the last IPSC. The prominent effect of the slow calcium chelator EGTA-AM in our experiments, suggests a loose coupling between presynaptic Ca^{2+} channels and the Ca^{2+} sensor, possibly in a form of microdomains (Meinrenken et al., 2002; Eggermann et al., 2012; Vyleta and Jonas, 2014). The Ca^{2+} dependance of release machinery was, however, not in focus of the present study. Alongside transmitter rebinding and spillover, asynchronous release is a major mechanism contributing to activity-dependent changes in inhibitory duration.

EFFICACY OF SLOW INHIBITION

Neurons in the auditory brainstem generate APs with an extraordinary temporal accuracy required for the computation of sound source location (for review see, Grothe et al., 2010). In the binaural nuclei of the superior olivary complex, the fast and mainly glycinergic inhibition may contribute by providing high precision phasic suppression of excitatory conductance (Awatramani et al., 2004; Magnusson et al., 2005; Chirila et al., 2007; Couchman et al., 2010; Roberts et al., 2013, 2014; Myoga et al., 2014). The monaural neurons in the mammalian cochlear nucleus, such as bushy cells of the AVCN and the granule cells of the DCN, on the other hand, utilize slow inhibition characterized by an activity-dependent conductance build-up (Balakrishnan et al., 2009; Xie and Manis, 2013). *In vivo*, the onset of acoustically evoked inhibition on SBCs is delayed compared to the excitation (Kuenzel et al., 2011; Nerlich et al., 2014) which cannot be solely explained by the polysynaptic inhibitory pathway causing a delay of just a few milliseconds (Smith and Rhode, 1989; Wickesberg and Oertel, 1990; Saint Marie et al., 1991; Ostapoff et al., 1997; Campagnola and Manis, 2014). Rather, the new data suggest that the slow time course of inhibition is predominantly determined by the receptor kinetics and transmitter clearance during short stimuli, whereas long duration or high frequency stimulation additionally engage spillover of glycine and asynchronous release of both glycine and GABA to prolong IPSCs. The contribution of these synaptic mechanisms can explain the slow onset of inhibition observed *in vivo*. With increasing sound intensity, the dynamic adjustment of inhibitory potency through synergistic glycine-GABA signaling (Nerlich et al., 2014) would ensure effective integration with strong and coincident excitatory inputs leading to non-monotonic rate-level functions and improved temporal precision of the SBC output (Kopp-Scheinpflug et al., 2002; Dehmel et al., 2010; Kuenzel et al., 2011). Consistent with this hypothesis, a modeling study of SBC inhibition with fast IPSC kinetics as those measured in AVCN T-stellate cells impaired the temporal precision of spiking (Xie and Manis, 2013). Thus, the activity-dependance of slow inhibition seems to be a critical factor for precise temporal processing in SBCs.

ACKNOWLEDGMENTS

This work was supported by the DFG grants MI 954/2-1 (Ivan Milenkovic, Jana Nerlich), MI 954/1-1 (Ivan Milenkovic), RU 390/19-1 (Rudolf Rübsamen, Jana Nerlich), GRK 1097 (Jana Nerlich, C.K.), the NIH grant NIH/NIDCD R01-DC008989 (R. Michael Burger, Jana Nerlich), and a DAAD scholarship to Jana Nerlich. The authors thank Stefan N. Oline for helpful comments on an earlier version of the manuscript.

REFERENCES

Apostolides, P. F., and Trussell, L. O. (2013). Rapid, activity-independent turnover of vesicular transmitter content at a mixed glycine/GABA synapse. *J. Neurosci.* 33, 4768–4781. doi: 10.1523/JNEUROSCI.5555-12.2013

Apostolides, P. F., and Trussell, L. O. (2014). Chemical synaptic transmission onto superficial stellate cells of the mouse dorsal cochlear nucleus. *J. Neurophysiol.* 111, 1812–1822. doi: 10.1152/jn.00821.2013

Atluri, P. P., and Regehr, W. G. (1996). Determinants of the time course of facilitation at the granule cell to Purkinje cell synapse. *J. Neurosci.* 16, 5661–5671.

Atluri, P. P., and Regehr, W. G. (1998). Delayed release of neurotransmitter from cerebellar granule cells. *J. Neurosci.* 18, 8214–8227.

Awatramani, G. B., Turecek, R., and Trussell, L. O. (2004). Inhibitory control at a synaptic relay. *J. Neurosci.* 24, 2643–2647. doi: 10.1523/jneurosci.5144-03.2004

Awatramani, G. B., Turecek, R., and Trussell, L. O. (2005). Staggered development of GABAergic and glycinergic transmission in the MNTB. *J. Neurophysiol.* 93, 819–828. doi: 10.1152/jn.00798.2004

Balakrishnan, V., Kuo, S. P., Roberts, P. D., and Trussell, L. O. (2009). Slow glycinergic transmission mediated by transmitter pooling. *Nat. Neurosci.* 12, 286–294. doi: 10.1038/nn.2265

Beato, M. (2008). The time course of transmitter at glycinergic synapses onto motoneurons. *J. Neurosci.* 28, 7412–7425. doi: 10.1523/JNEUROSCI.0581-08.2008

Bedet, C., Isambert, M. F., Henry, J. P., and Gasnier, B. (2000). Constitutive phosphorylation of the vesicular inhibitory amino acid transporter in rat central nervous system. *J. Neurochem.* 75, 1654–1663. doi: 10.1046/j.1471-4159.2000.0751654.x

Best, A. R., and Regehr, W. G. (2009). Inhibitory regulation of electrically coupled neurons in the inferior olive is mediated by asynchronous release of GABA. *Neuron* 62, 555–565. doi: 10.1016/j.neuron.2009.04.018

Borst, J. G. (2010). The low synaptic release probability in vivo. *Trends Neurosci.* 33, 259–266. doi: 10.1016/j.tins.2010.03.003

Bradaïa, A., Schlichter, R., and Trouslard, J. (2004). Role of glial and neuronal glycine transporters in the control of glycinergic and glutamatergic synaptic transmission in lamina X of the rat spinal cord. *J. Physiol.* 559(Pt. 1), 169–186. doi: 10.1113/jphysiol.2004.068858

Campagnola, L., and Manis, P. B. (2014). A map of functional synaptic connectivity in the mouse anteroventral cochlear nucleus. *J. Neurosci.* 34, 2214–2230. doi: 10.1523/JNEUROSCI.4669-13.2014

Campos, M. L., de Cabo, C., Wisden, W., Juiz, J. M., and Merlo, D. (2001). Expression of GABA(A) receptor subunits in rat brainstem auditory pathways: cochlear nuclei, superior olivary complex and nucleus of the lateral lemniscus. *Neuroscience* 102, 625–638. doi: 10.1016/s0306-4522(00)00525-x

Capogna, M., and Pearce, R. A. (2011). GABA A, slow: causes and consequences. *Trends Neurosci.* 34, 101–112. doi: 10.1016/j.tins.2010.10.005

Chanda, S., and Xu-Friedman, M. A. (2010). A low-affinity antagonist reveals saturation and desensitization in mature synapses in the auditory brain stem. *J. Neurophysiol.* 103, 1915–1926. doi: 10.1152/jn.00751.2009

Chen, S., and Diamond, J. S. (2002). Synaptically released glutamate activates extrasynaptic NMDA receptors on cells in the ganglion cell layer of rat retina. *J. Neurosci.* 22, 2165–2173.

Chen, C., and Regehr, W. G. (1999). Contributions of residual calcium to fast synaptic transmission. *J. Neurosci.* 19, 6257–6266.

Chéry, N., and de Koninck, Y. (1999). Junctional versus extrajunctional glycine and GABA(A) receptor-mediated IPSCs in identified lamina I neurons of the adult rat spinal cord. *J. Neurosci.* 19, 7342–7355.

Chirila, F. V., Rowland, K. C., Thompson, J. M., and Spirou, G. A. (2007). Development of gerbil medial superior olive: integration of temporally delayed excitation and inhibition at physiological temperature. *J. Physiol.* 584(Pt. 1), 167–190. doi: 10.1113/jphysiol.2007.137976

Coleman, W. L., Fischl, M. J., Weimann, S. R., and Burger, R. M. (2011). GABAergic and glycinergic inhibition modulate monaural auditory response properties in the avian superior olivary nucleus. *J. Neurophysiol.* 105, 2405–2420. doi: 10.1152/jn.01088.2010

Couchman, K., Grothe, B., and Felmy, F. (2010). Medial superior olivary neurons receive surprisingly few excitatory and inhibitory inputs with balanced strength and short-term dynamics. *J. Neurosci.* 30, 17111–17121. doi: 10.1523/JNEUROSCI.1760-10.2010

Dehmel, S., Kopp-Scheinpflug, C., Weick, M., Dörrscheidt, G. J., and Rübsamen, R. (2010). Transmission of phase-coupling accuracy from the auditory nerve to spherical bushy cells in the Mongolian gerbil. *Hear. Res.* 268, 234–249. doi: 10.1016/j.heares.2010.06.005

Diamond, J. S. (2001). Neuronal glutamate transporters limit activation of NMDA receptors by neurotransmitter spillover on CA1 pyramidal cells. *J. Neurosci.* 21, 8328–8338.

Dugué, G. P., Dumoulin, A., Triller, A., and Dieudonné, S. (2005). Target-dependent use of co-released inhibitory transmitters at central synapses. *J. Neurosci.* 25, 6490–6498. doi: 10.1523/jneurosci.1500-05.2005

Dumoulin, A., Triller, A., and Dieudonné, S. (2001). IPSC kinetics at identified GABAergic and mixed GABAergic and glycinergic synapses onto cerebellar Golgi cells. *J. Neurosci.* 21, 6045–6057.

Eggermann, E., Bucurenciu, I., Goswami, S. P., and Jonas, P. (2012). Nanodomain coupling between Ca^{2+} channels and sensors of exocytosis at fast mammalian synapses. *Nat. Rev. Neurosci.* 13, 7–21. doi: 10.1038/nrn3125

Eyre, M. D., Renzi, M., Farrant, M., and Nusser, Z. (2012). Setting the time course of inhibitory synaptic currents by mixing multiple GABA(A) receptor α subunit isoforms. *J. Neurosci.* 32, 5853–5867. doi: 10.1523/JNEUROSCI.6495-11.2012

Farrant, M., and Nusser, Z. (2005). Variations on an inhibitory theme: phasic and tonic activation of GABA(A) receptors. *Nat. Rev. Neurosci.* 6, 215–229. doi: 10.1038/nrn1625

Fischl, M. J., Weimann, S. R., Kearse, M. G., and Burger, R. M. (2014). Slowly emerging glycinergic transmission enhances inhibition in the sound localization pathway of the avian auditory system. *J. Neurophysiol.* 111, 565–572. doi: 10.1152/jn.00640.2013

Friauf, E., Hammerschmidt, B., and Kirsch, J. (1997). Development of adult-type inhibitory glycine receptors in the central auditory system of rats. *J. Comp. Neurol.* 385, 117–134. doi: 10.1002/(sici)1096-9861(19970818)385:1<117::aid-cne7>3.0.co;2-5

Gai, Y., and Carney, L. H. (2008). Influence of inhibitory inputs on rate and timing of responses in the anteroventral cochlear nucleus. *J. Neurophysiol.* 99, 1077–1095. doi: 10.1152/jn.00708.2007

Gingrich, K. J., Roberts, W. A., and Kass, R. S. (1995). Dependence of the GABAA receptor gating kinetics on the alpha-subunit isoform: implications for structure-function relations and synaptic transmission. *J. Physiol.* 489(Pt. 2), 529–543.

Goda, Y., and Stevens, C. F. (1994). Two components of transmitter release at a central synapse. *Proc. Natl. Acad. Sci. U S A* 91, 12942–12946. doi: 10.1073/pnas.91.26.12942

González-Forero, D., and Alvarez, F. J. (2005). Differential postnatal maturation of GABAA, glycine receptor and mixed synaptic currents in Renshaw cells and ventral spinal interneurons. *J. Neurosci.* 25, 2010–2023. doi: 10.1523/jneurosci.2383-04.2005

Grothe, B., Pecka, M., and McAlpine, D. (2010). Mechanisms of sound localization in mammals. *Physiol. Rev.* 90, 983–1012. doi: 10.1152/physrev.00026.2009

Hefft, S., and Jonas, P. (2005). Asynchronous GABA release generates long-lasting inhibition at a hippocampal interneuron-principal neuron synapse. *Nat. Neurosci.* 8, 1319–1328. doi: 10.1038/nn1542

Husson, Z., Rousseau, C. V., Broll, I., Zeilhofer, H. U., and Dieudonné, S. (2014). Differential GABAergic and glycinergic inputs of inhibitory interneurons and purkinje cells to principal cells of the cerebellar nuclei. *J. Neurosci.* 34, 9418–9431. doi: 10.1523/JNEUROSCI.0401-14.2014

Isaacson, J. S., and Walmsley, B. (1996). Amplitude and time course of spontaneous and evoked excitatory postsynaptic currents in bushy cells of the anteroventral cochlear nucleus. *J. Neurophysiol.* 76, 1566–1571.

Jonas, P., Bischofberger, J., and Sandkühler, J. (1998). Corelease of two fast neurotransmitters at a central synapse. *Science* 281, 419–424. doi: 10.1126/science.281.5375.419

Jones, M. V., and Westbrook, G. L. (1996). The impact of receptor desensitization on fast synaptic transmission. *Trends Neurosci.* 19, 96–101. doi: 10.1016/s0166-2236(96)80037-3

Joris, P. X., Carney, L. H., Smith, P. H., and Yin, T. C. (1994). Enhancement of neural synchronization in the anteroventral cochlear nucleus. I. Responses to tones at the characteristic frequency. *J. Neurophysiol.* 71, 1022–1036.

Keller, A. F., Coull, J. A., Chery, N., Poisbeau, P., and De Koninck, Y. (2001). Region-specific developmental specialization of GABA-glycine cosynapses in laminas I-II of the rat spinal dorsal horn. *J. Neurosci.* 21, 7871–7880.

Keros, S., and Hablitz, J. J. (2005). Subtype-specific GABA transporter antagonists synergistically modulate phasic and tonic GABAA conductances in rat neocortex. *J. Neurophysiol.* 94, 2073–2085. doi: 10.1152/jn.00520.2005

Kopp-Scheinpflug, C., Dehmel, S., Dörrscheidt, G. J., and Rübsamen, R. (2002). Interaction of excitation and inhibition in anteroventral cochlear nucleus neurons that receive large endbulb synaptic endings. *J. Neurosci.* 22, 11004–11018.

Kramer, F., Griesemer, D., Bakker, D., Brill, S., Franke, J., Frotscher, E., et al. (2014). Inhibitory glycinergic neurotransmission in the mammalian auditory brainstem upon prolonged stimulation: short-term plasticity and synaptic reliability. *Front. Neural Circuits* 8:14. doi: 10.3389/fncir.2014.00014

Kuenzel, T., Borst, J. G., and van der Heijden, M. (2011). Factors controlling the input-output relationship of spherical bushy cells in the gerbil cochlear nucleus. *J. Neurosci.* 31, 4260–4273. doi: 10.1523/JNEUROSCI.5433-10.2011

Kuhlmann, L., Burkitt, A. N., Paolini, A., and Clark, G. M. (2002). Summation of spatiotemporal input patterns in leaky integrate-and-fire neurons: application to neurons in the cochlear nucleus receiving converging auditory nerve fiber input. *J. Comput. Neurosci.* 12, 55–73. doi: 10.1023/A:1014994113776

Kullmann, D. M., Ruiz, A., Rusakov, D. M., Scott, R., Semyanov, A., and Walker, M. C. (2005). Presynaptic, extrasynaptic and axonal GABAA receptors in the CNS: where and why? *Prog. Biophys. Mol. Biol.* 87, 33–46. doi: 10.1016/j.pbiomolbio.2004.06.003

Kuo, S. P., Bradley, L. A., and Trussell, L. O. (2009). Heterogeneous kinetics and pharmacology of synaptic inhibition in the chick auditory brainstem. *J. Neurosci.* 29, 9625–9634. doi: 10.1523/JNEUROSCI.0103-09.2009

Lu, T., Rubio, M. E., and Trussell, L. O. (2008). Glycinergic transmission shaped by the corelease of GABA in a mammalian auditory synapse. *Neuron* 57, 524–535. doi: 10.1016/j.neuron.2007.12.010

Lu, T., and Trussell, L. O. (2000). Inhibitory transmission mediated by asynchronous transmitter release. *Neuron* 26, 683–694. doi: 10.1016/s0896-6273(00)81204-0

Magnusson, A. K., Kapfer, C., Grothe, B., and Koch, U. (2005). Maturation of glycinergic inhibition in the gerbil medial superior olive after hearing onset. *J. Physiol.* 568(Pt. 2), 497–512. doi: 10.1113/jphysiol.2005.094763

McIntire, S. L., Reimer, R. J., Schuske, K., Edwards, R. H., and Jorgensen, E. M. (1997). Identification and characterization of the vesicular GABA transporter. *Nature* 389, 870–876.

Meinrenken, C. J., Borst, J. G., and Sakmann, B. (2002). Calcium secretion coupling at calyx of held governed by nonuniform channel-vesicle topography. *J. Neurosci.* 22, 1648–1667.

Monsivais, P., Yang, L., and Rubel, E. W. (2000). GABAergic inhibition in nucleus magnocellularis: implications for phase locking in the avian auditory brainstem. *J. Neurosci.* 20, 2954–2963.

Myoga, M. H., Lehnert, S., Leibold, C., Felmy, F., and Grothe, B. (2014). Glycinergic inhibition tunes coincidence detection in the auditory brainstem. *Nat. Commun.* 5:3790. doi: 10.1038/ncomms4790

Nerlich, J., Kuenzel, T., Keine, C., Korenic, A., Rübsamen, R., and Milenkovic, I. (2014). Dynamic fidelity control to the central auditory system: synergistic glycine/GABAergic inhibition in the cochlear nucleus. *J. Neurosci.* 34, 11604–11620. doi: 10.1523/jneurosci.0719-14.2014

Nicol, M. J., and Walmsley, B. (2002). Ultrastructural basis of synaptic transmission between endbulbs of Held and bushy cells in the rat cochlear nucleus. *J. Physiol.* 539(Pt. 3), 713–723. doi: 10.1113/jphysiol.2001.012972

Nusser, Z., Sieghart, W., and Somogyi, P. (1998). Segregation of different GABAA receptors to synaptic and extrasynaptic membranes of cerebellar granule cells. *J. Neurosci.* 18, 1693–1703.

O'Brien, J. A., and Berger, A. J. (1999). Cotransmission of GABA and glycine to brain stem motoneurons. *J. Neurophysiol.* 82, 1638–1641.

Ostapoff, E. M., Benson, C. G., and Saint Marie, R. L. (1997). GABA- and glycine-immunoreactive projections from the superior olivary complex to the cochlear nucleus in guinea pig. *J. Comp. Neurol.* 381, 500–512. doi: 10.1002/(sici)1096-9861(19970519)381:4<500::aid-cne9>3.0.co;2-6

Otis, T. S., Wu, Y. C., and Trussell, L. O. (1996). Delayed clearance of transmitter and the role of glutamate transporters at synapses with multiple release sites. *J. Neurosci.* 16, 1634–1644.

Overstreet, L. S., and Westbrook, G. L. (2003). Synapse density regulates independence at unitary inhibitory synapses. *J. Neurosci.* 23, 2618–2626.

Paolini, A. G., FitzGerald, J. V., Burkitt, A. N., and Clark, G. M. (2001). Temporal processing from the auditory nerve to the medial nucleus of the trapezoid body in the rat. *Hear. Res.* 159, 101–116. doi: 10.1016/s0378-5955(01)00327-6

Piechotta, K., Weth, F., Harvey, R. J., and Friauf, E. (2001). Localization of rat glycine receptor alpha1 and alpha2 subunit transcripts in the developing auditory brainstem. *J. Comp. Neurol.* 438, 336–352. doi: 10.1002/cne.1319.abs

Protti, D. A., Gerschenfeld, H. M., and Llano, I. (1997). GABAergic and glycinergic IPSCs in ganglion cells of rat retinal slices. *J. Neurosci.* 17, 6075–6085.

Roberts, M. T., Seeman, S. C., and Golding, N. L. (2013). A mechanistic understanding of the role of feedforward inhibition in the mammalian sound localization circuitry. *Neuron* 78, 923–935. doi: 10.1016/j.neuron.2013.04.022

Roberts, M. T., Seeman, S. C., and Golding, N. L. (2014). The relative contributions of MNTB and LNTB neurons to inhibition in the medial superior olive assessed through single and paired recordings. *Front. Neural Circuits* 8:49. doi: 10.3389/fncir.2014.00049

Rousseau, F., Aubrey, K. R., and Supplisson, S. (2008). The glycine transporter GlyT2 controls the dynamics of synaptic vesicle refilling in inhibitory spinal cord neurons. *J. Neurosci.* 28, 9755–9768. doi: 10.1523/jneurosci.0509-08.2008

Rousseau, C. V., Dugué, G. P., Dumoulin, A., Mugnaini, E., Dieudonné, S., and Diana, M. A. (2012). Mixed inhibitory synaptic balance correlates with glutamatergic synaptic phenotype in cerebellar unipolar brush cells. *J. Neurosci.* 32, 4632–4644. doi: 10.1523/jneurosci.5122-11.2012

Russier, M., Kopysova, I. L., Ankri, N., Ferrand, N., and Debanne, D. (2002). GABA and glycine co-release optimizes functional inhibition in rat brainstem motoneurons in vitro. *J. Physiol.* 541(Pt. 1), 123–137. doi: 10.1113/jphysiol.2001.016063

Ryugo, D. K., and Sento, S. (1991). Synaptic connections of the auditory nerve in cats: relationship between endbulbs of held and spherical bushy cells. *J. Comp. Neurol.* 305, 35–48. doi: 10.1002/cne.903050105

Saint Marie, R. L., Benson, C. G., Ostapoff, E. M., and Morest, D. K. (1991). Glycine immunoreactive projections from the dorsal to the anteroventral cochlear nucleus. *Hear. Res.* 51, 11–28. doi: 10.1016/0378-5955(91)90003-r

Sato, K., Kuriyama, H., and Altschuler, R. A. (1995). Expression of glycine receptor subunits in the cochlear nucleus and superior olivary complex using non-radioactive in-situ hybridization. *Hear. Res.* 91, 7–18. doi: 10.1016/0378-5955(95)00156-5

Seddik, R., Schlichter, R., and Trouslard, J. (2007). Corelease of GABA/glycine in lamina-X of the spinal cord of neonatal rats. *Neuroreport* 18, 1025–1029. doi: 10.1097/wnr.0b013e3281667c0c

Smith, P. H., and Rhode, W. S. (1989). Structural and functional properties distinguish two types of multipolar cells in the ventral cochlear nucleus. *J. Comp. Neurol.* 282, 595–616. doi: 10.1002/cne.902820410

Song, I., Volynski, K., Brenner, T., Ushkaryov, Y., Walker, M., and Semyanov, A. (2013). Different transporter systems regulate extracellular GABA from vesicular and non-vesicular sources. *Front. Cell. Neurosci.* 7:23. doi: 10.3389/fncel.2013.00023

Szabadics, J., Tamás, G., and Soltesz, I. (2007). Different transmitter transients underlie presynaptic cell type specificity of GABAA,slow and GABAA,fast. *Proc. Natl. Acad. Sci. U S A* 104, 14831–14836. doi: 10.1073/pnas.0707204104

Takahashi, T., Momiyama, A., Hirai, K., Hishinuma, F., and Akagi, H. (1992). Functional correlation of fetal and adult forms of glycine receptors with developmental changes in inhibitory synaptic receptor channels. *Neuron* 9, 1155–1161. doi: 10.1016/0896-6273(92)90073-m

Tang, Z.-Q., Dinh, E. H., Shi, W., and Lu, Y. (2011). Ambient GABA-activated tonic inhibition sharpens auditory coincidence detection via a depolarizing shunting mechanism. *J. Neurosci.* 31, 6121–6131. doi: 10.1523/jneurosci.4733-10.2011

Tang, Z.-Q., and Lu, Y. (2012). Two GABAA responses with distinct kinetics in a sound localization circuit. *J. Physiol.* 590(Pt. 16), 3787–3805. doi: 10.1113/jphysiol.2012.230136

Thomas, C. G., Tian, H., and Diamond, J. S. (2011). The relative roles of diffusion and uptake in clearing synaptically released glutamate change during early postnatal development. *J. Neurosci.* 31, 4743–4754. doi: 10.1523/jneurosci.5953-10.2011

Todd, A. J., Watt, C., Spike, R. C., and Sieghart, W. (1996). Colocalization of GABA, glycine and their receptors at synapses in the rat spinal cord. *J. Neurosci.* 16, 974–982.

Verdoorn, T. A. (1994). Formation of heteromeric gamma-aminobutyric acid type A receptors containing two different alpha subunits. *Mol. Pharmacol.* 45, 475–480.

Veruki, M. L., Gill, S. B., and Hartveit, E. (2007). Spontaneous IPSCs and glycine receptors with slow kinetics in wide-field amacrine cells in the mature rat retina. *J. Physiol.* 581(Pt. 1), 203–219. doi: 10.1113/jphysiol.2006.127316

Vyleta, N. P., and Jonas, P. (2014). Loose coupling between Ca2+ channels and release sensors at a plastic hippocampal synapse. *Science* 343, 665–670. doi: 10.1126/science.1244811

Wang, P., and Slaughter, M. M. (2005). Effects of GABA receptor antagonists on retinal glycine receptors and on homomeric glycine receptor alpha subunits. *J. Neurophysiol.* 93, 3120–3126. doi: 10.1152/jn.01228.2004

Wentzel, P. R., De Zeeuw, C. I., Holstege, J. C., and Gerrits, N. M. (1993). Colocalization of GABA and glycine in the rabbit oculomotor nucleus. *Neurosci. Lett.* 164, 25–29. doi: 10.1016/0304-3940(93)90848-f

Wickesberg, R. E., and Oertel, D. (1990). Delayed, frequency-specific inhibition in the cochlear nuclei of mice: a mechanism for monaural echo suppression. *J. Neurosci.* 10, 1762–1768.

Williams, S. R., Buhl, E. H., and Mody, I. (1998). The dynamics of synchronized neurotransmitter release determined from compound spontaneous IPSCs in rat dentate granule neurones in vitro. *J. Physiol.* 510(Pt. 2), 477–497. doi: 10.1111/j.1469-7793.1998.477bk.x

Wojcik, S. M., Katsurabayashi, S., Guillemin, I., Friauf, E., Rosenmund, C., Brose, N., et al. (2006). A shared vesicular carrier allows synaptic corelease of GABA and glycine. *Neuron* 50, 575–587. doi: 10.1016/j.neuron.2006.04.016

Xie, R., and Manis, P. B. (2013). Target-specific IPSC kinetics promote temporal processing in auditory parallel pathways. *J. Neurosci.* 33, 1598–1614. doi: 10.1523/jneurosci.2541-12.2013

Xie, R., and Manis, P. B. (2014). GABAergic and glycinergic inhibitory synaptic transmission in the ventral cochlear nucleus studied in VGAT channelrhodopsin-2 mice. *Front. Neural Circuits* 8:84. doi: 10.3389/fncir.2014.00084

Xu-Friedman, M. A., and Regehr, W. G. (2000). Probing fundamental aspects of synaptic transmission with strontium. *J. Neurosci.* 20, 4414–4422.

Xu-Friedman, M. A., and Regehr, W. G. (2005). Dynamic-clamp analysis of the effects of convergence on spike timing. II. Few synaptic inputs. *J. Neurophysiol.* 94, 2526–2534. doi: 10.1152/jn.01308.2004

15

Development of glycinergic innervation to the murine LSO and SPN in the presence and absence of the MNTB

Stefanie C. Altieri[1,2], Tianna Zhao[1], Walid Jalabi[3] and Stephen M. Maricich[1]*

[1] Richard King Mellon Foundation Institute for Pediatric Research and Department of Pediatrics, University of Pittsburgh, Pittsburgh, PA, USA
[2] Department of Otolaryngology, University of Pittsburgh, Pittsburgh, PA, USA
[3] Department of Pediatrics, Case Western Reserve University, Cleveland, OH, USA

Correspondence:
Stephen M. Maricich, Richard King Mellon Foundation Institute for Pediatric Research and Department of Pediatrics, University of Pittsburgh, Pittsburgh, PA 15224, USA
e-mail: stephen.maricich@chp.edu

Neurons in the superior olivary complex (SOC) integrate excitatory and inhibitory inputs to localize sounds in space. The majority of these inhibitory inputs have been thought to arise within the SOC from the medial nucleus of the trapezoid body (MNTB). However, recent work demonstrates that glycinergic innervation of the SOC persists in *Egr2; En1*^{CKO} mice that lack MNTB neurons, suggesting that there are other sources of this innervation (Jalabi et al., 2013). To study the development of MNTB- and non-MNTB-derived glycinergic SOC innervation, we compared immunostaining patterns of glycine transporter 2 (GlyT2) at several postnatal ages in control and *Egr2; En1*^{CKO} mice. GlyT2 immunostaining was present at birth (P0) in controls and reached adult levels by P7 in the superior paraolivary nucleus (SPN) and by P12 in the lateral superior olive (LSO). In *Egr2; En1*^{CKO} mice, glycinergic innervation of the LSO developed at a similar rate but was delayed by one week in the SPN. Conversely, consistent reductions in the number of GlyT2$^+$ boutons located on LSO somata were seen at all ages in *Egr2; En1*^{CKO} mice, while these numbers reached control levels in the SPN by adulthood. Dendritic localization of GlyT2+ boutons was unaltered in both the LSO and SPN of adult *Egr2; En1*^{CKO} mice. On the postsynaptic side, adult *Egr2; En1*^{CKO} mice had reduced glycine receptor α1 (GlyRα1) expression in the LSO but normal levels in the SPN. GlyRα2 was not expressed by LSO or SPN neurons in either genotype. These findings contribute important information for understanding the development of MNTB- and non-MNTB-derived glycinergic pathways to the mouse SOC.

Keywords: hearing, deafness, mouse models, brain development, auditory system

INTRODUCTION

The pontine superior olivary complex (SOC) is the first central auditory region that receives significant bilateral acoustic information, and it is the primary site for detecting interaural level and timing differences (ILDs and ITDs) critical for sound localization. The neural pathways involved in these processes have been described in detail over the past few decades (Kandler et al., 2009). A critical player in both ILD and ITD detection is the medial nucleus of the trapezoid body (MNTB), which receives glutamatergic input from the contralateral cochlear nucleus (CN) and sends inhibitory projections to ipsilateral SOC nuclei. One major MNTB target is the lateral superior olive (LSO), which participates in ILD processing by integrating these inhibitory inputs with excitatory inputs from the ipsilateral CN (Boudreau and Tsuchitani, 1968; Moore and Caspary, 1983; Spangler et al., 1985; Sanes and Rubel, 1988; Helfert et al., 1989; Bledsoe et al., 1990; Wu and Kelly, 1991, 1992, 1995; Srinivasan et al., 2004). A second major target is the superior paraolivary nucleus (SPN), which also receives excitatory input from contralateral CN neurons (Friauf and Ostwald, 1988; Helfert et al., 1989; Thompson and Thompson, 1991; Schofield, 1995). The SPN encodes temporal sound features and has been proposed to function in sound localization, rhythm coding, gap detection and/or as a discontinuity detector (Behrend et al., 2002; Dehmel et al., 2002; Kulesza et al., 2003, 2007; Kadner et al., 2006; Kadner and Berrebi, 2008; Felix et al., 2014).

The primary neurotransmitter produced by the MNTB is glycine (Moore and Caspary, 1983; Peyret et al., 1987; Wenthold et al., 1987; Aoki et al., 1988; Helfert et al., 1989; Adams and Mugnaini, 1990). Studies done in many species demonstrate that glycinergic projections to SOC neurons develop during late embryogenesis and mature during the first two weeks of postnatal life, during which their action switches from depolarizing to hyperpolarizing (Wenthold et al., 1987; Helfert et al., 1989; Bledsoe et al., 1990; Sanes and Siverls, 1991; Kandler and Friauf, 1995; Kandler and Gillespie, 2005; Löhrke et al., 2005). In the rat, this switch is mirrored by the appearance and maturation of immunoreactivity for the glycine transporter type 2 (GlyT2; Friauf et al., 1999). Glycinergic network development in the SOC has not been well-studied in mice, where there is functional evidence for faster maturation of the auditory brainstem compared to other species (Ehret, 1976; Kullmann and Kandler, 2001). Understanding these pathways in mice is valuable given the wealth of genetic tools available to manipulate auditory regions for functional and behavioral investigations.

Recent work suggests that glycinergic projections to the SOC arise from additional sources other than the MNTB. Specifically, glycinergic innervation of the SOC is maintained in transgenic mice that lack MNTB neurons secondary to $Egr2^{Cre}$-mediated conditional deletion of the *En1* gene in rhombomeres 3 and 5 (*Egr2*; $En1^{CKO}$ mice; Jalabi et al., 2013). These inhibitory projections are functional but exhibit prolonged inhibitory postsynaptic current (IPSC) decay time constants in both LSO and SPN neurons compared to those seen in control mice. The mechanisms that underlie these differences, as well as the development of these alternative glycinergic projections, have not been studied. Surprisingly, sound localization ability in *Egr2*; $En1^{CKO}$ mice is relatively preserved, suggesting that remarkable plasticity exists in the developing auditory brainstem.

In this study, we sought to characterize the postnatal development and localization of glycinergic inputs to the LSO and SPN using immunohistochemistry for GlyT2. We also analyzed expression patterns of glycine receptor subtypes Glyα1 and Glyα2 in adult control and *Egr2*; $En1^{CKO}$ mice to see if differences between the two might explain the altered IPSC decay kinetics. Our findings demonstrate that mice lacking MNTB neurons have alterations in the time course of somatic glycinergic innervation in the SPN and in the amount of somatic innervation in the LSO, while dendritic localization of glycinergic terminals is unaltered in both regions. Furthermore, decreased expression of the adult glycine receptor isoform, GlyRα1, was found in the LSO but not SPN of *Egr2*; $En1^{CKO}$ mice.

MATERIALS AND METHODS

ANIMALS

$Egr2^{Cre/+}$ mice (Voiculescu et al., 2000) on a C57BL/6J background were mated with $En1^{flox/flox}$ mice (Sgaier et al., 2007) on a mixed background to produce mice of four genotypes: $Egr2^{+/+}$; $En1^{+/flox}$, $Egr2^{+/+}$; $En1^{flox/flox}$, $Egr2^{Cre/+}$; $En1^{+/flox}$ and $Egr2^{Cre/+}$; $En1^{flox/flox}$ (*Egr2*; $En1^{CKO}$; Jalabi et al., 2013). As no differences were seen previously between the control genotypes, we used only $Egr2^{+/+}$; $En1^{flox/flox}$ mice as controls in this study. Brother-sister matings of $Egr2^{+/+}$; $En1^{flox/flox}$ mice and $Egr2^{Cre/+}$; $En1^{flox/flox}$ mice were used to produce offspring. Postnatal day 0 (P0, day of birth), P3, P7, P12, and P14 mice of both sexes were used for early postnatal experiments, while 8–10 month-old female mice were used for adult experiments ($N = 2$ mice/genotype at each age). Mice were maintained and housed on a 12:12 light:dark cycle with access to food and water *ad libitum*. All procedures were approved by the Case Western Reserve University and University of Pittsburgh Institutional Animal Care and Use Committees.

TISSUE HARVESTING AND PROCESSING

Mice were deeply anesthetized with 300 mg/kg Avertin and transcardially perfused with ice-cold 4% paraformaldehyde (PFA). Whole brains were removed and post-fixed overnight at 4°C in 4% PFA. Following post-fixation, brains were cryoprotected in 30% sucrose for 48 h. Brains were then embedded in Tissue-Tek O.C.T. compound (Sakura Finetek, Torrance, CA, USA), quickly frozen and stored at −80°C before sectioning. Brains were sectioned in the coronal plane at 10 μm thickness using a CM1950 cryostat (Leica, Buffalo Grove, IL, USA). Sections were collected onto Superfrost/Plus slides (Thermo Fisher Scientific), dried overnight and stored in −80°C prior to use. Slide sets with 50 μm (adult) or 30 μm (young postnatal) separation between sections were prepared to allow systematic sampling through the SOC, and each set was immunostained with a different antibody

IMMUNOHISTOCHEMISTRY

Slides containing sections through the SOC were rehydrated in 1× PBS for 5 min and then incubated in blocking solution (0.3% Triton X-100, 3% donkey serum in 1× PBS) for 1 h. Primary antibodies were diluted in blocking solution and incubated overnight at 4°C. The following primary antibodies and concentrations were used: guinea-pig anti-glycine transporter 2 (GlyT2) polyclonal antibody (Millipore, Temecula, CA) at 1:1000; chicken anti-MAP2 polyclonal antibody (Abcam Inc., Cambridge, MA, USA) at 1:10000; rabbit anti-glycine receptor alpha 1 (GlyRα1) polyclonal antibody (Millipore, Temecula, CA, USA) at 1:1000; goat anti-glycine receptor alpha 2 (GlyRα2) polyclonal antibody at 1:500 (Santa Cruz Biotechnology, Dallas,TX). Slides were washed 3 × 5 min in 1× PBS. Secondary antibodies were diluted in blocking solution at 1:500 and incubated on the slides for 1 h at room temperature. The following secondary antibodies were used: Alexa Fluor 594-AffiniPure donkey anti-guinea pig, Alexa Fluor 488-AffiniPure donkey anti-chicken, Alexa Fluor 488-AffiniPure donkey anti-rabbit and Alexa Fluor 488-AffiniPure donkey anti-goat (Jackson ImmunoResearch, West Grove, PA). All slides were counterstained with DAPI. Following secondary antibody incubation, slides were washed 3 × 5 min in 1× PBS. In some cases, slides were counterstained with NeuroTrace Green Fluorescent Nissl (Life Technologies, Grand Island, NY) at a concentration of 1:100 diluted in 1× PBS for 30 min at room temperature. Slides were washed an additional 3 × 5 min in 1× PBS and then mounted with ProLong Gold (Life Technologies, Grand Island, NY). Slides were imaged using a Leica DM5500B epifluorescence microscope or an inverted Zeiss Axio Observer on a PerkinElmer Ultra*VIEW* VoX spinning disk confocal with a Hamamatsu C9100-13 camera and Volocity software.

BOUTON COUNTS AND LOCALIZATION

GlyT2+ boutons located on LSO and SPN neuron somata of P7, P12 and P14 mice were counted on six sections/side ($N = 12$ sections/mouse) on photographs taken at 60 μm increments on a Leica DM5500B epifluorescence microscope. For adult mice, bilateral LSO and SPN images across 10 sections/side ($N = 20$ sections/mouse) at 50 μm increments were used for counting. Images were processed using ImageJ 1.47V (NIH), and the number of boutons on all neuronal soma with an identifiable nucleus were counted and reported as mean puncta per neuron ± SEM. For analyzing localization of glycinergic innervation in the LSO or SPN, boutons were measured by distance from the cell body using Volocity software. The origin of the dendrite (0 μm distance from the soma) was defined as the region where the soma narrowed to form a distinct process. Neurons with an identifiable nucleus and visible dendrites at least 10 μm in length were used for analysis ($N = 12$ dendrites/genotype/brain region). Glycine receptor α1 isoform (GlyRα1) clusters were quantified by counting the numbers of immunopositive puncta located on

LSO or SPN neuronal somata ($N = 4$ sections/mouse at 50 μm increments).

STATISTICAL ANALYSIS

The number of boutons on LSO or SPN neuronal somata were compared using non-parametric Mann–Whitney *U* tests for genotype comparisons at the same age and Kruskal–Wallis tests with Dunn's multiple comparisons for age effects within a genotype. The number of boutons located in 5 μm segments up to 15 μm from the cell soma and the number of GlyRα1+ puncta were compared using Mann–Whitney tests. All statistical analyses were performed using GraphPad Prism software (La Jolla, CA, USA).

RESULTS

DEVELOPMENT OF GLYCINERGIC PROJECTIONS TO THE SOC OF *Egr2; En1*^{CKO} MICE AND CONTROL LITTERMATES DIFFERS IN TEMPORAL PATTERNING AND QUANTITY

We immunostained for GlyT2 to label glycinergic projections (Friauf et al., 1999) to the LSO and SPN throughout postnatal development starting on the day of birth (P0). In agreement with previous reports (Jursky and Nelson, 1996; Friauf et al., 1999), diffuse GlyT2 immunoreactivity was present in the LSO of littermate control and *Egr2; En1*^{CKO} mice at P0 and P3 (**Figures 1A–D′**). By P7, distinct boutons were present on cell somata (**Figures 1E–F′**). The number of boutons/soma increased between P7 and P12 in controls ($P < 0.04$) then remained constant at P14 and in adulthood (9.40 ± 0.19 vs. 10.47 ± 0.16 vs. 10.63 ± 0.17 vs. 10.47 ± 0.15, respectively; $N = 57$–168 soma from 12 to 20 LSO sections/mouse, $N = 2$ mice/age; $P < 0.001$ for age effects). The numbers of GlyT2+ boutons/soma also increased with age in *Egr2; En1*^{CKO} mice ($P < 0.001$), but were consistently 20–30% lower than control values at P7, P12, P14, and adulthood (6.73 ± 0.23 vs. 7.35 ± 0.20 vs. 7.86 ± 0.18 vs. 8.25 ± 0.16; $N = 39$–102 soma from 12 to 20 LSO sections/mouse, $N = 2$ mice/age; **Figures 1E–M**). Thus, glycinergic innervation to the LSO in *Egr2; En1*^{CKO} mice developed following a similar time course to that seen in littermate controls, but never reached control levels.

Similar to the LSO, diffuse GlyT2+ labeling was present in the SPN of P0 and P3 littermate controls and *Egr2; En1*^{CKO} mice (**Figures 2A–D′**). In control mice, the number of boutons/soma remained constant at P7, P12, P14, and adulthood, suggesting that maturation was achieved by the end of the first postnatal week (11.94 ± 0.23, vs. 12.27 ± 0.22 vs. 12.86 ± 0.25 vs. 13.02 ± 0.22, respectively, $N = 49$–81 soma from 12 to 20 SPN sections/mouse, $N = 2$ mice/age; $P = 0.06$ for age effects). In *Egr2; En1*^{CKO} mice, the number of boutons/soma gradually increased from P7 through P14 when numbers were similar to adults (8.63 ± 0.27, 9.30 ± 0.24, 11.92 ± 0.27, 12.03 ± 0.22, respectively, $N = 36$–81 soma from 12 to 20 SPN sections/mouse, $N = 2$ mice/age; $P < 0.001$ for age effects). While the numbers of boutons/soma were reduced by 25–30% compared to littermate controls at P7–P14, no differences were detected in adults, suggesting that development of glycinergic inputs to the SPN is simply delayed in *Egr2; En1*^{CKO} mice (**Figures 2E–M**).

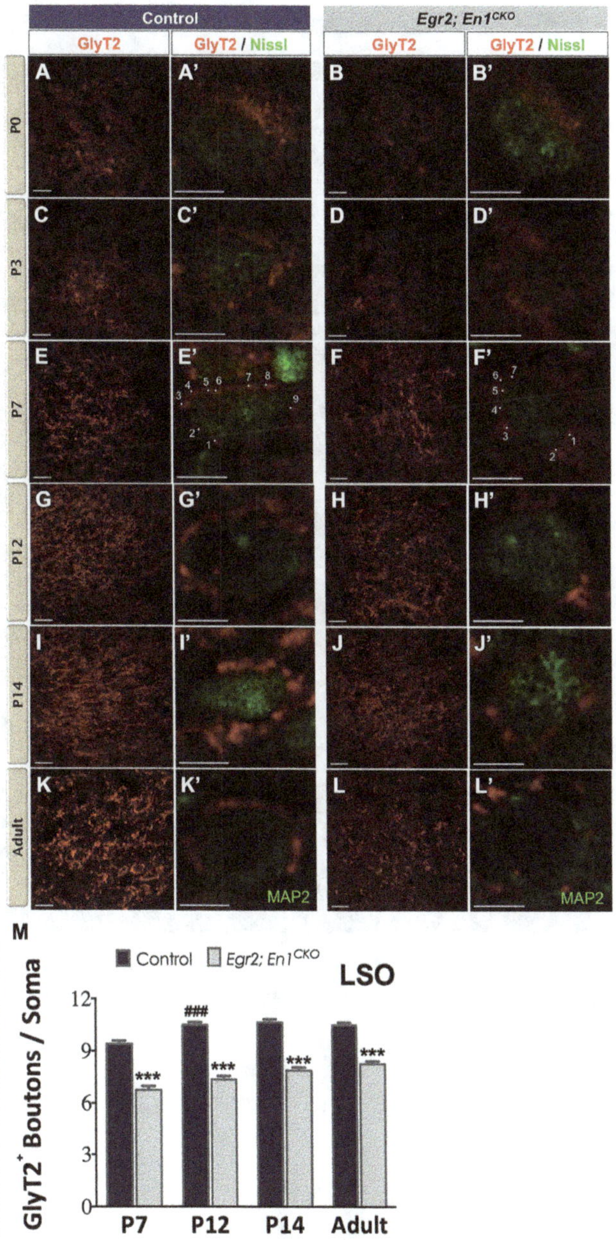

FIGURE 1 | Development of glycinergic innervation to the LSO of control and *Egr2; En1*^{CKO} mice. Diffuse GlyT2 immunoreactivity was detected as early as P0 in control **(A,A′)** and *Egr2; En1*^{CKO} mice **(B,B′)**. Slight increases in staining intensity were seen in P3 control **(C,C′)** and *Egr2; En1*^{CKO} mice **(D,D′)**. By P7, boutons located on LSO neuronal somata were easily discernible in both control **(E,E′)** and mutant mice **(F,F′)**, albeit to a lesser extent in the latter. Individual boutons are shown with dots and numbers. By P12, levels of glycinergic innervation were increased in control mice **(G,G′)** but remained constant in *Egr2; En1*^{CKO} mice **(H,H′)** compared to P7. Compared to controls **(I,I′,K,K′)**, *Egr2; En1*^{CKO} mice had reduced glycinergic innervation at two weeks of age and in adulthood **(J,J′, L,L′)**. The number of GlyT2^{+} boutons was counted in P7 and older mice when boutons were easily recognizable. Reductions in somatic GlyT2+ bouton number occurred in *Egr2; En1*^{CKO} mice compared to control littermates at all ages examined **(M)**. Data are represented as mean ± SEM. Higher magnification images of individual neurons are shown in **(A′–L′)**. Scale bars: 20 μm **(A–D)**; 26 μm **(E–L)**; 8 μm **(A′–L′)**. $^{***}P < 0.001$ vs. age-matched controls, $^{\#\#\#}P < 0.001$ vs. genotype-matched P7 mice.

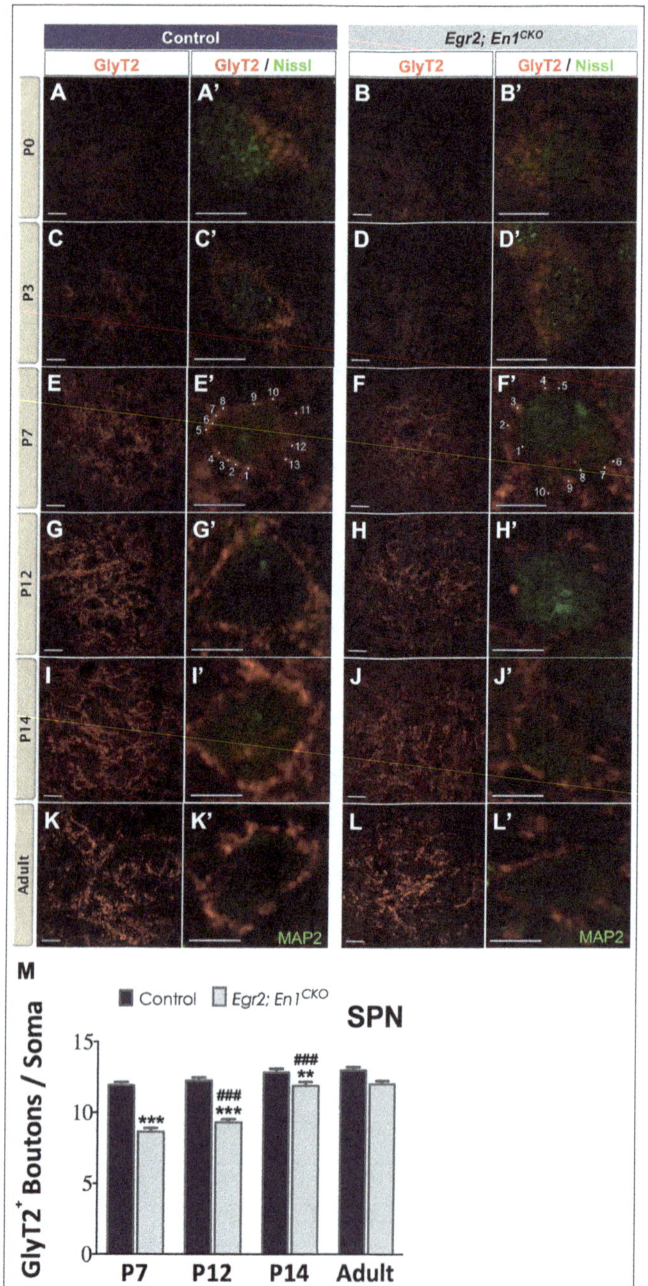

FIGURE 2 | Development of glycinergic innervation to the SPN of control and *Egr2; En1*^{CKO} mice. Diffuse GlyT2 staining was present at birth in control **(A,A′)** and *Egr2; En1*^{CKO} mice **(B,B′)**. Staining intensity increased by P3 in control **(C,C′)** and *Egr2; En1*^{CKO} mice **(D,D′)**. Identifiable boutons were first seen at P7 in control **(E,E′)** and *Egr2; En1*^{CKO} **(F,F′)** mice. Individual boutons are shown with dots and numbers. Staining intensity was also higher in control **(G,G′)** compared to *Egr2; En1*^{CKO} mice **(H,H′)** at P12. However, levels were comparable in control and *Egr2; En1*^{CKO} mice at P14 **(I,I′,J,J′)** and adulthood **(K,K′,L,L′)**. **(M)** GlyT2+ bouton number located on SPN neuronal somata did not change from P7-adulthood in control mice. Bouton numbers were reduced at from P7–P14 in *Egr2; En1*^{CKO} mice, but were similar to controls in adulthood. Data are represented as mean ± SEM. Higher magnification images of individual neurons are shown in **(A′–L′)**. Scale bars: 20 μm **(A–D)**; 26 μm **(E–L)**; 8 μm **(A′–L′)**. $^{**}P < 0.01$, $^{***}P < 0.001$ vs. age-matched controls and $^{###}P < 0.001$ vs. P7 or P12 *Egr2; En1*^{CKO} mice.

DENDRITIC LOCALIZATION OF GLYCINERGIC INNERVATION IS UNALTERED IN *Egr2; En1*^{CKO} MICE

We next examined whether *Egr2; En1*^{CKO} mice exhibited alterations in glycinergic innervation of LSO and SPN neuron dendrites by co-immunostaining for GlyT2 and microtubule-associated protein 2 (MAP2; **Figures 3A–D‴**). The overall distribution of boutons along the proximal 15 μm of LSO and SPN neuron dendrites was similar in littermate control and *Egr2; En1*^{CKO} mice (**Figures 3E–G**). Furthermore, the number of boutons binned into 5 μm segments up to 15 μm from the cell soma was also similar (LSO – Control: 0–5 μm – 2.67 ± 0.47, 5–10 μm – 2.58 ± 0.36, and 10–15 μm – 1.67 ± 0.31; *Egr2; En1*^{CKO} mice: 0–5 μm – 1.58 ± 0.40, 5–10 μm – 2.17 ± 0.42, and 10–15 μm – 2.17 ± 0.27; $P = 0.10$, $P = 0.65$, and $P = 0.26$, respectively and SPN – Control: 0–5 μm – 2.00 ± 0.35, 5–10 μm – 2.67 ± 0.36, and 10–15 μm – 2.92 ± 0.29; *Egr2; En1*^{CKO} mice: 0–5 μm – 1.82 ± 0.42, 5–10 μm – 2.46 ± 0.28, and 10–15 μm – 2.27 ± 0.36; $P = 0.50$, $P = 0.87$, and $P = 0.13$, respectively; **Figures 3H,I** insets and data not shown). Taken together, these data indicate that the number and location of dendritic GlyT2^{+} boutons is similar in control and *Egr2; En1*^{CKO} mice.

Egr2; En1^{CKO} MICE HAVE REDUCED SOMATIC EXPRESSION OF THE GlyRα1 GLYCINE RECEPTOR SUBUNIT IN LSO BUT NOT SPN NEURONS

We previously reported that glycinergic IPSC decay time constants were >2.5-fold slower in LSO and SPN neurons of *Egr2; En1*^{CKO} mice compared to littermate controls (Jalabi et al., 2013). We hypothesized that differences in the number or subunit composition of glycine receptors expressed by LSO and SPN neurons might explain these differences. Therefore, we examined expression patterns of two well-characterized glycine receptor subtypes, the adult-like isoform (GlyRα1) and the purported developmental isoform (GlyRα2). Punctate GlyRα1 immunoreactivity was present in LSO and SPN neurons of both genotypes (**Figures 4A–H**). However, the number of GlyRα1+ clusters/soma was significantly higher in LSO neurons of control vs. *Egr2; En1*^{CKO} mice (23.78 ± 1.07 vs. 13.91 ± 0.97; $N = 21$–29 soma from 4 nuclei/mouse, $N = 2$ mice/genotype, $P < 0.001$; **Figure 4I**). No difference was found in SPN neurons (control: 24.03 ± 1.85 vs. *Egr2; En1*^{CKO} mice: 20.93 ± 1.41; $N = 17$–27 soma from four nuclei/mouse, $N = 2$ mice/genotype, $P = 0.08$; **Figure 4J**). In both control and *Egr2; En1*^{CKO} mice, typical GlyRα1 rosettes (Hruskova et al., 2012) could be identified and glycinergic receptors were apposed to GlyT2$_{+}$ boutons (**Figures 4A‴,B‴,C‴,D‴,G′,H′**). GlyRα2 expression was not present in LSO (**Figures 4K–L‴**) or SPN (data not shown) neurons in control or *Egr2; En1*^{CKO} mice. This suggests that a failure to switch to the adult isoform (fast decay kinetics) from the developmental isoform (slower decay kinetics) does not account for altered IPSC kinetics in these mice.

DISCUSSION

Our data demonstrate that glycinergic innervation measured by GlyT2 immunoreactivity in the mouse LSO and SPN follows a similar developmental time course to that seen in other rodents such as guinea pigs and rats (Wenthold et al., 1987; Helfert et al., 1989, 1992; Friauf et al., 1999). Gradual increases in GlyT2 expression

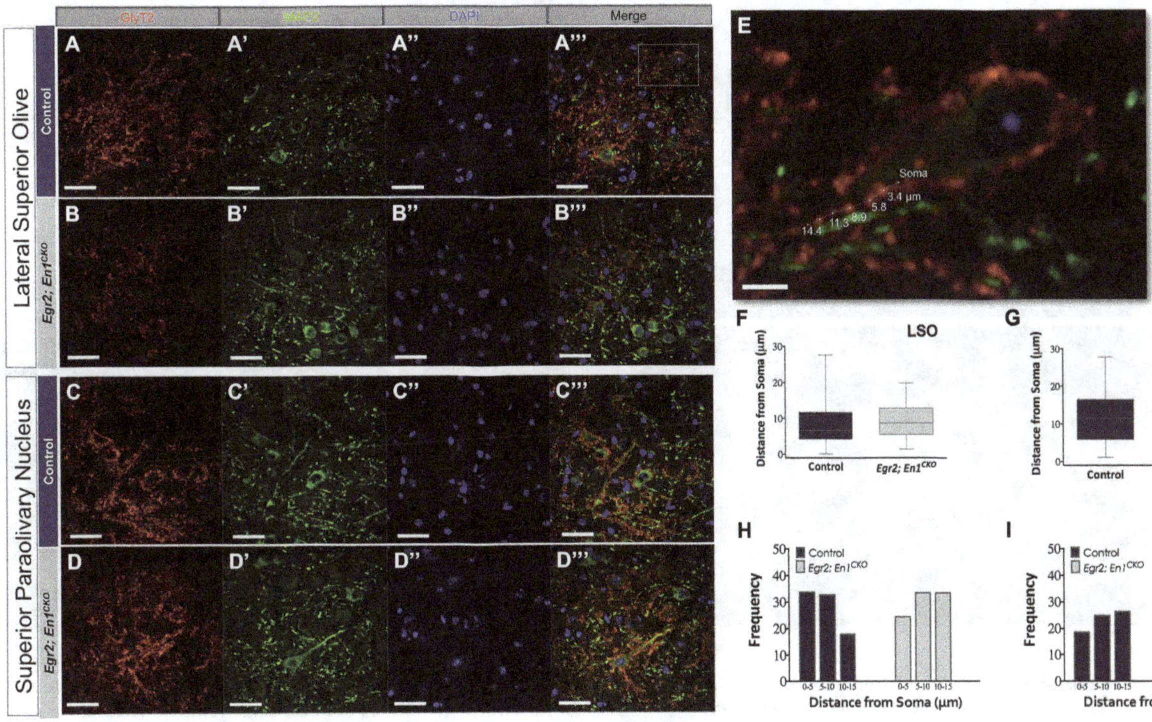

FIGURE 3 | Dendritic localization of GlyT2$^+$ boutons is unchanged in adult *Egr2; En1*^{CKO} mice. GlyT2+ boutons were present on MAP2+ dendrites of LSO and SPN neurons in adult control **(A–A‴,C–C‴)** and *Egr2; En1*^{CKO} mice **(B–B‴,D–D‴)**. **(E)** Area outlined by the white box in **(A‴)**. Distance of GlyT2$^+$ boutons from neuronal soma was measured as shown. Box plots depicting the median and distribution of bouton distance from cell somata in LSO **(F)** and SPN **(G)**. Whiskers are representative of minimum and maximum distance values. Data were further analyzed by looking at proximal vs. distal localization by determining the frequency (percentage) of boutons in 5 μm increments for dendrites in the LSO **(H)** and SPN **(I)**; no significant differences were present between control and *Egr2; En1*^{CKO} mice. Scale bars: 33 μm **(A–D‴)**; 16 μm **(E)**.

and the formation of distinct somatic boutons during the first postnatal week coincide with the timeframe of synaptic pruning and strengthening of connections arising from the MNTB during the transient excitatory period of these developing networks (Kim and Kandler, 2003). Adult-like GlyT2 expression occurs sooner in the SPN than in the LSO, and both mature in advance of hearing onset (Willott, 2001). This pattern coincides with the earlier functional maturation of SPN neurons demonstrated by their earlier switch from depolarizing (excitatory) to hyperpolarizing (inhibitory) glycinergic post-synaptic responses, which occurs by birth in the SPN but not until P3–P5 in the LSO (Kullmann and Kandler, 2001; Löhrke et al., 2005). One difference between rats and mice is that the intensity of GlyT2 immunoreactivity reaches maximum levels at P10 in the rat (Friauf et al., 1999), while in mice it is maximal in the adult (**Figures 1K–L′** and **2K–L′**).

Our data provide insights into the development of glycinergic SOC innervation in the absence of MNTB neurons. In the LSO, the number of GlyT2+ boutons/soma increases at a similar rate from P7 to adulthood but is consistently 20–30% lower in *Egr2; En1*^{CKO} than controls. This suggests that the developmental time course of GlyT2 immunoreactivity is similar in both genotypes. Conversely, glycinergic development is delayed in the SPN, as the number of glycinergic boutons/SPN neuron soma does not reach adult levels until P14 in *Egr2; En1*^{CKO} mice, 7 days after controls. However, the number of boutons/soma is similar in adult *Egr2; En1*^{CKO} and littermate control mice, suggesting that development is simply delayed rather than permanently altered as it is in the LSO. GlyT2 function is theorized to influence the development of inhibitory networks in the SOC because its expression precedes synapse maturation in multiple central auditory regions (Kandler and Friauf, 1995; Ehrlich et al., 1998; Friauf et al., 1999). Thus, reduced levels of GlyT2 expression in the LSO and SPN of *Egr2; En1*^{CKO} mice during early postnatal development could contribute to persistent changes in glycinergic circuitry and function in these mice.

The number and distribution of GlyT2+ boutons on the dendrites of LSO and SPN neurons is similar in adult *Egr2; En1*^{CKO} mice and littermate controls (**Figure 3**). This is consistent with the interpretation that non-MNTB-derived glycinergic projections normally target the dendrites, and ectopically expands to LSO and SPN neuronal somata only in the absence of competition from MNTB-derived projections. Alternatively, this could occur if improper refinement and/or synaptic pruning of distally located boutons takes place in the absence of MNTB-derived projections. For example, developmentally regulated activity-dependent relocation of inhibitory inputs from dendrites to cell somata occurs in medial superior olive (MSO) neurons of animals with well-developed low frequency hearing (Kapfer et al., 2002); whether a similar process occurs in the LSO of animals that rely on

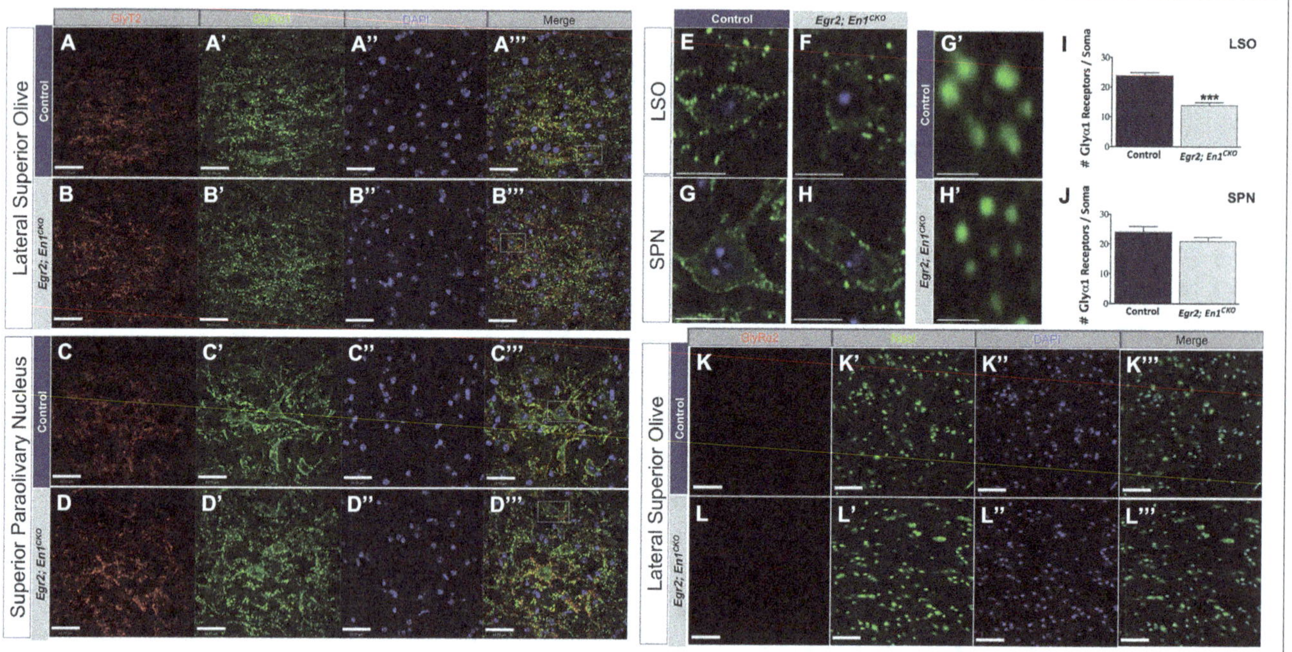

FIGURE 4 | Glycine receptor isoform expression patterns, but not receptor number, are similar in LSO and SPN neurons of adult control and *Egr2; En1*^{CKO} mice. Adult control and *Egr2; En1*^{CKO} mouse brain sections through the LSO **(A,B)** and SPN **(C,D)** were immunostained for GlyT2 **(A–D)** and the glycine receptor isoform alpha 1 (GlyRα1; **A′–D′**). **(E–H)** Higher magnification images showing punctate staining on LSO **(E,F)** and SPN **(G,H)** neuronal somata and dendrites are shown in control **(E,G)** and *Egr2; En1*^{CKO} **(F,H)** mice. **(G′,H′)** High magnification images of typical GlyRα1 rosettes. Counts of GlyRα1+ puncta per LSO **(I)** or SPN **(J)** neuronal soma revealed decreased numbers in the LSO, but not SPN, of *Egr2; En1*^{CKO} compared to control mice. Data are represented as mean $\pm$ SEM. Glycine receptor alpha 2 (GlyRα2) was not expressed by LSO neurons in adult control **(K)** or *Egr2; En1*^{CKO} mice **(L)**. DAPI **(A–D″,K″,L″)** and Nissl **(K′,L′)** counterstains are also shown. Scale bars: 33 μm **(A–D,K,L)**; 12 μm **(E–H)**; 2.3 μm **(G′,H′)**. $^{***}P < 0.001$ vs. control.

high-frequency hearing (like the mouse) is not known. A third possibility is that MNTB- and non-MNTB-derived glycinergic inputs normally intermingle on cell somata and dendrites, and that the non-MNTB-derived innervation expands in both locations in the absence of MNTB neurons. Identification of the source of the non-MNTB-derived innervation followed by labeling of its projections is necessary to distinguish between these possibilities. Regardless, changes in glycinergic bouton localization cannot cause the altered IPSC kinetics seen in LSO and SPN neurons of *Egr2; En1*^{CKO} mice (Jalabi et al., 2013).

We also examined GlyR subunit expression in the LSO and SPN of adult control and *Egr2; En1*^{CKO} mice. Glycine receptors are multimeric proteins composed of 2 alpha and 3 beta subunits (Lynch, 2009; Dutertre et al., 2012; Yang et al., 2012). Alpha subunits contain the ligand binding pocket and come in four isoforms (GlyRα1-α4), each of which confers different functional channel properties (Pfeiffer et al., 1982). We focused on GlyRα1 and GlyRα2 because these receptors are expressed by developing and/or mature SOC neurons of other species (Friauf et al., 1997; Piechotta et al., 2001), and they confer fast and slow IPSC decay kinetics to the GlyR, respectively (Takahashi et al., 1992; Bormann et al., 1993; Singer et al., 1998; Weiss et al., 2008). Our finding that GlyRα1 was highly expressed by LSO and SPN neurons of adult mice agrees with previous studies in adult rats (Sato et al., 1995; Friauf et al., 1997; Piechotta et al., 2001). GlyRα1 expression was detected in the LSO of *Egr2; En1*^{CKO} mice, but the number of receptor clusters per neuronal cell body was reduced compared to controls. This reduction, along with the reduced number of GlyT2+ boutons, may contribute to the decreased IPSC amplitudes seen in LSO neurons of these mice (Jalabi et al., 2013). Our hypothesis that maintained expression of GlyRα2, which is normally expressed only during embryonic and postnatal ages (Becker et al., 1988; Akagi et al., 1991; Malosio et al., 1991; Sato et al., 1995; Kungel and Friauf, 1997; Piechotta et al., 2001), might explain the aberrant IPSC decay kinetics proved to be incorrect as GlyRα2 was not expressed by LSO or SPN neurons in adult control or *Egr2; En1*^{CKO} mice. We did not examine GlyRα4 because it is minimally expressed in the CNS (Harvey et al., 2000) and therefore is unlikely to contribute to the altered electrophysiological responses seen in *Egr2; En1*^{CKO} mice. Similarly, we did not examine β subunit distribution as alterations in its expression are predicted to affect glycine receptor trafficking and clustering (Kneussel and Betz, 2000), which appear to be unaffected in *Egr2; En1*^{CKO} mice (**Figures 4E′,F′**). Future studies could examine GlyRα3 expression, which shows similar kinetics to GlyRα1 and is expressed in the auditory brainstem, albeit at lower levels (Sato et al., 1995).

Taken together, our findings demonstrate dynamic developmental reprogramming of the SOC glycinergic circuitry in the absence of the MNTB. Identifying the source(s) of this non-MNTB-derived innervation in *Egr2; En1*^{CKO} mice in conjunction with experiments to measure function and expression of receptors at critical developmental time points is necessary to clarify factors that lead to persistent changes. The striking ability of this system to compensate in the absence of the MNTB has potential clinical implications that might be important for understanding altered central auditory function in autism, where neuron number is lower in many SOC subnuclei (Rosenblum et al., 1980; Wong and Wong, 1991; Maziade et al., 2000; Kulesza, 2008; Kulesza et al., 2011), and in age-related hearing loss (Grimsley and Sivaramakrishnan, 2014).

ACKNOWLEDGMENTS

We are grateful for the assistance and insightful comments on the preparation of this manuscript provided by members of the Maricich Lab. We also extend thanks to Dr. Timothy Sanders at Children's Hospital of Pittsburgh (Pittsburgh, PA, USA) and his laboratory for the use of their confocal microscope, and to Dr. Gary Landreth at Case Western Reserve University for supplying laboratory space to Walid Jalabi. This work was supported by the Richard King Mellon Institute for Pediatric Research at the University of Pittsburgh (Stephen M. Maricich), the National Institute on Deafness and other Communication Disorders (NIDCD) of the National Institutes of Health under award number T32DC004199 NIH (Stefanie C. Altieri), and NIDCD F32DC011982 (Walid Jalabi).

REFERENCES

Adams, J. C., and Mugnaini, E. (1990). Immunocytochemical evidence for inhibitory and disinhibitory circuits in the superior olive. *Hear. Res.* 49, 281–298. doi: 10.1016/0378-5955(90)90109-3

Akagi, H., Hirai, K., and Hishinuma, F. (1991).Cloning of a glycine receptor subtype expressed in rat brain and spinal cord during a specific period of neuronal development. *FEBS Lett.* 281, 160–166. doi: 10.1016/0014-5793(91)80383-E

Aoki, E., Semba, R., Keino, H., Kato, K., and Kashiwamata, S. (1988). Glycine-like immunoreactivity in the rat auditory pathway. *Brain Res.* 442, 63–71. doi: 10.1016/0006-8993(88)91432-1

Becker, C. M., Hoch, W., and Betz, H. (1988). Glycine receptor heterogeneity in rat spinal cord during postnatal development. *EMBO J.* 7, 3717–3726.

Behrend, O., Brand, A., Kapfer, C., and Grothe, B. (2002). Auditory response properties in the superior paraolivary nucleus of the gerbil. *J. Neurophysiol.* 87, 2915–2928.

Bledsoe, S. C., Snead, C. R., Helfert, R. H., Prasad, V., Wenthold, R. J., and Altschuler, R. A. (1990). Immunocytochemical and lesion studies support the hypothesis that the projection from the medial nucleus of the trapezoid body to the lateral superior olive is glycinergic. *Brain Res.* 517, 189–194. doi: 10.1016/0006-8993(90)91025-C

Bormann, J., Rundström, N., Betz, H., and Langosch, D. (1993). Residues within transmembrane segment M2 determine chloride conductance of glycine receptor homo- and hetero-oligomers. *EMBO J.* 12, 3729–3737.

Boudreau, J. C., and Tsuchitani, C. (1968). Binaural interaction in the cat superior olive S segment. *J. Neurophysiol.* 31, 442–454. doi: 10.1121/1.2144209

Dehmel, S., Kopp-Scheinpflug, C., Dörrscheidt, G. J., and Rübsamen, R. (2002). Electrophysiological characterization of the superior paraolivary nucleus in the *Mongolian gerbil. Hear. Res.* 172, 18–36. doi: 10.1016/S0378-5955(02)00353-2

Dutertre, S., Becker, C.-M., and Betz, H. (2012). Inhibitory glycine receptors: an update. *J. Biol. Chem.* 287, 40216–40223. doi: 10.1074/jbc.R112.408229

Ehret, G. (1976). Development of absolute auditory thresholds in the house mouse (*Mus musculus*). *J. Am. Audiol. Soc.* 1, 179–184.

Ehrlich, I., Ilic, V., Lohmann, C., and Friauf, E. (1998). Development of glycinergic transmission in organotypic cultures from auditory brain stem. *Neuroreport* 9, 2785–2790. doi: 10.1097/00001756-199808240-00019

Felix, R. A., Magnusson, A. K., and Berrebi, A. S. (2014). The superior paraolivary nucleus shapes temporal response properties of neurons in the inferior colliculus. *Brain Struct. Funct.* doi: 10.1007/s00429-014-0815-8 [Epub ahead of print].

Friauf, E., Aragón, C., Löhrke, S., Westenfelder, B., and Zafra, F. (1999). Developmental expression of the glycine transporter GLYT2 in the auditory system of rats suggests involvement in synapse maturation. *J. Comp. Neurol.* 412, 17–37. doi: 10.1002/(SICI)1096-9861(19990913)412:1<17::AbreakID-CNE2>3.0.CO;2-E

Friauf, E., Hammerschmidt, B., and Kirsch, J. (1997). Development of adult-type inhibitory glycine receptors in the central auditory system of rats. *J. Comp. Neurol.* 385, 117–134. doi: 10.1002/(SICI)1096-9861(19970818)385:1<117::AID-CNE7>3.0.CO;2-5

Friauf, E., and Ostwald, J. (1988). Divergent projections of physiologically characterized rat ventral cochlear nucleus neurons as shown by intra-axonal injection of horseradish peroxidase. *Exp. Brain Res.* 73, 263–284. doi: 10.1007/BF00248219

Grimsley, C. A., and Sivaramakrishnan, S. (2014). Postnatal developmental changes in the medial nucleus of the trapezoid body in a mouse model of auditory pathology. *Neurosci. Lett.* 559, 152–157. doi: 10.1016/j.neulet.2013.11.051

Harvey, R. J., Schmieden, V., Holst Von, A., Laube, B., Rohrer, H., and Betz, H. (2000). Glycine receptors containing the alpha4 subunit in the embryonic sympathetic nervous system, spinal cord and male genital ridge. *Eur. J. Neurosci.* 12, 994–1001. doi: 10.1046/j.1460-9568.2000.00993.x

Helfert, R. H., Bonneau, J. M., Wenthold, R. J., and Altschuler, R. A. (1989). GABA and glycine immunoreactivity in the guinea pig superior olivary complex. *Brain Res.* 501, 269–286. doi: 10.1016/0006-8993(89)90644-6

Helfert, R. H., Juiz, J. M., Bledsoe, S. C., Bonneau, J. M., Wenthold, R. J., and Altschuler, R. A. (1992). Patterns of glutamate, glycine, and GABA immunolabeling in four synaptic terminal classes in the lateral superior olive of the guinea pig. *J. Comp. Neurol.* 323, 305–325. doi: 10.1002/cne.903230302

Hruskova, B., Trojanova, J., Kulik, A., Kralikova, M., Pysanenko, K., Bures, Z., et al. (2012). Differential distribution of glycine receptor subtypes at the rat calyx of held synapse. *J. Neurosci.* 32, 17012–17024. doi: 10.1523/JNEUROSCI.1547-12.2012

Jalabi, W., Kopp-Scheinpflug, C., Allen, P. D., Schiavon, E., Digiacomo, R. R., Forsythe, I. D., et al. (2013). Sound localization ability and glycinergic innervation of the superior olivary complex persist after genetic deletion of the medial nucleus of the trapezoid body. *J. Neurosci.* 33, 15044–15049. doi: 10.1523/JNEUROSCI.2604-13.2013

Jursky, F., and Nelson, N. (1996). Developmental expression of the glycine transporters GLYT1 and GLYT2 in mouse brain. *J. Neurochem.* 67, 336–344. doi: 10.1046/j.1471-4159.1996.67010336.x

Kadner, A., and Berrebi, A. S. (2008). Encoding of temporal features of auditory stimuli in the medial nucleus of the trapezoid body and superior paraolivary nucleus of the rat. Neuroscience 151, 868–887. doi: 10.1016/j.neuroscience.2007.11.008

Kadner, A., Kulesza, R. J., and Berrebi, A. S. (2006). Neurons in the medial nucleus of the trapezoid body and superior paraolivary nucleus of the rat may play a role in sound duration coding. *J. Neurophysiol.* 95, 1499–1508. doi: 10.1152/jn.00902.2005

Kandler, K., Clause, A., and Noh, J. (2009). Tonotopic reorganization of developing auditory brainstem circuits. *Nat. Neurosci.* 12, 711–717. doi: 10.1038/nn.2332

Kandler, K., and Friauf, E. (1995). Development of glycinergic and glutamatergic synaptic transmission in the auditory brainstem of perinatal rats. *J. Neurosci.* 15, 6890–6904.

Kandler, K., and Gillespie, D. C. (2005). Developmental refinement of inhibitory sound-localization circuits. *Trends Neurosci.* 28, 290–296. doi: 10.1016/j.tins.2005.04.007

Kapfer, C., Seidl, A. H., Schweizer, H., and Grothe, B. (2002). Experience-dependent refinement of inhibitory inputs to auditory coincidence-detector neurons. *Nat. Neurosci.* 5, 247–253. doi: 10.1038/nn810

Kim, G., and Kandler, K. (2003). Elimination and strengthening of glycinergic/GABAergic connections during tonotopic map formation. *Nat. Neurosci.* 6, 282–290. doi: 10.1038/nn1015

Kneussel, M., and Betz, H. (2000). Clustering of inhibitory neurotransmitter receptors at developing postsynaptic sites: the membrane activation model. *Trends Neurosci.* 23, 429–435. doi: 10.1016/S0166-2236(00)01627-1

Kulesza, R. J. (2008). Cytoarchitecture of the human superior olivary complex: nuclei of the trapezoid body and posterior tier. *Hear. Res.* 241, 52–63. doi: 10.1016/j.heares.2008.04.010

Kulesza, R. J., Kadner, A., and Berrebi, A. S. (2007). Distinct roles for glycine and GABA in shaping the response properties of neurons in the superior paraolivary nucleus of the rat. *J. Neurophysiol.* 97, 1610–1620. doi: 10.1152/jn.00613.2006

Kulesza, R. J., Lukose, R., and Stevens, L. V. (2011). Malformation of the human superior olive in autistic spectrum disorders. *Brain Res.* 1367, 360–371. doi: 10.1016/j.brainres.2010.10.015

Kulesza, R. J., Spirou, G. A., and Berrebi, A. S. (2003). Physiological response properties of neurons in the superior paraolivary nucleus of the rat. *J. Neurophysiol.* 89, 2299–2312. doi: 10.1152/jn.00547.2002

Kullmann, P. H., and Kandler, K. (2001). Glycinergic/GABAergic synapses in the lateral superior olive are excitatory in neonatal C57Bl/6J mice. *Brain Res. Dev. Brain Res.* 131, 143–147. doi: 10.1016/S0165-3806(01)00271-1

Kungel, M., and Friauf, E. (1997). Physiology and pharmacology of native glycine receptors in developing rat auditory brainstem neurons. *Brain Res. Dev. Brain Res.* 102, 157–165. doi: 10.1016/S0165-3806(97)00087-4

Löhrke, S., Srinivasan, G., Oberhofer, M., Doncheva, E., and Friauf, E. (2005). Shift from depolarizing to hyperpolarizing glycine action occurs at different perinatal ages in superior olivary complex nuclei. *Eur. J. Neurosci.* 22, 2708–2722. doi: 10.1111/j.1460-9568.2005.04465.x

Lynch, J. W. (2009). Native glycine receptor subtypes and their physiological roles. *Neuropharmacology* 56, 303–309. doi: 10.1016/j.neuropharm.2008.07.034

Malosio, M. L., Marquèze-Pouey, B., Kuhse, J., and Betz, H. (1991). Widespread expression of glycine receptor subunit mRNAs in the adult and developing rat brain. *EMBO J.* 10, 2401–2409.

Maziade, M., Mérette, C., Cayer, M., Roy, M. A., Szatmari, P., Côté, R., et al. (2000). Prolongation of brainstem auditory-evoked responses in autistic probands and their unaffected relatives. *Arch. Gen. Psychiatry* 57, 1077–1083. doi: 10.1001/archpsyc.57.11.1077

Moore, M. J., and Caspary, D. M. (1983). Strychnine blocks binaural inhibition in lateral superior olivary neurons. *J. Neurosci.* 3, 237–242.

Peyret, D., Campistron, G., Geffard, M., and Aran, J. M. (1987). Glycine immunoreactivity in the brainstem auditory and vestibular nuclei of the guinea pig. *Acta Otolaryngol.* 104, 71–76. doi: 10.3109/00016488709109049

Pfeiffer, F., Graham, D., and Betz, H. (1982). Purification by affinity chromatography of the glycine receptor of rat spinal cord. *J. Biol. Chem.* 257, 9389–9393.

Piechotta, K., Weth, F., Harvey, R. J., and Friauf, E. (2001). Localization of rat glycine receptor alpha1 and alpha2 subunit transcripts in the developing auditory brainstem. *J. Comp. Neurol.* 438, 336–352. doi: 10.1002/cne.1319

Rosenblum, S. M., Arick, J. R., Krug, D. A., Stubbs, E. G., Young, N. B., and Pelson, R. O. (1980). Auditory brainstem evoked responses in autistic children. *J. Autism Dev. Disord.* 10, 215–225. doi: 10.1007/BF02408472

Sanes, D. H., and Rubel, E. W. (1988). The ontogeny of inhibition and excitation in the gerbil lateral superior olive. *J. Neurosci.* 8, 682–700.

Sanes, D. H., and Siverls, V. (1991). Development and specificity of inhibitory terminal arborizations in the central nervous system. *J. Neurobiol.* 22, 837–854. doi: 10.1002/neu.480220805

Sato, K., Kuriyama, H., and Altschuler, R. A. (1995). Expression of glycine receptor subunits in the cochlear nucleus and superior olivary complex using non-radioactive in-situ hybridization. *Hear. Res.* 91, 7–18. doi: 10.1016/0378-5955(95)00156-5

Schofield, B. R. (1995). Projections from the cochlear nucleus to the superior paraolivary nucleus in guinea pigs. *J. Comp. Neurol.* 360, 135–149. doi: 10.1002/cne.903600110

Sgaier, S. K., Lao, Z., Villanueva, M. P., Berenshteyn, F., Stephen, D., Turnbull, R. K., et al. (2007). Genetic subdivision of the tectum and cerebellum into functionally related regions based on differential sensitivity to engrailed proteins. *Development* 134, 2325–2335. doi: 10.1242/dev.000620

Singer, J. H., Talley, E. M., Bayliss, D. A., and Berger, A. J. (1998). Development of glycinergic synaptic transmission to rat brain stem motoneurons. *J. Neurophysiol.* 80, 2608–2620.

Spangler, K. M., Warr, W. B., and Henkel, C. K. (1985). The projections of principal cells of the medial nucleus of the trapezoid body in the cat. *J. Comp. Neurol.* 238, 249–262. doi: 10.1002/cne.902380302

Srinivasan, G., Friauf, E., and Löhrke, S. (2004). Functional glutamatergic and glycinergic inputs to several superior olivary nuclei of the rat revealed by optical imaging. Neuroscience 128, 617–634. doi: 10.1016/j.neuroscience.2004.06.012

Takahashi, T., Momiyama, A., Hirai, K., Hishinuma, F., and Akagi, H. (1992). Functional correlation of fetal and adult forms of glycine receptors with developmental changes in inhibitory synaptic receptor channels. *Neuron* 9, 1155–1161. doi: 10.1016/0896-6273(92)90073-M

Thompson, A. M., and Thompson, G. C. (1991). Projections from the posteroventral cochlear nucleus to the superior olivary complex in guinea pig: light and EM observations with the PHA-L method. *J. Comp. Neurol.* 311, 495–508. doi: 10.1002/cne.903110405

Voiculescu, O., Charnay, P., and Schneider-Maunoury, S. (2000). Expression pattern of a Krox-20/Cre knock-in allele in the developing hindbrain, bones, and peripheral nervous system. *Genesis* 26, 123–126. doi: 10.1002/(SICI)1526-968X(200002)26:2<123::AID-GENE7>3.0.CO;2-O

Weiss, J., O'Sullivan, G. A., Heinze, L., Chen, H.-X., Betz, H., and Wässle, H. (2008). Glycinergic input of small-field amacrine cells in the retinas of wild-type and glycine receptor deficient mice. *Mol. Cell. Neurosci.* 37, 40–55. doi: 10.1016/j.mcn.2007.08.012

Wenthold, R. J., Huie, D., Altschuler, R. A., and Reeks, K. A. (1987). Glycine immunoreactivity localized in the cochlear nucleus and superior olivary complex. Neuroscience 22, 897–912. doi: 10.1016/0306-4522(87)92968-X

Willott, J. F. (2001). *Handbook of Mouse Auditory Research.* Boca Raton, FL: CRC Press.

Wong, V., and Wong, S. N. (1991). Brainstem auditory evoked potential study in children with autistic disorder. *J. Autism Dev. Disord.* 21, 329–340. doi: 10.1201/9781420038736

Wu, S. H., and Kelly, J. B. (1991). Physiological properties of neurons in the mouse superior olive: membrane characteristics and postsynaptic responses studied in vitro. *J. Neurophysiol.* 65, 230–246. doi: 10.1007/BF02207329

Wu, S. H., and Kelly, J. B. (1992). Synaptic pharmacology of the superior olivary complex studied in mouse brain slice. *J. Neurosci.* 12, 3084–3097.

Wu, S. H., and Kelly, J. B. (1995). Inhibition in the superior olivary complex: pharmacological evidence from mouse brain slice. *J. Neurophysiol.* 73, 256–269.

Yang, Z., Taran, E., Webb, T. I., and Lynch, J. W. (2012). Stoichiometry and subunit arrangement of α1β glycine receptors as determined by atomic force microscopy. *Biochemistry* 51, 5229–5231. doi: 10.1021/bi300063m

16

GABAergic and glycinergic inhibitory synaptic transmission in the ventral cochlear nucleus studied in VGAT channelrhodopsin-2 mice

Ruili Xie[1] and Paul B. Manis[1,2]*

[1] Department of Otolaryngology/Head and Neck Surgery, University of North Carolina at Chapel Hill, Chapel Hill, NC, USA
[2] Department of Cell Biology and Physiology, University of North Carolina at Chapel Hill, Chapel Hill, NC, USA

***Correspondence:**
Paul B. Manis, Department of Otolaryngology/Head and Neck Surgery, University of North Carolina at Chapel Hill, G127 Physician's Office Building, CB#7070, 170 Manning Drive, Chapel Hill, NC 27599-7070, USA
e-mail: pmanis@med.unc.edu

Both glycine and GABA mediate inhibitory synaptic transmission in the ventral cochlear nucleus (VCN). In mice, the time course of glycinergic inhibition is slow in bushy cells and fast in multipolar (stellate) cells, and is proposed to contribute to the processing of temporal cues in both cell types. Much less is known about GABAergic synaptic transmission in this circuit. Electrical stimulation of the auditory nerve or the tuberculoventral pathway evokes little GABAergic synaptic current in brain slice preparations, and spontaneous GABAergic miniature synaptic currents occur infrequently. To investigate synaptic currents carried by GABA receptors in bushy and multipolar cells, we used transgenic mice in which channelrhodopsin-2 and EYFP is driven by the vesicular GABA transporter (VGAT-ChR2-EYFP) and is expressed in both GABAergic and glycinergic neurons. Light stimulation evoked action potentials in EYFP-expressing presynaptic cells, and evoked inhibitory postsynaptic potentials (IPSPs) in non-expressing bushy and planar multipolar cells. Less than 10% of the IPSP amplitude in bushy cells arose from GABAergic synapses, whereas 40% of the IPSP in multipolar neurons was GABAergic. In voltage clamp, glycinergic IPSCs were significantly slower in bushy neurons than in multipolar neurons, whereas there was little difference in the kinetics of the GABAergic IPSCs between two cell types. During prolonged stimulation, the ratio of steady state vs. peak IPSC amplitude was significantly lower for glycinergic IPSCs. Surprisingly, the reversal potentials of GABAergic IPSCs were negative to those of glycinergic IPSCs in both bushy and multipolar neurons. In the absence of receptor blockers, repetitive light stimulation was only able to effectively evoke IPSCs up to 20 Hz in both bushy and multipolar neurons. We conclude that local GABAergic release within the VCN can differentially influence bushy and multipolar cells.

Keywords: IPSC, target-specific inhibition, bushy, multipolar, stellate

INTRODUCTION

Inhibition plays multiple roles in sensory information processing that depend on the spatial arrangement of inhibitory circuits relative to the sensory map, and the time course of synaptic currents. Thus, inhibition can shape sensory response areas, as well as define the temporal patterns and rates of ongoing responses. In the auditory brainstem, local and projection circuits utilize both glycine and GABA as transmitters. For example, descending pathways from subnuclei of the superior olivary complex to the cochlear nuclei include both glycincergic and GABAergic components (Ostapoff et al., 1997). Local circuits within the cochlear nuclei can be glycinergic, GABAergic, or utilize both transmitters (Kolston et al., 1992). In the ventral cochlear nucleus (VCN), the synaptically mediated conductances and kinetics of glycine receptors have been extensively studied (Wu and Oertel, 1986; Harty and Manis, 1996; Ferragamo et al., 1998; Harty and Manis, 1998; Xie and Manis, 2013). The glycinergic synaptic conductances of the two principal cell types in the VCN, the bushy and multipolar cells, have very different kinetics (Xie and Manis, 2013), suggesting a critical role for the time course of inhibition in auditory processing by the cochlear nuclei. Whether there are also differences in $GABA_A$ synaptic currents between these two principal cell types is not known.

Synaptically-mediated conductances associated exclusively with $GABA_A$ receptors have been difficult to detect in the VCN, possibly because such synapses are small and relatively rare compared to glycinergic synapses (Juiz et al., 1996). Electrical stimulation of the auditory nerve or the tuberculoventral pathway from the dorsal cochlear nucleus (DCN) evokes little or no GABAergic synaptic current in VCN neurons in brain slices (Xie and Manis, 2013), and spontaneous GABAergic miniature synaptic currents are observed infrequently when glycinergic receptors are blocked with strychnine. However, in VCN slices, $GABA_A$ conductances can be activated pharmacologically (Wu and Oertel, 1986; Milenković et al., 2007), and block of GABA receptors suggests a role in gating polysynaptic activity (Ferragamo et al., 1998). Furthermore, neurotransmitter binding suggests that GABA receptors are present in the VCN (Frostholm and Rotter, 1986; Juiz et al., 1994). Anatomical studies have revealed GAD-positive terminals on the soma and proximal dendrites of most cochlear nucleus neurons (Adams and Mugnaini, 1987; Moore and Moore, 1987; Roberts and Ribak, 1987; Saint Marie et al., 1989). Iontophoresis of GABA and muscimol *in vivo* has clearly demonstrated that GABA receptor activation can inhibit the acoustic responses of VCN neurons (Caspary et al., 1979, 1994; Palombi and Caspary, 1992; Ebert and Ostwald, 1995a,b; Backoff et al., 1999). A common theme is that GABA suppresses spontaneous activity more than evoked activity. GABA antagonists also modify the responses to sinusoidally amplitude-modulated tones and to tones in noise (Backoff et al., 1999; Gai and Carney, 2008), suggesting a functional role for GABA in enhancing information about envelopes, and in spectral processing in circuits of the VCN. The robust and fairly consistent effects seen *in vivo* however stand in contrast to an absence of synaptically-evoked GABA responses in *in vitro* experiments.

There are two potential explanations for the differences between the *in vitro* and *in vivo* evidence for $GABA_A$ mediated synaptic inhibition in the VCN. First, *in vivo*, pharmacological agonists and antagonists can activate or inactivate the GABAergic circuits, because all of the incoming pathways are intact and functional, regardless of whether they originate within the cochlear nuclei or from descending projections. In contrast, in brain slices, such circuits may be completely or partially missing because they arise from outside the nucleus, or because the fibers run in different planes than the primary slice orientation. Thus, the receptors would remain functional, but stimulation at an appropriate site to activate specific axons from the extrinsic circuits may be difficult to achieve. Second, there are few GABAergic neurons in the VCN, and few GABAergic neurons from the surrounding granule cell regions or the DCN project into the VCN, so local stimulation of the auditory nerve root region or the DCN is not likely to consistently reveal GABAergic inhibition. In the present study, we have used a mouse line in which channelrhodopsin-2 (ChR2) is expressed in neurons under control of the vesicular GABA transporter (VGAT) promoter. VGAT is expressed in glycinergic, GABAergic, and mixed GABAergic-glycinergic synapses (Dumoulin et al., 1999), and is expressed by both glycinergic and GABAergic neurons in the cochlear nuclei (Wang et al., 2009). As a result, in the VGAT-ChR2 mice, optical stimulation can be used to selectively stimulate both local neurons, as well as axons of VGAT-ChR2 expressing distantly-located cells that may project into the nuclei. Using this approach, we have characterized and compared the GABAergic and glycinergic synaptic potentials and conductances in VCN bushy and planar multipolar cells.

MATERIALS AND METHODS

VGAT-ChR2-EYFP mice (B6.Cg-Tg(Slc32a1-COP4*H134R/EYFP)8Gfng/J; (Zhao et al., 2011)) were purchased from Jackson Laboratories (stock #014548) and maintained in our breeding colony. The mice incorporate a BAC transgene that expresses ChR2 and enhanced yellow fluorescent protein (EYFP) under the control of the VGAT promoter. Because ChR2 is fused to EYFP, EYFP fluorescence directly reports the cellular localization of ChR2 (see **Figure 1**). All animal procedures were approved by the University of North Carolina Internal Animal Concerns and Use Committee (IACUC).

Slice preparation follows the approach used in our recent studies (Wang and Manis, 2005; Xie and Manis, 2013). Mice were anesthetized with an intraperitoneal injection of 100 mg/kg ketamine and 10 mg/kg xylazine, decapitated, and the brain dissected and placed in a warmed (34°C) artificial cereberospinal fluid (ACSF) solution. The ACSF contained (in mM): 122 NaCl, 3 KCl, 1.25 NaH_2PO_4, 25 $NaHCO_3$, 20 glucose, 3 myo-inositol, 2 sodium pyruvate, 0.4 ascorbic acid, 2.5 $CaCl_2$, and 1.5 $MgSO_4$, saturated with 95% O_2-5% CO_2. After taking a thin slice that removes the external granule cell layer over the anterior VCN, a single 350 μm thick parasagittal slice of the cochlear nuclei that includes the VCN and DCN was cut and incubated in ACSF at 34°C for about 1 h before recordings commenced. During recording, slices were placed in a fast-flow chamber (Warner Instruments) on a fixed stage (34°C), and visualized under both brightfield and fluorescence optics (Zeiss FS2 microscope). Fluorescence illumination to detect cells expressing EYFP was provided by a 505 nm LED (Phillips).

Some experiments were performed on a separate recording system that permitted 2-photon illumination as well as wide-field fluorescence. For the overall evaluation of EYFP expression, standard fluorescence (1-photon) was imaged using illumination from a 530 nm LED (Phillips Luxeon) through a standard Zeiss filter set. Images were captured with a Photometrics EM512 CCD camera. For 2-photon illumination, a custom system built around a Ti-Sapphire laser (Coherent Chameleon Ultra II) was coupled through a Pockels cell (Conoptics) and scan mirrors (Cambridge 6210 H) into a modified epi-illumination train on a Zeiss FS2 microscope through a dichroic mirror (FF670-SDi01, Semrock) and a 630 × 0.90 nA water immersion objective (Zeiss). The collected fluorescence was passed through a short-pass filter (FF01-680/SP-25, Semrock), followed by a narrowband filter (FF03-525/50–25 or FF02-617/73–25; Semrock) depending on the fluorophore to be detected. The fluorescence was detected by a cooled Ga-As photomultiplier (Hamamatsu H7422P50) and amplified with a custom wide-band current-to-voltage converter before being digitized.

Photostimulation in these experiments was provided by gating the light from a 470 nm LED coupled through the epi-illumination ports of the microscopes. The light from the LED was passed through a lens and a pair of dichroic mirrors. The lens was adjusted so that the illumination was visually uniform at the specimen plane. Photostimulation took place through a 40 × 0.75 nA objective, focused on the cell of interest. To measure the illuminated area, we soaked a strip of nitrocellulose filter paper (Schleicher and Schuell) with a ~1% solution of Lucifer Yellow Cadeverine Biotin X (Life Technologies) in water, then dried the paper, and sandwiched it between two coverslips. The illumination from the objective was used to bleach the dye over about 5 min, after which a low-magnification image of the

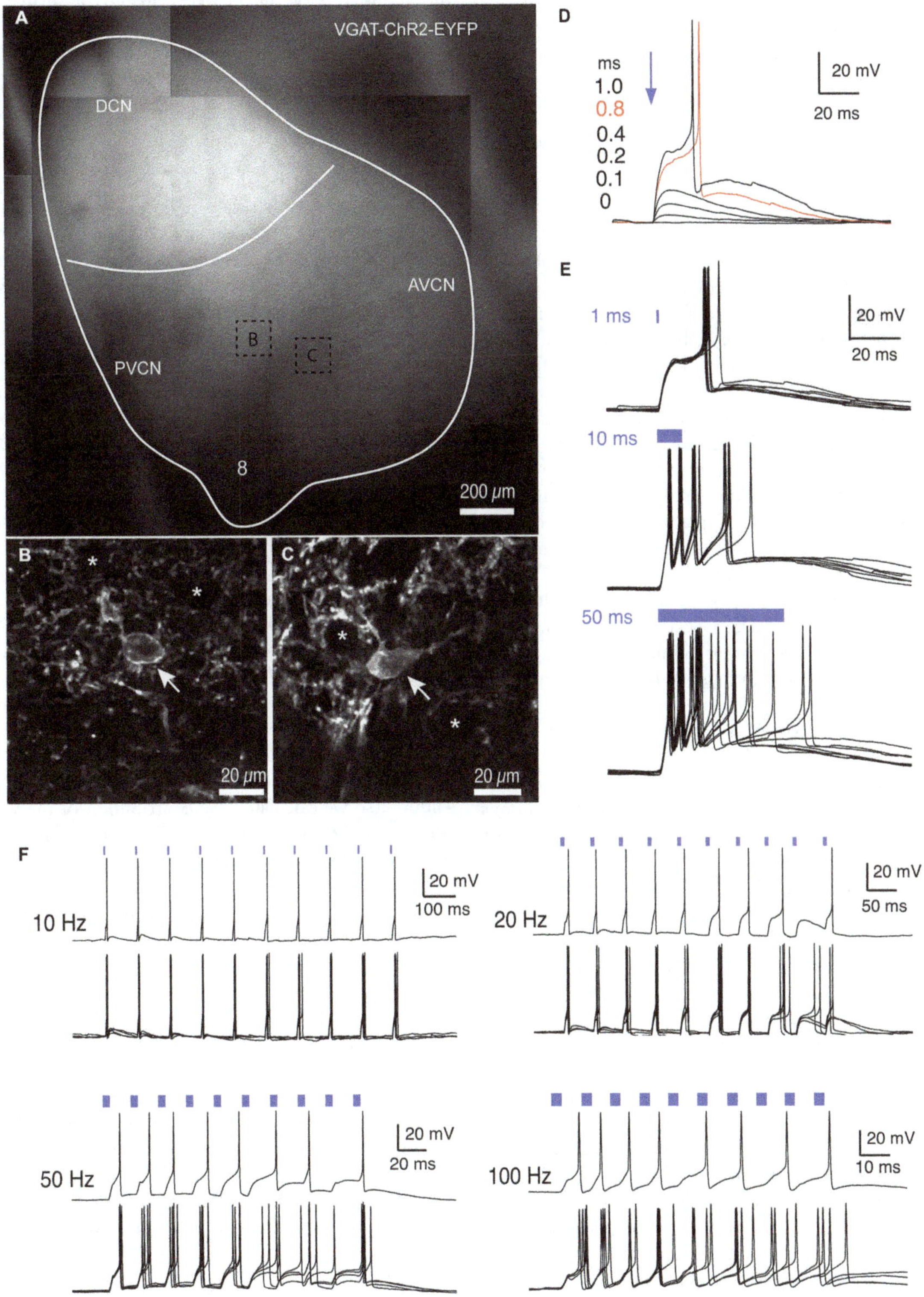

FIGURE 1 | Photostimulation drives excitatory responses in EYFP expressing cells in VGAT-ChR2-EYFP mice. (A) Expression pattern of ChR2 in cochlear nucleus as visualized by EYFP fluorescence. Notice that expression is absent in the 8th nerve root region, moderate in anteroventral cochlear nucleus (AVCN) and posteroventral cochlear nucleus (PVCN), and high in the DCN. The image is a mosaic assembled from different areas of the cochlear nuclei. **(B–C)** Multiphoton images of EYFP expressing cells from areas as marked in **(A)**. Expression of the EYFP-ChR2 construct is present in both membrane and cytoplasm. Arrows mark expressing neurons. Asterisks mark non-expressing cells whose soma is surrounded by expressing terminals. **(D)** Example responses from an EYFP-ChR2 expressing cell to different durations of 470 nm illumination from 0 (no light) to 1.0 ms.

(*Continued*)

FIGURE 1 | Continued
The threshold of the light duration was 0.8 ms in this cell, which evoked an action potential as shown in red. All sub-threshold traces are averages of 5–10 trials; traces with spikes are single trials. **(E)** Longer duration illumination reliably evoked a single spike or trains of spikes (same cell in **(D)**). Each plot shows the responses to 5–10 trials. **(F)** Ten 2-ms light pulses at 10, 20, 50, and 100 Hz evoke trains of spikes. Top: single trial; bottom: superimposed traces from four trials. Note that tonic firing is evoked at higher frequencies, although the cell no longer entrains to individual flashes.

bleached spot was digitized, and the diameter of the bleached area measured. The diameter of the circular area illuminated with the 40X objective was 780 μm at the focal plane. Because cells were recorded from the center of the visible field, the illumination was roughly centered over the cell. The incident light at the specimen plane was ~0.8 mW (Newport 1917-R power meter with 818UV/DB detector), corresponding to an irradiance of ~1.7 mW/mm^2. For a few experiments we used a 63X objective to record the photostimulation evoked response patterns in ChR2-expressing neurons (**Figure 1**). For this objective, the diameter of the illuminated area at the focal plane was measured to be 280 μm, and the total incident power was 0.110 mW, corresponding to an irradiance of ~2.1 mW/mm^2.

Whole-cell tight seal recordings were made with Multiclamp 700A and B amplifiers, using KG-33 glass (King Glass, Claremont, CA) or 1.2 mm glass (Sutter). Pipettes were backfilled with one of three electrode solutions, and had open tip resistances of 4–7 MOhms. The K-gluconate based electrode solution used for current clamp recordings contained (in mM): 126 K-gluconate, 6 KCl, 2 NaCl, 10 HEPES, 0.2 EGTA, 4 Mg-ATP, 0.3 Tris-GTP, and 10 Tris-phosphocreatine, with pH adjusted to 7.2 with KOH. Two different Cs-based electrode solutions were used for voltage clamp recordings. One had a low chloride concentration (8 mM; calculated $E_{Cl} = -71.1$ mV), and contained (in mM): 130 $CsMetSO_3$, 5 CsCl, 5 EGTA, 10 HEPES, 4 MgATP, 0.3 Tris-GTP, 10 Tris-phosphocreatine, and 3 QX-314 (chloride salt), with pH adjusted to 7.2 with CsOH. The second Cs-based electrode solution had high chloride concentration (38 mM; calculated $E_{Cl} = -31.1$ mV) and contained (in mM): 105 $CsMetSO_3$, 35 CsCl, 5 EGTA, 10 HEPES, 4 MgATP, 0.3 Tris-GTP, 10 Tris-phosphocreatine, and 3 QX-314 (chloride salt), with pH adjusted to 7.2 with CsOH. For voltage clamp recordings, compensation of >75% was applied on-line. Junction potentials are calculated to be −12 mV for the K-gluconate based electrode solution, −8 mV for the Cs-based electrode solution with 8 mM chloride and −7 mV for the Cs-based electrode solution with 38 mM chloride. All reported voltages have been corrected for the appropriate junction potentials. Cells were characterized in current clamp by their firing patterns, and morphologically by their patterns of dendritic branching when filled with Lucifer Yellow or AlexaFluor (594, 488). Cells recorded in voltage clamp were identified by their dendritic branching patterns in conjunction with the time course of sIPSCs (Xie and Manis, 2013). Cells with 1–2 short, stout dendrites and a profusion of fine dendrites at the end of each primary dendrite were classified as bushy cells. Cells which had 2–5 long primary dendrites that were oriented parallel to the fascicles of the auditory nerve fibers were classified as planar multipolar (T-stellate) cells. Cells that had 2–5 long primary dendrites, at least some of which crossed the fascicles of auditory nerve fibers at an oblique angle were classified as radiate multipolar cells.

ANALYSIS

IPSC decay time constants were calculated by fitting the decay phase of IPSCs with single or double exponential functions. Double exponential fits were used only when the χ^2 value from single exponential fits. Weighted decay time constants (τ_w) were calculated from double exponential fits as previous described (Xie and Manis, 2013) using the following function: $\tau_w = A_1{}^*\tau_1 + A_2{}^*\tau_2$, where A_1 and A_2 are the normalized amplitude of each component and $A_1 + A_2 = 1$.

Reversal potentials were measured using Cs^+ electrodes containing 38 mM Cl^-. For these measurements, cells were held in voltage-clamp at −57 mV, and stepped from −107 to +13 mV (corrected for a −7 mV junction potential) in 10 mV steps for 750–850 ms. A 20 ms maximal light flash was delivered 600 ms after the onset of the voltage step. The presentation of voltages was randomized, and the entire sequence was repeated four times, with a 10 s interval between trials. Reversal potentials were measured in control solution, following exposure to 2 μM strychnine, and following the addition of both 10 μM SR95531 and 2 μM strychnine. No evoked currents were seen with the combination of strychnine and SR95531, except in one radiate multipolar cell, where light-evoked ChR2 currents reversing at +4 mV were observed (data from this cell is not included in the multipolar population analyzed in the Results section). Not all voltage-gated currents were blocked with the Cs^+ electrode solution, so we calculated the contribution of the voltage-gated current to the overall response. To accomplish this, the time course of voltage-gated current for each trace, beginning 200 ms before the light flash, and ending 150–250 ms after the flash onset, excluding a 100 ms window starting at the time of the flash, was fit to a cubic polynomial. The estimated current during the flash was then interpolated from the polynomial fit, and subtracted from the evoked response. The evoked response was calculated as the mean current over 16 ms beginning 4 ms after the flash onset. The command voltage was corrected for the uncompensated portion of the series resistance (compensation of 75% was used, and the uncompensated series resistance ranged from 1.3 to 2.5 MΩ) and the total (unsubtracted) current. The resulting current-voltage relationship, which often exhibited a modest outward rectification, was then fit to a cubic spline function. The reversal potential was calculated from the zero current intercept, and the synaptic conductance was calculated from the slope at −60 mV.

REAGENTS

Strychnine (2 μM, Sigma-Aldrich) was bath applied to block glycine receptors. SR95531 (10 μM, Sigma-Aldrich) was bath applied to block $GABA_A$ receptors. CNQX (5 μM, Tocris Bioscience) was bath applied to block AMPA receptors. Tetrodotoxin (1 μM, Sigma-Aldrich) was used to block voltage-gated sodium channels. All salts used to make the ACSF were purchased from Sigma-Aldrich.

SOFTWARE AND STATISTICAL ANALYSIS

All recordings, control of optical stimulation and both CCD and laser imaging, were made using custom software, Acq4 (Campagnola et al., 2014). Data were analyzed using Igor Pro (version 6.3.4.0, WaveMetrics), and custom routines in Acq4 using the Python libraries numpy (version 1.8.0)[1] and scipy (version 0.13.3).[2] Statistical analyses were performed using GraphPad Prism (GraphPad Software Version 5.01 and 6.0, San Diego, CA). Group results were compared using unpaired or paired student's t-tests, or using a two-way repeated measures ANOVA. Data are presented as mean ± standard deviation.

RESULTS

PHOTOSTIMULATION GENERATES DEPOLARIZATION AND SPIKES IN eYFP EXPRESSING CELLS IN VGAT-ChR2-eYFP MICE

We examined the expression pattern of ChR2-eYFP in the cochlear nucleus of the VGAT-ChR2-EYFP mice. As ChR2 is expressed in conjunction with EYFP, the expression can be visualized under 505–530 nm light that excites EYFP (**Figures 1A–C**). As shown in **Figure 1A**, the expression was high in the DCN, moderate in the anteroventral cochlear nucleus (AVCN) and posteroventral cochlear nucleus (PVCN), and very low in the auditory nerve root area. This pattern is consistent with the distribution of inhibitory neurons in the cochlear nuclei, in which DCN contains the most inhibitory neurons including cartwheel and tuberculoventral neurons, AVCN and PVCN only contain scattered inhibitory (radiate multipolar, or D-stellate) neurons, and the auditory nerve area is made up of excitatory nerve fibers with few inhibitory neurons. Multiphoton imaging of individual neurons expressing EYFP in the AVCN and PVCN (**Figures 1B,C**, arrows) revealed the ChR2 construct in both the cell membrane and cytoplasm. The majority of the neurons in the AVCN and PVCN, however, do not express ChR2 as shown by the dark cells (marked with asterisks) in **Figures 1B,C**. These non-expressing cells are likely excitatory neurons including bushy and planar multipolar (T-stellate) neurons. Interestingly, the soma of these neurons is often surrounded by a ring of fluorescent terminals, suggesting that these cells receive synaptic inputs from expressing inhibitory neurons.

We next studied how expressing neurons in the AVCN respond to photostimulation using light pulses at 470 nm with different durations (**Figures 1D,E**), delivered through a 63X objective focused on the recorded cell. Current clamp recordings were obtained using standard K-gluconate electrode solution. Light pulses with different durations (**Figure 1D**) evoked depolarization and action potentials in the expressing neurons. The size of the depolarization increased with increasing light duration until it reached action potential threshold. The threshold duration of light ranged from 0.4 to 1.0 ms with an average of 0.8 ± 0.3 ms (n = 4). Suprathreshold light pulses reliably drove spikes in expressing neurons, and prolonged light pulses (10 and 50 ms in **Figure 1E**) generated multiple spikes. Expressing neurons were also able to fire trains of spikes in response to trains of brief light pulses at 10–100 Hz (**Figure 1F**), although entrainment was only seen for the first few pulses at 50 and 100 Hz, after which firing continued at a lower rate than the pulse rate. In contrast, non-expressing neurons always responded to light pulses with IPSPs and never responded with EPSPs, depolarization or action potentials. These results suggests that inhibitory neurons expressing VGAT can be selectively stimulated, and further that non-expressing cells are excitatory neurons that receive inhibitory input from the expressing cells.

[1]www.numpy.org
[2]www.scipy.org

THE STRENGTH OF GABAergic RELATIVE TO GLYCINERGIC INHIBITION IS LARGER IN MULTIPOLAR THAN BUSHY CELLS

We next characterized the light evoked inhibitory responses using current clamp recordings from non-expressing neurons in AVCN. All non-expressing neurons were classified into two cell types based on their characteristic firing patterns to depolarizing current injections. Bushy neurons fire only one or a few transient spikes after the onset of the depolarizing current injection (**Figure 2A**), while multipolar (stellate) neurons fire tonically throughout the duration of the current injection (**Figure 2D**). The multipolar neurons are primarily planar multipolar (T-stellate) neurons, because these are excitatory neurons that do not express ChR2 in this mouse.

Brief 470 nm light pulses evoked IPSPs in both bushy and multipolar neurons (**Figures 2B,E**). In bushy neurons, light pulses of different durations evoked IPSPs that decayed very rapidly (**Figure 2B**). In contrast, light evoked IPSPs in the multipolar cells were longer lasting (**Figure 2E**). The average half-width of the IPSPs evoked by 20 ms light pulse was 15.25 ± 6.0 ms (n = 6) in bushy cells, but was 27.5 ± 8.4 ms (n = 6) in multipolar neurons (**Figure 2G**; unpaired t-test: t_{10} = 2.92, p = 0.015). The shorter IPSP half-width in bushy neurons is likely due to their faster membrane time constant compared to multipolar neurons (Manis and Marx, 1991; Francis and Manis, 2000; Xie and Manis, 2013).

We then isolated the glycinergic and GABAergic components of the light evoked IPSPs using strychnine and SR95531. Under control condition, 20 ms light pulses evoked IPSPs with similar amplitude in both bushy (−9.3 ± 3.8 mV, n = 6) and multipolar neurons (−7.6 ± 3.1 mV, n = 6) (**Figure 2H**; unpaired t-test: t_{10} = 0.89, p = 0.393). Bath application of 2 μM strychnine reduced IPSP amplitudes by 93.9 ± 4.3% (n = 6) in bushy neurons, but only by 59.5 ± 19.9% (n = 5) in multipolar neurons (**Figures 2C,F**; unpaired t-test: t_9 = 4.18, p = 0.0024). The remaining IPSPs in both cell types were fully blocked with a subsequent application of 10 μM SR95531 in the presence of strychnine. Previously, only glycinergic IPSPs have been seen (Wu and Oertel, 1986; Xie and Manis, 2013) following electrical stimulation. Thus, our new results demonstrate the presence of functional synaptically-evoked GABAergic IPSPs in VCN neurons in slices.

THE TIME COURSE OF GABAergic INHIBITION IS SIMILAR IN BUSHY AND MULTIPOLAR NEURONS

In a separate population of cells, we investigated the kinetics of the light evoked synaptic currents under voltage clamp (**Figure 3**). Recordings were made using Cs-based electrode solution (8 mM Cl^-) with 3 mM QX-314 to block potassium and sodium channels

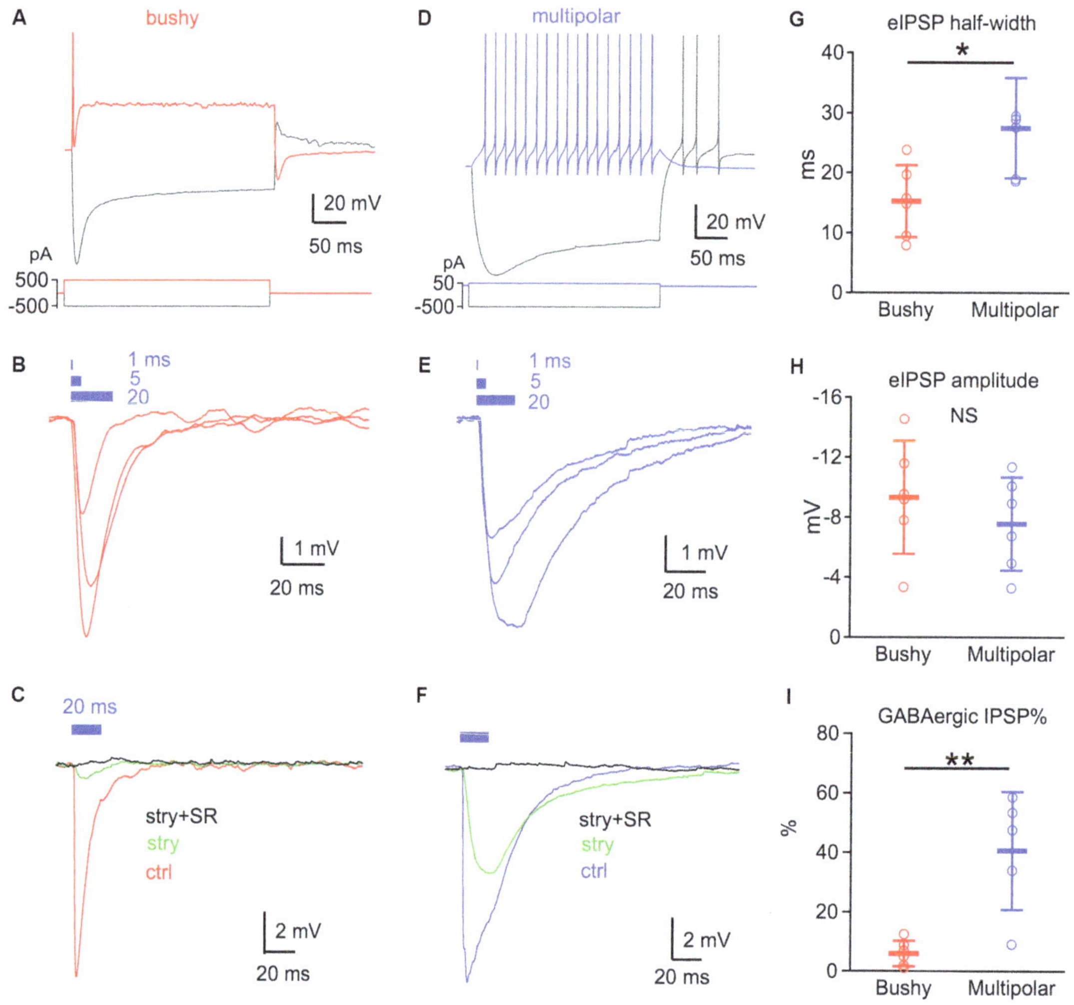

FIGURE 2 | GABAergic inhibition is weak in bushy but strong in multipolar neurons. **(A)** Discharge pattern of a bushy neuron to direct current injection. The bushy neuron fires only one or a few spikes with depolarizing current injections. **(B)** Light pulses at different durations evoke brief IPSP responses in bushy neurons. Each trace is an average of six trials. Blue bars on top mark the timing of the light pulses with duration of 1, 5 and 20 ms. **(C)** Strychnine (stry) blocks the majority of the IPSP evoked by 20 ms light pulses in bushy neurons. Addition of SR95531 (stry+SR) fully blocks light evoked IPSPs. Traces are averages of 10 trials. Data in **(A–C)** are from the same bushy neuron. **(D)** Discharge pattern of an example multipolar neuron to direct current injections. Multipolar neurons fire a regular train of spikes throughout the current injection. **(E)** Light pulses at durations of 1, 5 and 20 ms evoke IPSPs in multipolar neurons. Note that the IPSPs have a wider half-width than those of bushy neurons in **(B)**. **(F)** Strychnine only blocks about half of light evoked IPSP. The remainder of the current is fully blocked by the further addition of SR95531. Data in **(D–F)** are from the same multipolar neuron. **(G–I)** Summary data of the eIPSP half-width **(G)**, eIPSP amplitude **(H)** and percentage of GABAergic IPSP **(I)**. * $p < 0.05$; ** $p < 0.01$. Data is plotted as mean ± S.D.

and improve clamp quality. Cells were held at +42 mV so that the IPSCs were large and outward. Light pulses of 1 or 2 ms were used to evoke repeatable single spikes in presynaptic inputs (**Figures 1D,E**), to help minimize the possibility that the kinetics of evoked IPSCs were contaminated by multiple synaptic events.

The amplitudes of light evoked IPSCs in bushy and multipolar neurons were not different under control conditions, similar to the results for IPSPs. The peak IPSC amplitude was 2.65 ± 1.15 nA ($n = 7$) in bushy neurons and 2.10 ± 2.02 nA ($n = 5$) in multipolar neurons (**Figure 3C**; unpaired t-test: $t_{10} = 0.60$, $p = 0.56$). As shown in **Figures 3A,B**, strychnine blocked most of the IPSC in both bushy and multipolar neurons. We measured the amplitude of the GABAergic IPSCs (in the presence of strychnine) and of the glycinergic IPSCs (computed as the difference between control IPSCs and strychnine-resistant IPSCs). There was no significant difference in the glycinergic IPSC amplitudes (bushy: 2.60 ± 1.13 nA, $n = 7$; multipolar: 1.96 ± 1.98 nA, $n = 5$; **Figure 3C**; unpaired t-test: $t_{10} = 0.71$, $p = 0.49$) between two cell types. However, the GABAergic IPSCs were significantly smaller in bushy neurons (50 ± 24 pA, $n = 7$) than in multipolar neurons (137 ± 61 pA, $n = 5$) (**Figure 3C**; unpaired t-test: $t_{10} = 3.50$, $p = 0.0057$), consistent with the IPSP data (**Figure 2I**). The small percentage of GABAergic IPSC components measured here with short light

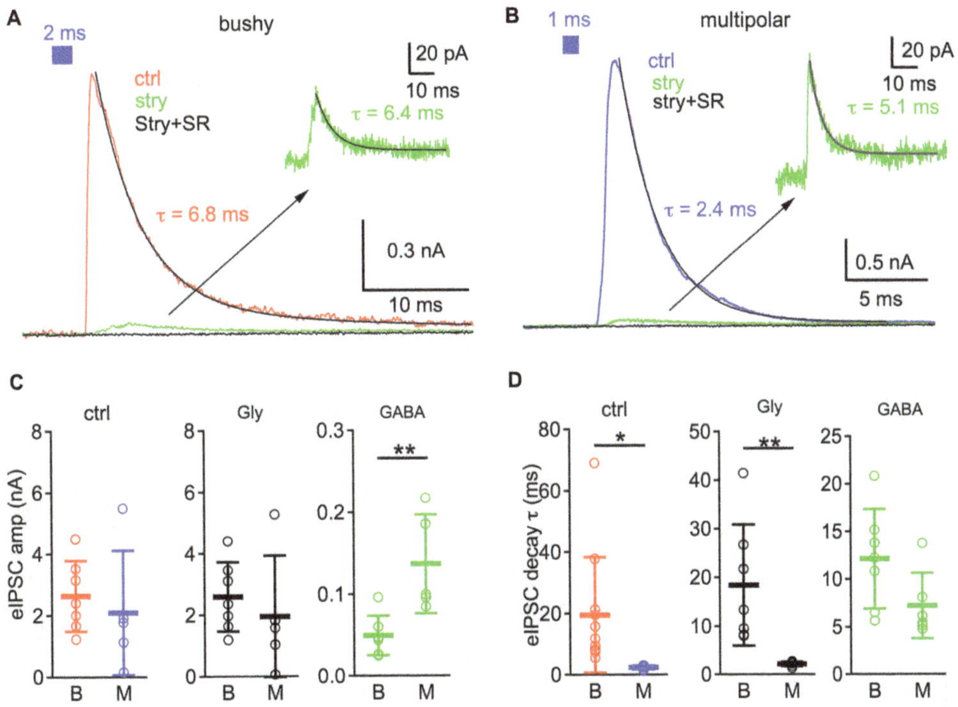

FIGURE 3 | Kinetics of GABAergic and glycinergic IPSCs in bushy and multipolar neurons. (A) A 2 ms light pulse (blue bar on top) evokes IPSCs in a bushy neuron. The IPSC is mostly blocked by strychnine (stry) and is fully blocked by a combination of strychnine and SR95531 (Stry + SR). Inset: magnified IPSC trace after strychnine block. The weighted decay time constants of the IPSCs are obtained by fitting the IPSC decay with double exponential functions (black curves) under both control and stry conditions. **(B)** 1 ms light pulse evokes IPSCs in a multipolar neuron. Plots are organized the same as in **(A)**. Decay time constants of IPSCs are obtained by fitting the IPSC decay with single exponential functions (black curves). Traces in both **(A)** and **(B)** are averages of 10 trials. **(C)** Comparison of the light evoked IPSC amplitudes between bushy and multipolar neurons including the control IPSC amplitude (ctrl), glycinergic IPSC component (Gly), and GABAergic IPSC component (GABA). Abcissa: B: bushy neurons; M: multipolar neurons. **(D)** Comparison of the eIPSC decay time constants. * $p < 0.05$; ** $p < 0.01$. Data is plotted as mean ± S.D.

pulses (compare to IPSP components in **Figure 2I**) suggests that GABAergic inhibition is more effectively activated with long light stimulation, which is also demonstrated in **Figure 4**.

We next measured the decay phase of IPSCs by fitting with double exponential functions in bushy neurons (**Figure 3A**) and single exponential functions in multipolar neurons (**Figure 3B**). Weighted decay time constants were then calculated in bushy cells for comparison. As shown in **Figure 3D**, light evoked IPSCs under control conditions were significantly slower in bushy neurons (weighted decay time constant: 19.5 ± 18.9 ms, $n = 11$) than multipolar neurons (decay time constant: 2.4 ± 0.7 ms, $n = 6$) (unpaired t-test: $t_{15} = 2.19$, $p = 0.045$). This difference persisted when pharmacologically isolated glycinergic IPSCs were measured (bushy glycinergic IPSC decay: 18.4 ± 12.5 ms, $n = 7$; multipolar glycinergic IPSC decay: 2.1 ± 0.5, $n = 6$; unpaired t-test: $t_{11} = 3.19$, $p = 0.0087$). The fast kinetics of glycinergic IPSCs in multipolar cells is consistent with our previous observations with electrically evoked IPSCs and spontaneous mIPSCs (Xie and Manis, 2013). In the presence of strychnine, the isolated GABAergic component showed a trend for bushy cells (12.2 ± 5.2 ms, $n = 7$) to have a slower decay time constant than the multipolar neurons (7.2 ± 3.4, $n = 6$), however, the difference was not statistically significant (**Figure 3D**; unpaired t-test: $t_{11} = 1.97$, $p = 0.074$). The results suggest that GABAergic inhibition in bushy and multipolar neurons, unlike glycinergic inhibition (Xie and Manis, 2013), does not have widely different kinetics in bushy and multipolar cells.

GLYCINERGIC IPSCs ARE PHASIC WHEREAS GABAergic IPSCs HAVE A LARGE TONIC COMPONENT IN RESPONSE TO SUSTAINED ILLUMINATION

We further studied the IPSC kinetics in response to longer duration illumination. Glycinergic and GABAergic IPSCs were pharmacologically isolated with strychnine and SR95531 as above. As shown in **Figures 4A,B**, both glycinergic IPSCs and GABAergic IPSCs peaked in amplitude shortly after the onset of the light stimulation. The amplitude of glycinergic IPSCs, however, decayed rapidly, whereas GABAergic IPSCs showed less decay and exhibited sustained currents until the end of the light stimulation.

To quantify the magnitude of the current decrease (which we term "sustained current ratio"), we calculated the peak and steady state IPSC amplitudes in response to 50 ms light pulses. The steady state IPSC amplitude was measured from the average current during the last 10 ms of the stimulation. The sustained current ratio of the IPSCs was then calculated as the steady state

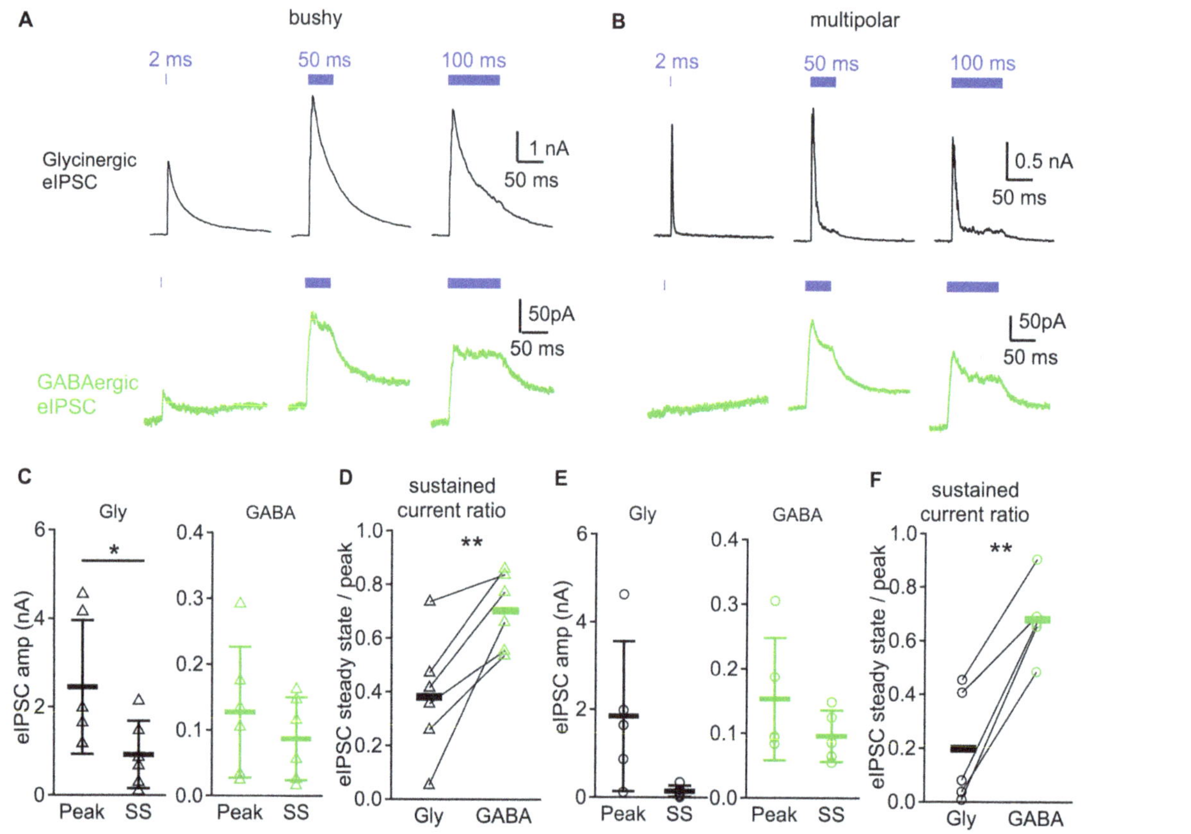

FIGURE 4 | Glycinergic IPSCs are phasic compared to GABAergic IPSCs in response to sustained illumination. (A) IPSC responses evoked by different durations of light (2, 50, and 100 ms) in a bushy neuron. Notice that the glycinergic IPSCs peak shortly after the onset of the light pulse and decay rapidly even though the illumination is still on, whereas GABAergic IPSCs show little decay in amplitude. **(B)** Light evoked IPSC responses in a multipolar neuron. Traces in both **(A)** and **(B)** are averages of 10 trials. **(C)** Summary of the IPSC peak amplitudes (peak) and steady state amplitudes (SS) in bushy neurons. In **(C-F)**: Gly: glycinergic IPSCs; GABA: GABAergic IPSCs. **(D)** Summary of the sustained current ratio in bushy neurons. **(E)** Summary of the IPSC peak amplitudes and steady state amplitudes in multipolar neurons. **(F)** Summary of the sustained current ratio in multipolar neurons. In **(D)** and **(F)**: each connected pair represents a single neuron; black bar marks the average of the group. * $p < 0.05$; ** $p < 0.01$.

divided by the peak IPSC amplitude. As shown in **Figure 4C**, glycinergic IPSCs in bushy neurons showed significantly larger peak amplitudes (2.45 ± 1.51 nA, $n = 6$) than steady state IPSC amplitudes (0.93 ± 0.76 nA, $n = 6$) (paired t-test: $t_5 = 3.95$, $p = 0.011$). In contrast, there was no significant difference in the GABAergic IPSCs between the peak (127 ± 99 pA, $n = 6$) and steady state amplitudes (87 ± 63 pA, $n = 6$) (paired t-test: $t_5 = 2.12$, $p = 0.088$). The computed sustained current ratio was significantly smaller for glycinergic IPSCs (0.38 ± 0.23, $n = 6$) than for GABAergic IPSCs (0.70 ± 0.14, $n = 6$) (**Figure 4D**; paired t-test: $t_5 = 4.51$, $p = 0.0063$). In multipolar neurons, the glycinergic IPSC had a peak amplitude of 1.85 ± 1.71 nA ($n = 5$) and a steady state amplitude of 0.15 ± 0.13 nA ($n = 5$) (**Figure 4E**; paired t-test: $t_4 = 2.22$, $p = 0.090$). The GABAergic IPSC had peak amplitude of 153 ± 95 pA ($n = 5$) and steady state amplitude of 96 ± 40 pA ($n = 5$) (**Figure 4E**; Wilcoxon matched pairs test: $p = 0.063$). Although the steady state and peak amplitudes were not significantly different for either glycinergic or GABAergic IPSC components of the multipolar neurons, there was a significant difference in the sustained current ratio between the two (**Figure 4F**; glycinergic IPSC: 0.20 ± 0.22; GABAergic IPSC: 0.68 ± 0.15, $n = 5$; paired t-test: $t_4 = 7.71$, $p = 0.0015$). Therefore, in both bushy and multipolar neurons, glycinergic IPSCs decrease more over time than GABAergic IPSCs in response to sustained illumination.

GABAergic AND GLYCINERGIC IPSCs HAVE DIFFERENT REVERSAL POTENTIALS IN MULTIPOLAR NEURONS

It is known that both GABAergic and glycinergic IPSCs are associated with an increased permeability for chloride ions across the membrane (Eccles et al., 1977; Wu and Oertel, 1986; Bormann et al., 1987; Harty and Manis, 1996). Therefore, we would expect that both types of IPSCs should have the same reversal potentials, close to the equilibrium potential for chloride. In this study, however, we surprisingly found that the glycinergic IPSCs and GABAergic IPSCs possess different reversal potentials.

The difference in the reversal potential between glycinergic and GABAergic IPSCs was initially observed as different directions of currents in three different multipolar neurons when recorded

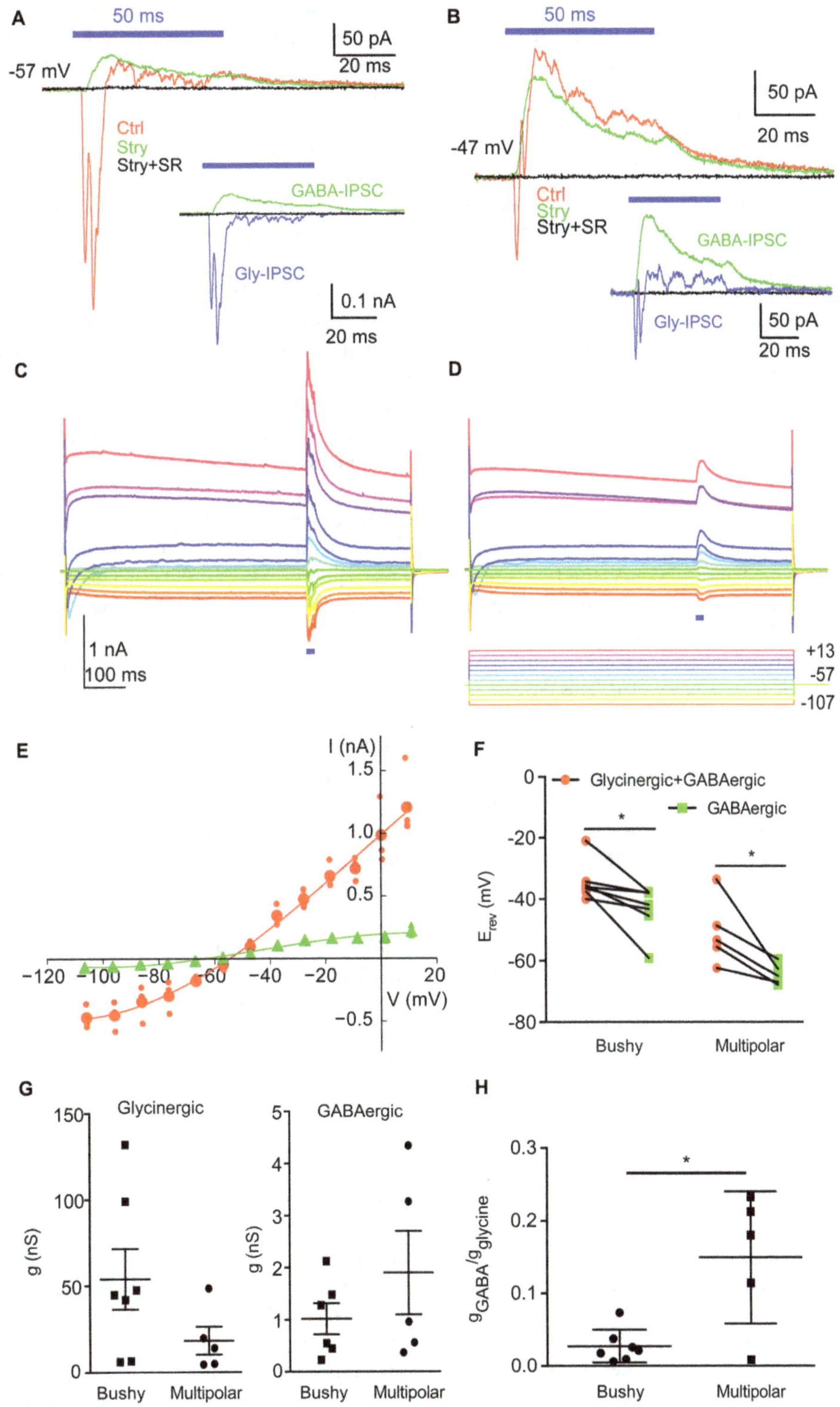

FIGURE 5 | GABAergic and glycinergic IPSCs show different reversal potentials in multipolar neurons. (A) Multipolar neuron held at −57 mV using 38 mM Cl^- electrode solution. IPSC traces show currents in control solution (red), in strychnine (stry, green), and in both strychnine and SR95531 (stry + SR, black). Inset: Isolated glycinergic IPSC (blue), GABAergic IPSC (green), and complete block in stry + SR (black). The glycinergic IPSC is inward, whereas the GABAergic IPSC is outward, suggesting different IPSC reversal potentials. **(B)** IPSCs recorded at holding potential of −47 mV from the same neuron as in **(A)**. Traces in **(A)** and **(B)** are the averages of 20 trials.

(*Continued*)

FIGURE 5 | Continued
(C) Response to a 20 ms light flash (blue bar below traces) in a voltage-clamped multipolar cell with 38 mM $[Cl^-]_i$ at different voltage steps. The light-evoked currents are superimposed on unblocked currents. Each trace is the average of four trials; peaks of capacitative transients at onset and offset of voltage steps have been clipped. **(D)** Same cell as in **(C)**, in the presence of 2 μM strychnine to isolate the GABAergic component. Voltage steps are indicated below the traces. Current and voltage scales are the same in **(C)** and **(D)**. **(E)** Current-voltage relationship of the light-evoked current (see Section Materials and Methods for analysis details). Large red circles: mean of currents across four trials in control conditions; small circles show responses for individual trials. Red line: cubic spline fit to the data. Large green triangles: responses in the presence of strychnine; small triangles show responses for individual trials. Green line: cubic spline fit to the data. **(F)** Reversal potentials measured as in **(E)** for, for total (glycinergic + GABAergic) currents, and isolated GABAergic currents. Measurements made sequentially in the same cell are connected. Asterisk indicates ANOVA post tests, $p < 0.05$. **(G)** Conductance at −60 mV in individual cells. **(H)** Ratio of GABAergic to glycinergic conductance at −60 mV for individual cells (asterisk, $p < 0.05$).

using Cs-based electrode solution containing 38 mM Cl^- (**Figure 5**). At a holding potential of −57 mV, the IPSCs of one multipolar neuron (**Figure 5A**) under control conditions showed an initial inward current followed by mixed inward and outward currents. When the glycinergic IPSCs were blocked with strychnine, an outward GABAergic IPSC was revealed. This IPSC in turn was completely blocked by the subsequent addition of SR95531, confirming that it was mediated by $GABA_A$ receptors. The isolated glycinergic IPSC was entirely inward at this holding potential. Similar features were also apparent in this cell when held at −47 mV (**Figure 5B**). These results suggest that the reversal potentials of the glycinergic and GABAergic IPSCs are different.

To further clarify the differences in reversal potentials, we made systematic measurements of light-evoked currents at different membrane potentials under control conditions, and in the presence of strychnine alone, and with strychnine and SR95531. Recordings were made using Cs-based electrode solution (38 mM Cl^-), from 5 multipolar cells and 7 bushy cells in a separate series of experiments. An example of the responses to the voltage steps in the control solution, and the superimposed light evoked response is shown in **Figure 5C** for one of the multipolar cells. Even with Cs^+ in the pipette, modest outward currents were evoked by depolarizing voltage steps, and small inward I_h currents were observed with hyperpolarizing voltage steps. The voltage-gated currents were subtracted from the light-evoked current as described in the Section Materials and Methods, to measure the isolated current-voltage relationship of the synaptic conductance shown in 5E (red circles). For this cell, the control reversal potential, estimated by interpolation, was −55.6 mV. After the addition of strychnine, the currents were smaller (**Figure 5D**), and the reversal potential shifted negative to −68.0 mV (**Figure 5E**, green triangles). As above, the strychnine-insensitive current was blocked by 10 μM SR95531. A summary of the reversal potentials across all cells tested is shown in **Figure 5F**. A two-way repeated measures ANOVA revealed no interaction between cell types ($F_{1,10} = 1.011$, $p = 0.34$), consistent with the observation that the reversal for GABAergic IPSCs was always negative to that of glycinergic IPSCs in both cell types. The comparison between cell types revealed a significant difference ($F_{1,10} = 27.48$, $p = 0.0004$), as did the comparison between the reversals of GABAergic and glycinergic IPSCs ($F_{1,10} = 22.05$, $p = 0.0008$). Sidak's multiple comparison corrected post-tests revealed that the reversal potentials for both glycinergic and GABAergic IPSCs were significantly different in bushy cells ($t_{10} = 2.859$, $p = 0.034$; mean difference −8.8 mV, standard error = 3.1) and in multipolar cells ($t_{10} = 3.732$, $p = 0.0078$; mean difference −13.7 mV, standard error = 3.67).

The glycinergic conductance, measured as the slope of the current-voltage relationship at −60 mV, could be quite large in bushy cells (**Figure 5G**), but this difference was not significantly different than the conductance in multipolar cells (unpaired t-test, $t_{10} = 1.395$, $p = 0.19$). The GABAergic conductance similarly was not significantly different between the two cell types (unpaired t-test, assuming unequal variances, $t_{4.81} = 1.087$, $p = 0.33$). **Figure 5H** compares the ratios of the GABAergic to glycinergic conductance in individual cells, and reveals a significant difference between cell types (unpaired t-test assuming unequal variances, multipolar ratio 0.15 ± 0.09, bushy ratio 0.027 ± 0.023, $t_{4.36} = 2.936$, $p = 0.038$). This difference is consistent with the larger maximal GABA currents measured in multipolar cells shown in **Figure 3**. From these observations, we conclude that GABAergic IPSCs reverse at a potential negative to glycinergic IPSCs in both bushy and multipolar cells. These results also show that that the reversal for glycinergic IPSCs in bushy cells is not different than that expected from the equilibrium potential for Cl^- (one-sample t-test, −35.4 ± 6.8 vs. −31.1 mV, $t_6 = 1.668$, $p = 0.15$), whereas that for glycinergic IPSCs in multipolar cells is significantly negative to the expected reversal potential (one-sample t-test, −50.8 ± 10.7 vs. −31.1 mV, $t_4 = 4.098$, $p = 0.015$).

GABAergic IPSCs ARE BLOCKED BY TETRODOTOXIN

The GABAergic IPSCs did not often show large rapidly-decaying current events typically seen with the glycinergic IPSCs, which raised a question regarding whether the IPSCs arose from action-potential evoked release, or simply from ChR2 mediated depolarization of presynaptic terminals, and subsequent asynchronous release. To address this, we tested three cells (all multipolar cells). Recordings were made in control solutions, followed by the addition of 2 μM strychnine to isolate the GABAergic component. Examples of traces for a cell held at +13 and −107 mV are shown in **Figure 6**. The isolated GABAergic component (green traces) was completely blocked by the addition of 1 μM TTX to the bath (black trace). The same result was obtained in the other two cells. These experiments indicate that the light evoked GABAergic IPSC requires presynaptic action potentials that initiate transmitter release, and is that ChR2-mediated depolarization of presynaptic terminals alone is not sufficient to drive release.

LIGHT EVOKED INHIBITON ONLY ENTRAINS FOR LOW FREQUENCIES

Under physiological conditions, many neurons in the the auditory system fire at relatively high rates. However, light evoked firing in inhibitory neurons in this VGAT-ChR2-EYFP mouse may not

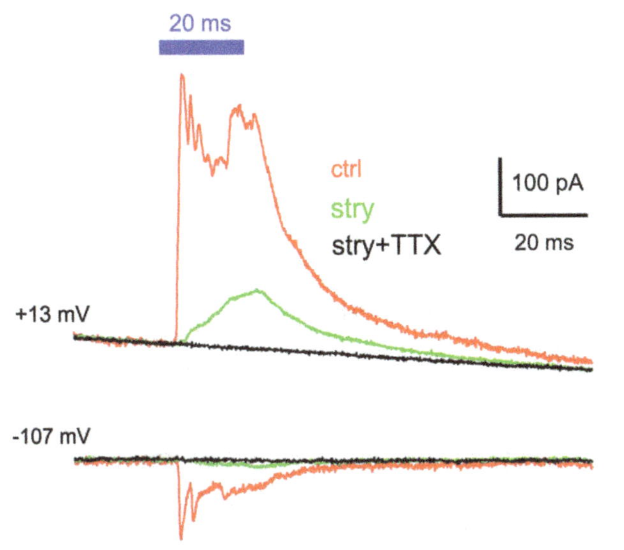

FIGURE 6 | GABAergic IPSCs are blocked by tetrodotoxin. Cells were tested in control conditions (red traces), in the presence of 2 μM strychnine to isolate the GABAergic IPSC (green trace), and in the presence of both strychnine and 1 μM tetrodotoxin to block action potential evoked release. No IPSC was evident in the presence of tetrodotoxin in any of the three cells tested, indicating that voltage-gated sodium channel activation is required for GABA release in response to ChR2 activation.

be able to follow high rates due to desensitization of ChR2 currents (Lin et al., 2009). We therefore tested the effectiveness of the light evoked inhibitory synaptic transmission with repeated stimulation. Ten light pulses of 1–2 ms duration were presented at frequencies of 10, 20, 50 and 100 Hz to drive inhbitory synaptic transmission onto bushy and multipolar neurons. Cells were held at −57 mV while using a Cs-based electrode solution with 38 mM chloride. No strychnine or GABAzine was used in this set of experiments, and excitatory transmission was blocked by including 5 μM CNQX in the bath. Under these conditions (brief light pulse stimulation), the IPSCs were only inward as the outward GABAergic IPSCs were masked by the larger glycinergic IPSCs (**Figures 7A,B**).

At low frequencies, 10 and 20 Hz, the brief pulses of light evoked a sustained train of IPSCs in both bushy (**Figure 7A**) and multipolar neurons (**Figure 7B**). The IPSCs became smaller during the trains in both cell types (**Figures 7C,D**), likely because of synaptic depression of the currents. At higher frequencies, such as 50 and 100 Hz, however, light pulses only evoked IPSCs in response to the first few stimuli, and failed to consistently drive synaptic currents later in the trains (**Figures 7C,D**).

DISCUSSION

Cochlear nucleus neurons receive both glycinergic and GABAergic inhibition from multiple sources. Glycinergic inhibition arises from local radiate multipolar (D-stellate) neurons within AVCN (Smith and Rhode, 1989; Arnott et al., 2004), tuberculoventral neurons in the DCN (Wickesberg and Oertel, 1990; Saint Marie et al., 1991; Wickesberg et al., 1991; Ostapoff et al., 1997), as well as neurons in the superior olivary complex (Ostapoff et al., 1997). GABAergic inhibition to the AVCN mostly comes from the descending projections from the superior olivary complex. Our results demonstrate that evoked glycinergic and GABAergic inhibition can be identified in bushy and multipolar neurons of the VCN using optical stimulation. The results also demonstrate that GABAergic inhibition is more prominent in multipolar cells than in bushy cells, but that the time course of the synaptic conductance is similar. This differs from the results for glycinergic inhibition, which is much faster in multipolar cells, and slower in bushy cells, both when evoked optically (this study and (Campagnola and Manis, 2014)) and electrically (Xie and Manis, 2013). Furthermore we find that the reversal potentials for glycinergic and GABAergic currents are different in both multipolar and bushy neurons.

METHOD AND LIMITATIONS

VGAT is expressed in all cells that use glycine and GABA as a neurotransmitter (Dumoulin et al., 1999; Wang et al., 2009). We have used a pharmacological approach to characterize the synaptic conductances produced by each transmitter in the VCN. Because the VGAT-ChR2-EYFP mouse expresses ChR2 in all cells that express VGAT, all inhibitory cells should be light-sensitive. As is apparent from the spatial distribution of EYFP, which is part of the ChR2 construct in these mice, ChR2 is present not only in cell bodies, but in the dendrites, axons, and synaptic terminals of all VGAT expressing cells (**Figure 1**). As a result, light impinging on any part of the cell could excite it and ultimately result in transmitter release at terminals. Previous work with similar constructs shows that the threshold for excitation varies with the region of the cell that is illuminated, and that generally the soma will be the lowest-threshold region (Katzel et al., 2011). However, variation in expression, channel density, and illumination factors mean that the stimulation is likely to be relatively non-specific unless other controls are available (spatial and pharmacological). In the present experiments, illumination was limited to an area of the cochlear nuclei surrounding the recorded cell, since (for most experiments) the illumination was provided through the 40X objective. This area was approximately 780 μm in diameter, and so included a large region of the cochlear nuclei. The stimulated elements may include not only presynaptic neurons located in the slice (for example, radiate multipolar cells), but also the terminals of cells whose cell bodies are further away or even no longer present in the slice. This is an advantage in that we were able to observe synaptically-mediated GABA conductances that likely arose from pathways not included in the slice. Unfortunately, it is not clear what the source of these inputs might be. In future experiments, the use of a slice preparation in which the lateral and/or ventral nuclei of the trapezoid body is included would in principal allow a more selective activation of those inhibitory inputs, without potential co-activation of other excitatory pathways as might be engaged with electrical stimulation. Laser scanning mapping (Katzel et al., 2011; Campagnola and Manis, 2014) would also be

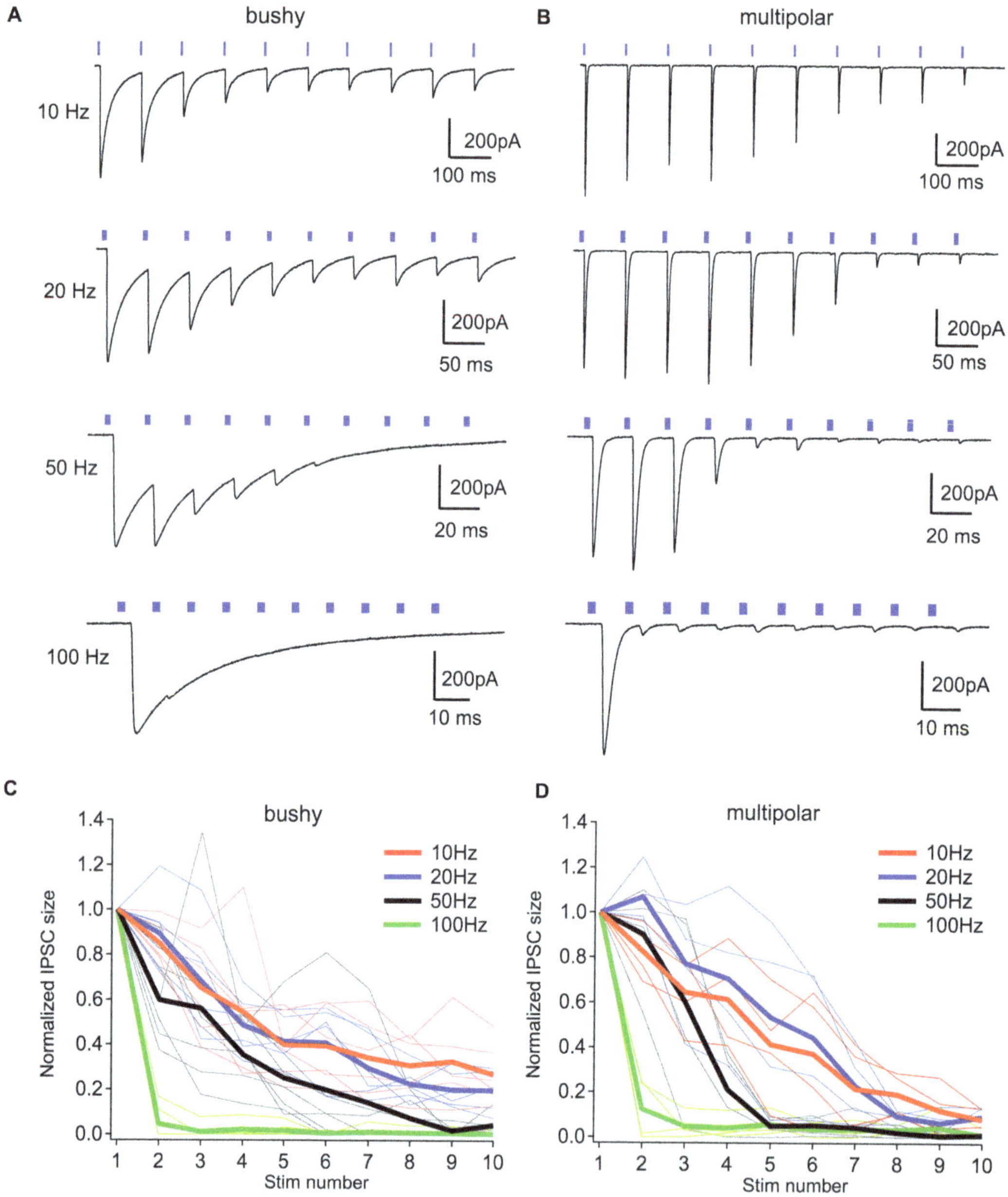

FIGURE 7 | Light evoked inhibiton only entrains for low frequencies. **(A)** Example IPSCs to light trains consisting of ten 2-ms pulses. Notice that IPSCs are only effectively evoked throughout the trains at 20 Hz in this neuron. At 50 and 100 Hz, light failed to evoke IPSCs in the later phase of the trains. **(B)** Example IPSCs to light trains in a multipolar neuron. **(C)** Normalized IPSC amplitudes through the light stimulus trains at different frequencies in bushy neurons. **(D)** Normalized IPSC amplitudes through the light stimulus trains at different frequencies in multipolar neurons. In **(C, D)**, thin lines show individual neurons; thick lines are group averages for each frequency.

advantageous to provide better localization of source cells in such studies.

A second limitation is that only relatively low rates of stimulation can be used with ChR2, due to its desensitization with repeated or prolonged light exposure (Lin et al., 2009). This limits the ability to reliably stimulate pathways at high rates, and partially explains why we see strong depression of the synaptic responses even at relatively low frequencies (**Figure 7**) compared to electrical stimulation, where responses up to 400 Hz can be studied (Xie and Manis, 2013). The use of mice expressing newer and faster ChR2 constructs (Lin, 2012) could be used to stimulate at higher rates. Nonetheless, the present study showed that this mouse is useful in utilizing photostimulation to study the neural circuitry and inhibitory synaptic transmission in local brain regions.

SYNAPTICALLY EVOKED GABAergic CONDUCTANCES

Maximal GABAergic currents and conductances were larger in multipolar neurons than in bushy cells. Unlike the time course of glycinergic inhibition (Xie and Manis, 2013), there was not a clear difference in the time course of the GABAergic synaptic currents between cell types. However, we did observe a difference in the sustained IPSCs with long-duration illumination between glycinergic and GABAergic conductances, which could reflect the relatively fast desensitization of glycine receptors (Harty and Manis, 1998) compared to the slower desensitization of $GABA_A$ receptors (Frosch et al., 1992). These observations, together with the differential innervation of bushy and multipolar cells from sources within the cochlear nucleus (Campagnola and Manis, 2014), suggest that different sources and kinds of inhibition are selectively targeted to bushy and multipolar cells.

There are two additional potential mechanisms for the observed differences in the sustained IPSC responses. The first is that glycinergic and GABAergic inhibition come from different presynaptic sources. The optical stimulation could result in phasic firing in glycinergic neurons, even for sustained illumination, whereas the GABAergic source neurons could fire more tonically. In this case, the time course of the glycinergic and GABAergic IPSCs would be inherited from the presynaptic firing pattern. The available recordings from the presynaptic cells within the VCN that express ChR2 however suggests that they have sustained firing during prolonged illumination (**Figure 1**). However, the firing pattern could be different for terminals of descending GABAergic inputs. The second potential mechanism is that the response to thes prolonged illumination is not due to action potential evoked release in the GABAergic inhibitory neurons (or their axons), but rather results from sustained depolarization of the synaptic terminals, leading to a tonic release. However, we found that TTX blocked the GABAergic IPSCs (**Figure 6**), indicating that the IPSCs resulted from an action-potential dependent release of transmitter.

Although the glycinergic IPSCs reversed close to the expected Cl^- equilibrium potential in bushy cells, in multipolar neurons the reversal was surprisingly negative to the expected potential. Previous studies have shown that glycinergic (Wu and Oertel, 1986; Harty and Manis, 1996) and GABAergic (Wu and Oertel, 1986; Milenković et al., 2007) conductances in VCN neurons are mediated via a change in Cl^- conductance. There are two potential mechanisms that could contribute to a difference between the expected and measured equilibrium potentials. First, this could result from the limitations of space-clamp with single-electrode voltage clamp methods, if the inhibitory synapses are located remotely from the cell body. With a single-electrode voltage clamp, errors are introduced into the measurement of remote synaptic currents, and these errors increase with distance from the synapse to the somatic recording site (Spruston et al., 1993). Such errors can affect the estimation of reversal potentials, since the distant synaptic sites can be at a significantly different voltage than the soma. Second, recent evidence suggests that impermeant negative charges associated with intracellular phosphoproteins and surface glycoproteins can significantly affect the equilibrium for Cl^- (Glykys et al., 2014), and so the local ionic environment near the receptors may not be the same as that expected from the intracellular and extracellular ion concentrations.

We also unexpectedly observed a difference between the reversal potentials for glycinergic and GABAergic IPSCs. GABAergic IPSCs reversed at a potential 9 mV negative to glycinergic IPSCs in bushy cells, and 14 mV negative in multipolar cells. There are a number of potential causes for this difference. First, GABA receptors have different ionic permeability than glycine receptors for ions other than Cl^-. In particular, of the anionic species in the ACSF and intracellularly, HCO_3^- is more highly permeable in GABA than glycine receptors (Bormann et al., 1987). A difference in the local pH or in HCO_3^- handling near the receptors could influence the balance of anionic species permeating the open receptor, and this could affect the reversal, as has been shown for activity-dependent shifts in cartwheel cells (Kim and Trussell, 2009). Second, the glycinergic and GABAergic synapses could have different spatial distributions, so that, again, the voltages could be different for receptors at different locations. A spatial separation between GABA and glycine receptors has been qualitatively indicated in multipolar neurons (Juiz et al., 1989, 1996). Here, glycine receptors were found mostly on the proximal dendrites, whereas GABA receptors were mostly observed in remote, medium and small caliber dendrites, some of which could belong to multipolar cells. Evidence for a similar spatial separation between GABA and glycine receptors may also hold for AVCN bushy neurons. Glycine receptors are primarily found on the soma of the bushy cells (Altschuler et al., 1986; Wenthold et al., 1988). In contrast, GABA receptors were not seen opposing axosomatic terminals in bushy cells (Juiz et al., 1989, 1996), and were reported to be present at low levels (Lim et al., 2000). Furthermore, VGAT positive puncta have been seen in alignment with bushy-cell dendrites (Gomez-Nieto and Rubio, 2009), suggesting the possibility of dendritic GABAergic synapses. Finally, as $[Cl^-]_i$ has been shown to vary in different compartments of some neurons (Duebel et al., 2006; Szabadics et al., 2006; Glykys et al., 2014), spatial segregation of GABAergic and glycinergic synapses could result in synapses faced with different ionic environments, and thus have different reversal potentials. A distal location for the GABAergic synapses would also be consistent with the slower and smaller IPSCs that we observed.

SUMMARY

Neurons of the cochlear nuclei receive both glycinergic and GABAergic inhibition from multiple sources. Although the synaptic properties and function of the glycinergic inhibition in the AVCN has been well studied, the synaptic function of GABAergic inhibition is less well understood because it is weaker and largely arises from sources outside the CN. In this exploratory study, we used cochlear nucleus slices from transgenic VGAT-ChR2-EYFP mouse and photostimulation to activate inhibitory neurons to study both glycinergic and GABAergic inhibition. We found that multipolar neurons receive stronger GABAergic inhibition than bushy cells, and that the time course of inhibition for both cell types was slow relative to the fast glycinergic inhibition in multipolar cells. Lastly, we observed differences in the reversal potentials for glycinergic and GABAergic IPSCs that may be consistent with different spatial distributions of receptors in the cells.

ACKNOWLEDGMENTS

We thank Heather O'Donohue and Megan Kratz for maintaining the mouse colony and genotyping, Luke Campagnola and Megan Kratz for developing the 2-photon imaging system and the data acquisition program, and Dr. Patricia Maness (UNC) for introducing us to the VGAT-ChR2-EYFP mice. This work was supported by NIDCD grant R01 DC004551 to Paul B. Manis.

REFERENCES

Adams, J. C., and Mugnaini, E. (1987). Patterns of glutamate decarboxylase immunostaining in the feline cochlear nuclear complex studied with silver enhancement and electron microscopy. *J. Comp. Neurol.* 262, 375–401. doi: 10.1002/cne.902620305

Altschuler, R. A., Betz, H., Parakkal, M. H., Reeks, K. A., and Wenthold, R. J. (1986). Identification of glycinergic synapses in the cochlear nucleus through immunocytochemical localization of the postsynaptic receptor. *Brain Res.* 369, 316–320. doi: 10.1016/0006-8993(86)90542-1

Arnott, R. H., Wallace, M. N., Shackleton, T. M., and Palmer, A. R. (2004). Onset neurones in the anteroventral cochlear nucleus project to the dorsal cochlear nucleus. *J. Assoc. Res. Otolaryngol.* 5, 153–170. doi: 10.1007/s10162-003-4036-8

Backoff, P. M., Shadduck Palombi, P., and Caspary, D. M. (1999). Gamma-aminobutyric acidergic and glycinergic inputs shape coding of amplitude modulation in the chinchilla cochlear nucleus. *Hear. Res.* 134, 77–88. doi: 10.1016/s0378-5955(99)00071-4

Bormann, J., Hamill, O. P., and Sakmann, B. (1987). Mechanism of anion permeation through channels gated by glycine and gamma-aminobutyric acid in mouse cultured spinal neurones. *J. Physiol.* 385, 243–286.

Campagnola, L., Kratz, M. B., and Manis, P. B. (2014). ACQ4: an open-source software platform for data acquisition and analysis in neurophysiology research. *Front. Neuroinform.* 8:3. doi: 10.3389/fninf.2014.00003

Campagnola, L., and Manis, P. B. (2014). A map of functional synaptic connectivity in the mouse anteroventral cochlear nucleus. *J. Neurosci.* 34, 2214–2230. doi: 10.1523/jneurosci.4669-13.2014

Caspary, D. M., Backoff, P. M., Finlayson, P. G., and Palombi, P. S. (1994). Inhibitory inputs modulate discharge rate within frequency receptive fields of anteroventral cochlear nucleus neurons. *J. Neurophysiol.* 72, 2124–2133.

Caspary, D. M., Havey, D. C., and Faingold, C. L. (1979). Effects of microiontophoretically applied glycine and GABA on neuronal response patterns in the cochlear nuclei. *Brain Res.* 172, 179–185. doi: 10.1016/0006-8993(79)90909-0

Duebel, J., Haverkamp, S., Schleich, W., Feng, G., Augustine, G. J., Kuner, T., et al. (2006). Two-photon imaging reveals somatodendritic chloride gradient in retinal ON-type bipolar cells expressing the biosensor Clomeleon. *Neuron* 49, 81–94. doi: 10.1016/j.neuron.2005.10.035

Dumoulin, A., Rostaing, P., Bedet, C., Levi, S., Isambert, M. F., Henry, J. P., et al. (1999). Presence of the vesicular inhibitory amino acid transporter in GABAergic and glycinergic synaptic terminal boutons. *J. Cell Sci.* 112(Pt. 6), 811–823.

Ebert, U., and Ostwald, J. (1995a). GABA alters the discharge pattern of chopper neurons in the rat ventral cochlear nucleus. *Hear. Res.* 91, 160–166. doi: 10.1016/0378-5955(96)83100-5

Ebert, U., and Ostwald, J. (1995b). GABA can improve acoustic contrast in the rat ventral cochlear nucleus. *Exp. Brain Res.* 104, 310–322. doi: 10.1007/bf00242016

Eccles, J., Nicoll, R. A., Oshima, T., and Rubia, F. J. (1977). The anionic permeability of the inhibitory postsynaptic membrane of hippocampal pyramidal cells. *Proc. R. Soc. Lond. B Biol. Sci.* 198, 345–361. doi: 10.1098/rspb.1977.0102

Ferragamo, M. J., Golding, N. L., and Oertel, D. (1998). Synaptic inputs to stellate cells in the ventral cochlear nucleus. *J. Neurophysiol.* 79, 51–63.

Francis, H. W., and Manis, P. B. (2000). Effects of deafferentation on the electrophysiology of ventral cochlear nucleus neurons. *Hear. Res.* 149, 91–105. doi: 10.1016/s0378-5955(00)00165-9

Frosch, M. P., Lipton, S. A., and Dichter, M. A. (1992). Desensitization of GABA-activated currents and channels in cultured cortical neurons. *J. Neurosci.* 12, 3042–3053.

Frostholm, A., and Rotter, A. (1986). Autoradiographic localization of receptors in the cochlear nucleus of the mouse. *Brain Res. Bull.* 16, 189–203. doi: 10.1016/0361-9230(86)90033-x

Gai, Y., and Carney, L. H. (2008). Influence of inhibitory inputs on rate and timing of responses in the anteroventral cochlear nucleus. *J. Neurophysiol.* 99, 1077–1095. doi: 10.1152/jn.00708.2007

Glykys, J., Dzhala, V., Egawa, K., Balena, T., Saponjian, Y., Kuchibhotla, K. V., et al. (2014). Local impermeant anions establish the neuronal chloride concentration. *Science* 343, 670–675. doi: 10.1126/science.1245423

Gomez-Nieto, R., and Rubio, M. E. (2009). A bushy cell network in the rat ventral cochlear nucleus. *J. Comp. Neurol.* 516, 241–263. doi: 10.1002/cne.22139

Harty, T. P., and Manis, P. B. (1996). Glycine-evoked currents in acutely dissociated neurons of the guinea pig ventral cochlear nucleus. *J. Neurophysiol.* 75, 2300–2311.

Harty, T. P., and Manis, P. B. (1998). Kinetic analysis of glycine receptor currents in ventral cochlear nucleus. *J. Neurophysiol.* 79, 1891–1901.

Juiz, J. M., Albin, R. L., Helfert, R. H., and Altschuler, R. A. (1994). Distribution of GABAA and GABAB binding sites in the cochlear nucleus of the guinea pig. *Brain Res.* 639, 193–201. doi: 10.1016/0006-8993(94)91730-2

Juiz, J. M., Helfert, R. H., Bonneau, J. M., Wenthold, R. J., and Altschuler, R. A. (1996). Three classes of inhibitory amino acid terminals in the cochlear nucleus of the guinea pig. *J. Comp. Neurol.* 373, 11–26. doi: 10.1002/(sici)1096-9861(19960909)373:1<11::aid-cne2>3.0.co;2-g

Juiz, J. M., Helfert, R. H., Wenthold, R. J., De Blas, A. L., and Altschuler, R. A. (1989). Immunocytochemical localization of the GABAA/benzodiazepine receptor in the guinea pig cochlear nucleus: evidence for receptor localization heterogeneity. *Brain Res.* 504, 173–179. doi: 10.1016/0006-8993(89)91620-x

Katzel, D., Zemelman, B. V., Buetfering, C., Wolfel, M., and Miesenbock, G. (2011). The columnar and laminar organization of inhibitory connections to neocortical excitatory cells. *Nat. Neurosci.* 14, 100–107. doi: 10.3410/f.7498957.7793055

Kim, Y., and Trussell, L. O. (2009). Negative shift in the glycine reversal potential mediated by a Ca2+- and pH-dependent mechanism in interneurons. *J. Neurosci.* 29, 11495–11510. doi: 10.1523/jneurosci.1086-09.2009

Kolston, J., Osen, K. K., Hackney, C. M., Ottersen, O. P., and Storm-Mathisen, J. (1992). An atlas of glycine- and GABA-like immunoreactivity and colocalization in the cochlear nuclear complex of the guinea pig. *Anat. Embryol. (Berl)* 186, 443–465. doi: 10.1007/bf00185459

Lim, R., Alvarez, F. J., and Walmsley, B. (2000). GABA mediates presynaptic inhibition at glycinergic synapses in a rat auditory brainstem nucleus. *J. Physiol.* 525(Pt. 2), 447–459. doi: 10.1111/j.1469-7793.2000.t01-1-00447.x

Lin, J. Y. (2012). Optogenetic excitation of neurons with channelrhodopsins: light instrumentation, expression systems and channelrhodopsin variants. *Prog. Brain Res.* 196, 29–47. doi: 10.1016/b978-0-444-59426-6.00002-1

Lin, J. Y., Lin, M. Z., Steinbach, P., and Tsien, R. Y. (2009). Characterization of engineered channelrhodopsin variants with improved properties and kinetics. *Biophys. J.* 96, 1803–1814. doi: 10.1016/j.bpj.2008.11.034

Manis, P. B., and Marx, S. O. (1991). Outward currents in isolated ventral cochlear nucleus neurons. *J. Neurosci.* 11, 2865–2880.

Milenković, I., Witte, M., Turecek, R., Heinrich, M., Reinert, T., and Rübsamen, R. (2007). Development of chloride-mediated inhibition in neurons of the anteroventral cochlear nucleus of gerbil (Meriones unguiculatus). *J. Neurophysiol.* 98, 1634–1644. doi: 10.1152/jn.01150.2006

Moore, J. K., and Moore, R. Y. (1987). Glutamic acid decarboxylase-like immunoreactivity in brainstem auditory nuclei of the rat. *J. Comp. Neurol.* 260, 157–174. doi: 10.1002/cne.902600202

Ostapoff, E. M., Benson, C. G., and Saint Marie, R. L. (1997). GABA- and glycine-immunoreactive projections from the superior olivary complex to the cochlear nucleus in guinea pig. *J. Comp. Neurol.* 381, 500–512. doi: 10.1002/(sici)1096-9861(19970519)381:4<500::aid-cne9>3.0.co;2-6

Palombi, P. S., and Caspary, D. M. (1992). GABAA receptor antagonist bicuculline alters response properties of posteroventral cochlear nucleus neurons. *J. Neurophysiol.* 67, 738–746.

Roberts, R. C., and Ribak, C. E. (1987). GABAergic neurons and axon terminals in the brainstem auditory nuclei of the gerbil. *J. Comp. Neurol.* 258, 267–280. doi: 10.1002/cne.902580207

Saint Marie, R. L., Benson, C. G., Ostapoff, E. M., and Morest, D. K. (1991). Glycine immunoreactive projections from the dorsal to the anteroventral cochlear nucleus. *Hear. Res.* 51, 11–28. doi: 10.1016/0378-5955(91)90003-r

Saint Marie, R. L., Morest, D. K., and Brandon, C. J. (1989). The form and distribution of GABAergic synapses on the principal cell types of the ventral cochlear nucleus of the cat. *Hear. Res.* 42, 97–112. doi: 10.1016/0378-5955(89)90120-2

Smith, P. H., and Rhode, W. S. (1989). Structural and functional properties distinguish two types of multipolar cells in the ventral cochlear nucleus. *J. Comp. Neurol.* 282, 595–616. doi: 10.1002/cne.902820410

Spruston, N., Jaffe, D. B., Williams, S. H., and Johnston, D. (1993). Voltage- and space-clamp errors associated with the measurement of electrotonically remote synaptic events. *J. Neurophysiol.* 70, 781–802.

Szabadics, J., Varga, C., Molnar, G., Olah, S., Barzo, P., and Tamas, G. (2006). Excitatory effect of GABAergic axo-axonic cells in cortical microcircuits. *Science* 311, 233–235. doi: 10.1126/science.1121325

Wang, Y., and Manis, P. B. (2005). Synaptic transmission at the cochlear nucleus endbulb synapse during age-related hearing loss in mice. *J. Neurophysiol.* 94, 1814–1824. doi: 10.1152/jn.00374.2005

Wang, Y., Kakizaki, T., Sakagami, H., Saito, K., Ebihara, S., Kato, M., et al. (2009). Fluorescent labeling of both GABAergic and glycinergic neurons in vesicular GABA transporter (VGAT)-venus transgenic mouse. *Neuroscience* 164, 1031–1043. doi: 10.1016/j.neuroscience.2009.09.010

Wenthold, R. J., Parakkal, M. H., Oberdorfer, M. D., and Altschuler, R. A. (1988). Glycine receptor immunoreactivity in the ventral cochlear nucleus of the guinea pig. *J. Comp. Neurol.* 276, 423–435. doi: 10.1002/cne.902760307

Wickesberg, R. E., and Oertel, D. (1990). Delayed, frequency-specific inhibition in the cochlear nuclei of mice: a mechanism for monaural echo suppression. *J. Neurosci.* 10, 1762–1768.

Wickesberg, R. E., Whitlon, D., and Oertel, D. (1991). Tuberculoventral neurons project to the multipolar cell area but not to the octopus cell area of the posteroventral cochlear nucleus. *J. Comp. Neurol.* 313, 457–468. doi: 10.1002/cne.903130306

Wu, S. H., and Oertel, D. (1986). Inhibitory circuitry in the ventral cochlear nucleus is probably mediated by glycine. *J. Neurosci.* 6, 2691–2706.

Xie, R., and Manis, P. B. (2013). Target-specific IPSC kinetics promote temporal processing in auditory parallel pathways. *J. Neurosci.* 33, 1598–1614. doi: 10.1523/jneurosci.2541-12.2013

Zhao, S., Ting, J. T., Atallah, H. E., Qiu, L., Tan, J., Gloss, B., et al. (2011). Cell type-specific channelrhodopsin-2 transgenic mice for optogenetic dissection of neural circuitry function. *Nat. Methods* 8, 745–752. doi: 10.1038/nmeth.1668

17

Nitric oxide signaling modulates synaptic inhibition in the superior paraolivary nucleus (SPN) via cGMP-dependent suppression of KCC2

Lina Yassin*[1], *Susanne Radtke-Schuller*[1], *Hila Asraf*[2], *Benedikt Grothe*[1], *Michal Hershfinkel*[2], *Ian D. Forsythe*[3] and *Cornelia Kopp-Scheinpflug*[1]

[1] *Division of Neurobiology, Department Biology II, Ludwig-Maximilians-University Munich, Planegg-Martinsried, Germany*
[2] *Department of Physiology and Cell Biology, Faculty of Health Sciences, Ben-Gurion University of the Negev, Beer-Sheva, Israel*
[3] *Department of Cell Physiology and Pharmacology, University of Leicester, Leicester, UK*

Correspondence:
Cornelia Kopp-Scheinpflug, Division of Neurobiology, Department Biology II, Ludwig-Maximilians-University Munich, Großhaderner Strasse 2, 82152 Planegg-Martinsried, Germany
e-mail: cks@bio.lmu.de

Glycinergic inhibition plays a central role in the auditory brainstem circuitries involved in sound localization and in the encoding of temporal action potential firing patterns. Modulation of this inhibition has the potential to fine-tune information processing in these networks. Here we show that nitric oxide (NO) signaling in the auditory brainstem (where activity-dependent generation of NO is documented) modulates the strength of inhibition by changing the chloride equilibrium potential. Recent evidence demonstrates that large inhibitory postsynaptic currents (IPSCs) in neurons of the superior paraolivary nucleus (SPN) are enhanced by a very low intracellular chloride concentration, generated by the neuronal potassium chloride co-transporter (KCC2) expressed in the postsynaptic neurons. Our data show that modulation by NO caused a 15 mV depolarizing shift of the IPSC reversal potential, reducing the strength of inhibition in SPN neurons, without changing the threshold for action potential firing. Regulating inhibitory strength, through cGMP-dependent changes in the efficacy of KCC2 in the target neuron provides a postsynaptic mechanism for rapidly controlling the inhibitory drive, without altering the timing or pattern of the afferent spike train. Therefore, this NO-mediated suppression of KCC2 can modulate inhibition in one target nucleus (SPN), without influencing inhibitory strength of other target nuclei (MSO, LSO) even though they are each receiving collaterals from the same afferent nucleus (a projection from the medial nucleus of the trapezoid body, MNTB).

Keywords: nitric oxide, KCC2, post-inhibitory rebound, gap-detection, auditory brainstem

INTRODUCTION

The superior olivary complex (SOC) consists of groups of highly specialized brainstem nuclei that compute various acoustic features in sound location processing. Irrespective of the specific task, such as detecting differences in interaural time (medial superior olive; MSO), interaural intensity (lateral superior olive; LSO), or processing transient temporal information (superior paraolivary nucleus; SPN), glycinergic inhibition mediated by the medial nucleus of the trapezoid body (MNTB) is a key component of the afferent input to each of these nuclei (Grothe et al., 2010; Johnston et al., 2010). Thus, the MNTB is the major inhibitory hub within the SOC, with individual MNTB neurons providing collateral projections to multiple, functionally diverse targets (Banks and Smith, 1992; Sommer et al., 1993) where they serve fast and temporally precise inhibition, similar to the role of fast spiking inhibitory interneurons in other brain circuits (Bartos et al., 2002; Tepper et al., 2004). This common source of afferent inhibition (the MNTB) raises the question of what mechanisms are available to modulate the synaptic responses of the individual postsynaptic targets which serve differing roles in these diverse computational functions.

One key parameter of inhibitory strength is the chloride electrochemical gradient, which is the driving force for the hyperpolarizing action of synaptic inhibition and is determined by the intracellular chloride concentration. Early in development the sodium-potassium-chloride co-transporter type 1 (NKCC1) maintains a high intracellular chloride ($[Cl^-]_i$) concentration in most neurons and hence Cl^--mediated synaptic events are depolarizing (Cherubini et al., 2011; Friauf et al., 2011; but see Balakrishnan et al., 2003 for an exception). It is postulated that early in development, inhibitory synapses generate excitatory postsynaptic potentials (EPSPs) that act to stabilize synapse formation, and that as neurons mature there is a switch to expression of neuronal potassium chloride co-transporter type 2 (KCC2), driving a low $[Cl^-]_i$ and supporting hyperpolarizing IPSPs (Kandler and Gillespie, 2005). The trafficking, cell surface expression and transport-activity of KCC2 are closely controlled by neuronal activity (Fiumelli et al., 2005; Wake et al., 2007) with increased KCC2 activity caused by protein oligomerization and changes in phosphorylation (Casula et al., 2001; Blaesse et al., 2006; Chamma et al., 2012). As $[Cl^-]_i$ declines, the driving force favors influx of Cl^- ions which strengthens IPSPs and synaptic inhibition (Lohrke et al., 2005; Friauf et al., 2011; Ben-Ari et al., 2012). In mature neurons, KCC2 can be down-regulated under pathophysiological conditions, reducing the effectiveness of inhibition and causing hyperexcitability (Wake et al., 2007; Hewitt et al., 2009; Boulenguez et al., 2010). A variety of mechanisms modulate KCC2 activity and it is unclear which messengers mediate particular physiological responses, but one potential candidate is nitric oxide (NO).

NO is a gaseous messenger molecule involved in the regulation of synaptic transmission and neuronal function (Garthwaite, 2008). In neurons it is generated by neuronal nitric oxide synthase (nNOS) (Garthwaite and Boulton, 1995). Local NO may also reflect activity in blood vessels (from endothelial or eNOS) or inducible NO synthase (iNOS), with increased NO being associated with inflammatory and neurodegenerative diseases (Steinert et al., 2010; Nakamura et al., 2013) as well as following prolonged synaptic activity (Brenman et al., 1996; Holscher, 1997; Steinert et al., 2008, 2011). NO binds to its intracellular receptor, soluble guanylyl cyclase (sGC) leading to raised intracellular cGMP, which in turn interacts with multiple kinases and phosphatases (Francis et al., 2010).

Given the evidence for activity-dependent NO generation in neural cells (Garthwaite et al., 1988; Brenman et al., 1996; Steinert et al., 2008) and expression of KCC2 and nNOS in the SOC (Reuss and Riemann, 2000; Reuss et al., 2000; Balakrishnan et al., 2003; Lohrke et al., 2005; Blaesse et al., 2006) we asked if these signaling pathways might converge to adjust MNTB-mediated inhibition to the needs of the postsynaptic target neurons during specific stimulus conditions. Our results provide evidence that NO signaling can powerfully modulate the strength of inhibitory synaptic transmission by changing the Cl^- equilibrium potential via cGMP-dependent regulation of KCC2.

MATERIALS AND METHODS

IN VITRO PREPARATIONS

All experimental procedures were approved by the Bavarian district government and were done according to the European Communities Council Directive (2010/63/EU). C57Bl6 mice and Mongolian gerbils (*Meriones unguiculatus*) (P12–P21) were killed by decapitation and coronal brainstem slices (200 μm-thick) containing the SOC were cut in a high sucrose, low-sodium artificial cerebral spinal fluid (ACSF) at ~0°C. Slices were maintained in a normal ACSF at 37°C for 30–45 min, after which they were stored at room temperature (~20°C) in a continually recycling slice-maintenance chamber. Composition of the normal ACSF was (mM): NaCl 125, KCl 2.5, $NaHCO_3$ 26, glucose 10, NaH_2PO_4 1.25, sodium pyruvate 2, myo-inositol 3, $CaCl_2$ 2, $MgCl_2$ 1, and ascorbic acid 0.5; pH was 7.4, bubbled with 95% O_2, 5% CO_2. For the low-sodium ACSF, NaCl was replaced by 200 mM sucrose, and $CaCl_2$ and $MgCl_2$ concentrations were changed to 0.5 and 6 mM, respectively. Experiments were conducted at physiological temperature with the recording chamber being continuously perfused with ACSF at a rate of 1–2 ml min^{-1}. An inline feedback temperature controller and heated stage were used to maintain chamber temperature at 36 ± 1°C (TC344B, Warner Instruments, Hamden, CT, USA).

PATCH-CLAMP

Whole-cell patch-clamp and current-clamp recordings were made from visually identified SOC neurons (Olympus BX51WI microscope) using an EPC10/2 HEKA amplifier, sampling at 50 kHz and filtering at 10 kHz. Patch pipettes were pulled from borosilicate glass capillaries (GC150F-7.5, OD: 1.5 mm; Harvard Apparatus, Edenbridge, UK) using a DMZ Universal puller (Zeitz). Their resistance was ~3.5 MΩ when filled with a patch solution containing (mM): K-gluconate 97.5, KCl 32.5, HEPES 40, EGTA 5, $MgCl_2$ 1, Na_2phosphocreatine 5, pH was adjusted to 7.2 with KOH. Stated voltages are corrected for a liquid junction potential of −11 mV. Whole-cell series resistances were compensated by 50–80% and recordings in which the series resistance changed more than 2–3 MΩ were omitted from analysis. Synaptic currents were evoked by afferent fiber stimulation with a concentric bipolar electrode (FHC) driven by voltage pulses generated by the HEKA amplifier and post-amplified by a linear stimulus isolator (Pulse Stimulator AM-2100). Glutamatergic currents were blocked (50 μM D-AP5, 20 μM DNQX), GABAergic currents were blocked by 10 μM SR95531 and glycinergic currents were confirmed by blockade with 1 μM strychnine. The NO was applied via the NO donor sodium nitroprusside (SNP; 100 μM) which was prepared immediately before use. sGC was blocked with 1H-[1,2,4]Oxadiazolo[4,3-a]quinoxalin-1-one (ODQ, 1 μM).

IMMUNOCYTOCHEMISTRY

The brains of four Mongolian gerbils (*Meriones unguiculatus*) and four C57Bl6 mice (both aged 2–3 month) were perfusion-fixed with 4% paraformaldehyde, cryoprotected with 22.5% sucrose overnight and shock frozen in CO_2 snow. Coronal brainstem sections were cut with a cryostat (40 μm thick; LEICA CM 3050S) and collected in phosphate buffered saline 0.05 M, pH 7.4 (PBS). After washing, non-specific binding sites were saturated with a blocking solution containing 1% BSA, 0.3% Triton X-100, and 0.1% saponin in PBS, for 1 h at room temperature and incubated in the primary antibody mix (diluted in blocking solution) for two nights at 4°C. The specificity of the primary antibodies used has been previously published for rodents and relevant publications are indicated for the respective antibodies. The primary antibodies used were: [rabbit anti-KCC2 1:500, Millipore, 07-432 (Kopp-Scheinpflug et al., 2011)], guinea pig anti-GlyT2 [1:500 Millipore, AB1773 (Hassfurth et al., 2010)], mouse monoclonal anti NOS-B1 [1:200, Sigma N2280 (Coote and Rees, 2008)], chicken anti-Map2 [1:1000, Neuromics, CH22103 (Kapfer et al., 2002)]. Subsequently, the sections were washed and incubated with the appropriate secondary antibodies: Alexa488 donkey anti-rabbit (1:300, Molecular Probes A21206), Cy3 donkey anti-guinea pig (1:300, Chemicon AP193C), Alexa488 donkey anti-mouse (1:300, Invitrogen A21202), Alexa 647 donkey-anti-chicken (1:300, Dianova 115-605-205). For the NADPH-d staining, sections were processed as described by Vincent and Kimura (1992).

IMAGE ACQUISITION

To image the NADPH-d stain in bright-field microscopy and to visualize immunohistochemical labeling, the sections were viewed with a VS120 S1 microscope [Olympus BX61VST with software dotSlide® (Olympus)]. For overviews in **Figure 1A** and in enlarged images of the immunohistochemical labeling, confocal optical sections were acquired with a Leica TCS SP confocal laser-scanning microscope (Leica Microsystems, Mannheim, Germany) equipped with a Plan 10.0×/NA 0.40 and a Plan 63×/NA1.32 oil immersion objective. After stack acquisition and Z chromatic shift correction between color channels, RGB stacks, montages of RGB optical sections, and maximum-intensity projections were assembled into tables using ImageJ (1.39q Wayan Rasband, National Institutes of Health, USA) and Adobe Photoshop CS6 (Adobe Systems, San Jose, CA) software; figure images were arranged using CorelDRAW X6 (Corel Corporation, Ottawa, Ontario, Canada).

MEASUREMENT OF KCC2 ACTIVITY

Human neuroblastoma SHSY-5Y cells were grown in DMEM containing 10% fetal bovine serum at 37°C in a humidified atmosphere containing 5% CO_2. Cells were seeded on 10 mm glass coverslips 48 h prior to the experiment. SHSY-5Y cells were loaded with the pH sensitive fluorescent dye BCECF-AM (0.5 μM, 12 min. 2′,7′-bis-(2-carboxyethyl)-5-(and-6)-carboxyfluorescein acetoxymethyl ester; TefLabs) in a Ringer's solution (composition in mM: NaCl 120, MgCl 0.8, KCl 5.4, CaCl 1.8, HEPES 20, glucose 15) containing 0.1% BSA. Coverslips were placed in a perfusion chamber and imaged using 440/470 nm excitation filters and a bandpass emission filter at 535 nm (Chroma Technology) as described before (Hershfinkel et al., 2009). To monitor KCC2 activity we used the NH_4Cl/BCECF paradigm (Hershfinkel et al., 2009). In absence of extracellular K^+, NH_4Cl (5 mM) added to the extracellular solution results in equilibrium between NH_3 and NH_4^+. This is disrupted as NH_3 rapidly diffuses through the membrane, binds H^+ within the cytoplasm and causes alkalinization of the cells, which is detected by an increase in BCECF fluorescence (**Figure 5A**). In the absence of K^+, the remaining extracellular NH_4^+ serves as a surrogate potassium ion and is transported into the cell by KCC2 via reverse transport (Chorin et al., 2011). The NH_4^+ influx changes the equilibrium between NH_3 and NH_4^+ within the cells, releasing H^+, and leading to acidification and a decrease of BCECF fluorescence. The rate of acidification is proportional to KCC2 activity, and blocking KCC2 in mature neurons blocks this transport and the acidification, leading to a prolonged alkalinization of the cells (Hershfinkel et al., 2009). Baseline KCC2 activity in SHSY-5Y cells is low, so the cells were initially incubated in low-osmolarity Ringer's solution containing only 100 mM NaCl for 5 min. Subsequently, baseline fluorescence was achieved and NH_4Cl (5 mM) was added to the superfusion, nominally K^+-free, Ringer's solution. The acidification rate, representing KCC2 activity, was calculated for a minimum of 20 cells/coverslip in each experiment. Rates were averaged across 5–10 independent measurements. As indicated, SNP (300 μM) was added for 45 min, at a concentration not toxic to these cells (Wagle and Singh, 2000) in the presence or absence of ODQ (1 μM) or the cell permeable Zn^{2+} chelator N,N,N′,N′-tetrakis (2-pyridalmethyl) ethylenediamine (TPEN, 10 μM). Statistical analyses were performed using analysis of variance with *post-hoc* comparisons.

DATA ANALYSIS AND STATISTICAL METHODS

Data analysis was conducted with IgorPro 5.0 and custom written macros were employed. Statistical analyses of the data were performed with SigmaStat/SigmaPlot™ (SPSS Science, Chicago, IL). Results are reported as mean ± s.e.m.; *n* being the number of neurons recorded from at least three different animals. Statistical comparisons between different data sets were made using unpaired Student's *t*-test, while before and after comparisons were made by the paired Student's *t*-test. Differences were considered statistically significant at $p < 0.05$.

RESULTS

The neuronal glycine transporter type 2 (GlyT2) labels the inhibitory synaptic terminals around the respective target neurons, where it is responsible for the re-uptake of glycine from the synaptic cleft. Thus, GlyT2 is a reliable marker for neuron populations that receive strong glycinergic inputs. In the auditory brainstem, GlyT2 labeled neurons in the LSO, MSO, and SPN which all receive powerful inhibition from the MNTB (**Figure 1**). The labeling pattern of all three structures is comparable between mouse (**Figure 1A**) and gerbil (**Figure 1B**). The MSO is smaller in mouse compared to gerbil, as is expected for an animal with a small head and little low-frequency hearing. The immunohistochemistry also shows that KCC2 is expressed postsynaptically in the LSO, MSO and SPN of both mouse and gerbil and this mirrors the presynaptic labeling for GlyT2 (**Figure 1** insets).

KCC2 ACTIVITY LEVELS DIFFER BETWEEN BRAINSTEM NUCLEI

It is not possible to determine the activity and effectiveness of the KCC2 transporter in these different nuclei by measuring protein expression alone. KCC2 activity was monitored by measuring changes in the reversal potential of glycinergic synaptic currents evoked in response to electrical stimulation of the MNTB (and pharmacologically isolated by blocking glutamatergic and GABAergic components with 50 μM D-AP5, 20 μM DNQX, and 10 μM SR95531, respectively). The reversal potentials of the glycinergic currents, $E_{glycine}$, were measured before (closed triangles in **Figure 1C**) and after blocking KCC2 activity with furosemide (0.5 mM; open circles in **Figure 1C**). In whole-cell patch recording, dialysis of the intracellular solution with the pipette solution enabled the introduction of a high intracellular chloride concentration (34.5 mM) that should maximize KCC2 activity in order to restore the usually low intracellular chloride concentration in LSO, MSO, and SPN neurons (Lohrke et al., 2005). The activity of KCC2 in these neurons is evident from the deviation of the measured IPSC reversal potential from the calculated reversal potential based on the internal and external chloride concentrations using the Nernst equation ($E_{calc} = -46$ mV; dotted line in **Figure 1E**). More negative deviations from E_{calc} toward more hyperpolarized reversal potentials provide an estimate for the activity of KCC2 that is driving this displacement. Blocking KCC2 by bath application of furosemide (0.5 mM) consistently shifted $E_{glycine}$ toward more positive voltages near the

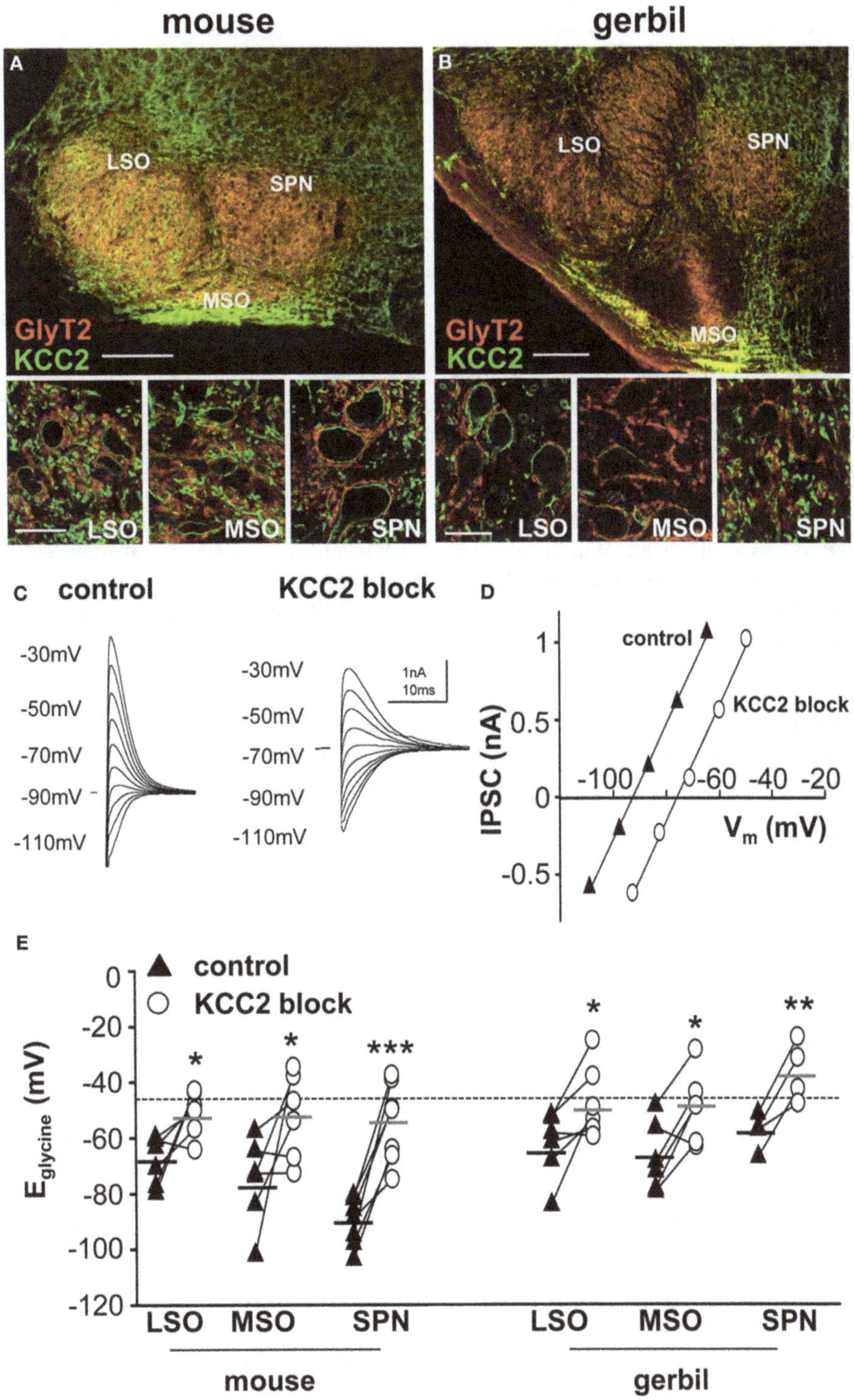

FIGURE 1 | KCC2 mirrors the expression of GlyT2 in the superior olivary complex. Overview of mouse **(A)** and gerbil **(B)** SOC and enlarged images of LSO, MSO, and SPN double-labeled for GlyT2 (red), and KCC2 (green). Scale bars: 200 μm in overviews, 25 μm in magnified images. **(C)** Glycinergic IPSCs were evoked in a mouse SPN neuron by electrical stimulation of the MNTB. The command potentials ranged from −120 to −30 mV in steps of 10 mV. The IPSC reversal potential changed from −90 mV in control conditions (closed triangles in panel **D**) to −70 mV after the blockade of KCC2 (open circles in panel **D**) with furosemide. Stimulus artifacts were removed for clarity. **(D)** Current-voltage relationship for the IPSCs shown in **(C)**. The parallel shift of the curves indicates a sole change in reversal potential without changing the conductance. **(E)** IPSC reversal potentials were depolarized after blockade of KCC2. The deviations from the calculated reversal potential (black dotted line) are indicative of KCC2 activity levels and suggest that KCC2 is most active in the mouse SPN. The small black and grey horizontal lines represent the mean value of the respective control and the furosemide data sets. *$p \leq 0.05$, **$p \leq 0.01$ and ***$p \leq 0.001$.

calculated Nernst potential (**Figure 1D**). This shift was now measured for neurons in LSO, MSO and SPN in both mouse and gerbil (**Figure 1E**). Though there was a significant depolarizing shift in $E_{glycine}$ for all three nuclei in both mouse and gerbil, the largest and most consistent shift in $E_{glycine}$ was seen in the neurons of mouse SPN (**Table 1**).

NITRIC OXIDE AS AN ADDITIONAL (VOLUME) TRANSMITTER IN AUDITORY BRAINSTEM SIGNAL PROCESSING

MNTB neurons express nNOS and generate the messenger molecule NO in an activity-dependent manner (Steinert et al., 2008, 2011). Here we show that nNOS is expressed in MNTB and SPN neurons of mice and gerbils (**Figures 2A,B**). Not all neurons in the SPN seem to express nNOS, but since NO acts as a volume transmitter it can affect even the nNOS negative neurons. Besides somatic nNOS staining, there is also a strong nNOS-positive labeling of the neuropil of the SOC nuclei. NADPH, a necessary coenzyme for the generation of NO has been used to successfully label nNOS positive neuronal somata as well as their axons (Luth et al., 1995; Reuss et al., 2000). Within the auditory brainstem NADPH positive somata are labeled in the MNTB and in the SPN (**Figures 2C,D**), corroborating the nNOS staining (**Figures 2A,B**). Similar to the nNOS staining there is heavily labeled neuropil in the LSO, MSO, and also the SPN, suggesting NO might be involved in local signal processing throughout the auditory brainstem. Although the labeling appeared weaker in the gerbil SOC this could reflect the lower specificity of the nNOS antibody that is based on the mouse sequence.

NO SIGNALING SUPPRESSES KCC2 ACTIVITY IN A cGMP DEPENDENT MANNER

Sustained synaptic stimulation causes generation of NO within the SOC (Steinert et al., 2008, 2011). Here, endogenous NO release was mimicked by bath application of the NO-donor (SNP; 100 μM) and its effect on KCC2 activity was measured. Strong KCC2 activity drives the negative $E_{glycine}$ (Lohrke et al., 2005) in mature mammalian auditory brainstem neurons. Within the nuclei of the SOC in mouse and gerbil, mouse SPN neurons showed the largest deviation from calculated reversal potential for glycine (**Figure 1C**), suggesting that KCC2 activity is strongest in the SPN. Therefore, SPN neurons might support an activity-dependent mechanism that allows down-regulation of KCC2, but this seems to be less essential in the MSO and LSO. To test this hypothesis, the effect of NO on KCC2 activity in mouse LSO, MSO and SPN was measured before and during the application of NO. NO did not affect KCC2 activity in MSO or LSO neurons, but caused a depolarizing shift in $E_{glycine}$ from -83.7 ± 5.4 mV to -67.3 ± 4.5 mV ($n = 10$, $p = 0.002$; **Figures 3A–C**), in the SPN consistent with suppression of KCC2. The IPSC current-voltage relationship showed a parallel shift (**Figure 3B**) and the glycinergic conductance did not change significantly during the NO application ($IPSG_{control}$: 39.1 ± 9.1 nS; $IPSG_{NO}$: 36.7 ± 8.5 nS; $n = 10$; $P = 0.57$). These results indicate that there was no direct effect of NO signaling on the glycine receptors nor was there a major influence on presynaptic glycine release (**Figure 3D**).

The messenger molecule NO can mediate its action either via s-nitrosylation of proteins or by generation of cGMP and downstream activation of kinases or phosphatases (**Figure 4A**). To test between these mechanisms, ODQ (1 μM) was used to specifically block sGC. Indeed, the presence of ODQ in the bath resulted in stable $E_{glycine}$ values even during the additional application of the NO-donor (**Figures 4B,C**; control-$E_{glycine}$: -73.0 ± 5.2 mV; ODQ-$E_{glycine}$: -73.1 ± 5.6 mV; ODQ/NO-$E_{glycine}$: -69.5 ± 5.6 mV; $n = 10$; $P = 0.809$; ANOVA) suggesting that NO modulation of KCC2 is mediated via a sGC/cGMP-dependent signaling. We also analyzed the amplitudes during ODQ-conditioning and following perfusion of ODQ/NO. The change in amplitude was only about 10 percent and was not significant in ANOVA testing against the control condition (ODQ: $11 \pm 8\%$; ODQ/NO: $9 \pm 8\%$; $p = 0.17$).

A direct test for NO regulation of KCC2, was achieved by monitoring KCC2-dependent NH_4^+ transport in SHSY-5Y neuroblastoma cells, which express endogenous KCC2 (Chorin et al., 2011). Using the NH_4Cl paradigm, KCC2 activity is represented by acidification following reversed activity of KCC2 that is inducing NH_4^+ transport into the cells (see Materials and Methods). Under control conditions, NH_4^+-induced acidification rate of $-1.7 \pm 0.1 \times 10^{-4} \Delta F_{440}/F_{470}$/s ($n = 5$), was monitored (**Figure 5A**). Application of the NO-donor SNP (300 μM) resulted in down-regulation of KCC2 activity by about 2-fold to $-0.80 \pm 0.07 \times 10^{-4}$ $\Delta F_{440}/F_{470}$/s ($n = 13$; **Figure 5B**). This confirms that KCC2 activity is suppressed by NO (**Figure 5B**). In cortical neurons an increase in the intracellular zinc concentration has been shown to cause consistent KCC2-suppression (Hershfinkel et al., 2009). To test for a change in intracellular Zn^{2+} in the present experiment, a membrane permeable Zn^{2+} chelator (TPEN; 10 μM) was used to chelate intracellular Zn^{2+} prior to the application of SNP while KCC2-dependent NH_4^+-induced acidification rate was monitored in the cells. Interestingly, chelating intracellular Zn^{2+} completely

Table 1 | Suppression of KCC2-activity measured as shift in $E_{glycine}$ by 0.5 mM furosemide across different nuclei and species.

	Mouse			Gerbil		
	LSO	MSO	SPN	LSO	MSO	SPN
Control $E_{glycine}$	-68.6 ± 8.7 mV	-75.8 ± 15.7 mV	-90.6 ± 8.6 mV	-62.9 ± 4.9 mV	-67.4 ± 12.4 mV	-58.1 ± 3.03 mV
Furosemide $E_{glycine}$	-51.0 ± 8.2 mV	-52.2 ± 15.4 mV	-54.5 ± 14.3 mV	-47.0 ± 13.7 mV	-49.0 ± 12.8 mV	-36.4 ± 5.4 mV
Δ $E_{glycine}$	**17.6 mV**	**23.6 mV**	**36.2 mV**	**15.9 mV**	**18.4 mV**	**21.7 mV**
n	6	6	7	6	6	4
Significance	$p = 0.037$	$p = 0.025$	$p \leq 0.001$	$p = 0.035$	$p = 0.018$	$p = 0.014$

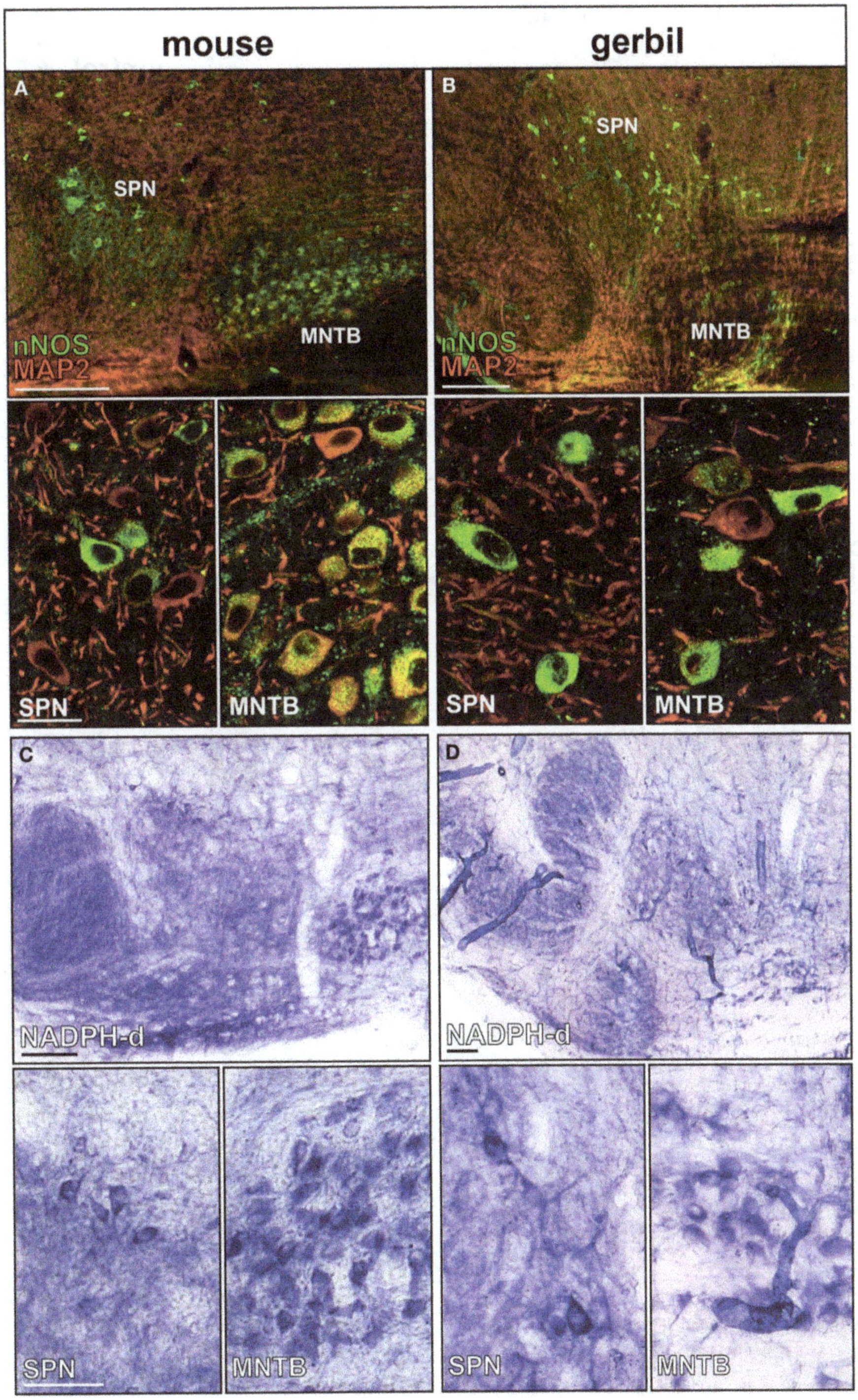

FIGURE 2 | nNOS expression in SPN and MNTB of mouse and gerbil. Double-staining of **(A)** mouse and **(B)** gerbil SOC for MAP2 (red) and nNOS (green); insets show the respective high magnification images of SPN and MNTB. Histochemical staining of NADPH-diaphorase activity in the SOC of **(C)** mouse and **(D)** gerbil. High-magnification images of SPN and MNTB neurons show NADPH-d positive neurons in both nuclei confirming the nNOS staining. Scale bars: 200 μm in overviews, 25 μm in magnified images.

blocked the effect of SNP ($-1.7 \pm 0.2 \times 10^{-4}$ $\Delta F_{440}/F_{470}$/s; $n = 7$), suggesting that increased concentrations of intracellular Zn^{2+} are involved in the NO-dependent attenuation of KCC2 activity in the SHSY-5Y cells (**Figure 5B**). To determine whether the increase in intracellular Zn^{2+} was caused by s-nitrosylation or by sGC/cGMP mediated signaling, the sGC inhibitor 1 μM ODQ was applied prior to and during the SNP and again the suppressive effect of the SNP was reversed to $-1.3 \pm 0.1 \times 10^{-4}$ $\Delta F_{440}/F_{470}$/s

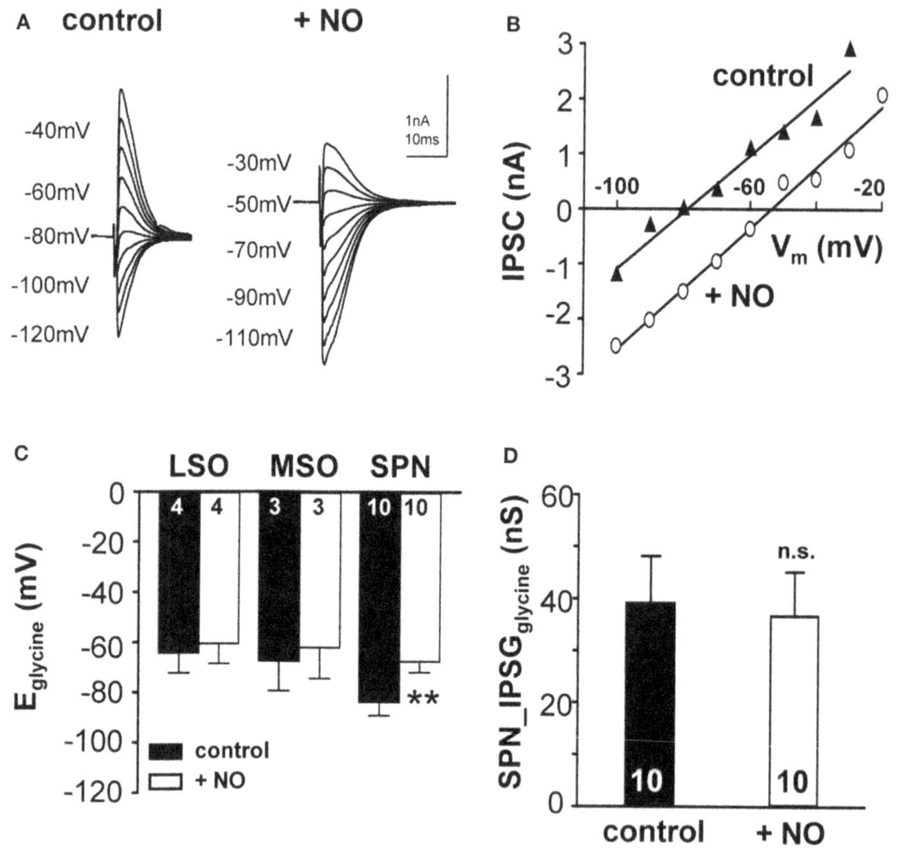

FIGURE 3 | Nitric oxide suppresses KCC2 activity. (A) Glycinergic IPSCs were evoked in a mouse SPN neuron by electrical stimulation of the MNTB. The command potentials ranged from −120 to −30 mV in steps of 10 mV. The IPSC reversal potential changed from −80 mV in control conditions to −50 mV after the modulation of KCC2 activity by NO signaling. **(B)** Current–voltage relationship for the SPN-IPSCs shown in **(A)**. The parallel shift of the curves indicates a sole change in reversal potential without changing the conductance. **(C)** Average data show a significant depolarizing shift in IPSC reversal potential following NO application in the SPN, but not in LSO or MSO. **(D)** The overall glycinergic conductance in SPN neurons is unchanged by NO, indicating no change in the glycine receptor or the glycine release to be involved. $^{**}p \leq 0.01$.

($n = 7$), consistent with the hypothesis that the rise in $[Zn^{2+}]_i$ is downstream of sGC/cGMP/PKG in causing suppression of KCC2 (**Figure 5B**). Both, ODQ and also TPEN prevented the NO-mediated suppression of KCC2 (**Figures 5A,B**). If however, furosemide was applied in addition to ODQ and TPEN, KCC2 activity was again reduced due to a direct interaction between KCC2 and furosemide (**Figures 5A,B**).

NO SUPPRESSES IPSPs AND OFFSET FIRING WITHOUT CHANGING INTRINSIC ACTION POTENTIAL THRESHOLD

NO mediated suppression of KCC2 reduces the IPSP-driven membrane hyperpolarization from -80.1 ± 2.2 mV to -68.6 ± 1.6 mV ($n = 7$; $p \leq 0.001$; **Figure 6A**). The typical offset/rebound firing pattern of SPN neurons in response to sound requires the evoked IPSPs to hyperpolarize the membrane potential to about −80 mV (Kopp-Scheinpflug et al., 2011). Following NO signaling, inhibitory synaptic inputs will no longer generate rebound firing (**Figure 6B**). The SPN firing response to MNTB-evoked IPSP trains was compared in the presence of low (control) or high NO (**Figure 6B**). In control conditions, the trace shows a burst of offset action potentials at the end of the stimulus train, but after raising NO in the test condition, only smaller IPSPs were generated which did not trigger offset firing at the end of the train.

This NO-mediated change in SPN firing could reflect a change in postsynaptic intrinsic excitability, as observed in the MNTB (Steinert et al., 2008), so somatic injection of hyperpolarizing and depolarizing currents were used (**Figure 6C**) to test neuronal excitability. The mean rate-level functions measured under control conditions completely overlapped with that measured during the raised NO condition, indicating that there was no significant change in intrinsically evoked action potential firing. Action potential number and current threshold were the same before and during application of NO (**Figures 6C–F**). This result corroborates the finding that NO-mediated suppression of KCC2 is the mechanism mediating the change in the neuronal firing in the SPN, rather than any direct action of NO on action potential generation.

PHYSIOLOGICAL RELEVANCE: NO REDUCES GAP-DETECTION ABILITY OF SPN NEURONS

SPN neurons receive a range of synaptic projections and express a suite of voltage-gated ionic conductances that enable these

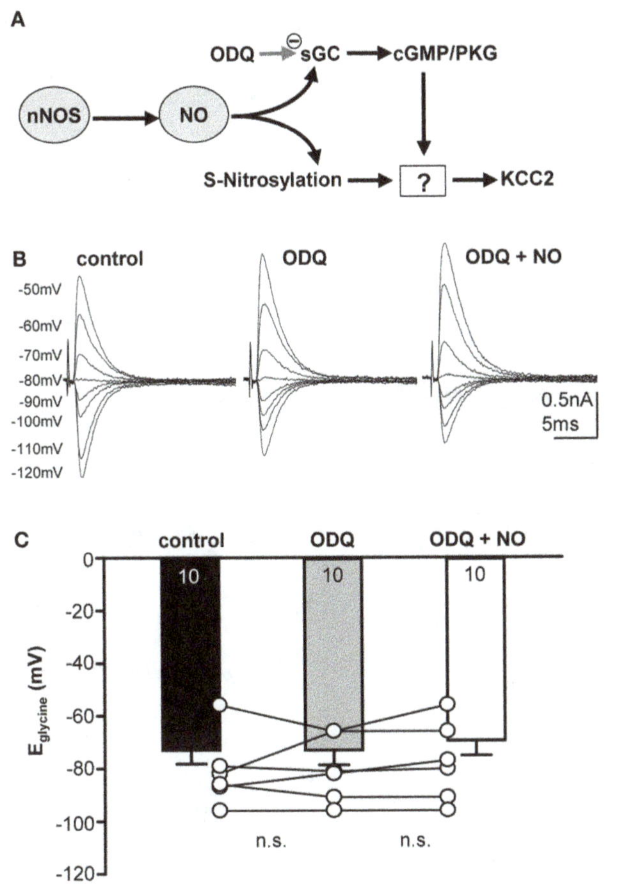

FIGURE 4 | Nitrergic signaling acting on KCC2 is cGMP-dependent. **(A)** Cartoon of possible intracellular signaling mechanisms by NO. **(B)** Glycinergic IPSCs were evoked in a mouse SPN neuron by electrical stimulation of the MNTB. The command potentials ranged from −120 to −50 mV in steps of 10 mV. Blockade of sGC with ODQ prevents the depolarizing shift of the reversal potential normally observed following NO application. **(C)** Average data show that ODQ prevents the NO-mediated depolarizing shift in $E_{glycine}$. There is no significant change between the three conditions.

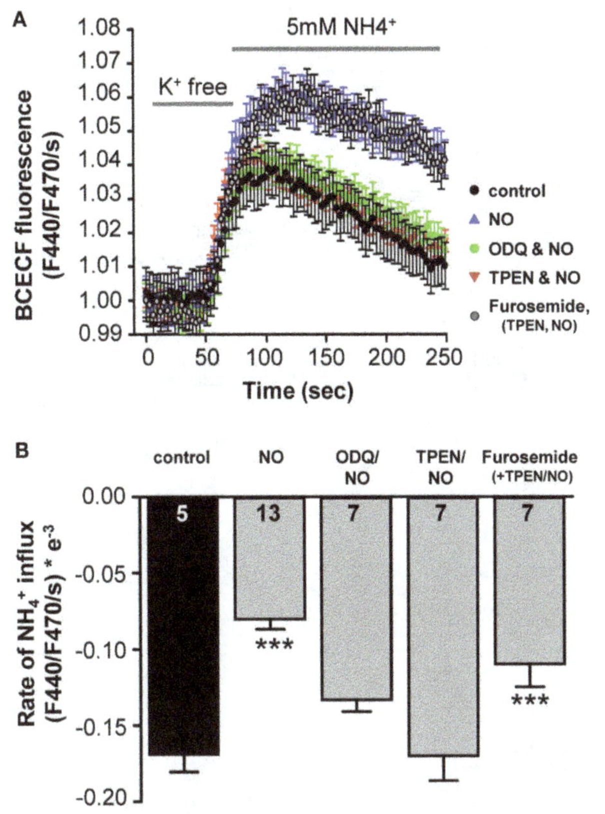

FIGURE 5 | NO-mediated suppression of KCC2 requires intracellular cGMP and Zinc. **(A)** KCC2 activity was monitored with the pH-sensitive dye BCECF in SHSY-5Y cells that express endogenous KCC2. Cells were incubated for 5 min with K^+ free extracellular solution, and the rate of intracellular pH change following application of NH_4Cl (5 mM) was monitored (see Materials and Methods). **(A,B)** Plots of NH_4^+- mediated acidification rates (mean ± s.e.m.) in control, treated with NO, NO+ODQ, NO+TPEN, or ODQ+TPEN+furosemide. Significance was assessed using a One-Way ANOVA. Ns are given in the bars. $^{***}p \leq 0.001$.

neurons to integrate their inputs and fire rebound action potentials at the end of an IPSP train (Kopp-Scheinpflug et al., 2011). This in turn allows computation of auditory gap-detection (Kadner and Berrebi, 2008). We used a gap-detection paradigm to explore how this physiological mechanism is influenced by NO signaling. Gap-detection on a cellular level was determined by current-clamp recording from SPN neurons during synaptic stimulation of the inhibitory inputs from the MNTB. Two 100 Hz stimulus trains of 100 ms duration each were separated by gaps of 20, 30, 40, 50, or 60 ms (each gap-protocol was repeated 10 times). At the gap, short-latency offset action potentials were generated (**Figure 7A**) in the SPN neurons, with action potential numbers proportional to gap-duration (**Figure 7C**). In the control condition (low-NO), all gaps evoked action potentials and gaps of 20 ms or longer were reliably detected with success rates greater than 50%. However, following bath application of NO, gap-detection thresholds increased, so that only longer gaps triggered action potentials (**Figures 7B,C**) and gap-detection for durations shorter than 60 ms was disabled (**Figure 7D**).

DISCUSSION

The MNTB is a common source of glycinergic inhibition, but this innervation is performing different functions in each of the target nuclei. Given that individual MNTB neurons are projecting to multiple nuclei and firing patterns are the same for each target, it is important to understand how the inhibitory synaptic strength can be independently modulated in each target nucleus to fine-tune local synaptic actions. Conventionally two options are considered: presynaptic modulation of transmitter release and postsynaptic modulation of receptor activation and/or receptor kinetics. Here we demonstrate a third option—namely modulation of the IPSC reversal potential. Our results show that the gaseous messenger molecule NO can serve as a control device of inhibitory synaptic strength by controlling $E_{Cl}/E_{glycine}$ in the postsynaptic target neurons via cGMP-dependent suppression of the potassium-chloride co-transporter type 2 (KCC2).

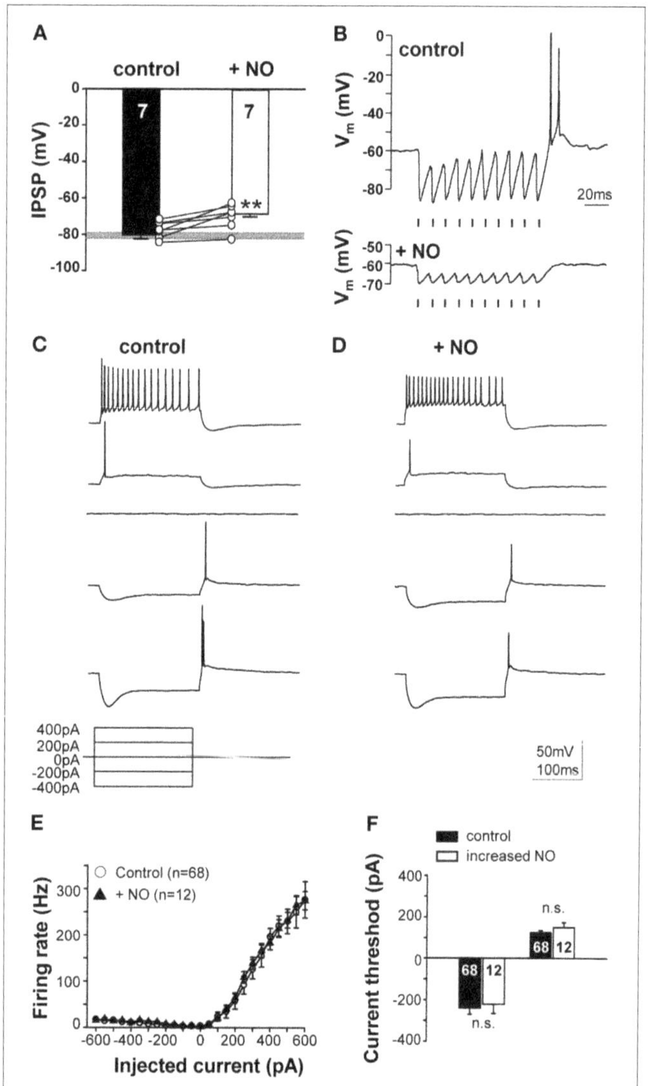

FIGURE 6 | NO suppresses IPSPs and offset firing without changing intrinsic action potential threshold. **(A)** Suppression of KCC2 causes synaptically-evoked IPSPs to be less hyperpolarizing. The grey bar indicates the voltage threshold for generating rebound action potentials (-80.4 ± 1.5 mV; $n = 71$). **(B)** Glycinergic IPSPs in response to 100 Hz pulse trains (indicated by the mark below the recordings) evoked rebound action potentials at the end of the train in the control condition (upper trace). Application of NO (lower trace) reduced the IPSP amplitudes and did not result in rebound firing. Stimulus artifacts were removed for clarity. **(C)** Current-clamp responses to hyperpolarizing and depolarizing current injections revealed similar firing patterns in the control and **(D)** the NO condition. **(E)** Input–output functions did not differ between control and NO conditions. **(F)** Injection of similar magnitude currents evoked similar rebound firing (or firing in response to depolarization) for both conditions, indicating no significant change in action potential threshold. $^{**}p \leq 0.01$.

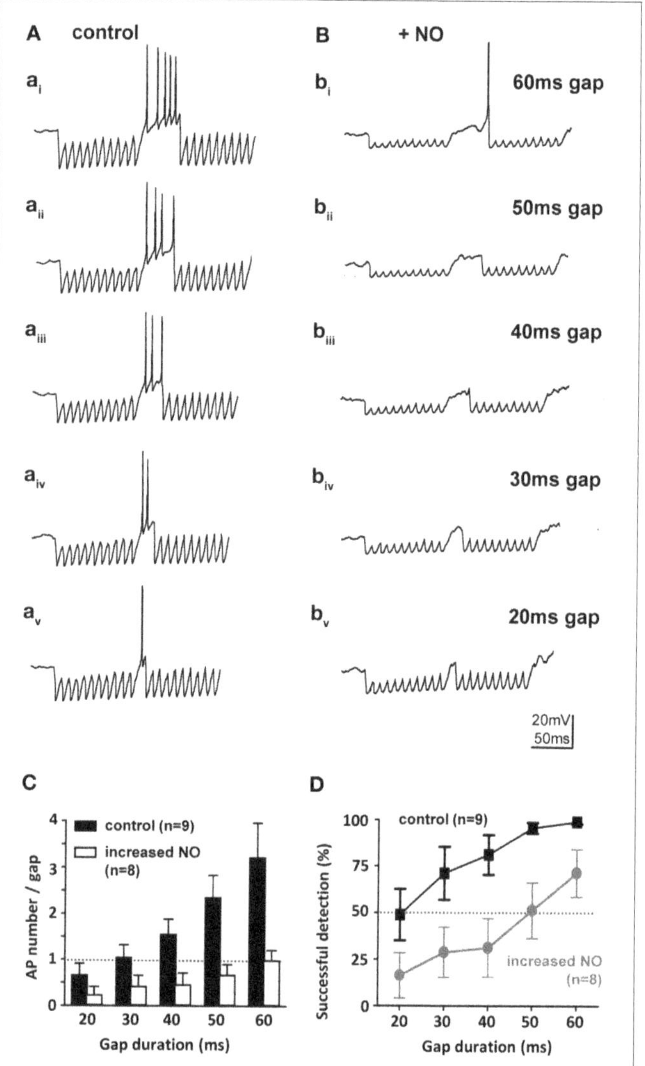

FIGURE 7 | Nitric oxide suppresses gap-detection on a cellular level. **(A)** Mouse SPN neurons show offset firing in responses to gaps of different durations (60–20 ms) embedded in trains of electrically evoked IPSPs. **(B)** Bath application of an NO donor reduced the number of action potentials per gap and delayed the action potential within the gap so that only longer gaps were detected. Stimulus artifacts were removed for clarity. **(C)** The number of evoked action potentials increased with gap duration in controls (black bars), but was never more than one with NO (white bars). **(D)** Repetitive stimulation (10 IPSP trains) was used to estimate gap-detection success, which is plotted here as % offset action potentials against gap duration. Threshold was defined as 50% success (dashed line); controls (black) reliably detected gaps of 20 ms or longer, but following NO, gap-detection thresholds increased to 60 ms or longer. Data plotted as mean ± s.e.m. (n indicated on the respective graph).

KCC2 drives a low internal chloride concentration, hence increasing the hyperpolarizing action of inhibition. KCC2 is present throughout the central nervous system, but is particularly highly expressed in the hippocampus, hypothalamus, brainstem, and motor neurons of the spinal cord (Vinay and Jean-Xavier, 2008; Blaesse et al., 2009). Developmental up-regulation of KCC2 expression strengthens hyperpolarizing inhibition (Cherubini et al., 2011; Friauf et al., 2011). Consequently, acquired loss of KCC2 function in mature neurons will lead to hyperexcitability and seizures due to less hyperpolarizing inhibitory inputs (Wake et al., 2007; Vinay and Jean-Xavier, 2008; Boulenguez et al., 2010; Arion and Lewis, 2011). Deficient KCC2 activity has been described following neuronal damage such as physical trauma or ischemia and the following mechanisms are suggested to be involved: transcriptional regulation via neurotrophin receptor activation (Rivera et al., 2002, 2004), post-translational regulation via changes in the phosphorylation state of KCC2 (Blaesse et al., 2009; Chamma et al., 2013) and activity-dependent down-regulation after NMDA-receptor activation and calcium influx (Ginsberg, 2008; Lee et al., 2011). Previous experiments in the auditory brainstem show that activation of NMDA receptors in the MNTB causes the necessary calcium influx that triggers the activation of nNOS and thus the generation of NO (Steinert et al., 2008). As a volume transmitter NO can then act on the surrounding neurons of LSO, MSO, and SPN. The SPN itself also expresses nNOS [**Figure 2**; (Reuss, 1998; Reuss et al., 2000)], providing a further local source of NO in the SPN. Here, we studied the link between NO and the mechanism by which KCC2 is down-regulated. Our present data show that NO-mediated KCC2 suppression is absent if sGC is blocked, suggesting that KCC is suppressed via a cGMP-dependent mechanism (**Figure 4**). An additional possible downstream mechanism is the NO-mediated recruitment of intracellular Zn^{2+} that suppresses KCC2 activity (Hershfinkel et al., 2009). NO can trigger increase in $[Zn^{2+}]_i$ in at least two different ways; either via cGMP/PKG-dependent release from internal stores (Jang et al., 2007) or via s-nitrosylation of metallothioneins (Zhang et al., 2004). Our ODQ-data support the NO-cGMP pathway leading to Zn^{2+}-mediated suppression of KCC2.

In the central nervous system NO is generally thought to act as a retrograde volume transmitter that modulates transmitter release presynaptically (for a recent reviews see Hardingham et al., 2013). Here we show a postsynaptic mechanism which mediates a parallel shift in the IPSC current-voltage relationship that is inconsistent with a presynaptic change in transmitter release. Instead we demonstrate that this regulation in inhibitory strength is mediated by modulation of the chloride equilibrium potential and does not involve the glycine receptors directly. It is interesting to note that this mechanism is likely to be unique to inhibitory synaptic transmission, since changing the sodium or potassium equilibrium potential would interfere with action potential generation, propagation and waveform.

SIGNIFICANCE OF KCC2 SUPPRESSION FOR INFORMATION PROCESSING IN THE SPN

The present study employs a mouse model for *in vitro* demonstration of NO-mediated regulation of sound offset encoding/gap-detection mechanisms in the auditory brainstem. Brief gaps in sound determine sound rhythms (Felix et al., 2011; Kopp-Scheinpflug et al., 2011) and suggest a correlation between gap-detection and speech perception (Snell et al., 2002; Frisina et al., 2006). Although information about sound offsets and gaps is processed in the auditory cortex, it is derived from subcortical computations (Scholl et al., 2010). Gaps in sound are reliably encoded in the SPN in the auditory brainstem (Kadner and Berrebi, 2008; Kopp-Scheinpflug et al., 2011) by a mechanism that requires three elements: large glycinergic IPSPs, driven by an extreme negative chloride reversal potential (E_{Cl}), combined with a large hyperpolarization-activated non-specific cationic current (I_H), and a T-type calcium conductance (I_{TCa}) (Kopp-Scheinpflug et al., 2011). Our present data show that NO negatively modulates KCC2 which can lead to the following cascade of events: less hyperpolarized IPSPs cause less activation of I_H (HCN channels) and do not provide sufficient hyperpolarization to enable recovery of I_{TCa} (low-threshold calcium channels) from inactivation; therefore the typical offset firing/gap detection in SPN neurons is restricted by NO. The loss of temporal resolution (as measured by gap-detection) is a prevalent dilemma in models of ageing, hearing loss and neurodegeneration. At the same time individuals with inflammatory and neurodegenerative diseases often show increased levels of NO in nervous system tissue (Sweeten et al., 2004; Steinert et al., 2010). Effective modulators of gap-detection thresholds would provide an important mechanism which would influence higher levels of processing. Attempts to improve gap-detection by facilitating GABAergic inhibition have failed (Gleich and Strutz, 2011) which is consistent with the *glycinergic*/KCC2 mechanism as described here. Facilitation of KCC2 (e.g., by NO-scavengers) could be considered for future treatments as a means to enhance local inhibition in the brain.

SIGNIFICANCE OF KCC2 SUPPRESSION FOR BINAURAL INFORMATION PROCESSING IN THE MSO AND LSO

In both, the interaural level difference processing LSO as well as in the interaural time difference processing MSO, the balance of excitation and MNTB-mediated inhibition is crucial for adjusting the binaural sensitivity of single neurons as well as the population output (Grothe et al., 2010). Traditionally considered to be rather static, the binaural sensitivity of both, LSO and MSO, has recently been shown to be surprisingly dynamic (Magnusson et al., 2008; Hassfurth et al., 2010; Fischl et al., 2012; Stange et al., 2013). Modulation via NO may superimpose these adaptations on the binaural system by globally adjusting synaptic sensitivity to changing levels of acoustic exposure. However, according to our present study, NO-mediated suppression of KCC2 activity results in a weakening of the main inhibitory input to SPN neurons. In contrast, KCC2 activity in LSO and MSO neurons is not affected, suggesting a different role of NO than suppressing inhibition.

In summary, our results show that the NO synthesizing enzyme nNOS is expressed in the SOC where NO can be generated in an activity-dependent manner. Future studies should aim at identifying the significance of NO as a volume transmitter in the auditory brainstem in an *in vivo* preparation. NO can act as a powerful modulator of inhibitory transmission by suppressing KCC2. This novel mechanism of activity-dependent modulation of the equilibrium potential could be widely utilized in other areas of the nervous system to control local inhibitory strength.

AUTHOR CONTRIBUTIONS

Lina Yassin: conducted electrophysiological experiments and analyzed data, Susanne Radtke-Schuller: conducted immunohistochemistry, Hila Asraf: conducted KCC2 measurements, Benedikt Grothe: interpreted data and jointly wrote manuscript, Michal Hershfinkel: designed KCC2 measurements, interpreted data and jointly wrote manuscript, Ian D. Forsythe: conceived project jointly with Cornelia Kopp-Scheinpflug, interpreted data and jointly wrote manuscript. Cornelia Kopp-Scheinpflug: conceived project, conducted experiments, analyzed and interpreted data, wrote manuscript.

ACKNOWLEDGMENT

This research was funded by the Medical Research Council, UK; the Israel Science Foundation (513/09); the Graduate School for Systemic Neurosciences and the DFG (KO2207/3-1).

REFERENCES

Arion, D., and Lewis, D. A. (2011). Altered expression of regulators of the cortical chloride transporters NKCC1 and KCC2 in schizophrenia. *Arch. Gen. Psychiatry* 68, 21–31. doi: 10.1001/archgenpsychiatry.2010.114

Balakrishnan, V., Becker, M., Lohrke, S., Nothwang, H. G., Guresir, E., and Friauf, E. (2003). Expression and function of chloride transporters during development of inhibitory neurotransmission in the auditory brainstem. *J. Neurosci.* 23, 4134–4145.

Banks, M. I., and Smith, P. H. (1992). Intracellular recordings from neurobiotin-labeled cells in brain slices of the rat medial nucleus of the trapezoid body. *J. Neurosci.* 12, 2819–2837.

Bartos, M., Vida, I., Frotscher, M., Meyer, A., Monyer, H., Geiger, J. R., et al. (2002). Fast synaptic inhibition promotes synchronized gamma oscillations in hippocampal interneuron networks. *Proc. Natl. Acad. Sci. U.S.A.* 99, 13222–13227. doi: 10.1073/pnas.192233099

Ben-Ari, Y., Khalilov, I., Kahle, K. T., and Cherubini, E. (2012). The GABA excitatory/inhibitory shift in brain maturation and neurological disorders. *Neuroscientist* 18, 467–486. doi: 10.1177/1073858412438697

Blaesse, P., Airaksinen, M. S., Rivera, C., and Kaila, K. (2009). Cation-chloride cotransporters and neuronal function. *Neuron* 61, 820–838. doi: 10.1016/j.neuron.2009.03.003

Blaesse, P., Guillemin, I., Schindler, J., Schweizer, M., Delpire, E., Khiroug, L., et al. (2006). Oligomerization of KCC2 correlates with development of inhibitory neurotransmission. *J. Neurosci.* 26, 10407–10419. doi: 10.1523/JNEUROSCI.3257-06.2006

Boulenguez, P., Liabeuf, S., Bos, R., Bras, H., Jean-Xavier, C., Brocard, C., et al. (2010). Down-regulation of the potassium-chloride cotransporter KCC2 contributes to spasticity after spinal cord injury. *Nat. Med.* 16, 302–307. doi: 10.1038/nm.2107

Brenman, J. E., Chao, D. S., Gee, S. H., McGee, A. W., Craven, S. E., Santillano, D. R., et al. (1996). Interaction of nitric oxide synthase with the postsynaptic density protein PSD-95 and alpha1-syntrophin mediated by PDZ domains. *Cell* 84, 757–767. doi: 10.1016/S0092-8674(00)81053-3

Casula, S., Shmukler, B. E., Wilhelm, S., Stuart-Tilley, A. K., Su, W., Chernova, M. N., et al. (2001). A dominant negative mutant of the KCC1 K-Cl cotransporter: both N- and C-terminal cytoplasmic domains are required for K-Cl cotransport activity. *J. Biol. Chem.* 276, 41870–41878. doi: 10.1074/jbc.M107155200

Chamma, I., Chevy, Q., Poncer, J. C., and Levi, S. (2012). Role of the neuronal K-Cl co-transporter KCC2 in inhibitory and excitatory neurotransmission. *Front. Cell. Neurosci.* 6:5. doi: 10.3389/fncel.2012.00005

Chamma, I., Heubl, M., Chevy, Q., Renner, M., Moutkine, I., Eugene, E., et al. (2013). Activity-dependent regulation of the K/Cl transporter KCC2 membrane diffusion, clustering, and function in hippocampal neurons. *J. Neurosci.* 33, 15488–15503. doi: 10.1523/JNEUROSCI.5889-12.2013

Cherubini, E., Griguoli, M., Safiulina, V., and Lagostena, L. (2011). The depolarizing action of GABA controls early network activity in the developing hippocampus. *Mol. Neurobiol.* 43, 97–106. doi: 10.1007/s12035-010-8147-z

Chorin, E., Vinograd, O., Fleidervish, I., Gilad, D., Herrmann, S., Sekler, I., et al. (2011). Upregulation of KCC2 activity by zinc-mediated neurotransmission via the mZnR/GPR39 receptor. *J. Neurosci.* 31, 12916–12926. doi: 10.1523/JNEUROSCI.2205-11.2011

Coote, E. J., and Rees, A. (2008). The distribution of nitric oxide synthase in the inferior colliculus of guinea pig. *Neuroscience* 154, 218–225. doi: 10.1016/j.neuroscience.2008.02.030

Felix, R. A. 2nd., Fridberger, A., Leijon, S., Berrebi, A. S., and Magnusson, A. K. (2011). Sound rhythms are encoded by postinhibitory rebound spiking in the superior paraolivary nucleus. *J. Neurosci.* 31, 12566–12578. doi: 10.1523/JNEUROSCI.2450-11.2011

Fischl, M. J., Combs, T. D., Klug, A., Grothe, B., and Burger, R. M. (2012). Modulation of synaptic input by GABAB receptors improves coincidence detection for computation of sound location. *J. Physiol.* 590, 3047–3066. doi: 10.1113/jphysiol.2011.226233

Fiumelli, H., Cancedda, L., and Poo, M. M. (2005). Modulation of GABAergic transmission by activity via postsynaptic Ca2+-dependent regulation of KCC2 function. *Neuron* 48, 773–786. doi: 10.1016/j.neuron.2005.10.025

Francis, S. H., Busch, J. L., Corbin, J. D., and Sibley, D. (2010). cGMP-dependent protein kinases and cGMP phosphodiesterases in nitric oxide and cGMP action. *Pharmacol. Rev.* 62, 525–563. doi: 10.1124/pr.110.002907

Friauf, E., Rust, M. B., Schulenborg, T., and Hirtz, J. J. (2011). Chloride cotransporters, chloride homeostasis, and synaptic inhibition in the developing auditory system. *Hear. Res.* 279, 96–110. doi: 10.1016/j.heares.2011.05.012

Frisina, S. T., Mapes, F., Kim, S., Frisina, D. R., and Frisina, R. D. (2006). Characterization of hearing loss in aged type II diabetics. *Hear. Res.* 211, 103–113. doi: 10.1016/j.heares.2005.09.002

Garthwaite, J. (2008). Concepts of neural nitric oxide-mediated transmission. *Eur. J. Neurosci.* 27, 2783–2802. doi: 10.1111/j.1460-9568.2008.06285.x

Garthwaite, J., and Boulton, C. L. (1995). Nitric oxide signaling in the central nervous system. *Annu. Rev. Physiol.* 57, 683–706. doi: 10.1146/annurev.ph.57.030195.003343

Garthwaite, J., Charles, S. L., and Chess-Williams, R. (1988). Endothelium-derived relaxing factor release on activation of NMDA receptors suggests role as intercellular messenger in the brain. *Nature* 336, 385–388. doi: 10.1038/336385a0

Ginsberg, M. D. (2008). Neuroprotection for ischemic stroke: past, present and future. *Neuropharmacology* 55, 363–389. doi: 10.1016/j.neuropharm.2007.12.007

Gleich, O., and Strutz, J. (2011). The Effect of gabapentin on gap detection and forward masking in young and old gerbils. *Ear Hear.* 32, 741–749. doi: 10.1097/AUD.0b013e318222289f

Grothe, B., Pecka, M., and McAlpine, D. (2010). Mechanisms of sound localization in mammals. *Physiol. Rev.* 90, 983–1012. doi: 10.1152/physrev.00026.2009

Hardingham, N., Dachtler, J., and Fox, K. (2013). The role of nitric oxide in pre-synaptic plasticity and homeostasis. *Front. Cell. Neurosci.* 7:190. doi: 10.3389/fncel.2013.00190

Hassfurth, B., Grothe, B., and Koch, U. (2010). The mammalian interaural time difference detection circuit is differentially controlled by GABAB receptors during development. *J. Neurosci.* 30, 9715–9727. doi: 10.1523/JNEUROSCI.1552-10.2010

Hershfinkel, M., Kandler, K., Knoch, M. E., Dagan-Rabin, M., Aras, M. A., Abramovitch-Dahan, C., et al. (2009). Intracellular zinc inhibits KCC2 transporter activity. *Nat. Neurosci.* 12, 725–727. doi: 10.1038/nn.2316

Hewitt, S. A., Wamsteeker, J. I., Kurz, E. U., and Bains, J. S. (2009). Altered chloride homeostasis removes synaptic inhibitory constraint of the stress axis. *Nat. Neurosci.* 12, 438–443. doi: 10.1038/nn.2274

Holscher, C. (1997). Nitric oxide, the enigmatic neuronal messenger: its role in synaptic plasticity. *Trends Neurosci.* 20, 298–303. doi: 10.1016/S0166-2236(97)01065-5

Jang, Y., Wang, H., Xi, J., Mueller, R. A., Norfleet, E. A., and Xu, Z. (2007). NO mobilizes intracellular Zn^{2+} via cGMP/PKG signaling pathway and prevents mitochondrial oxidant damage in cardiomyocytes. *Cardiovasc. Res.* 75, 426–433. doi: 10.1016/j.cardiores.2007.05.015

Johnston, J., Forsythe, I. D., and Kopp-Scheinpflug, C. (2010). Going native: voltage-gated potassium channels controlling neuronal excitability. *J. Physiol.* 588, 3187–3200. doi: 10.1113/jphysiol.2010.191973

Kadner, A., and Berrebi, A. S. (2008). Encoding of temporal features of auditory stimuli in the medial nucleus of the trapezoid body and superior paraolivary nucleus of the rat. *Neuroscience* 151, 868–887. doi: 10.1016/j.neuroscience.2007.11.008

Kandler, K., and Gillespie, D. C. (2005). Developmental refinement of inhibitory sound-localization circuits. *Trends Neurosci.* 28, 290–296. doi: 10.1016/j.tins.2005.04.007

Kapfer, C., Seidl, A. H., Schweizer, H., and Grothe, B. (2002). Experience-dependent refinement of inhibitory inputs to auditory coincidence-detector neurons. *Nat. Neurosci.* 5, 247–253. doi: 10.1038/nn810

Kopp-Scheinpflug, C., Tozer, A. J., Robinson, S. W., Tempel, B. L., Hennig, M. H., and Forsythe, I. D. (2011). The sound of silence: ionic mechanisms encoding sound termination. *Neuron* 71, 911–925. doi: 10.1016/j.neuron.2011.06.028

Lee, H. H., Deeb, T. Z., Walker, J. A., Davies, P. A., and Moss, S. J. (2011). NMDA receptor activity downregulates KCC2 resulting in depolarizing GABAA receptor-mediated currents. *Nat. Neurosci.* 14, 736–743. doi: 10.1038/nn.2806

Lohrke, S., Srinivasan, G., Oberhofer, M., Doncheva, E., and Friauf, E. (2005). Shift from depolarizing to hyperpolarizing glycine action occurs at different perinatal ages in superior olivary complex nuclei. *Eur. J. Neurosci.* 22, 2708–2722. doi: 10.1111/j.1460-9568.2005.04465.x

Luth, H. J., Hedlich, A., Hilbig, H., Winkelmann, E., and Mayer, B. (1995). Postnatal development of NADPH-diaphorase/nitric oxide synthase positive nerve cells in the visual cortex of the rat. *J. Hirnforsch.* 36, 313–328.

Magnusson, A. K., Park, T. J., Pecka, M., Grothe, B., and Koch, U. (2008). Retrograde GABA signaling adjusts sound localization by balancing excitation and inhibition in the brainstem. *Neuron* 59, 125–137. doi: 10.1016/j.neuron.2008.05.011

Nakamura, T., Tu, S., Akhtar, M. W., Sunico, C. R., Okamoto, S., and Lipton, S. A. (2013). Aberrant protein s-nitrosylation in neurodegenerative diseases. *Neuron* 78, 596–614. doi: 10.1016/j.neuron.2013.05.005

Reuss, S. (1998). Nitric oxide synthase in the auditory brain stem. *Neuroreport* 9, 3643–3646.

Reuss, S., and Riemann, R. (2000). Distribution and projections of nitric oxide synthase neurons in the rodent superior olivary complex. *Microsc. Res. Tech.* 51, 318–329. doi: 10.1002/1097-0029(20001115)51:4%3C318::AID-JEMT3%3E3.0.CO;2-Y

Reuss, S., Schaeffer, D. F., Laages, M. H., and Riemann, R. (2000). Evidence for increased nitric oxide production in the auditory brain stem of the aged dwarf hamster (*Phodopus sungorus*): an NADPH-diaphorase histochemical study. *Mech. Ageing Dev.* 112, 125–134. doi: 10.1016/S0047-6374(99)00082-2

Rivera, C., Li, H., Thomas-Crusells, J., Lahtinen, H., Viitanen, T., Nanobashvili, A., et al. (2002). BDNF-induced TrkB activation down-regulates the K+-Cl- cotransporter KCC2 and impairs neuronal Cl- extrusion. *J. Cell Biol.* 159, 747–752. doi: 10.1083/jcb.200209011

Rivera, C., Voipio, J., Thomas-Crusells, J., Li, H., Emri, Z., Sipila, S., et al. (2004). Mechanism of activity-dependent downregulation of the neuron-specific K-Cl cotransporter KCC2. *J. Neurosci.* 24, 4683–4691. doi: 10.1523/JNEUROSCI.5265-03.2004

Scholl, B., Gao, X., and Wehr, M. (2010). Nonoverlapping sets of synapses drive on responses and off responses in auditory cortex. *Neuron* 65, 412–421. doi: 10.1016/j.neuron.2010.01.020

Snell, K. B., Mapes, F. M., Hickman, E. D., and Frisina, D. R. (2002). Word recognition in competing babble and the effects of age, temporal processing, and absolute sensitivity. *J. Acoust. Soc. Am.* 112, 720–727. doi: 10.1121/1.1487841

Sommer, I., Lingenhohl, K., and Friauf, E. (1993). Principal cells of the rat medial nucleus of the trapezoid body: an intracellular *in vivo* study of their physiology and morphology. *Exp. Brain Res.* 95, 223–239. doi: 10.1007/BF00229781

Stange, A., Myoga, M. H., Lingner, A., Ford, M. C., Alexandrowa, O., Felmy, F., et al. (2013). Adaptation in sound localization: from GABAB receptor-mediated synaptic modulation to perception. *Nat. Neurosci.* 16, 1840–1847. doi: 10.1038/nn.3548

Steinert, J. R., Chernova, T., and Forsythe, I. D. (2010). Nitric oxide signaling in brain function, dysfunction, and dementia. *Neuroscientist* 16, 435–452. doi: 10.1177/1073858410366481

Steinert, J. R., Kopp-Scheinpflug, C., Baker, C., Challiss, R. A., Mistry, R., Haustein, M. D., et al. (2008). Nitric oxide is a volume transmitter regulating postsynaptic excitability at a glutamatergic synapse. *Neuron* 60, 642–656. doi: 10.1016/j.neuron.2008.08.025

Steinert, J. R., Robinson, S. W., Tong, H., Haustein, M. D., Kopp-Scheinpflug, C., and Forsythe, I. D. (2011). Nitric oxide is an activity-dependent regulator of target neuron intrinsic excitability. *Neuron* 71, 291–305. doi: 10.1016/j.neuron.2011.05.037

Sweeten, T. L., Posey, D. J., Shankar, S., and McDougle, C. J. (2004). High nitric oxide production in autistic disorder: a possible role for interferon-gamma. *Biol. Psychiatry* 55, 434–437. doi: 10.1016/j.biopsych.2003.09.001

Tepper, J. M., Koos, T., and Wilson, C. J. (2004). GABAergic microcircuits in the neostriatum. *Trends Neurosci.* 27, 662–669. doi: 10.1016/j.tins.2004.08.007

Vinay, L., and Jean-Xavier, C. (2008). Plasticity of spinal cord locomotor networks and contribution of cation-chloride cotransporters. *Brain Res. Rev.* 57, 103–110. doi: 10.1016/j.brainresrev.2007.09.003

Vincent, S. R., and Kimura, H. (1992). Histochemical mapping of nitric oxide synthase in the rat brain. *Neuroscience* 46, 755–784. doi: 10.1016/0306-4522(92)90184-4

Wagle, A., and Singh, J. P. (2000). Fibroblast growth factor protects nitric oxide-induced apoptosis in neuronal SHSY-5Y cells. *J. Pharmacol. Exp. Ther.* 295, 889–895.

Wake, H., Watanabe, M., Moorhouse, A. J., Kanematsu, T., Horibe, S., Matsukawa, N., et al. (2007). Early changes in KCC2 phosphorylation in response to neuronal stress result in functional downregulation. *J. Neurosci.* 27, 1642–1650. doi: 10.1523/JNEUROSCI.3104-06.2007

Zhang, Y., Wang, H., Li, J., Jimenez, D. A., Levitan, E. S., Aizenman, E., et al. (2004). Peroxynitrite-induced neuronal apoptosis is mediated by intracellular zinc release and 12-lipoxygenase activation. *J. Neurosci.* 24, 10616–10627. doi: 10.1523/JNEUROSCI.2469-04.2004

Permissions

All chapters in this book were first published by Frontiers; hereby published with permission under the Creative Commons Attribution License or equivalent. Every chapter published in this book has been scrutinized by our experts. Their significance has been extensively debated. The topics covered herein carry significant findings which will fuel the growth of the discipline. They may even be implemented as practical applications or may be referred to as a beginning point for another development.

The contributors of this book come from diverse backgrounds, making this book a truly international effort. This book will bring forth new frontiers with its revolutionizing research information and detailed analysis of the nascent developments around the world.

We would like to thank all the contributing authors for lending their expertise to make the book truly unique. They have played a crucial role in the development of this book. Without their invaluable contributions this book wouldn't have been possible. They have made vital efforts to compile up to date information on the varied aspects of this subject to make this book a valuable addition to the collection of many professionals and students.

This book was conceptualized with the vision of imparting up-to-date information and advanced data in this field. To ensure the same, a matchless editorial board was set up. Every individual on the board went through rigorous rounds of assessment to prove their worth. After which they invested a large part of their time researching and compiling the most relevant data for our readers.

The editorial board has been involved in producing this book since its inception. They have spent rigorous hours researching and exploring the diverse topics which have resulted in the successful publishing of this book. They have passed on their knowledge of decades through this book. To expedite this challenging task, the publisher supported the team at every step. A small team of assistant editors was also appointed to further simplify the editing procedure and attain best results for the readers.

Apart from the editorial board, the designing team has also invested a significant amount of their time in understanding the subject and creating the most relevant covers. They scrutinized every image to scout for the most suitable representation of the subject and create an appropriate cover for the book.

The publishing team has been an ardent support to the editorial, designing and production team. Their endless efforts to recruit the best for this project, has resulted in the accomplishment of this book. They are a veteran in the field of academics and their pool of knowledge is as vast as their experience in printing. Their expertise and guidance has proved useful at every step. Their uncompromising quality standards have made this book an exceptional effort. Their encouragement from time to time has been an inspiration for everyone.

The publisher and the editorial board hope that this book will prove to be a valuable piece of knowledge for researchers, students, practitioners and scholars across the globe.

List of Contributors

Matthew J. Fischl and R. Michael Burger
Department of Biological Sciences, Lehigh University, Bethlehem, PA, USA

Daniel T. Case
Neuroscience Graduate Program, McMaster University, Hamilton, ON, Canada

Javier Alamilla
Department of Psychology, Neuroscience and Behaviour, McMaster University, Hamilton, ON, Canada

Deda C. Gillespie
Neuroscience Graduate Program, McMaster University, Hamilton, ON, Canada
Department of Psychology, Neuroscience and Behaviour, McMaster University, Hamilton, ON, Canada

Miloslav Sedlacek and Stephan D. Brenowitz
Section on Synaptic Transmission, National Institute on Deafness and Other Communication Disorders, National Institutes of Health, Bethesda, MD, USA

Michael T. Roberts, Stephanie C. Seeman and Nace L. Golding
Department of Neuroscience, Center for Learning and Memory, The University of Texas at Austin, Austin, TX, USA

Vibhakar C. Kotak
Center for Neural Science, New York University, New York, USA

Dan H. Sanes
Center for Neural Science, New York University, New York, USA
Department of Biology, New York University, New York, USA

William R. Hamlet and Yong Lu
Department of Anatomy and Neurobiology, College of Medicine, Northeast Ohio Medical University, Rootstown, OH, USA
School of Biomedical Sciences, Kent State University, Kent, OH, USA

Yu-Wei Liu and Zheng-Quan Tang
Department of Anatomy and Neurobiology, College of Medicine, Northeast Ohio Medical University, Rootstown, OH, USA

Kanthaiah Koka and Daniel J. Tollin
Department of Physiology and Biophysics, University of Colorado School of Medicine, Aurora, CO, USA

Harunori Ohmori
Department of Physiology and Neurobiology, Faculty of Medicine, Kyoto University, Kyoto, Japan

Otto Albrecht, Anna Dondzillo, Florian Mayer and Achim Klug
Department of Physiology and Biophysics, School of Medicine, University of Colorado, Aurora, CO, USA

John A. Thompson
Department of Neurosurgery, School of Medicine, University of Colorado, Aurora, CO, USA

Florian Kramer, Désirée Griesemer, Dennis Bakker, Sina Brill and Erik Frotscher
Animal Physiology Group, Department of Biology, University of Kaiserslautern, Kaiserslautern, Germany

Jürgen Franke
Chair for Applied Mathematical Statistics, Department of Mathematics, University of Kaiserslautern, Kaiserslautern, Germany
Center for Mathematical and Computational Modeling, University of Kaiserslautern, Kaiserslautern, Germany

Eckhard Friauf
Animal Physiology Group, Department of Biology, University of Kaiserslautern, Kaiserslautern, Germany
Center for Mathematical and Computational Modeling, University of Kaiserslautern, Kaiserslautern, Germany

Johana Trojanova, Michaela Kralikova, Josef Syka and Rostislav Turecek
Department of Auditory Neuroscience, Laboratory of Synaptic Transmission, Institute of Experimental Medicine, Academy of Sciences of the Czech Republic, Prague, Czech Republic

Akos Kulik
Department of Physiology II, University of Freiburg, Freiburg, Germany
BIOSS Centre for Biological Signalling Studies, University of Freiburg, Freiburg, Germany

Jiri Janacek
Department of Biomathematics, Institute of Physiology, Academy of Sciences of the Czech Republic, Prague, Czech Republic

Pierre F. Apostolides and Laurence O. Trussell
Oregon Hearing Research Center and Vollum Institute, Oregon Health and Science University, Portland, OR, USA

Jana Nerlich, Christian Keine and Rudolf Rübsamen
Department of Neurobiology, Faculty of Biosciences, Pharmacy and Psychology, University of Leipzig, Leipzig, Germany

Ivan Milenkovic
Department of Physiology, Faculty of Medicine, Carl Ludwig Institute for Physiology, University of Leipzig, Leipzig, Germany

Stefanie C. Altieri
Richard King Mellon Foundation Institute for Pediatric Research and Department of Pediatrics, University of Pittsburgh, Pittsburgh, PA, USA
Department of Otolaryngology, University of Pittsburgh, Pittsburgh, PA, USA

Tianna Zhao and Stephen M. Maricich
Richard King Mellon Foundation Institute for Pediatric Research and Department of Pediatrics, University of Pittsburgh, Pittsburgh, PA, USA

Walid Jalabi
Department of Pediatrics, Case Western Reserve University, Cleveland, OH, USA

Ruili Xie
Department of Otolaryngology/Head and Neck Surgery, University of North Carolina at Chapel Hill, Chapel Hill, NC, USA

Paul B. Manis
Department of Otolaryngology/Head and Neck Surgery, University of North Carolina at Chapel Hill, Chapel Hill, NC, USA
Department of Cell Biology and Physiology, University of North Carolina at Chapel Hill, Chapel Hill, NC, USA

Lina Yassin, Susanne Radtke-Schuller, Michael Pecka, Benedikt Grothe and Cornelia Kopp-Scheinpflug
Division of Neurobiology, Department Biology II, Ludwig-Maximilians-University Munich, Planegg-Martinsried, Germany

Hila Asraf and Michal Hershfinkel
Department of Physiology and Cell Biology, Faculty of Health Sciences, Ben-Gurion University of the Negev, Beer-Sheva, Israel

Ian D. Forsythe
Department of Cell Physiology and Pharmacology, University of Leicester, Leicester, UK

Index

A

Action Potentials, 57-63, 67, 85, 149, 220

Afterhyperpolarization, 56-58, 170

Analysis Of Variance, 77, 177, 214

Anterograde Tracing, 117-118

Anteroventral Cochlear Nucleus, 30, 52, 64-65, 105-106, 115, 155, 175, 186-187, 199, 201, 210-211

Archosaurs, 14-15, 17-18, 28

Asynchronous Release, 87, 175-177, 180, 182-186

Auditory Brainstem, 11-13, 19, 29-30, 32-35, 38-39, 53, 64-65, 68, 73, 76, 78, 83, 88-89, 107, 110, 115-116, 121, 128-130, 132, 151, 153, 168, 184, 186-187, 189-190, 194-197, 210, 212, 216, 221-222

Auditory Nerve Fibers, 41-48, 51, 91, 97-99, 104, 109, 153, 168-169, 200

Auditory System, 12, 30, 39-40, 43, 52, 65, 73-74, 84, 88-89, 94, 104, 109, 114-115, 132, 145, 147, 150, 152-153, 163, 175, 187, 189, 195

B

Binaural Sensitivity, 21, 221

Brain Slice Preparation, 2, 68-69

C

Calyx Of Held, 22, 29, 32, 39, 54, 59, 61, 63-65, 89-90, 95, 104, 106-107, 117, 129-132, 144, 151-156, 158, 160, 162-165, 178, 187, 195

Characteristic Frequency, 30, 64, 77, 91, 95, 110, 115, 187

Cochlear Nucleus, 11-12, 19, 29-30, 32, 35, 41-44, 46, 51-52, 55-56, 58, 64-68, 88-90, 104-108, 115, 117, 121, 125, 129, 131, 150-151, 153, 155, 166-169, 172-176, 183, 186-189, 195-199, 201, 207, 209-211

Cochlear Nucleus-superior Olive, 55

Contralateral Auditory Nerves, 54, 63

Coupling Coefficients, 169, 171

Cross-suppression, 1-2, 9

D

Desensitization, 9, 12, 51, 152, 180, 185-187, 207, 209-210

Directional Transfer Functions, 90, 101, 106

Dorsal Cochlear Nucleus, 41, 44, 51-52, 65-66, 105, 107, 166, 169, 173-174, 176, 186, 197

E

Electrical Synapses, 166, 172

Electrophysiology, 34, 42, 55, 120, 126, 128, 133, 167

Excitatory Postsynaptic Potentials, 54

F

Firing Rates, 26, 57, 62, 113, 134, 172, 183-185

Fusiform Cells, 41, 43-45, 49-50, 52, 167-173

G

Gap Junctions, 166, 169-174

Globular Bushy Cells, 53, 61-64, 90, 107, 117, 121

Glutamate Receptors, 12, 65, 69, 71-72, 86, 89, 113, 115, 164

Glutamatergic Transmission, 2, 43, 70, 73

Glutamic Acid Decarboxylase, 125, 167, 210

Glycine, 1-12, 14, 33-39, 43, 47, 57, 65, 67, 73, 75, 104, 106-107, 120-121, 125-126, 129-130, 134, 148-149, 151-155, 159, 162-168, 171, 173, 175-177, 179-181, 183-190, 192, 194-197, 200, 207, 209-211, 214, 216, 218, 221, 223

Glycine Transporter, 12, 125, 130, 151, 163, 167-168, 179, 188-190, 195, 214

Glycinergic Inhibition, 12, 28, 41, 89, 104, 117, 129, 151, 186-187, 197, 201, 203, 207, 209, 212, 219

Green Fluorescent Protein, 117-118, 131, 165, 174

H

Hippocampus, 37, 50, 67, 73, 87-88, 147, 150, 152, 164, 220, 222

I

Immunohistochemistry, 117, 119, 125, 154, 190

Immunostaining, 119, 189, 192, 210

Inhibitory Postsynaptic Current, 67, 175

Inhibitory Postsynaptic Potentials, 53, 75, 79, 81, 197

Innervation, 29, 39, 44-46, 51, 109, 125, 129, 189-195, 209, 219

Interaural Difference Cues, 109, 114

Interaural Level Differences, 16, 28, 67

Interaural Phase Difference, 110, 115

Interaural Time Differences, 16, 30, 65, 88, 106, 115

Interneurons, 41-44, 47-48, 52, 109, 114, 153, 164, 166-169, 173, 187, 210, 212

Intersynaptic Pooling, 175, 178

L

Lateral Superior Olive, 12, 19, 30-31, 33, 39-40, 67, 73-74, 88, 90, 106-107, 115, 132, 150, 153, 189, 195-196, 212

M

Medial Superior Olive, 19, 29-32, 53-54, 64-66, 87-89, 106-107, 109, 115-116, 150, 186-188, 193

Meriones Unguiculatus, 69, 210, 213
Morganucodon, 19, 28, 31

N
Neocortex, 51-52, 67, 140, 147, 150-152, 164
Neurotransmission, 12, 33, 36, 38-39, 64-66, 106, 115, 132, 140-141, 143-144, 146, 148, 151, 153, 164, 187, 222
Nucleus Laminaris, 1, 12-13, 18, 31-32, 75, 77-78, 88-89, 109, 114-116, 146, 152

P
Paraformaldehyde, 92, 118, 155, 167, 190, 213
Patch-clamp Recordings, 37, 133
Phasic Inhibition, 11, 76, 87, 109, 113-114, 176
Phosphatase Activity, 1-2
Phosphate Buffered Saline, 118, 167, 213
Phosphorylation, 7, 186, 213, 221, 223
Photostimulation, 198-201, 208-209

Postsynaptic Membrane, 1-2, 67, 210
Pressure-gradient Receiver, 17-18
Presynaptic Terminal, 183, 185

R

Random Spectral Shape, 90-91, 94, 108
Repeated-measures, 77, 177
Retrograde Tracing, 117-118, 127

S
Sauropsids, 14, 16-17, 28
Short-term Depression, 34, 41-42, 47-48, 60, 132-133, 135, 152-153
Sound Localization, 1, 10-12, 14-19, 21-22, 24-25, 27-31, 39, 53, 60, 64-65, 67, 73, 76, 88-90, 100, 104-107, 114-115, 129-130, 151-153, 175, 187-190, 195, 212, 222-223
Spectral Coding, 97, 99-100, 104-105
Spherical Bushy Cells, 90, 175, 186-188
Stellate Cells, 42, 66, 166-169, 171-174, 186
Striatum, 33, 37, 164
Strontium, 39, 183-184, 188
Strychnine, 1, 3-6, 11, 30, 43-44, 47, 49-50, 57, 73, 104, 121, 126, 134, 159, 167-168, 184, 196, 198, 200-203, 205-207, 213
Superficial Stellate Cell, 166
Superior Olivary Complex, 12, 30-31, 39, 58, 64-65, 73, 106-107, 119, 130-131, 153, 163, 186-189, 195-197, 207, 210, 212, 223
Synaptic Attenuation, 132-133, 139, 141, 148, 151
Synaptic Plasticity, 12, 39, 41-43, 47-48, 50-52, 65, 72-73, 107, 113, 130, 132, 151-153, 168, 173, 222

T
Tonic Inhibition, 23, 76, 89, 109, 175, 188
Transmitter Rebinding, 176, 179, 183, 185
Trapezoid Body, 19, 31, 33, 39, 53-54, 59, 64-65, 67, 74, 88, 90-92, 105-107, 115, 117, 119-120, 129-132, 150, 153, 155, 163-164, 187, 189, 195-196, 207, 212, 222-223
Tuberculoventral Cell, 44, 47-48, 50-51

V
Ventral Cochlear Nucleus, 150, 176

www.ingramcontent.com/pod-product-compliance
Lightning Source LLC
LaVergne TN
LVHW060551210926
848485LV00005B/1296